NURSING RESEARCH

9TH EDITION

NURSING RESEARCH

Methods and Critical Appraisal for Evidence-Based Practice

Geri LoBiondo-Wood, PhD, RN, FAAN

Professor and Coordinator, PhD in Nursing Program
University of Texas Health Science Center at Houston
School of Nursing
Houston, Texas

Judith Haber, PhD, RN, FAAN

The Ursula Springer Leadership Professor in Nursing
New York University
Rory Meyers College of Nursing
New York, New York

ELSEVIER

ELSEVIER

3251 Riverport Lane
St. Louis, Missouri 63043

NURSING RESEARCH: METHODS AND CRITICAL APPRAISAL
FOR EVIDENCE-BASED PRACTICE, NINTH EDITION ISBN: 978-0-323-43131-6

Notices

Knowledge and best practice in this field are constantly changing. As new research and experience broaden our understanding, changes in research methods, professional practices, or medical treatment may become necessary.

Practitioners and researchers must always rely on their own experience and knowledge in evaluating and using any information, methods, compounds, or experiments described herein. In using such information or methods they should be mindful of their own safety and the safety of others, including parties for whom they have a professional responsibility.

With respect to any drug or pharmaceutical products identified, readers are advised to check the most current information provided (i) on procedures featured or (ii) by the manufacturer of each product to be administered, to verify the recommended dose or formula, the method and duration of administration, and contraindications. It is the responsibility of practitioners, relying on their own experience and knowledge of their patients, to make diagnoses, to determine dosages and the best treatment for each individual patient, and to take all appropriate safety precautions.

To the fullest extent of the law, neither the Publisher nor the authors, contributors, or editors assume any liability for any injury and/or damage to persons or property as a matter of products liability, negligence or otherwise, or from any use or operation of any methods, products, instructions, or ideas contained in the material herein.

Previous editions copyrighted 2014, 2010, 2006, 2002, 1998, 1994, 1990, 1986.

Library of Congress Cataloging-in-Publication Data

Names: LoBiondo-Wood, Geri, editor. | Haber, Judith, editor.
Title: Nursing research : methods and critical appraisal for evidence-based practice / [edited by] Geri LoBiondo-Wood, Judith Haber.
Other titles: Nursing research (LoBiondo-Wood)
Description: 9th edition. | St. Louis, Missouri : Elsevier, [2018] | Includes bibliographical references and index.
Identifiers: LCCN 2017008727 | ISBN 9780323431316 (pbk. : alk. paper)
Subjects: | MESH: Nursing Research—methods | Research Design | Evidence-Based Nursing—methods
Classification: LCC RT81.5 | NLM WY 20.5 | DDC 610.73072—dc23 LC record available at https://lccn.loc.gov/2017008727

Executive Content Strategist: Lee Henderson
Content Development Manager: Lisa Newton
Content Development Specialist: Melissa Rawe
Publishing Services Manager: Jeff Patterson
Book Production Specialist: Carol O'Connell
Design Direction: Renee Duenow

Printed in China

Last digit is the print number: 9 8 7 6 5 4 3 2

ABOUT THE AUTHORS

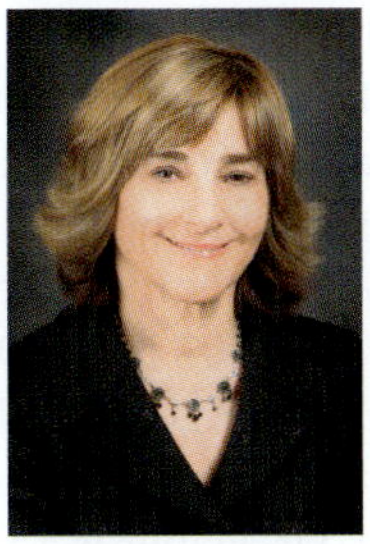

Geri LoBiondo-Wood, PhD, RN, FAAN, is Professor and Coordinator of the PhD in Nursing Program at the University of Texas Health Science Center at Houston, School of Nursing (UTHSC-Houston) and former Director of Research and Evidence-Based Practice Planning and Development at the MD Anderson Cancer Center, Houston, Texas. She received her Diploma in Nursing at St. Mary's Hospital School of Nursing in Rochester, New York; Bachelor's and Master's degrees from the University of Rochester; and a PhD in Nursing Theory and Research from New York University. Dr. LoBiondo-Wood teaches research and evidence-based practice principles to undergraduate, graduate, and doctoral students. At MD Anderson Cancer Center, she developed and implemented the Evidence-Based Resource Unit Nurse (EB-RUN) Program. She has extensive national and international experience guiding nurses and other health care professionals in the development and utilization of research. Dr. LoBiondo-Wood is an Editorial Board member of *Progress in Transplantation* and a reviewer for *Nursing Research, Oncology Nursing Forum,* and *Oncology Nursing.* Her research and publications focus on chronic illness and oncology nursing. Dr. Wood has received funding from the Robert Wood Johnson Foundation Future of Nursing Scholars program for the past several years to fund full-time doctoral students.

Dr. LoBiondo-Wood has been active locally and nationally in many professional organizations, including the Oncology Nursing Society, Southern Nursing Research Society, the Midwest Nursing Research Society, and the North American Transplant Coordinators Organization. She has received local and national awards for teaching and contributions to nursing. In 1997, she received the Distinguished Alumnus Award from New York University, Division of Nursing Alumni Association. In 2001 she was inducted as a Fellow of the American Academy of Nursing and in 2007 as a Fellow of the University of Texas Academy of Health Science Education. In 2012 she was appointed as a Distinguished Teaching Professor of the University of Texas System and in 2015 received the John McGovern Outstanding Teacher Award from the University of Texas Health Science Center at Houston School of Nursing.

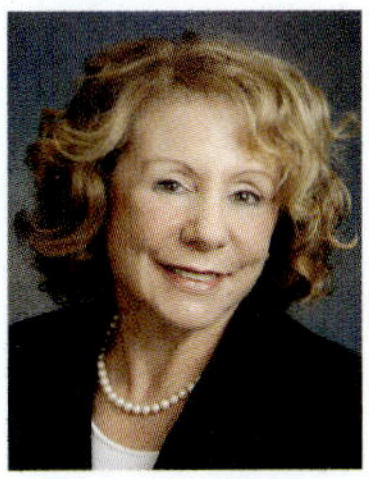

Judith Haber, PhD, RN, FAAN, is the Ursula Springer Leadership Professor in Nursing at the Rory Meyers College of Nursing at New York University. She received her undergraduate nursing education at Adelphi University in New York, and she holds a Master's degree in Adult Psychiatric–Mental Health Nursing and a PhD in Nursing Theory and Research from New York University. Dr. Haber is internationally recognized as a clinician and educator in psychiatric–mental health nursing. She was the editor of the award-winning classic textbook, *Comprehensive Psychiatric* Nursing, published for eight editions and translated into five languages. She has extensive clinical experience in psychiatric nursing, having been an advanced practice psychiatric nurse in private practice for over 30 years, specializing in treatment of families coping with the psychosocial impact of acute and chronic illness. Her NIH-funded program of research addressed physical and psychosocial adjustment to illness, focusing specifically on women with breast cancer and their partners and, more recently, breast cancer survivorship and lymphedema prevention and risk reduction. Dr. Haber is also committed to an interprofessional program of clinical scholarship related to interprofessional education and improving oral-systemic health outcomes and is the Executive Director of a national nursing oral health initiative, the *Oral Health Nursing Education and Practice (OHNEP)* program, funded by the DentaQuest and Washington Dental Service Foundations.

Dr. Haber is the recipient of numerous awards, including the 1995 and 2005 APNA Psychiatric Nurse of the Year Award, the 2005 APNA Outstanding Research Award, and the 1998 ANA Hildegarde Peplau Award. She received the 2007 NYU Distinguished Alumnae Award, the 2011 Distinguished Teaching Award, and the 2014 NYU Meritorious Service Award. In 2015, Dr. Haber received the Sigma Theta Tau International Marie Hippensteel Lingeman Award for Excellence in Nursing Practice. Dr. Haber is a Fellow in the American Academy of Nursing and the New York Academy of Medicine. Dr. Haber has consulted, presented, and published widely on evidence-based practice, interprofessional education and practice, as well as oral-systemic health issues.

CONTRIBUTORS

Terri Armstrong, PhD, ANP-BC, FAANP
Senior Investigator, Neuro-oncology Branch
Center for Cancer Research
National Cancer Institute
National Institutes of Health
Bethesda, Maryland

Julie Barroso, PhD, ANP, RN, FAAN
Professor and Department Chair
Medical University of South Carolina
Charleston, South Carolina

Carol Bova, PhD, RN, ANP
Professor of Nursing and Medicine
Graduate School of Nursing
University of Massachusetts
Worcester, Massachusetts

Dona Rinaldi Carpenter, EdD, RN
Professor and Chair
University of Scranton
Department of Nursing
Scranton, Pennsylvania

Maja Djukic, PhD, RN
Assistant Professor
Rory Meyers College of Nursing
New York University
New York, New York

Mei R. Fu, PhD, RN, FAAN
Associate Professor
Rory Meyers College of Nursing
New York University
New York, New York

Mattia J. Gilmartin, PhD, RN
Senior Research Scientist
Executive Director, NICHE Program
Rory Meyers College of Nursing
New York University
New York, New York

Deborah J. Jones, PhD, MS, RN
Margaret A. Barnett/PARTNERS Professorship
Associate Dean for Professional Development and Faculty Affairs
Associate Professor
University of Texas Health Science Center at Houston
School of Nursing
Houston, Texas

Carl Kirton, DNP, RN, MBA
Chief Nursing Officer
University Hospital
Newark, New Jersey;
Adjunct Faculty
Rory Meyers College of Nursing
New York University
New York, New York

Barbara Krainovich-Miller, EdD, RN, PMHCNS-BC, ANEF, FAAN
Professor
Rory Meyers College of Nursing
New York University
New York, New York

Elaine Larson, PhD, RN, FAAN, CIC
Anna C. Maxwell Professor of Nursing Research
Associate Dean for Research
Columbia University School of Nursing
New York, New York

Melanie McEwen, PhD, RN, CNE, ANEF
Professor
University of Texas Health Science Center at Houston
School of Nursing
Houston, Texas

Gail D'Eramo Melkus, EdD, ANP, FAAN
Florence & William Downs Professor in Nursing Research
Associate Dean for Research
Rory Meyers College of Nursing
New York University
New York, New York

Susan Sullivan-Bolyai, DNSc, CNS, RN, FAAN
Associate Professor
Rory Meyers College of Nursing
New York University
New York, New York

Marita Titler, PhD, RN, FAAN
Rhetaugh G. Dumas Endowed Professor
Department Chair
Department of Systems, Populations and Leadership
University of Michigan School of Nursing
Ann Arbor, Michigan

Mark Toles, PhD, RN
Assistant Professor
University of North Carolina at Chapel Hill
School of Nursing
Chapel Hill, North Carolina

REVIEWERS

Karen E. Alexander, PhD, RN, CNOR
Program Director RN-BSN
Assistant Professor
Department of Nursing
University of Houston Clear Lake-Pearland
Houston, Texas

Donelle M. Barnes, PhD, RN, CNE
Associate Professor
College of Nursing
University of Texas, Arlington
Arlington, Texas

Susan M. Bezek, PhD, RN, ACNP, CNE
Assistant Professor
Division of Nursing
Keuka College
Keuka Park, New York

Rose M. Kutlenios, PhD, MSN, MN, BSN
ANCC Board Certification, Adult Psychiatric/Mental Health Clinical Specialist
ANCC Board Certification, Adult Nurse Practitioner
Nursing Program Director and Associate Professor
Department of Nursing
West Liberty University
West Liberty, West Virginia

Shirley M. Newberry, PhD, RN, PHN
Professor
Department of Nursing
Winona State University
Winona, Minnesota

Sheryl Scott, DNP, RN, CNE
Assistant Professor and Chair
School of Nursing
Wisconsin Lutheran College
Milwaukee, Wisconsin

TO THE FACULTY

The foundation of the ninth edition of *Nursing Research: Methods and Critical Appraisal for Evidence-Based Practice* continues to be the belief that nursing research is integral to all levels of nursing education and practice. Over the past three decades since the first edition of this textbook, we have seen the depth and breadth of nursing research grow, with more nurses conducting research and using research evidence to shape clinical practice, education, administration, and health policy.

The National Academy of Medicine has challenged all health professionals to provide team-based care based on the best available scientific evidence. This is an exciting challenge. Nurses, as clinicians and interprofessional team members, are using the best available evidence, combined with their clinical judgment and patient preferences, to influence the nature and direction of health care delivery and document outcomes related to the quality and cost-effectiveness of patient care. As nurses continue to develop a unique body of nursing knowledge through research, decisions about clinical nursing practice will be increasingly evidence based.

As editors, we believe that all nurses need not only to understand the research process but also to know how to critically read, evaluate, and apply research findings in practice. We realize that understanding research, as a component of evidence-based practice and quality improvement practices, is a challenge for every student, but we believe that the challenge can be accomplished in a stimulating, lively, and learner-friendly manner.

Consistent with this perspective is an ongoing commitment to advancing implementation of evidence-based practice. Understanding and applying research must be an integral dimension of baccalaureate education, evident not only in the undergraduate nursing research course but also threaded throughout the curriculum. The research role of baccalaureate graduates calls for evidence-based practice and quality improvement competencies; central to this are critical appraisal skills—that is, nurses should be competent research consumers.

Preparing students for this role involves developing their critical thinking skills, thereby enhancing their understanding of the research process, their appreciation of the role of the critiquer, and their ability to actually critically appraise research. An undergraduate research course should develop this basic level of competence, an essential requirement if students are to engage in evidence-informed clinical decision making and practice, as well as quality improvement activities.

The primary audience for this textbook remains undergraduate students who are learning the steps of the research process, as well as how to develop clinical questions, critically appraise published research literature, and use research findings to inform evidence-based clinical practice and quality improvement initiatives. This book is also a valuable resource for students at the master's, DNP, and PhD levels who want a concise review of the basic steps of the research process, the critical appraisal process, and the principles and tools for evidence-based practice and quality improvement.

This text is also an important resource for practicing nurses who strive to use research evidence as the basis for clinical decision making and development of evidence-based policies, protocols, and standards or who collaborate with nurse-scientists in conducting clinical research and evidence-based practice. Finally, this text is an important resource for considering how evidence-based practice, quality improvement, and interprofessional collaboration are essential competencies for students and clinicians practicing in a transformed health care system, where nurses and their interprofessional team members are accountable for the quality and cost-effectiveness of care provided to their patient population. Building on the success of the eighth edition, we reaffirm our commitment to introducing evidence-based practice, quality improvement processes, and research principles to baccalaureate students, thereby providing a cutting-edge, research consumer foundation for their clinical practice. *Nursing Research: Methods and Critical Appraisal for Evidence-Based Practice* prepares nursing students and practicing nurses to become knowledgeable nursing research consumers by doing the following:

- Addressing the essential evidence-based practice and quality improvement role of the nurse, thereby embedding evidence-based competencies in clinical practice.
- Demystifying research, which is sometimes viewed as a complex process.
- Using a user-friendly, evidence-based approach to teaching the fundamentals of the research process.
- Including an exciting chapter on the role of theory in research and evidence-based practice.
- Providing a robust chapter on systematic reviews and clinical guidelines.
- Offering two innovative chapters on current strategies and tools for developing an evidence-based practice.
- Concluding with an exciting chapter on quality improvement and its application to practice.
- Teaching the critical appraisal process in a user-friendly progression.
- Promoting a lively spirit of inquiry that develops critical thinking and critical reading skills, facilitating mastery of the critical appraisal process.
- Developing information literacy, searching, and evidence-based practice competencies that prepare students and nurses to effectively locate and evaluate the best research evidence.
- Emphasizing the role of evidence-based practice and quality improvement initiatives as the basis for informing clinical decisions that support nursing practice.
- Presenting numerous examples of recently published research studies that illustrate and highlight research concepts in a manner that brings abstract ideas to life for students. These examples are critical links that reinforce evidence-based concepts and the critiquing process.
- Presenting five published articles, including a meta-analysis, in the Appendices, the highlights of which are woven throughout the text as exemplars of research and evidence-based practice.
- Showcasing, in four new inspirational **Research Vignettes,** the work of renowned nurse researchers whose careers exemplify the links among research, education, and practice.
- Introducing new pedagogical *interprofessional education chapter features,* **IPE Highlights and IPE Critical Thinking Challenges** and quality improvement, **QSEN Evidence-Based Practice Tips.**
- Integrating stimulating pedagogical chapter features that reinforce learning, including **Learning Outcomes, Key Terms, Key Points, Critical Thinking Challenges, Helpful Hints, Evidence-Based Practice Tips, Critical Thinking Decision Paths,** and numerous tables, boxes, and figures.
- Featuring a revised section titled **Appraising the Evidence,** accompanied by an updated **Critiquing Criteria** box in each chapter that presents a step of the research process.

- Offering a student **Evolve site** with interactive review questions that provide chapter-by-chapter review in a format consistent with that of the NCLEX® Examination.
- Offering a **Student Study Guide** that promotes active learning and assimilation of nursing research content.
- Presenting **Faculty Evolve Resources** that include a test bank, TEACH lesson plans, PowerPoint slides with integrated audience response system questions, and an image collection. Evolve resources for both students and faculty also include a research article library with appraisal exercises for additional practice in reviewing and critiquing, as well as content updates.

The ninth edition of *Nursing Research: Methods and Critical Appraisal for Evidence-Based Practice* is organized into four parts. Each part is preceded by an introductory section and opens with an engaging Research Vignette by a renowned nurse researcher.

Part I, Overview of Research and Evidence-Based Practice, contains four chapters: Chapter 1, "Integrating Research, Evidence-Based Practice, and Quality Improvement Processes," provides an excellent overview of research and evidence-based practice processes that shape clinical practice. The chapter speaks directly to students and highlights critical reading concepts and strategies, facilitating student understanding of the research process and its relationship to the critical appraisal process. The chapter introduces a model evidence hierarchy that is used throughout the text. The style and content of this chapter are designed to make subsequent chapters user friendly. The next two chapters address foundational components of the research process. Chapter 2, "Research Questions, Hypotheses, and Clinical Questions," focuses on how research questions and hypotheses are derived, operationalized, and critically appraised. Students are also taught how to develop clinical questions that are used to guide evidence-based inquiry, including quality improvement projects. Chapter 3, "Gathering and Appraising the Literature," showcases cutting-edge information literacy content and provides students and nurses with the tools necessary to effectively search, retrieve, manage, and evaluate research studies and their findings. Chapter 4, "Theoretical Frameworks for Research," is a user-friendly theory chapter that provides students with an understanding of how theories provide the foundation of research studies and evidence-based practice projects.

Part II, Processes and Evidence Related to Qualitative Research, contains three interrelated qualitative research chapters. Chapter 5, "Introduction to Qualitative Research," provides an exciting framework for understanding qualitative research and the significant contribution of qualitative research to evidence-based practice. Chapter 6, "Qualitative Approaches to Research," presents, illustrates, and showcases major qualitative methods using examples from the literature as exemplars. This chapter highlights the questions most appropriately answered using qualitative methods. Chapter 7, "Appraising Qualitative Research," synthesizes essential components of and criteria for critiquing qualitative research reports using published qualitative research study.

Part III, Processes and Evidence Related to Quantitative Research, contains Chapters 8 to 18. This group of chapters delineates essential steps of the quantitative research process, with published clinical research studies used to illustrate each step. These chapters are streamlined to make the case for linking an evidence-based approach with essential steps of the research process. Students are taught how to critically appraise the strengths and weaknesses of each step of the research process in a synthesized critique of a study. The steps of the quantitative research process, evidence-based concepts, and critical appraisal criteria are synthesized in Chapter 18 using two published research studies, providing a model for appraising strengths and weaknesses of studies, and determining applicability to practice. Chapter 11, a unique chapter, addresses the use of the types of systematic reviews that support an evidence-based practice as well as the development and application of clinical guidelines.

Part IV, Application of Research: Evidence-Based Practice, contains three chapters that showcase evidence-based practice models and tools. Chapter 19, "Strategies and Tools for Developing an Evidence-Based Practice," is a revised, vibrant, user-friendly, evidence-based toolkit with exemplars that capture the essence of high-quality, evidence-informed nursing care. It "walks" students and practicing nurses through clinical scenarios and challenges them to consider the relevant evidence-based practice "tools" to develop and answer questions that emerge from clinical situations. Chapter 20, "Developing an Evidence-Based Practice," offers a dynamic presentation of important evidence-based practice models that promote evidence-based decision making. Chapter 21, "Quality Improvement," is an innovative, engaging chapter that outlines the quality improvement process with information from current guidelines. Together, these chapters provide an inspirational conclusion to a text that we hope motivates students and practicing nurses to advance their evidence-based practice and quality improvement knowledge base and clinical competence, positioning them to make important contributions to improving health care outcomes as essential members of interprofessional teams.

Stimulating critical thinking is a core value of this text. Innovative chapter features such as **Critical Thinking Decision Paths, Evidence-Based Practice Tips, Helpful Hints, Critical Thinking Challenges, IPE Highlights, and QSEN Evidence-Based Practice Tips** enhance critical thinking, promote the development of evidence-based decision-making skills, and cultivate a positive value about the importance of collaboration in promoting evidence-based, high quality and cost-effective clinical outcomes.

Consistent with previous editions, we promote critical thinking by including sections called **"Appraising the Evidence,"** which describe the critical appraisal process related to the focus of the chapter. **Critiquing Criteria** are included in this section to stimulate a systematic and evaluative approach to reading and understanding qualitative and quantitative research and evaluating its strengths and weaknesses. Extensive resources are provided on the Evolve site that can be used to develop critical thinking and evidence-based competencies.

The development and refinement of an evidence-based foundation for clinical nursing practice is an essential priority for the future of professional nursing practice. The ninth edition of *Nursing Research: Methods and Critical Appraisal for Evidence-Based Practice* will help students develop a basic level of competence in understanding the steps of the research process that will enable them to critically analyze research studies, judge their merit, and judiciously apply evidence in clinical practice. To the extent that this goal is accomplished, the next generation of nursing professionals will have a cadre of clinicians who inform their practice using theory, research evidence, and clinical judgment, as they strive to provide high-quality, cost-effective, and satisfying health care experiences in partnership with individuals, families, and communities.

Geri LoBiondo-Wood
Geri.L.Wood@uth.tmc.edu

Judith Haber
jh33@nyu.edu

TO THE STUDENT

We invite you to join us on an exciting nursing research adventure that begins as you turn the first page of the ninth edition of *Nursing Research: Methods and Critical Appraisal for Evidence-Based Practice.* The adventure is one of discovery! You will discover that the nursing research literature sparkles with pride, dedication, and excitement about the research dimension of professional nursing practice. Whether you are a student or a practicing nurse whose goal is to use research evidence as the foundation of your practice, you will discover that nursing research and a commitment to evidence-based practice positions our profession at the forefront of change. You will discover that evidence-based practice is integral to being an effective member of an interprofessional team prepared to meet the challenge of providing quality whole person care in partnership with patients, their families/significant others, as well as with the communities in which they live. Finally, you will discover the richness in the "Who," "What," "Where," "When," "Why," and "How" of nursing research and evidence-based practice, developing a foundation of knowledge and skills that will equip you for clinical practice and making a significant contribution to achieving the Triple Aim, that is, contributing to high quality and cost-effective patient outcomes associated with satisfying patient experiences!

We think you will enjoy reading this text. Your nursing research course will be short but filled with new and challenging learning experiences that will develop your evidence-based practice skills. The ninth edition of *Nursing Research: Methods and Critical Appraisal for Evidence-Based Practice* reflects cutting-edge trends for developing evidence-based nursing practice. The four-part organization and special features in this text are designed to help you develop your critical thinking, critical reading, information literacy, interprofessional, and evidence-based clinical decision-making skills, while providing a user-friendly approach to learning that expands your competence to deal with these new and challenging experiences. The companion Study Guide, with its chapter-by-chapter activities, serves as a self-paced learning tool to reinforce the content of the text. The accompanying Evolve website offers review questions to help you reinforce the concepts discussed throughout the book.

Remember that evidence-based practice skills are used in every clinical setting and can be applied to every patient population or clinical practice issue. Whether your clinical practice involves primary care or critical care and provides inpatient or outpatient treatment in a hospital, clinic, or home, you will be challenged to apply your evidence-based practice skills and use nursing research as the foundation for your evidence-based practice. The ninth edition of *Nursing Research: Methods and Critical Appraisal for Evidence-Based Practice* will guide you through this exciting adventure, where you will discover your ability to play a vital role in contributing to the building of an evidence-based professional nursing practice.

Geri LoBiondo-Wood
Geri.L.Wood@uth.tmc.edu

Judith Haber
jh33@nyu.edu

ACKNOWLEDGMENTS

No major undertaking is accomplished alone; there are those who contribute directly and those who contribute indirectly to the success of a project. We acknowledge with deep appreciation and our warmest thanks the help and support of the following people:

- Our students, particularly the nursing students at the University of Texas Health Science Center at Houston School of Nursing and the Rory Meyers College of Nursing at New York University, whose interest, lively curiosity, and challenging questions sparked ideas for revisions in the ninth edition.
- Our chapter contributors, whose passion for research, expertise, cooperation, commitment, and punctuality made them a joy to have as colleagues.
- Our vignette contributors, whose willingness to share evidence of their research wisdom made a unique and inspirational contribution to this edition.
- Our colleagues, who have taken time out of their busy professional lives to offer feedback and constructive criticism that helped us prepare this ninth edition.
- Our editors, Lee Henderson, Melissa Rawe, and Carol O'Connell, for their willingness to listen to yet another creative idea about teaching research in a meaningful way and for their expert help with manuscript preparation and production.
- Our families: Rich Scharchburg; Brian Wood; Lenny, Andrew, Abbe, Brett, and Meredith Haber; and Laurie, Bob, Mikey, Benjy, and Noah Goldberg for their unending love, faith, understanding, and support throughout what is inevitably a consuming—but exciting—experience.

Geri LoBiondo-Wood

Judith Haber

CONTENTS

NURSING RESEARCH

PART I

Overview of Research and Evidence-Based Practice

Research Vignette: Terri Armstrong

RESEARCH VIGNETTE

WITH A LITTLE HELP FROM MY FRIENDS

Terri Armstrong, PhD ANP-BC, FAANP, FAAN
Senior Investigator
Neuro-Oncology Branch
National Cancer Institute
National Institute of Health
Bethesda, Maryland

I grew up surrounded by family and strong role models of women working in health care in a small town in Ohio. When in college, the three most important women in my life (my mom, grandmother, and great-grandmother) were all diagnosed with cancer. This led me to seek out a nursing position in oncology, and over time, I was able to be actively involved in their care. This experience taught me so much and led to the desire to do more to make the daily lives of people with cancer better. After obtaining a master's in oncology and a postmaster's nurse practitioner, an opportunity to work with Dr. M. Gilbert, a well-known caring physician who specialized in the care and treatment of patients with central nervous system (CNS) tumors and a great mentor, became available, so my work with people with CNS tumors began.

After several years, I realized that the quality of life of the brain tumor patients and families was significantly impacted by the symptoms they experienced. Over 80% were unable to return to work from the time of diagnosis, and their daily lives (and those of their families) were often consumed with managing the neurologic and treatment-related symptoms. I realized that obtaining my PhD would be an important step to learn the skills I would need to try to find answers to solve the problems CNS tumor patients were facing.

At that time, many of the conceptual models identified solitary symptoms and their impact on the person. I learned from my experience and in caring for patients that symptoms seldom occurred in isolation and that the meaning the symptoms had for patients' daily lives was important, as was learning about the patients' perception of that impact. I developed a conceptual model to identify those relationships and guide my research (Armstrong, 2003). My focus since then has been on patient-centered outcomes research, focusing on the impact of symptoms on the illness trajectory, tolerance of therapy, and potential to influence survival. My work is never done in isolation. I have been fortunate to work with research teams, including those who work alongside me and important collaborators across disciplines and the world. Team research, in which the views of various disciplines are brought together, is important in every step of research—from the hypothesis to study design and finally interpretation of the results.

My work is interconnected, but I believe it can be categorized into three general areas:

1. Improving assessment and our understanding of the experience of patients with CNS tumors.

   Patients with primary brain tumors are highly symptomatic, with implications for functional status, and are used in making treatment decisions. I led a team that developed the M.D. Anderson Symptom Inventory for Brain Tumors (MDASI-BT) (Armstrong et al., 2005; Armstrong et al., 2006) and spinal cord tumors (MDASI-Spine) (Armstrong, Gning, et al., 2010). We have completed studies showing that symptoms are associated with tumor progression (Armstrong et al., 2011). We have also been able to quantify limitations of patients' functional status (Armstrong et al., 2015), in a way that caregivers report is congruent with the patient, and have found that electronic technology (such as iPads) can be used for this (Armstrong et al., 2012). Our work with the Collaborative Ependymoma Research Organization (CERN, www.cern-foundation.org) has allowed us to reach out to patients with this rarer tumor to understand the natural history and impact of the disease and its treatment on patients around the world (Armstrong, Vera-Bolanos, et al., 2010; Armstrong, Vera-Bolanos, & Gilbert, 2011). Based on these surveys, we have developed materials to inform patients and are launching an expansion of this project, in which we will evaluate risk factors (both based on history and genetics) for the occurrence of these tumors in both adults and children.

2. Incorporation of clinical outcomes assessment into brain tumor clinical trials.

Clinical trials often assess the impact of therapy on how the tumor appears on imaging or survival, but the impact on the person is often not assessed. I have been fortunate to work with Dr. M. Gilbert and Dr. J. Wefel to incorporate these outcomes into large clinical trials, providing clear evidence that it was feasible to incorporate patient outcomes measures and that the results of these evaluations could impact the interpretation of the clinical trial (Armstrong et al., 2013; Gilbert et al., 2014). As a result of my involvement in these efforts, I recently chaired a daylong workshop exploring the use of clinical outcomes assessments (COAs) in brain tumor trials, a workshop cosponsored by the FDA and the Jumpstarting Brain Tumor Drug Development (JSBTDD) consortia that also included members of the academic community, patient advocates, pharmaceutical industry, and the NIH. This successful workshop has resulted in a series of white papers that were recently published on the importance of including these in clinical trials (Armstrong, Bishof, et al., 2016; Helfer et al., 2016).

3. Identification of clinical and genomic predictors of toxicity.

Toxicity associated with treatment also impacts the patient. For example, Temozolomide, the most common agent used in the treatment of brain tumors, has a low overall incidence of myelotoxicity (impact on blood counts that help to fight infection or clot the blood). However, in the select patients who develop toxicity, there are significant clinical implications (treatment holds or cessation, and even death). I work with an interdisciplinary group that began to explore the clinical predictors of this toxicity and then explored associated genomic changes associated with risk (Armstrong et al., 2009). Currently, I am also working with a research team exploring risk factors and pathogenesis of radiation-induced fatigue and sleepiness, which is a major symptom in a large percentage of patients undergoing cranial radiotherapy for their brain tumor (Armstrong, Shade, et al., 2016). The ultimate goal of this part of my research is to begin to uncover phenotypes associated with symptoms and to uncover the underlying biologic processes, so that we can initiate measures prior to the occurrence of symptoms, rather than waiting for them to occur and then trying to mitigate them.

In addition to conducting focused outcomes research as outlined previously, I have over 25 years' dedication to the clinical care of persons with tumors of the CNS. This work is the best part of my job and is a critical linkage and inspiration in my research, with the goal of improving the daily life of patients and improving our understanding of the underlying biology of symptoms and experience that our patients have.

REFERENCES

Armstrong, T. S. (2003). Symptoms experience: a concept analysis. *Oncology Nursing Society, 30*(4), 601–606.

Armstrong, T. S., Cohen, M. Z., Eriksen, L., & Cleeland, C. (2005). Content validity of self-report measurement instruments: an illustration from the development of the Brain Tumor Module of the M. D. Anderson Symptom Inventory. *Oncology Nursing Society, 32*(3), 669–676.

Armstrong, T. S., Mendoza, T., Gning, I., et al. (2006). Validation of the M. D. Anderson Symptom Inventory Brain Tumor Module (MDASI-BT). *Journal of Neuro-Oncology, 80*(1), 27–35.

Armstrong, T. S., Cao, Y., Scheurer, M. E., et al. (2009). Risk analysis of severe myelotoxicity with temozolomide: The effects of clinical and genetic factors. *Neuro-Oncology, 11*(6), 825–832.

Armstrong, T. S., Gning, I., Mendoza, T. R., et al. (2010). Reliability and validity of the M. D. Anderson Symptom Inventory-Spine Tumor Module. *Journal of Neurosurgery Spine, 12*(4), 421–430.

Armstrong, T. S., Vera-Bolanos, E., Bekele, B. N., et al. (2010). Adult ependymal tumors: prognosis and the M. D. Anderson Cancer Center experience. *Neuro-Oncology, 12*(8), 862–870.

Armstrong, T. S., Vera-Bolanos, E., & Gilbert, M. R. (2011). Clinical course of adult patients with ependymoma: results of the Adult Ependymoma Outcomes Project. *Cancer, 117*(22), 5133–5141.

Armstrong, T. S., Vera-Bolanos, E., Gning, I., et al. (2011). The impact of symptom interference using the MD Anderson Symptom Inventory-Brain Tumor Module (MDASI-BT) on prediction of recurrence in primary brain tumor patients. *Cancer, 117*(14), 3222–3228.

Armstrong, T. S., Wefel, J. S., Gning, I., et al. (2012). Congruence of primary brain tumor patient and caregiver symptom report. *Cancer, 118*(20), 5026–5037.

Armstrong, T. S., Wefel, J. S., Wang, M., et al. (2013). Net clinical benefit analysis of radiation therapy oncology group 0525: a phase III trial comparing conventional adjuvant temozolomide with dose-intensive temozolomide in patients with newly diagnosed glioblastoma. *Journal of Clinical Oncology, 31*(32), 4076–4084.

Armstrong, T. S., Vera-Bolanos, E., Acquaye, A. A., et al. (2015). The symptom burden of primary brain tumors: evidence for a core set of tumor and treatment-related symptoms. *Neuro-Oncology, 18*(2), 252–260. Epub August 19, 2015.

Armstrong, T. S., Bishof, A. M., Brown, P. D., et al. (2016). Determining priority signs and symptoms for use as clinical outcomes assessments in trials including patients with malignant gliomas: panel 1 report. *Neuro-Oncology, 18*(Suppl. 2), ii1–ii12.

Armstrong, T. S., Shade, M. Y., Breton, G., et al. (2016). Sleep-wake disturbance in patients with brain tumors. *Neuro-Oncology*, in press.

Gilbert, M. R., Dignam, J. J., Armstrong, T. S., et al. (2014). A randomized trial of bevacizumab for newly diagnosed glioblastoma. *New England Journal of Medicine, 370*(8), 699–708.

Helfer, J. L., Wen, P. Y., Blakeley, J., et al. (2016). Report of the Jumpstarting Brain Tumor Drug Development Coalition and FDA clinical trials clinical outcome assessment endpoints workshop (October 15, 2014, Bethesda, MD). *Neuro-Oncology, 18*(Suppl. 2), ii26–ii36.

1

Integrating Research, Evidence-Based Practice, and Quality Improvement Processes

Geri LoBiondo-Wood and Judith Haber

Go to Evolve at **http://evolve.elsevier.com/LoBiondo/** for review questions, critiquing exercises, and additional research articles for practice in reviewing and critiquing.

LEARNING OUTCOMES

After reading this chapter, you should be able to do the following:

- State the significance of research, evidence-based practice, and quality improvement (QI).
- Identify the role of the consumer of nursing research.
- Define evidence-based practice.
- Define QI.
- Discuss evidence-based and QI decision making.
- Explain the difference between quantitative and qualitative research.
- Explain the difference between the types of systematic reviews.
- Identify the importance of critical reading skills for critical appraisal of research.
- Discuss the format and style of research reports/articles.
- Discuss how to use an evidence hierarchy when critically appraising research studies.

KEY TERMS

abstract
clinical guidelines
consensus guidelines
critical appraisal
critical reading
critique
evidence-based guidelines
evidence-based practice
integrative review
levels of evidence
meta-analysis
meta-synthesis
quality improvement
qualitative research
quantitative research
research
systematic review

We invite you to join us on an exciting nursing research adventure that begins as you read the first page of this chapter. The adventure is one of discovery! You will discover that the nursing research literature sparkles with pride, dedication, and excitement about this dimension of professional practice. As you progress through your educational program, you are taught how to ensure quality and safety in practice through acquiring knowledge of the various sciences and health care principles. A critical component of clinical knowledge is understanding research as it applies to practicing from a base of evidence.

Whether you are a student or a practicing nurse whose goal is to use **research** as the foundation of your practice, you will discover that **research**, **evidence-based practice**, and **quality improvement** (QI) positions our profession at the cutting edge of change and improvement in patient outcomes. You will also discover the cutting edge "who," "what," "where," "when," "why," and "how" of nursing research, and develop a foundation of evidence-based practice knowledge and competencies that will equip you for your clinical practice.

Your nursing research adventure will be filled with new and challenging learning experiences that develop your evidence-based practice skills. Your critical thinking, critical reading, and clinical decision-making skills will expand as you develop clinical questions, search the research literature, evaluate the research evidence found in the literature, and make clinical decisions about applying the "best available evidence" to your practice. For example, you will be encouraged to ask important clinical questions, such as, "What makes a telephone education intervention more effective with one group of patients with a diagnosis of congestive heart failure but not another?" "What is the effect of computer learning modules on self-management of diabetes in children?" "What research has been conducted in the area of identifying barriers to breast cancer screening in African American women?" "What is the quality of studies conducted on telehealth?" "What nursing-delivered smoking cessation interventions are most effective?" This book will help you begin your adventure into evidence-based practice by developing an appreciation of research as the foundation for evidence-based practice and QI.

NURSING RESEARCH, EVIDENCE-BASED PRACTICE, AND QUALITY IMPROVEMENT

Nurses are challenged to stay abreast of new information to provide the highest quality of patient care (Institute of Medicine [IOM], 2011). Nurses are challenged to expand their "comfort zone" by offering creative approaches to old and new health problems, as well as designing new and innovative programs that make a difference in the health status of our citizens. This challenge can best be met by integrating rapidly expanding research and evidence-based knowledge about biological, behavioral, and environmental influences on health into the care of patients and their families.

It is important to differentiate between research, evidence-based practice, and QI. **Research** is the systematic, rigorous, critical investigation that aims to answer questions about nursing phenomena. Researchers follow the steps of the scientific process, outlined in this chapter and discussed in detail in each chapter of this textbook. There are two types of research: quantitative and qualitative. The methods used by nurse researchers are the same methods used by other disciplines; the difference is that nurses study questions relevant to nursing practice. Published research studies are read and evaluated for use in clinical practice. Study findings provide evidence that is evaluated, and applicability to practice is used to inform clinical decisions.

Evidence-based practice is the collection, evaluation, and integration of valid research evidence, combined with clinical expertise and an understanding of patient and family values and preferences, to inform clinical decision making (Sackett et al., 2000). Research studies are gathered from the literature and assessed so that decisions about application to practice can be made, culminating in nursing practice that is evidence based. ➤ **Example:** To help you understand the importance of evidence-based practice, think about the systematic review and meta-analysis from Al-Mallah and colleagues (2015), which assessed the impact of nurse-led clinics on the mortality and morbidity of patients with cardiovascular disease (see Appendix E). Based on their synthesis of the literature, they put forth several conclusions regarding the implications for practice and further research for nurses working in the field of cardiovascular care.

QI is the systematic use of data to monitor the outcomes of care processes as well as the use of improvement methods to design and test changes in practice for the purpose of continuously improving the quality and safety of health care systems (Cronenwett et al., 2007). While research supports or generates new knowledge, evidence-based practice and QI uses currently available knowledge to improve health care delivery. When you first read about these three processes, you will notice they have similarities. Each begins with a question. The difference is that in a research study the question is tested with a design appropriate to the question and specific methodology (i.e., sample, instruments, procedures, and data analysis) used to test the research question and contribute to new, generalizable knowledge. In the evidence-based practice and QI processes, a question is used to search the literature for already completed studies in order to bring about improvements in care.

All nurses share a commitment to the advancement of nursing science by conducting research and using research evidence in practice. Research promotes accountability, which is one of the hallmarks of the nursing profession and a fundamental concept of the American Nurses Association (ANA) Code for Nurses (ANA, 2015). There is a consensus that the research role of the baccalaureate and master's graduate calls for **critical appraisal** skills. That is, nurses must be knowledgeable consumers of research, who can evaluate the strengths and weaknesses of research evidence and use existing standards to determine the merit and readiness of research for use in clinical practice. Therefore, to use research for an evidence-based practice and to practice using the highest quality processes, you do not have to conduct research; however, you do need to understand and appraise the steps of the research process in order to read the research literature critically and use it to inform clinical decisions.

As you venture through this text, you will see the steps of the research, evidence-based practice, and QI processes. The steps are systematic and relate to the development of evidence-based practice. Understanding the processes that researchers use will help you develop the assessment skills necessary to judge the soundness of research studies.

Throughout the chapters, terminology pertinent to each step is identified and illustrated with examples. Five published studies are found in the appendices and used as examples to illustrate significant points in each chapter. Judging the study's strength and quality, as well as its applicability to practice, is key. Before you can judge a study, it is important to understand the differences among studies. There are different study designs that you will see as you read through this text and the appendices. There are standards not only for critiquing the soundness of each step of a study, but also for judging the strength and quality of evidence provided by a study and determining its applicability to practice.

This chapter provides an overview of research study designs and appraisal skills. It introduces the overall format of a research article and provides an overview of the subsequent chapters in the book. It also introduces the QI and evidence-based practice processes, a level of evidence hierarchy model, and other tools for helping you evaluate the strength and quality of research evidence. These topics are designed to help you read research articles more effectively and with greater understanding, so that you can make evidence-based clinical decisions and contribute to quality and cost-effective patient outcomes.

TYPES OF RESEARCH: QUALITATIVE AND QUANTITATIVE

Research is classified into two major categories: qualitative and quantitative. A researcher chooses between these categories based on the question being asked. That is, a researcher may wish to test a cause-and-effect relationship, or to assess if variables are related, or may wish to discover and understand the meaning of an experience or process. A researcher would choose to conduct a **qualitative research** study if the question is about understanding the meaning of a human experience such as grief, hope, or loss. The meaning of an experience is based on the view that meaning varies and is subjective. The context of the experience also plays a role in qualitative research. That is, the experience of loss as a result of a miscarriage would be different than the experience of losing a parent.

Qualitative research is generally conducted in natural settings and uses data that are words or text rather than numeric to describe the experiences being studied. Qualitative studies are guided by research questions, and data are collected from a small number of subjects, allowing an in-depth study of a phenomenon. ➤ **Example:** vanDijk et al. (2016) explored how patients assign a number to their postoperative pain experience (see Appendix C). Although qualitative research is systematic in its method, it uses a subjective approach. Data from qualitative studies help nurses understand experiences or phenomena that affect patients; these data also assist in generating theories that lead clinicians to develop improved patient care and stimulate further research. Highlights of the general steps of qualitative studies and the journal format for a qualitative article are outlined in Table 1.1. Chapters 5 through 7 provide an in-depth view of qualitative research underpinnings, designs, and methods.

Whereas qualitative research looks for meaning, **quantitative research** encompasses the study of research questions and/or hypotheses that describe phenomena, test relationships,

TABLE 1.1 Steps of the Research Process and Journal Format: Qualitative Research

Research Process Steps and/or Format Issues	Usual Location in Journal Heading or Subheading
Identifying the phenomenon	Abstract and/or in introduction
Research question study purpose	Abstract and/or in beginning or end of introduction
Literature review	Introduction and/or discussion
Design	Abstract and/or in introductory section or under method section entitled "Design" or stated in method section
Sample	Method section labeled "Sample" or "Subjects"
Legal-ethical issues	Data collection or procedures section or in sample section
Data collection procedure	Data collection or procedures section
Data analysis	Methods section under subhead "Data Analysis" or "Data Analysis and Interpretation"
Results	Stated in separate heading: "Results" or "Findings"
Discussion and recommendation	Combined in separate section: "Discussion" or "Discussion and Implications"
References	At end of article

assess differences, seek to explain cause-and-effect relationships between variables, and test for intervention effectiveness. The numeric data in quantitative studies are summarized and analyzed using statistics. Quantitative research techniques are systematic, and the methodology is controlled. Appendices A, B, and D illustrate examples of different quantitative approaches to answering research questions. Table 1.2 indicates where each step of the research process can usually be located in a quantitative research article and where it is discussed in this text. Chapters 2, 3, and 8 through 18 describe processes related to quantitative research.

The primary difference is that a qualitative study seeks to interpret meaning and phenomena, whereas quantitative research seeks to test a hypothesis or answer research questions using statistical methods. Remember as you read research articles that, depending on the nature of the research problem, a researcher may vary the steps slightly; however, all of the steps should be addressed systematically.

TABLE 1.2 Steps of the Research Process and Journal Format: Quantitative Research

Research Process Steps and/or Format Issue	Usual Location in Journal Heading or Subheading	Text Chapter
Research problem	Abstract and/or in article introduction or separately labeled: "Problem"	2
Purpose	Abstract and/or in introduction, or end of literature review or theoretical framework section, or labeled separately: "Purpose"	2
Literature review	At end of heading "Introduction" but not labeled as such, or labeled as separate heading: "Literature Review," "Review of the Literature," or "Related Literature"; or not labeled or variables reviewed appear as headings or subheadings	3
TF and/or CF	Combined with "Literature Review" or found in separate section as TF or CF; or each concept used in TF or CF may appear as separate subheading	3, 4
Hypothesis/research questions	Stated or implied near end of introduction, may be labeled or found in separate heading or subheading: "Hypothesis" or "Research Questions"; or reported for first time in "Results"	2
Research design	Stated or implied in abstract or introduction or in "Methods" or "Methodology" section	8–10
Sample: type and size	"Size" may be stated in abstract, in methods section, or as separate subheading under methods section as "Sample," "Sample/Subjects," or "Participants"; "Type" may be implied or stated in any of previous headings described under size	12
Legal-ethical issues	Stated or implied in sections: "Methods," "Procedures," "Sample," or "Subjects"	13
Instruments	Found in sections: "Methods," "Instruments," or "Measures"	14
Validity and reliability	Specifically stated or implied in sections: "Methods," "Instruments," "Measures," or "Procedures"	15
Data collection procedure	In methods section under subheading "Procedure" or "Data Collection," or as separate heading: "Procedure"	14
Data analysis	Under subheading: "Data Analysis"	16
Results	Stated in separate heading: "Results"	16, 17
Discussion of findings and new findings	Combined with results or as separate heading: "Discussion"	17
Implications, limitations, and recommendations	Combined in discussion or as separate major headings	17
References	At end of article	4
Communicating research results	Research articles, poster, and paper presentations	1, 20

CF, Conceptual framework; *TF*, theoretical framework.

CRITICAL READING SKILLS

To develop an expertise in evidence-based practice, you will need to be able to critically read all types of research articles. As you read a research article, you may be struck by the difference in style or format of a research article versus a clinical article. The terms of a research article are new, and the content is different. You may also be thinking that the research article is hard to read or that it is technical and boring. You may simultaneously wonder, "How will I possibly learn to appraise all the steps of a research study, the terminology, and the process of evidence-based practice? I'm only on Chapter 1. This is not so easy; research is as hard as everyone says."

Remember that learning occurs with time and help. Reading research articles can be difficult and frustrating at first, but the best way to become a knowledgeable research consumer is to use **critical reading** skills when reading research articles. As a student, you are not expected to understand a research article or critique it perfectly the first time. Nor are you expected to develop these skills on your own. An essential objective of this book is to help you acquire critical reading skills so that you can use research in your practice. Becoming a competent critical thinker and reader of research takes time and patience.

Learning the research process further develops critical appraisal skills. You will gradually be able to read a research article and reflect on it by identifying assumptions, key concepts, and methods, and determining whether the conclusions are based on the study's findings. Once you have obtained this critical appraisal competency, you will be ready to synthesize the findings of multiple studies to use in developing an evidence-based practice. This will be a very exciting and rewarding process for you. Analyzing a study critically can require several readings. As you review and synthesize a study, you will begin an appraisal process to help you determine the study's worth. An illustration of how to use critical reading strategies is provided in Box 1.1, which contains an excerpt from the abstract, introduction, literature review, theoretical framework literature, and methods and procedure section of a quantitative study (Nyamathi et al., 2015) (see Appendix A). Note that in this article there is both a literature review and a theoretical framework section that clearly support the study's objectives and purpose. Also note that parts of the text from the article were deleted to offer a number of examples within the text of this chapter.

IPE HIGHLIGHT

Start an IPE Journal Club with students from other health professions programs on your campus. Select a research study to read, understand, and critically appraise together. It is always helpful to collaborate on deciding whether the findings are applicable to clinical practice.

STRATEGIES FOR CRITIQUING RESEARCH STUDIES

Evaluation of a research article requires a critique. A **critique** is the process of critical appraisal that objectively and critically evaluates a research report's content for scientific merit and application to practice. It requires some knowledge of the subject matter and knowledge of how to critically read and use critical appraisal criteria. You will find:

- Summarized examples of critical appraisal criteria for qualitative studies and an example of a qualitative critique in Chapter 7
- Summarized critical appraisal criteria and examples of a quantitative critique in Chapter 18

BOX 1.1 Example of Critical Appraisal Reading Strategies

Introductory Paragraphs, Study's Purpose and Aims	Globally, incarcerated populations encounter a host of public health care issues; two such issues—HAV and HBV diseases—are vaccine preventable. In addition, viral hepatitis disproportionately impacts the homeless because of increased risky sexual behaviors and drug use (Stein, Andersen, Robertson, & Gelberg, 2012), along with substandard living conditions (Hennessey, Bangsberg, Weinbaum, & Hahn, 2009). Purpose—Despite knowledge of awareness of risk factors for HBV infection, intervention programs designed to enhance completion of the three-series Twinrix HAV/HBV vaccine and identification of prognostic factors for vaccine completion have not been widely studied. The purpose of this study was to first assess whether seronegative parolees previously randomized to any one of three intervention conditions were more likely to complete the vaccine series as well as to identify the predictors of HAV/HBV vaccine completion.
Literature Review—Concepts Preventable disease vaccinations Homelessness	Despite the availability of the HBV vaccine, there has been a low rate of completion for the three-dose core of the accelerated vaccine series (Centers for Disease Control and Prevention, 2012). Among incarcerated populations, HBV vaccine coverage is low; in a study among jail inmates, 19% had past HBV infection, and 12% completed the HBV vaccination series (Hennessey, Kim, et al., 2009). Although HBV is well accepted behind bars—because of the lack of funding and focus on prevention as a core in the prison system—few inmates complete the series (Weinbaum, Sabin, & Santibanez, 2005). In addition, prevention may not be priority. Authors contend that, although the HBV vaccine is cost-effective, it is underutilized among high-risk (Rich et al., 2003) and incarcerated populations (Hunt & Saab, 2009). For homeless men on parole, vaccination completion may be affected by level of custody; generally, the higher the level of custody, the higher the risk an inmate poses.
Conceptual Framework	The comprehensive health seeking and coping paradigm (Nyamathi, 1989), adapted from a coping model (Lazarus & Folkman, 1984), and the health seeking and coping paradigm (Schlotfeldt, 1981) guided this study and the variables selected (see Fig. 1.1). The comprehensive health seeking and coping paradigm has been successfully applied by our team to improve our understanding of HIV and HBV/hepatitis C virus (HCV) protective behaviors and health outcomes among homeless adults (Nyamathi, Liu, et al., 2009)—many of whom had been incarcerated (Nyamathi et al., 2012).
Methods/Design	The study used a randomized clinical trial.
Specific Aims and Hypotheses	In this model, a number of factors are thought to relate to the outcome variable, completion of the HAV/HBV vaccine series. These factors include sociodemographic factors, situational factors, personal factors, social factors, and health seeking and coping responses.
Subject Recruitment and Accrual	An RCT where 600 male parolees participating in an RDT program were randomized into one of three intervention conditions aimed at assessing program efficacy on reducing drug use and recidivism at 6 and 12 months, as well as vaccine completion in eligible subjects. There were four inclusion criteria for recruitment purposes in assessing program efficacy on reducing drug use and recidivism: (1) history of drug use prior to their latest incarceration, (2) between ages of 18 and 60, (3) residing in the participating RDT program, and (4) designated as homeless as noted on the prison or jail discharge form.
Procedure	The study was approved by the University of California, Los Angeles Institutional Review Board and registered with clinical Trials.gov. Building upon previous studies, we developed varying levels of peer-coached and nurse-led programs designed to improve HAV/HBV vaccine receptivity at 12-month follow-up among homeless offenders recently released to parole. See Appendix A for details in the "Interventions" section.
Intervention Fidelity	Several strategies for treatment fidelity included study design, interventionist's training, and standardization of interventions. See the Interventions section in Appendix A.

HBA, Hepatitis A virus; *HBV,* hepatitis B virus; *RCT,* randomized clinical trial.

- An in-depth exploration of the criteria for evaluation required in quantitative research critiques in Chapters 8 through 18
- Criteria for qualitative research critiques presented in Chapters 5 through 7
- Principles for qualitative and quantitative research in Chapters 1 through 4

Critical appraisal criteria are the standards, appraisal guides, or questions used to assess an article. In analyzing a research article, you must evaluate each step of the research process and ask questions about whether each step meets the criteria. For instance, the critical appraisal criteria in Chapter 3 ask if "the literature review identifies gaps and inconsistencies in the literature about a subject, concept, or problem," and if "all of the concepts and variables are included in the review." These two questions relate to critiquing the research question and the literature review components of the research process. Box 1.1 lists several gaps identified in the literature by Nyamathi and colleagues (2015) and how the study intended to fill these gaps by conducting research for the stated objective and purpose (see Appendix A). Remember that when doing a critique, you are pointing out strengths as well as weaknesses. Standardized critical appraisal tools such as those from the Center for Evidence Based Medicine (CEBM) Critical Appraisal Tools (www.cebm.net/critical-appraisal) can be used to systematically appraise the strength and quality of evidence provided in research articles (see Chapter 20).

Critiquing can be thought of as looking at a completed jigsaw puzzle. Does it form a comprehensive picture, or is a piece out of place? What is the level of evidence provided by the study and the findings? What is the balance between the risks and benefits of the findings that contribute to clinical decisions? How can I apply the evidence to my patient, to my patient population, or in my setting? When reading several studies for synthesis, you must assess the interrelationship of the studies, as well as the overall strength and quality of evidence and applicability to practice. Reading for synthesis is essential in critiquing research. Appraising a study helps with the development of an evidence table (see Chapter 20).

OVERCOMING BARRIERS: USEFUL CRITIQUING STRATEGIES

Throughout the text, you will find features that will help refine the skills essential to understanding and using research in your practice. A Critical Thinking Decision Path related to each step of the research process in each chapter will sharpen your decision-making skills as you critique research articles. Look for Internet resources in chapters that will enhance your consumer skills. Critical Thinking Challenges, which appear at the end of each chapter, are designed to reinforce your critical reading skills in relation to the steps of the research process. Helpful Hints, designed to reinforce your understanding, appear at various points throughout the chapters. Evidence-Based Practice Tips, which will help you apply evidence-based practice strategies in your clinical practice, are provided in each chapter.

When you complete your first critique, congratulate yourself; mastering these skills is not easy. Best of all, you can look forward to discussing the points of your appraisal, because your critique will be based on objective data, not just personal opinion. As you continue to use and perfect critical analysis skills by critiquing studies, remember that these skills are an expected competency for delivering evidence-based and quality nursing care.

EVIDENCE-BASED PRACTICE AND RESEARCH

Along with gaining comfort while reading and critiquing studies, there is one final step: deciding how, when, and if to apply the studies to your practice so that your practice is evidence based. **Evidence-based practice** allows you to systematically use the best available evidence with the integration of individual clinical expertise, as well as the patient's values and preferences, in making clinical decisions (Sackett et al., 2000). Evidence-based practice involves processes and steps, as does the research process. These steps are presented throughout the text. Chapter 19 provides an overview of evidence-based practice steps and strategies.

When using evidence-based practice strategies, the first step is to be able to read a study and understand how each section is linked to the steps of the research process. The following section introduces you to the research process as presented in published articles. Once you read a study, you must decide which **level of evidence** the study provides and how well the study was designed and executed. Fig. 1.1 illustrates a model for determining the levels

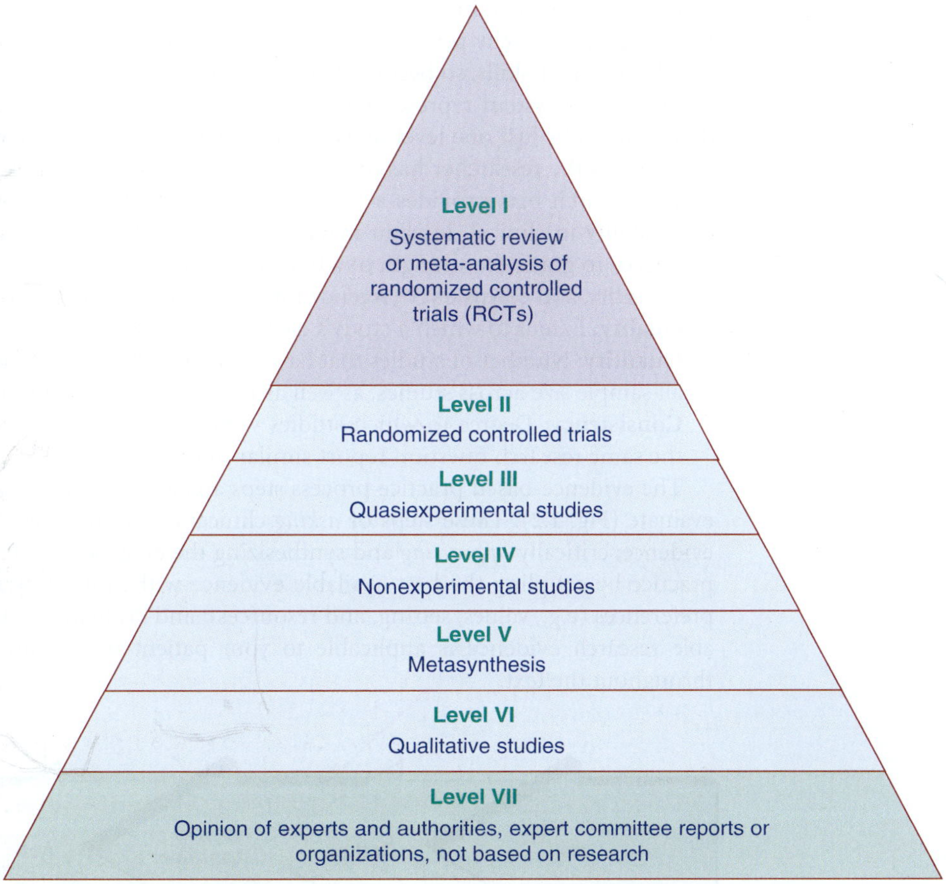

FIG 1.1 Levels of evidence: Evidence hierarchy for rating levels of evidence associated with a study's design. Evidence is assessed at a level according to its source.

of evidence associated with a study's design, ranging from systematic reviews of randomized clinical trials (RCTs) (see Chapters 9 and 10) to expert opinions. The rating system, or evidence hierarchy model, presented here is just one of many. Many hierarchies for assessing the relative worth of both qualitative and quantitative designs are available. Early in the development of evidence-based practice, evidence hierarchies were thought to be very inflexible, with systematic reviews or meta-analyses at the top and qualitative research at the bottom. When assessing a clinical question that measures cause and effect, this may be true; however, nursing and health care research are involved in a broader base of problem solving, and thus assessing the worth of a study within a broader context of applying evidence into practice requires a broader view.

The meaningfulness of an evidence rating system will become clearer as you read Chapters 8 through 11. ➤ **Example:** The Nyamathi et al. (2015) study is Level II because of its experimental, randomized control trial design, whereas the vanDijk et al. (2016) study is Level VI because it is a qualitative study. The level itself does not tell a study's worth; rather it is another tool that helps you think about a study's strengths and weaknesses and the nature of the evidence provided in the findings and conclusions. Chapters 7 and 18 will provide an understanding of how studies can be assessed for use in practice. You will use the evidence hierarchy presented in Fig. 1.1 throughout the book as you develop your research consumer skills, so become familiar with its content.

This rating system represents levels of evidence for judging the strength of a study's design, which is just one level of assessment that influences the confidence one has in the conclusions the researcher has drawn. Assessing the strength of scientific evidence or potential research bias provides a vehicle to guide evaluation of research studies for their applicability in clinical decision making. In addition to identifying the level of evidence, one needs to grade the strength of a body of evidence, incorporating the domains of quality, quantity, and consistency (Agency for Healthcare Research and Quality, 2002).

- **Quality:** Extent to which a study's design, implementation, and analysis minimize bias.
- **Quantity:** Number of studies that have evaluated the research question, including overall sample size across studies, as well as the strength of the findings from data analyses.
- **Consistency:** Degree to which studies with similar and different designs investigating the same research question report similar findings.

The evidence-based practice process steps are: ask, gather, assess and appraise, act, and evaluate (Fig. 1.2). These steps of *asking* clinical questions; identifying and *gathering* the evidence; critically *appraising* and synthesizing the evidence or literature; *acting* to change practice by coupling the best available evidence with your clinical expertise and patient preferences (e.g., values, setting, and resources); and *evaluating* if the use of the best available research evidence is applicable to your patient or organization will be discussed throughout the text.

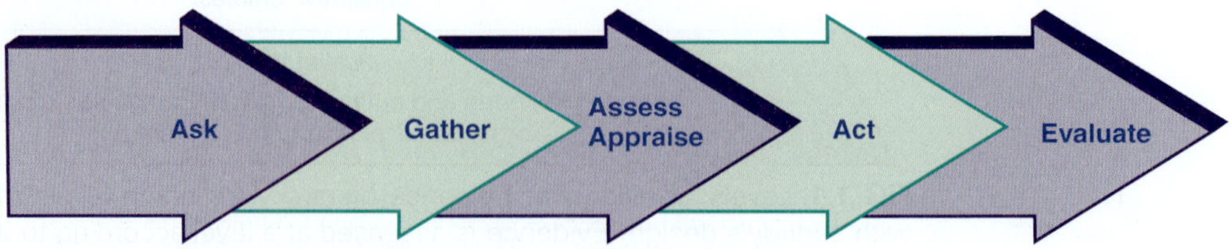

FIG 1.2 Evidence-based practice steps.

To maintain an evidence-based practice, studies are evaluated using specific criteria. Completed studies are evaluated for strength, quality, and consistency of evidence. Before one can proceed with an evidence-based project, it is necessary to understand the steps of the research process found in research studies.

RESEARCH ARTICLES: FORMAT AND STYLE

Before you begin reading research articles, it is important to understand their organization and format. Many journals publish research, either as the sole type of article or in addition to clinical or theoretical articles. Many journals have some common features but also unique characteristics. All journals have guidelines for manuscript preparation and submission. A review of these guidelines, which are found on a journal's website, will give you an idea of the format of articles that appear in specific journals.

Remember that even though each step of the research process is discussed at length in this text, you may find only a short paragraph or a sentence in an article that provides the details of the step. A publication is a shortened version of the researcher(s) completed work. You will also find that some researchers devote more space in an article to the results, whereas others present a longer discussion of the methods and procedures. Most authors give more emphasis to the method, results, and discussion of implications than to details of assumptions, hypotheses, or definitions of terms. Decisions about the amount of material presented for each step of the research process are bound by the following:

- A journal's space limitations
- A journal's author guidelines
- The type or nature of the study
- The researcher's decision regarding which component of the study is the most important

The following discussion provides a brief overview of each step of the research process and how it might appear in an article. It is important to remember that a quantitative research article will differ from a qualitative research article. The components of qualitative research are discussed in Chapters 5 and 6, and are summarized in Chapter 7.

Abstract

An **abstract** is a short, comprehensive synopsis or summary of a study at the beginning of an article. An abstract quickly focuses the reader on the main points of a study. A well-presented abstract is accurate, self-contained, concise, specific, nonevaluative, coherent, and readable. Abstracts vary in word length. The length and format of an abstract are dictated by the journal's style. Both quantitative and qualitative research studies have abstracts that provide a succinct overview of the study. An example of an abstract can be found at the beginning of the study by Nyamathi et al. (2015) (see Appendix A). Their abstract follows an outline format that highlights the major steps of the study. It partially reads as follows:

Purpose/Objective: "The study focused on completion of the HAV and HBV vaccine series among homeless men on parole. The efficacy of the three levels of peer counseling (PC) and nurse delivered intervention was compared at 12 month follow up."

In this example, the authors provide a view of the study variables. The remainder of the abstract provides a synopsis of the background of the study and the methods, results, and conclusions. The studies in Appendices A through D all have abstracts.

HELPFUL HINT

An abstract is a concise short overview that provides a reference to the research purpose, research questions, and/or hypotheses, methodology, and results, as well as the implications for practice or future research.

Introduction

Early in a research article, in a section that may or may not be labeled "Introduction," the researcher presents a background picture of the area researched and its significance to practice (see Chapter 2).

Definition of the Purpose

The purpose of the study is defined either at the end of the researcher's initial introduction or at the end of the "Literature Review" or "Conceptual Framework" section. The study's purpose may or may not be labeled (see Chapters 2 and 3), or it may be referred to as the study's aim or objective. The studies in Appendices A through D present specific purposes for each study in untitled sections that appear in the beginning of each article, as well as in the article's abstract.

Literature Review and Theoretical Framework

Authors of studies present the literature review and theoretical framework in different ways. Many research articles merge the "Literature Review" and the "Theoretical Framework." This section includes the main concepts investigated and may be called "Review of the Literature," "Literature Review," "Theoretical Framework," "Related Literature," "Background," "Conceptual Framework," or it may not be labeled at all (see Chapters 2 and 3). By reviewing Appendices A through D, you will find differences in the headings used. Nyamathi et al. (2015) (see Appendix A) use no labels and present the literature review but do have a section labeled theoretical framework, while the study in Appendix B has a literature review and a conceptual framework integrated in the beginning of the article. One style is not better than another; the studies in the appendices contain all the critical elements but present the elements differently.

HELPFUL HINT

Not all research articles include headings for each step or component of the research process, but each step is presented at some point in the article.

Hypothesis/Research Question

A study's research questions or hypotheses can also be presented in different ways (see Chapter 2). Research articles often do not have separate headings for reporting the "Hypotheses" or "Research Question." They are often embedded in the "Introduction" or "Background" section or not labeled at all (e.g., as in the studies in the appendices). If a study uses hypotheses, the researcher may report whether the hypotheses were or were not supported toward the end of the article in the "Results" or "Findings" section. Quantitative research studies have hypotheses or research questions. Qualitative research studies do not have hypotheses, but have research questions and purposes. The studies in Appendices A,

B, and D have hypotheses. The study in Appendix C does not, since it is a qualitative study; rather it has a purpose statement.

Research Design

The type of research design can be found in the abstract, within the purpose statement, or in the introduction to the "Procedures" or "Methods" section, or not stated at all (see Chapters 6, 9, and 10). For example, the studies in Appendices A, B, and D identify the design in the abstract.

One of your first objectives is to determine whether the study is qualitative (see Chapters 5 and 6) or quantitative (see Chapters 8, 9, and 10). Although the rigor of the critical appraisal criteria addressed do not substantially change, some of the terminology of the questions differs for qualitative versus quantitative studies. Do not get discouraged if you cannot easily determine the design. One of the best strategies is to review the chapters that address designs. The following tips will help you determine whether the study you are reading employs a quantitative design:

- Hypotheses are stated or implied (see Chapter 2).
- The terms *control* and *treatment group* appear (see Chapter 9).
- The terms *survey, correlational, case control,* or *cohort* are used (see Chapter 10).
- The terms *random* or *convenience* are mentioned in relation to the sample (see Chapter 12).
- Variables are measured by instruments or scales (see Chapter 14).
- Reliability and validity of instruments are discussed (see Chapter 15).
- Statistical analyses are used (see Chapter 16).

In contrast, qualitative studies generally do not focus on "numbers." Some qualitative studies may use standard quantitative terms (e.g., subjects) rather than qualitative terms (e.g., informants). Deciding on the type of qualitative design can be confusing; one of the best strategies is to review the qualitative chapters (see Chapters 5 through 7). Begin trying to link the study's design with the level of evidence associated with that design as illustrated in Fig. 1.1. This will give you a context for evaluating the strength and consistency of the findings and applicability to practice. Chapters 8 through 11 will help you understand how to link the levels of evidence with quantitative designs. A study may not indicate the specific design used; however, all studies inform the reader of the methodology used, which can help you decide the type of design the authors used to guide the study.

Sampling

The population from which the sample was drawn is discussed in the section "Methods" or "Methodology" under the subheadings of "Subjects" or "Sample" (see Chapter 12). Researchers should tell you both the population from which the sample was chosen and the number of subjects that participated in the study, as well as if they had subjects who dropped out of the study. The authors of the studies in the appendices discuss their samples in enough detail so that the reader is clear about who the subjects are and how they were selected.

Reliability and Validity

The discussion of the instruments used to study the variables is usually included in a "Methods" section under the subheading of "Instruments" or "Measures" (see Chapter 14). Usually each instrument (or scale) used in the study is discussed, as well as its reliability and validity (see Chapter 15). The studies in Appendices A, B, and D discuss each of the measures used in the "Methods" section under the subheading "Measures" or "Instruments." The reliability and validity of each measure is also presented.

In some cases, the reliability and validity of commonly used, established instruments in an article are not presented, and you are referred to other references.

Procedures and Collection Methods

The data collection procedures, or the individual steps taken to gather measurable data (usually with instruments or scales), are generally found in the "Procedures" section (see Chapter 14). In the studies in Appendices A through D, the researchers indicate how they conducted the study in detail under the subheading "Procedure" or "Instruments and Procedures." Notice that the researchers in each study included in the Appendices provided information that the studies were approved by an institutional review board (see Chapter 13), thereby ensuring that each study met ethical standards.

Data Analysis/Results

The data-analysis procedures (i.e., the statistical tests used and the results of descriptive and/or inferential tests applied in quantitative studies) are presented in the section labeled "Results" or "Findings" (see Chapters 16 and 17). Although qualitative studies do not use statistical tests, the procedures for analyzing the themes, concepts, and/or observational or print data are usually described in the "Method" or "Data Collection" section and reported in the "Results," "Findings," or "Data Analysis" section (see Appendix C and Chapters 5 and 6).

Discussion

The last section of a research study is the "Discussion" (see Chapter 17). In this section the researchers tie together all of the study's pieces and give a picture of the study as a whole. The researchers return to the literature reviewed and discuss how their study is similar to, or different from, other studies. Researchers may report the results and discussion in one section but usually report their results in separate "Results" and "Discussion" sections (see Appendices A through D). One particular method is no better than another. Journal and space limitations determine how these sections will be handled. Any new or unexpected findings are usually described in the "Discussion" section.

Recommendations and Implications

In some cases, a researcher reports the implications and limitations based on the findings for practice and education, and recommends future studies in a separate section labeled "Conclusions"; in other cases, this appears in several sections, labeled with such titles as "Discussion," "Limitations," "Nursing Implications," "Implications for Research and Practice," and "Summary." Again, one way is not better than the other—only different.

References

All of the references cited are included at the end of the article. The main purpose of the reference list is to support the material presented by identifying the sources in a manner that allows for easy retrieval. Journals use various referencing styles.

Communicating Results

Communicating a study's results can take the form of a published article, poster, or paper presentation. All are valid ways of providing data and have potential to effect high-quality patient care based on research findings. Evidence-based nursing care plans and QI practice protocols, guidelines, or standards are outcome measures that effectively indicate communicated research.

HELPFUL HINT

If you have to write a paper on a specific concept or topic that requires you to critique and synthesize the findings from several studies, you might find it useful to create an evidence table of the data (see Chapter 20). Include the following information: author, date, study type, design, level of evidence, sample, data analysis, findings, and implications.

SYSTEMATIC REVIEWS: META-ANALYSES, INTEGRATIVE REVIEWS, AND META-SYNTHESES

Systematic Reviews

Other article types that are important to understand for evidence-based practice are review articles. Review articles include **systematic reviews**, meta-analyses, integrative reviews (sometimes called narrative reviews), **meta-syntheses**, and meta-summaries. A **systematic review** is a summation and assessment of a group of research studies that test a similar research question. Systematic reviews are based on a clear question, a detailed plan which includes a search strategy, and appraisal of a group of studies related to the question. If statistical techniques are used to summarize and assess studies, the systematic review is labeled as a meta-analysis. A **meta-analysis** is a summary of a number of studies focused on one question or topic, and uses a specific statistical methodology to synthesize the findings in order to draw conclusions about the area of focus. An **integrative review** is a focused review and synthesis of research or theoretical literature in a particular focus area, and includes specific steps of literature integration and synthesis without statistical analysis; it can include both quantitative and qualitative articles (Cochrane Consumer Network, 2016; Uman, 2011; Whittemore, 2005). At times reviews use the terms *systematic review* and *integrative review* interchangeably. Both **meta-synthesis** and **meta-summary** are the synthesis of a number of qualitative research studies on a focused topic using specific qualitative methodology (Kastner et al., 2016; Sandelowski & Barrosos, 2007).

The components of review articles will be discussed in greater detail in Chapters 6, 11, and 20. These articles take a number of studies related to a clinical question and, using a specific set of criteria and methods, evaluate the studies as a whole. While they may vary somewhat in approach, these reviews all help to better inform and develop evidence-based practice. The meta-analysis in Appendix E is an example of a systematic review that is a meta-analysis.

CLINICAL GUIDELINES

Clinical guidelines are systematically developed statements or recommendations that serve as a guide for practitioners. Two types of clinical guidelines will be discussed throughout this text: consensus, or expert-developed guidelines, and evidence-based guidelines. **Consensus guidelines**, or expert-developed guidelines, are developed by an agreement of experts in the field. **Evidence-based guidelines** are those developed using published research findings. Guidelines are developed to assist in bridging practice and research and are developed by professional organizations, government agencies, institutions, or convened expert panels. Clinical guidelines provide clinicians with an algorithm for clinical management or decision making for specific diseases (e.g., breast cancer) or treatments (e.g., pain management). Not all clinical guidelines are well developed and, like research, must be assessed before implementation. Though they are systematically developed and make explicit recommendations for practice, clinical guidelines may be formatted differently. Guidelines for practice are becoming more important as third party and government payers are requiring practices to be based on evidence. Guidelines should present scope and purpose of the practice, detail who the development group included, demonstrate scientific rigor, be clear in its presentation, demonstrate clinical applicability, and demonstrate editorial independence (see Chapter 11).

QUALITY IMPROVEMENT

As a health care provider, you are responsible for continuously improving the quality and safety of health care for your patients and their families through systematic redesign of health care systems in which you work. The Institute of Medicine (2001) defined quality health care as care that is safe, effective, patient-centered, timely, efficient, and equitable. Therefore, the goal of QI is to bring about measurable changes across these six domains by applying specific methodologies within a care setting. While several QI methods exist, the core steps for improvement commonly include the following:

- Conducting an assessment
- Setting specific goals for improvement
- Identifying ideas for changing current practice
- Deciding how improvements in care will be measured
- Rapidly testing practice changes
- Measuring improvements in care
- Adopting the practice change as a new standard of care

Chapter 21 focuses on building your competence to participate in and lead QI projects by providing an overview of the evolution of QI in health care, including the nurse's role in meeting current regulatory requirements for patient care quality. Chapter 19 discusses QI models and tools, such as cause-and-effect diagrams and process mapping, as well as skills for effective teamwork and leadership that are essential for successful QI projects.

As you venture through this textbook, you will be challenged to think not only about reading and understanding research studies, but also about applying the findings to your practice. Nursing has a rich legacy of research that has grown in depth and breadth. Producers of research and clinicians must engage in a joint effort to translate findings into practice that will make a difference in the care of patients and families.

KEY POINTS

- Research provides the basis for expanding the unique body of scientific evidence that forms the foundation of evidence-based nursing practice. Research links education, theory, and practice.

- As consumers of research, nurses must have a basic understanding of the research process and critical appraisal skills to evaluate research evidence before applying it to clinical practice.
- Critical appraisal is the process of evaluating the strengths and weaknesses of a research article for scientific merit and application to practice, theory, or education; the need for more research on the topic or clinical problem is also addressed at this stage.
- Critical appraisal criteria are the measures, standards, evaluation guides, or questions used to judge the worth of a research study.
- Critical reading skills will enable you to evaluate the appropriateness of the content of a research article, apply standards or critical appraisal criteria to assess the study's scientific merit for use in practice, or consider alternative ways of handling the same topic.
- A level of evidence model is a tool for evaluating the strength (quality, quantity, and consistency) of a research study and its findings.
- Each article should be evaluated for the study's strength and consistency of evidence as a means of judging the applicability of findings to practice.
- Research articles have different formats and styles depending on journal manuscript requirements and whether they are quantitative or qualitative studies.
- Evidence-based practice and QI begin with the careful reading and understanding of each article contributing to the practice of nursing, clinical expertise, and an understanding of patient values.
- QI processes are aimed at improving clinical care outcomes for patients and better methods of system performance.

CRITICAL THINKING CHALLENGES

- IPE How might nurses discuss the differences between evidence-based practice and research with their colleagues in other professions?
- From your clinical practice, discuss several strategies nurses can undertake to promote evidence-based practice.
- What are some strategies you can use to develop a more comprehensive critique of an evidence-based practice article?
- A number of different components are usually identified in a research article. Discuss how these sections link with one another to ensure continuity.
- How can QI data be used to improve clinical practice?

REFERENCES

Agency for Healthcare Research and Quality. (2002). Systems to rate the strength of scientific evidence. *File inventory, Evidence Report/Technology Assessment No. 47*, AHRQ Publication No. 02-E016.

Al-Mallah, M. H., Farah, I., Al-Madani, W., et al. (2015). The impact of nurse-led clinics on the mortality and mortality of patients with cardiovascular diseases: A systematic review and meta-analysis. *Journal of Cardiovascular Nursing*, *31*(1), 89–95. doi:10.1097/JCN.0000000000000224.

American Nurses Association (ANA). (2015). *Code of ethics for nurses for nurses with interpretive statements*. Washington, DC: The Association.

Cochrane Consumer Network, The Cochrane Library, 2016, retrieved online. www.cochranelibrary.com.

Cronenwett, L., Sherwood, G., Barnsteiner, J., et al. (2007). Quality and safety education for nurses. *Nursing Outlook*, *55*(3), 122–131.

Institute of Medicine [IOM]. (2011). *The future of nursing: Leading change, advancing health.* Washington, DC: National Academic Press.

Institute of Medicine Committee on Quality of Health Care in America. (2001). *Crossing the quality chasm: A new health system for the 21st century*. Washington, DC: National Academy Press.

Kastner, M., Antony, J., Soobiah, C., et al. (2016). Conceptual recommendations for selecting the most appropriate knowledge synthesis method to answer research questions related to complex evidence. *Journal of Clinical Epidemiology*, *73*, 43–49.

Nyamathi, A., Salem, B. E., Zhang, S., et al. (2015). Nursing case management, peer coaching, and hepatitus A and B vaccine completion among homeless men recently released on parole. *Nursing Research*, *64*, 177–189, doi:10.1097/NNR.0000000000000083.

Sackett, D. L., Straus, S., Richardson, S., et al. (2000). *Evidence-based medicine: How to practice and teach EBM* (2nd ed.). London: Churchill Livingstone.

Sandelowski, M., & Barroso, J. (2007). *Handbook of Qualitative Research*, New York, NY: Springer Pub. Co.

Uman, L.S. (2011). Systematic reviews and meta-analyses. *Journal of the Canadian Academy of Child and Adolescent Psychiatry*, *20*(1), 57–59.

vanDijk, J. F. M., Vervoot, S. C. J. M., vanWijck, A. J. M., et al. (2016). Postoperative patients' perspectives on rating pain: A qualitative study. *International Journal of Nursing Studies*, *53*, 260–269.

Whittemore, R. (2005). Combining evidence in nursing research. *Nursing Research*, *54*(1), 56–62.

Go to Evolve at **http://evolve.elsevier.com/LoBiondo/** for review questions, critiquing exercises, and additional research articles for practice in reviewing and critiquing.

2

Research Questions, Hypotheses, and Clinical Questions

Judith Haber

Go to Evolve at **http://evolve.elsevier.com/LoBiondo/** for review questions, critiquing exercises, and additional research articles for practice in reviewing and critiquing.

LEARNING OUTCOMES

After reading this chapter, you should be able to do the following:

- Describe how the research question and hypothesis relate to the other components of the research process.
- Describe the process of identifying and refining a research question or hypothesis.
- Discuss the appropriate use of research questions versus hypotheses in a research study.
- Identify the criteria for determining the significance of a research question or hypothesis.
- Discuss how the purpose, research question, and hypothesis suggest the level of evidence to be obtained from the findings of a research study.
- Discuss the purpose of developing a clinical question.
- Discuss the differences between a research question and a clinical question in relation to evidence-based practice.
- Apply critiquing criteria to the evaluation of a research question and hypothesis in a research report.

KEY TERMS

clinical question
complex hypothesis
dependent variable
directional hypothesis
hypothesis
independent variable
nondirectional hypothesis
population
purpose
research hypothesis
research question
statistical hypothesis
testability
theory
variable

At the beginning of this chapter, you will learn about research questions and hypotheses from the perspective of a researcher, which, in the second part of this chapter, will help you generate your own clinical questions that you will use to guide the development of evidence-based practice projects. From a clinician's perspective, you must understand the research question and hypothesis as it aligns with the rest of a study. As a practicing nurse, developing clinical questions (see Chapters 19, 20, and 21) is the first step of the evidence-based practice process for quality improvement programs like those that decrease risk for development of pressure ulcers.

When nurses ask questions such as, "Why are things done this way?" "I wonder what would happen if . . . ?" "What characteristics are associated with . . . ?" or "What is the effect of ____ on patient outcomes?", they are often well on their way to developing a research question or hypothesis. Research questions are usually generated by situations that emerge from practice, leading nurses to wonder about the effectiveness of one intervention versus another for a specific patient population.

The research question or hypothesis is a key preliminary step in the research process. The **research question** tests a measureable relationship to be examined in a research study. The **hypothesis** predicts the outcome of a study.

Hypotheses can be considered intelligent hunches, guesses, or predictions that provide researchers with direction for the research design and the collection, analysis, and interpretation of data. Hypotheses are a vehicle for testing the validity of the theoretical framework assumptions and provide a bridge between **theory** (a set of interrelated concepts, definitions, and propositions) and the real world (see Chapter 4).

For a clinician making an evidence-informed decision about a patient care issue, a clinical question, such as whether chlorhexidine or povidone-iodine is more effective in preventing central line catheter infections, would guide the nurse in searching and retrieving the best available evidence. This evidence, combined with clinical expertise and patient preferences, would provide an answer on which to base the most effective decision about patient care for this population.

Often the research questions or hypotheses appear at the beginning of a research article, but may be embedded in the purpose, aims, goals, or even the results section of the research report. This chapter provides you with a working knowledge of quantitative research questions and hypotheses. It also highlights the importance of clinical questions and how to develop them.

DEVELOPING AND REFINING A RESEARCH QUESTION: STUDY PERSPECTIVE

A researcher spends a great deal of time refining a research idea into a testable research question. Research questions or topics are not pulled from thin air. In Table 2.1, you will see that research questions can indicate that practical experience, critical appraisal of the scientific literature, or interest in an untested theory forms the basis for the development of a research idea. The research question should reflect a refinement of the researcher's initial thinking. The evaluator of a research study should be able to identify that the researcher has:

- Defined a specific question area
- Reviewed the relevant literature
- Examined the question's potential significance to nursing
- Pragmatically examined the feasibility of studying the research question

Defining the Research Question

Brainstorming with faculty or colleagues may provide valuable feedback that helps the researcher focus on a specific research question area. **Example:** ➤ Suppose a researcher told a colleague that her area of interest was health disparities about the effectiveness of peer

TABLE 2.1 How Practical Experience, Scientific Literature, and Untested Theory Influence the Development of a Research Idea

Area	Influence	Example
Clinical experience	Clinical practice provides a wealth of experience from which research problems can be derived. The nurse may observe a particular event or pattern and become curious about why it occurs, as well as its relationship to other factors in the patient's environment.	Health professionals observe that despite improvements in symptom management for cancer patients receiving chemotherapy, side effects remain highly prevalent. Symptoms such as nausea/vomiting, diarrhea, constipation, and fatigue are common, and patients report that they negatively affect functional status and quality of life, including costly and distressing hospitalizations. A study by Traeger et al. (2015) tested a model integrated into outpatient care for patients with breast cancer, lung cancer, and colorectal cancer, designed to reduce symptom burden to be delivered by each patient's oncology team nurse practitioner that included telephone follow-up, symptom assessment, advice, and triage according to actual clinical practice. The aim was to ensure optimal patient-NP management of side effects early in the course of care.
Critical appraisal of the scientific literature	Critical appraisal of studies in journals may indirectly suggest a clinical problem by stimulating the reader's thinking. The nurse may observe the outcome data from a single study or a group of related studies that provide the basis for developing a pilot study, quality improvement project, or clinical practice guideline to determine the effectiveness of this intervention in their setting.	At a staff meeting with members of an interprofessional team at a cancer center, it was noted that the center did not have a standardized clinical practice guideline for mucositis, a painful chemotherapy side effect involving the oral cavity that has a negative impact on nutrition, oral hygiene, and comfort. The team wanted to identify the most effective approaches for treating adults and children experiencing mucositis. Their search for, and critical appraisal of, existing research studies led the team to develop an interprofessional mucositis guideline that was relevant to their patient population and clinical setting (NYU Langone Medical Center, 2016).
Gaps in the literature	A research idea may also be suggested by a critical appraisal of the literature that identifies gaps in the literature and suggests areas for future study. Research ideas also can be generated by research reports that suggest the value of replicating a particular study to extend or refine the existing scientific knowledge base.	Obesity is a widely recognized risk factor for many conditions treated in primary care settings including type 2 diabetes, cardiovascular disease, hypertension, and osteoarthritis. Although weight and achieving a healthy weight for children and adults is a Healthy People 2020 goal and a national priority, the prevalence of obesity remains high, and there is little research on targeted interventions for weight loss in primary care settings. Therefore, the purpose of a study by Thabault, Burke, and Ades (2015) was to evaluate an NP-led motivational interviewing IBT program implemented in an adult primary care practice with obese patients to determine feasibility and acceptance of the intervention.
Interest in untested theory	Verification of a theory and its concepts provides a relatively uncharted area from which research problems can be derived. Inasmuch as theories themselves are not tested, a researcher may consider investigating a concept or set of concepts related to a nursing theory or a theory from another discipline. The researcher would pose questions like, "If this theory is correct, what kind of behavior would I expect to observe in particular patients and under which conditions?" "If this theory is valid, what kind of supporting evidence will I find?"	Bandura's (1997) health self-efficacy construct, an individual's confidence in the ability to perform a behavior, overcome barriers to that behavior, and exert control over the behavior through self-regulation and goal setting, was used by Richards, Ogata, and Cheng (2016) to investigate whether health-related self-efficacy provides the untested theoretical foundation for behavior change related to increasing physical activity using a dog walking (Dogs PAW) intervention.

IBT, Intensive behavioral therapy.

coaching or case management in improving health outcomes with challenging patient populations such as those who are homeless. The colleague may have asked, "What is it about the topic that specifically interests you?" This conversation may have initiated a chain of thought that resulted in a decision to explore the effectiveness of a nursing case management and peer coaching intervention on hepatitis A and B (HAV and HBV) vaccine completion rates among homeless men recently released on parole (Nyamathi et al., 2015) (see Appendix A). Fig. 2.1

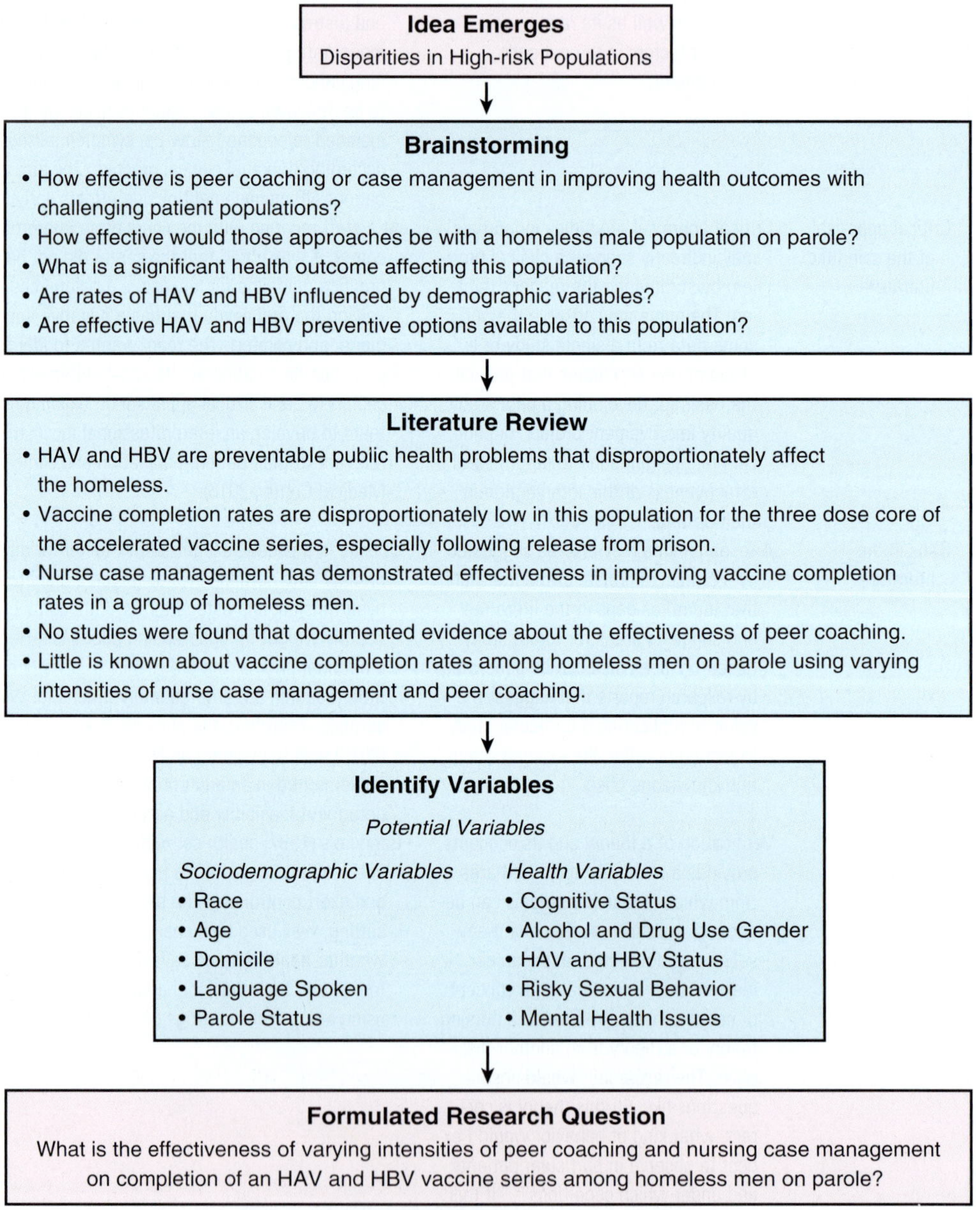

FIG 2.1 Development of a research question.

illustrates how a broad area of interest (health disparities, nursing case management, peer coaching) was narrowed to a specific research topic (effectiveness of nursing case management and peer coaching on HAV and HBV vaccine completion among homeless men recently released on parole).

QSEN EVIDENCE-BASED PRACTICE TIP

A well-developed research question guides a focused search for scientific evidence about assessing, diagnosing, treating, or providing patients with information about their prognosis related to a specific health problem.

Beginning the Literature Review

The literature review should reveal a relevant collection of studies and systematic reviews that have been critically examined. Concluding sections in such articles (i.e., the recommendations and implications for practice) often identify remaining gaps in the literature, the need for replication, or the need for additional knowledge about a particular research focus (see Chapter 3). In the previous example, the researcher may have conducted a preliminary review of books and journals for theories and research studies on factors apparently critical to vaccine completion rates for preventable health problems like HAV and HBV, as well as risk factors contributing to the disproportionate impact of HAV and HBV on the homeless, such as risky sexual activity, drug use, substandard living conditions, and older age. These factors, called variables, should be potentially relevant, of interest, and measurable.

QSEN EVIDENCE-BASED PRACTICE TIP

The answers to questions generated by qualitative data reflect evidence that may provide the first insights about a phenomenon that has not been previously studied.

Other variables, called *demographic variables,* such as race, ethnicity, gender, age, education, and physical and mental health status, are also suggested as essential to consider. **Example:** ➤ Despite the availability of the HAV and HBV vaccines, there has been a low completion rate for the three-dose core of the accelerated vaccine series, particularly following release from prison. This information can then be used to further define the research question and continue the search of the literature to identify effective intervention strategies reported in other studies with similar high-risk populations (e.g., homeless) that could be applied to this population. **Example:** ➤ One study documented the effectiveness of a nurse case management program in improving vaccine completion rates in a group of homeless adults, but no studies were found about the effectiveness of peer coaching. At this point, the researcher could write the tentative research question: "What is the effectiveness of peer coaching and nursing case management on completion of an HAV and HBV vaccine series among homeless men on parole?" You can envision the interrelatedness of the initial definition of the question area, the literature review, and the refined research question.

HELPFUL HINT

Reading the literature review or theoretical framework section of a research article helps you trace the development of the implied research question and/or hypothesis.

Examining Significance

When considering a research question, it is crucial that the researcher examine the question's potential significance for nursing. This is sometimes referred to as the "so what" question, because the research question should have the potential to contribute to and extend the scientific body of nursing knowledge. Guidelines for selecting research questions should meet the following criteria:

- Patients, nurses, the medical community in general, and society will potentially benefit from the knowledge derived from the study.
- Results will be applicable for nursing practice, education, or administration.
- Findings will provide support or lack of support for untested theoretical concepts.
- Findings will extend or challenge existing knowledge by filling a gap or clarifying a conflict in the literature.
- Findings will potentially provide evidence that supports developing, retaining, or revising nursing practices or policies.

If the research question has not met any of these criteria, the researcher is wise to extensively revise the question or discard it. **Example:** ➤ In the previously cited research question, the significance of the question includes the following facts:

- HAV and HBV are vaccine preventable.
- Viral hepatitis disproportionately impacts the homeless.
- Despite its availability, vaccine completion rates are low among high-risk and incarcerated populations.
- Accelerated vaccine programs have shown success in RCT studies.
- The use of nurse case management programs in accelerated vaccine programs also provides evidence of effectiveness.
- Little is known about vaccine completion among ex-offender populations on parole using varying intensities of nurse case management and peer coaches.
- This study sought to fill a gap in the related literature by assessing whether seronegative parolees randomized to one of three intervention conditions were more likely to complete the vaccine series as well as to identify predictors of HAV/HBV vaccine completion.

IPE HIGHLIGHT

It is helpful to collaborate with colleagues from other professions to identify an important clinical question that provides data for a quality improvement on your unit.

THE FULLY DEVELOPED RESEARCH QUESTION

When a researcher finalizes a research question, the following characteristics should be evident:

- It clearly identifies the variables under consideration.
- It specifies the population being studied.
- It implies the possibility of empirical testing.

Because each element is crucial to developing a satisfactory research question, the criteria will be discussed in greater detail. These elements can often be found in the introduction of the published article; they are not always stated in an explicit manner.

Variables

Researchers call the properties that they study "variables." Such properties take on different values. Thus a **variable**, as the name suggests, is something that varies. Properties that differ from each other, such as age, weight, height, religion, and ethnicity, are examples of variables. Researchers attempt to understand how and why differences in one variable relate to differences in another variable. **Example:** ➤ A researcher may be concerned about the variable of pneumonia in postoperative patients on ventilators in critical care units. It is a variable because not all critically ill postoperative patients on ventilators have pneumonia. A researcher may also be interested in what other factors can be linked to ventilator-acquired pneumonia (VAP). There is clinical evidence to suggest that elevation of the head of the bed and frequent oral hygiene are associated with decreasing risk for VAP. You can see that these factors are also variables that need to be considered in relation to the development of VAP in postoperative patients.

When speaking of variables, the researcher is essentially asking, "Is **X** related to **Y**? What is the effect of **X** on **Y**? How are $\mathbf{X_1}$ and $\mathbf{X_2}$ related to **Y**?" The researcher is asking a question about the relationship between one or more independent variables and a dependent variable. (*Note:* In cases in which multiple independent or dependent variables are present, subscripts are used to indicate the number of variables under consideration.)

An **independent variable**, usually symbolized by X, is the variable that has the presumed effect on the dependent variable. In experimental research studies, the researcher manipulates the independent variable (see Chapter 9). In nonexperimental research, the independent variable is not manipulated and is assumed to have occurred naturally before or during the study (see Chapter 10).

The **dependent variable**, represented by Y, varies with a change in the independent variable. The dependent variable is not manipulated. It is observed and assumed to vary with changes in the independent variable. Predictions are made from the independent variable to the dependent variable. It is the dependent variable that the researcher is interested in understanding, explaining, or predicting. **Example:** ➤ It might be assumed that the perception of pain intensity (the dependent variable) will vary in relation to a person's gender (the independent variable). In this case, we are trying to explain the perception of pain intensity in relation to gender (i.e., male or female). Although variability in the dependent variable is assumed to depend on changes in the independent variable, this does not imply that there is a causal relationship between X and Y, or that changes in variable X cause variable Y to change.

Table 2.2 presents a number of examples of research questions. Practice substituting other variables for the examples in Table 2.2. You will be surprised at the skill you develop in writing and critiquing research questions with greater ease.

Although one independent variable and one dependent variable are used in the examples, there is no restriction on the number of variables that can be included in a research question. Research questions that include more than one independent or dependent variable may be broken down into subquestions that are more concise.

Finally, it should be noted that variables are not inherently independent or dependent. A variable that is classified as independent in one study may be considered dependent in another study. **Example:** ➤ A nurse may review an article about depression that identifies depression in adolescents as predictive of risk for suicide. In this case, depression is the independent variable. When another article about the effectiveness of antidepressant

TABLE 2.2 Research Question Format

Type	Format	Example
Quantitative		
Correlational	Is there a relationship between **X** (independent variable) and **Y** (dependent variable) in the specified population?	Are there relationships between socio-demographic (age, willingness to receive HPV vaccination) and professional characteristics (education, belief that cervical cancer can be prevented by HPV vaccination) and overall knowledge about cervical cancer, HPV, and HPV vaccines?
Comparative	Is there a difference in **Y** (dependent variable) between people who have **X** characteristic (independent variable) versus those who do not have **X** characteristic?	Do female caregivers' appraisals of children's behavior differ by family type (level of hardiness and cohesiveness)?
Experimental	Is there a difference in **Y** (dependent variable) between Group A, who received **X** (independent variable), and Group B who did not receive **X**?	What is the difference in attitudes toward cancer pain management, pain intensity, pain relief, functional status, and quality of life in cancer patients who have received an educational intervention versus a coaching intervention versus usual care? (Thomas et al., 2012)
Qualitative		
Phenomenology	What is/was your lived experience of **X**?	What are parents' perceptions of circumstances influencing their own sleep when living with a severely ill child enrolled in HBHC? (Angelhoff, Edell-Gustafason, & Morelius, 2015)

HBHC, Hospital-based home care.

medication alone or in combination with cognitive behavioral therapy (CBT) in decreasing depression in adolescents is considered, change in depression is the dependent variable. Whether a variable is independent or dependent is a function of the role it plays in a particular study.

Population

The **population** is a well-defined set that has certain characteristics and is either clearly identified or implied in the research question. **Example:** ➤ In a retrospective cohort study studying the number of ED visits and hospitalizations in two different transition care programs, a research question may ask, "What is the differential effectiveness of nurse-led or physician-led intensive home visiting program providing transition care to patients with complex chronic conditions or receiving palliative care (Morrison, Palumbo, & Rambur, 2016)? Does a relationship exist between type of transition care model (nurse-led focused on chronic disease self-management or physician-led focused on palliative care and managing complex chronic conditions) and the number of ED visits and rehospitalizations 120 days pre- and posttransitional care interventions?" This question suggests that the population includes community-residing adults with complex chronic conditions or receiving palliative care who participated in either a nurse or physician-led transitional care program.

QSEN EVIDENCE-BASED PRACTICE TIP

Make sure that the population of interest and the setting have been clearly described so that if you were going to replicate the study, you would know exactly who the study population needed to be.

Testability

The research question must imply that it is **testable**, measurable by either qualitative or quantitative methods. **Example:** ➤ The research question "Should postoperative patients control how much pain medication they receive?" is stated incorrectly for a variety of reasons. One reason is that it is not testable; it represents a value statement rather than a research question. A scientific research question must propose a measureable relationship between an independent and a dependent variable. Many interesting and important clinical questions are not valid research questions because they are not amenable to testing.

> **HELPFUL HINT**
>
> Remember that research questions are used to guide all types of research studies but are most often used in exploratory, descriptive, qualitative, or hypothesis-generating studies.

The question "What are the relationships between vaccine completion rates among the ex-offender population and use of varying intensities of nurse case management and peer coaches?" is a testable research question. It illustrates the relationship between the variables, identifies the independent and dependent variables, and implies the testability of the research question. Table 2.3 illustrates how this research question is congruent with the three research question criteria.

This research question was originally derived from a general area of interest: health-seeking behavior and coping (HAV and HBV vaccine completion rates) in a high-risk population (ex-offenders on parole, homeless), factors related to vaccine completion (age, education, race/ethnicity, marital, and parental status), and potential strategies (nurse case management and peer coaching) to improve protective behaviors and health outcomes. The question crystallized further after a preliminary literature review (Nyamathi et al., 2015).

> **HELPFUL HINT**
>
> - Remember that research questions are often not explicitly stated. The reader has to infer the research question from the title of the report, the abstract, the introduction, or the purpose.
> - Using your focused question, search the literature for the best available answer to your clinical question.

TABLE 2.3 Components of the Research Question and Related Criteria

Variables	Population	Testability
Independent Variable • Nurse case management • Peer coaching • Age • Race/ethnicity • Marital and parental status education	• High-risk population of ex-offenders on parole and homeless	• Differential effect of nurse case management and peer coaching on HAV and HBV vaccine completion rates as evidence of health-seeking behavior and coping
Dependent Variable • HAV and HBV vaccine completion rates		

STUDY PURPOSE, AIMS, OR OBJECTIVES

The **purpose** of the study encompasses the aims or objectives the investigator hopes to achieve with the research. These three terms are synonymous. The researcher selects verbs to use in the purpose statement that suggest the planned approach to be used when studying the research question as well as the level of evidence to be obtained through the study findings. Verbs such as *discover, explore,* or *describe* suggest an investigation of an infrequently researched topic that might appropriately be guided by research questions rather than hypotheses. In contrast, verb statements indicating that the purpose is to test the effectiveness of an intervention or compare two alternative nursing strategies suggest a hypothesis-testing study for which there is an established knowledge base of the topic.

Remember that when the purpose of a study is to test the effectiveness of an intervention or compare the effectiveness of two or more interventions, the level of evidence is likely to have more strength and rigor than a study whose purpose is to explore or describe phenomena. Box 2.1 provides examples of purpose, aims, and objectives.

QSEN EVIDENCE-BASED PRACTICE TIP

The purpose, aims, or objectives often provide the most information about the intent of the research question and hypotheses, and suggest the level of evidence to be obtained from the findings of the study.

DEVELOPING THE RESEARCH HYPOTHESIS

Like the research question, hypotheses are often not stated explicitly in a research article. You will often find that hypotheses are embedded in the data analysis, results, or discussion section of the research report. Similarly, the population may not be explicitly stated, but will have been identified in the background, significance, and literature review. It is then up to you to figure out the hypotheses and population being tested. **Example:** ➤ In a study by Turner-Sack and colleagues (2016) (see Appendix B), the hypotheses are embedded in the "Data Analysis" and "Results" sections of the article. You must interpret that the statement, "Independent sample t-tests were conducted to compare the survivors, siblings, and parents on measures of psychological distress, life satisfaction, posttraumatic growth (PTG), and that of their matched parents" to understand that it represents hypotheses used to compare psychological functioning, PTG, coping, and cancer-related characteristics of adolescent cancer survivors' parents and siblings.

BOX 2.1 Examples of Purpose Statements

- The purpose of this study was to explore the relationship between future expectations, attitude toward use of violence to solve problems, and self-reported physical and relational bullying perpetration in a sample of seventh grade students (Stoddard, Varela, & Zimmerman, 2015). The aim of this study was to determine knowledge, awareness, and practices of Turkish hospital nurses in relation to cervical cancer, HPV, and HPV (Koc & Cinarli, 2015).
- The purposes of this longitudinal study with a sample composed of Hispanic, Black non-Hispanic, and White non-Hispanic bereaved parents were to test the relationships between spiritual/religious coping strategies and grief, mental health, and personal growth for mothers and fathers at 1 and 3 months after the infant/child's death in the NICU/PICU (Hawthorne et al., 2016). The goals of the current study were to examine psychological functioning and coping in parents and siblings of adolescent cancer survivors (Turner-Sack et al., 2016).

Hypotheses flow from the study's purpose, literature review, and theoretical framework. Fig. 2.2 illustrates this flow. A **hypothesis** is a declarative statement about the relationship between two or more variables. A hypothesis predicts an expected outcome of a study. Hypotheses are developed before the study is conducted because they provide direction for the collection, analysis, and interpretation of data.

HELPFUL HINT

When hypotheses are not explicitly stated by the author at the end of the introduction section or just before the methods section, they will be embedded or implied in the data analysis, results, or discussion section of a research article.

Relationship Statement

The first characteristic of a hypothesis is that it is a declarative statement that identifies the predicted relationship between two or more variables: the independent variable (**X**) and a dependent variable (**Y**). The direction of the predicted relationship is also specified in this statement. Phrases such as *greater than, less than, positively, negatively,* or *difference in* suggest the directionality that is proposed in the hypothesis. The following is an example of a directional hypothesis: "Nurse staff members' perceptions of transformational leadership among their nurse leaders (independent variable) is that it is negatively associated with nurse staff burnout (dependent variable)" (Lewis & Cunningham, 2016). The dependent and independent variables are explicitly identified, and the relational aspect of the prediction in the hypothesis is contained in the phrase "negatively associated with."

The nature of the relationship, either causal or associative, is also implied by the hypothesis. A causal relationship is one in which the researcher can predict that the independent variable (**X**) causes a change in the dependent variable (**Y**). In research, it is rare that one is in a firm enough position to take a definitive stand about a cause-and-effect relationship. **Example:** ➤ A researcher might hypothesize selected determinants of the decision-making

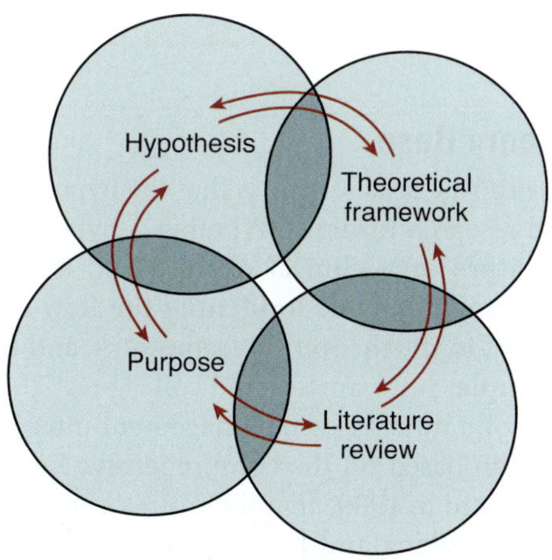

FIG 2.2 Interrelationships of purpose, literature review, theoretical framework, and hypothesis.

process, specifically expectation, socio-demographic factors, and decisional conflict would predict postdecision satisfaction and regret about their choice of treatment for breast cancer in Chinese-American women (Lee & Knobf, 2015). It would be difficult for a researcher to predict a cause-and-effect relationship, however, because of the multiple intervening variables (e.g., values, culture, role, support from others, personal resources, language literacy) that might also influence the subject's decision making about treatment for their breast cancer diagnosis.

Variables are more commonly related in noncausal ways; that is, the variables are systematically related but in an associative way. This means that the variables change in relation to each other. **Example:** ➤ There is strong evidence that asbestos exposure is related to lung cancer. It is tempting to state that there is a causal relationship between asbestos exposure and lung cancer. Do not overlook the fact, however, that not all of those who have been exposed to asbestos will have lung cancer, and not all of those who have lung cancer have had asbestos exposure. Consequently, it would be scientifically unsound to take a position advocating the presence of a causal relationship between these two variables. Rather, one can say only that there is an associative relationship between the variables of asbestos exposure and lung cancer, a relationship in which there is a strong systematic association between the two phenomena.

Testability

The second characteristic of a hypothesis is its **testability**. This means that the variables of the study must lend themselves to observation, measurement, and analysis. The hypothesis is either supported or not supported after the data have been collected and analyzed. The predicted outcome proposed by the hypothesis will or will not be congruent with the actual outcome when the hypothesis is tested.

HELPFUL HINT

When a hypothesis is **complex** (i.e., it contains more than one independent or dependent variable), it is difficult for the findings to indicate unequivocally that the hypothesis is supported or not supported. In such cases, the reader must infer which relationships are significant in the predicted direction from the findings or discussion section.

Theory Base

The third characteristic is that the hypothesis is consistent with an existing body of theory and research findings. Whether a hypothesis is arrived at on the basis of a review of the literature or a clinical observation, it must be based on a sound scientific rationale. You should be able to identify the flow of ideas from the research idea to the literature review, to the theoretical framework, and through the research question(s) or hypotheses. **Example:** ➤ Nyamathi and colleagues (2015) (see Appendix A) investigated the effectiveness of a nursing case management intervention in comparison to a peer coaching intervention based on the comprehensive health-seeking and coping paradigm developed by Nyamathi in 1989, adapted from a coping model by Lazarus and Folkman (1984), and the health-seeking and coping paradigm by Schlotfeldt (1981), which is a useful theoretical framework for case management, peer coaching interventions, and vaccine completion outcomes.

Wording the Hypothesis

As you read the scientific literature and become more familiar with it, you will observe that there are a variety of ways to word a hypothesis that are described in Tables 2.4 and 2.5. Information about hypotheses may be further clarified in the instruments, sample, or methods sections of a research report (see Chapters 12 and 15).

TABLE 2.4 Examples of How Hypotheses are Worded

Variables	Hypothesis	Type of Design; Level of Evidence Suggested
1. There Are Significant Differences in Self-reported Cancer Pain, Symptoms Accompanying Pain, and Functional Status According to Self-reported Ethnic Identity.		
IV: Ethnic identity	Nondirectional, research	Nonexperimental; Level IV
DV: Self-reported cancer pain		
DV: Symptoms accompanying pain		
DV: Functional status		
2. Individuals Who Participate in UC Plus BP Will Have a Greater Reduction in BP from Baseline to 12-month Follow-up than Individuals Who Receive UC Only.		
IV: TM	Directional, research	Experimental; Level II
IV: UC		
DV: Blood pressure		
3. There Will Be a Greater Decrease in State Anxiety Scores for Patients Receiving Structured Informational Videos Before Abdominal or Chest Tube Removal than for Patients Receiving Standard Information.		
IV: Preprocedure structured videotape information	Directional, research	Experimental; Level II
IV: Standard information		
DV: State anxiety		
4. Participants Randomly Assigned to the Intervention Group (Dog Walking Program) Will Show a Significant Increase in Physical Activity When Compared with Participants in the Control Group (No Dog Walking Program), and These Changes Will Remain 1 Year after the Start of the Intervention.		
IV: Dog walking intervention among dog owners	Directional, research	Experimental; Level II
IV: Control group—usual dog walking		
DV: Physical activity		
5. Nurses with High Social Support from Coworkers Will Have Lower Perceived Job Stress.		
IV: Social support	Directional, research	Nonexperimental; Level IV
DV: Perceived job stress		
6. There Will Be No Difference in Anesthetic Complication Rates Between Hospitals That Use CRNA for Obstetrical Anesthesia Versus Those That Use Anesthesiologists.		
IV: Type of anesthesia provider (CRNA or MD)	Null	Nonexperimental; Level IV
7. There Will Be No Significant Difference in the Duration of Patency of a 24-gauge Intravenous Lock in a Neonatal Patient When Flushed with 0.5 mL of Heparinized Saline (2 u/mL), Compared with 0.5 mL of 0.9% of Normal Saline.		
IV: Heparinized saline	Null	Experimental; Level II
IV: Normal saline		
DV: Duration of patency of intravenous lock		

BP, Blood pressure; *CRNA,* Certified Nurse Anesthetists; *DV,* dependent variable; *IV,* independent variable; *TM,* telemonitoring; *UC,* usual care.

TABLE 2.5 Examples of Statistical Hypotheses

Hypothesis	Variables	Type of Hypothesis	Type of Design Suggested
Oxygen inhalation by nasal cannula of up to 6 L/min does not affect oral temperature measurement taken with an electronic thermometer.	IV: Oxygen inhalation by nasal cannula DV: Oral temperature	Statistical; null	Experimental
There will be no difference in the performance accuracy of ANPs and FNPs in formulating accurate diagnoses and acceptable interventions for suspected cases of domestic violence.	IV: Nurse practitioner (ANP or FNP) category DV: Diagnosis and intervention performance accuracy	Statistical; null	Nonexperimental

ANPs, Adult nurse practitioners; *FNPs,* family nurse practitioners; *DV,* dependent variable; *IV,* independent variable.

Statistical Versus Research Hypotheses

You may observe that a hypothesis is further categorized as either a research or a statistical hypothesis. A **research hypothesis**, also known as a scientific hypothesis, consists of a statement about the expected relationship of the variables. A research hypothesis indicates what the outcome of the study is expected to be. A research hypothesis is also either directional or nondirectional. If the researcher obtains statistically significant findings for a research hypothesis, the hypothesis is supported. The examples in Table 2.4 represent research hypotheses.

A **statistical hypothesis**, also known as a null hypothesis, states that there is no relationship between the independent and dependent variables. The examples in Table 2.5 illustrate statistical hypotheses. If, in the data analysis, a statistically significant relationship emerges between the variables at a specified level of significance, the null hypothesis is rejected. Rejection of the statistical hypothesis is equivalent to acceptance of the research hypothesis.

Directional Versus Nondirectional Hypotheses

Hypotheses can be formulated directionally or nondirectionally. A **directional hypothesis** specifies the expected direction of the relationship between the independent and dependent variables. An example of a directional hypothesis is provided in a study by Parry and colleagues (2015) that investigated a novel noninvasive device to assess sympathetic nervous system functioning in patients with heart failure. The researchers hypothesized that participants with heart failure reduced ejection fraction (HFrEF), who have internal cardiac defibrillators or CRT pacemakers, will have a decrease in pre-ejection period (reflective of increased sympathetic nervous system activity) and decrease in left ventricular ejection time (reflective of an increased heart rate) with a postural change from sitting to standing.

In contrast, a **nondirectional hypothesis** indicates the existence of a relationship between the variables, but does not specify the anticipated direction of the relationship. **Example:** ➤ Rattanawiboon and colleagues (2016) evaluated the effectiveness of fluoride mouthwash delivery methods, swish, spray, or swab application, in raising salivary fluoride in comparison to conventional fluoride mouthwash, but did not predict which form of fluoride delivery would be most effective. Nurses who are learning to critically appraise research studies should be aware that both the directional and the nondirectional forms of hypothesis statements are acceptable.

RELATIONSHIP BETWEEN THE HYPOTHESIS AND THE RESEARCH DESIGN

Regardless of whether the researcher uses a statistical or a research hypothesis, there is a suggested relationship between the hypothesis, the design of the study, and the level of evidence provided by the results of the study. The type of design, experimental or nonexperimental (see Chapters 9 and 10), will influence the wording of the hypothesis. **Example:** ➤ When an experimental design is used, you would expect to see hypotheses that reflect relationship statements, such as the following:

- $\mathbf{X_1}$ is more effective than $\mathbf{X_2}$ on **Y**.
- The effect of $\mathbf{X_1}$ on **Y** is greater than that of $\mathbf{X_2}$ on **Y**.
- The incidence of **Y** will not differ in subjects receiving $\mathbf{X_1}$ and $\mathbf{X_2}$ treatments.
- The incidence of **Y** will be greater in subjects after $\mathbf{X_1}$ than after $\mathbf{X_2}$.

QSEN EVIDENCE-BASED PRACTICE TIP

Think about the relationship between the wording of the hypothesis, the type of research design suggested, and the level of evidence provided by the findings of a study using each kind of hypothesis. You may want to consider which type of hypothesis potentially will yield the strongest results applicable to practice.

Hypotheses reflecting experimental designs also test the effect of the experimental treatment (i.e., independent variable **X**) on the outcome (i.e., dependent variable **Y**). This suggests that the strength of the evidence provided by the results is Level II (experimental design) or Level III (quasi-experimental design).

In contrast, hypotheses related to nonexperimental designs reflect associative relationship statements, such as the following:

- **X** will be negatively related to **Y.**
- There will be a positive relationship between **X** and **Y**.

This suggests that the strength of the evidence provided by the results of a study that examined hypotheses with associative relationship statements would be at Level IV (nonexperimental design).

Table 2.6 provides an example of this concept. The Critical Thinking Decision Path will help you determine the type of hypothesis or research question presented in a study.

TABLE 2.6 Elements of a Clinical Question

Population	Intervention	Comparison Intervention	Outcome
Older adult hospitalized patients with indwelling urinary catheters	Daily nurse-led catheter rounds	No daily nurse-led catheter rounds	Decreased number of CAUTIs

CAUTIs, Catheter acquired urinary tract infections.

CRITICAL THINKING DECISION PATH

Determining the Use of a Hypothesis or Research Question

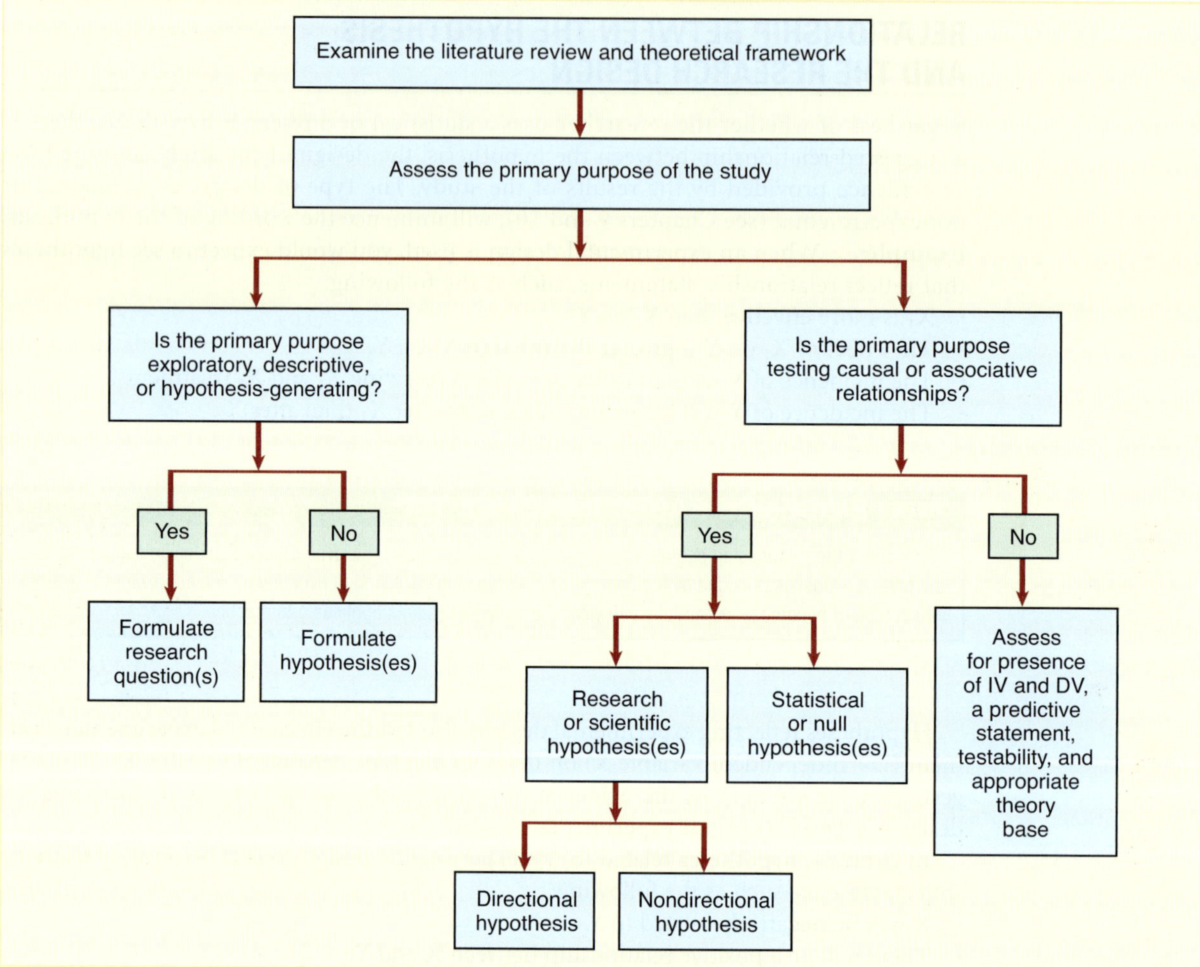

DEVELOPING AND REFINING A CLINICAL QUESTION: A CONSUMER'S PERSPECTIVE

Practicing nurses, as well as students, are challenged to keep their practice up to date by searching for, retrieving, and critiquing research articles that apply to practice issues that are encountered in their clinical setting (see Chapter 20). Practitioners strive to use the current best evidence from research when making clinical and health care decisions. As research consumers, you are not conducting research studies; however, your search for information from clinical practice is converted into focused, structured clinical questions that are the foundation of evidence-based practice and quality improvement projects. Clinical questions often arise from clinical situations for which there are no ready answers.

You have probably had the experience of asking, "What is the most effective treatment for . . . ?" or "Why do we still do it this way?"

Using similar criteria related to framing a research question, focused clinical questions form a basis for searching the literature to identify supporting evidence from research. **Clinical questions** have four components:

- Population
- Intervention
- Comparison
- Outcome

These components, known as PICO, provide an effective format for helping nurses develop searchable clinical questions. Box 2.2 presents each component of the clinical question.

The significance of the clinical question becomes obvious as research evidence from the literature is critically appraised. Research evidence is used together with clinical expertise and the patient's perspective to confirm, develop, or revise nursing standards, protocols, and policies that are used to plan and implement patient care (Cullum, 2000; Sackett et al., 2000; Thompson et al., 2004). Issues or questions can arise from multiple clinical and managerial situations. Using the example of catheter acquired urinary tract infections (CAUTIs), a team of staff nurses working on a medical unit in an acute care setting were reviewing their unit's quarterly quality improvement data and observed that the number of CAUTIs had increased by 25% over the past 3 months. The nursing staff reviewed the unit's standard of care and noted that although nurses were able to discontinue an indwelling catheter, according to a set of criteria and without a physician order, catheters were remaining in place for what they thought was too long and potentially contributing to an increase in the prevalence of CAUTIs. To focus the nursing staff's search of the literature, they developed the following question: Does the use of daily nurse-led catheter rounds in hospitalized older adults with indwelling urinary catheters lead to a decrease in CAUTIs? Sometimes it is helpful for nurses who develop clinical questions from a quality improvement perspective to consider three elements as they frame their focused question: (1) the situation, (2) the intervention, and (3) the outcome.

- The situation is the patient or problem being addressed. This can be a single patient or a group of patients with a particular health problem (e.g., hospitalized adults with indwelling urinary catheters).
- The intervention is the dimension of health care interest, and often asks whether a particular intervention is a useful treatment (e.g., daily nurse-led catheter rounds).

BOX 2.2 Components of a Clinical Question Using the PICO Format

Population: The individual patient or group of patients with a particular condition or health care problem (e.g., adolescents age 13–18 with type 1 insulin-dependent diabetes)

Intervention: The particular aspect of health care that is of interest to the nurse or the health team (e.g., a therapeutic [inhaler or nebulizer for treatment of asthma], a preventive [pneumonia vaccine], a diagnostic [measurement of blood pressure], or an organizational [implementation of a bar coding system to reduce medication errors] intervention)

Comparison intervention: Standard care or no intervention (e.g., antibiotic in comparison to ibuprofen for children with otitis media); a comparison of two treatment settings (e.g., rehabilitation center vs. home care)

Outcome: More effective outcome (e.g., improved glycemic control, decreased hospitalizations, decreased medication errors)

BOX 2.3 Examples of Clinical Questions

- Does using a Discharge Bundle combined with Teachback Methodology reduce pediatric readmissions? (Shermont et al., 2016)
- What is the most effective IV insulin practice guideline for cardiac surgery patients? (Westbrook et al., 2016)
- Does using a structured content and electronic nursing handover reduce patient clinical management errors? (Johnson et al., 2016)
- What is the impact of nursing teamwork on nurse-sensitive quality indicators? (Rahn, 2016)
- Do PCMH access and care coordination measures reflect the contributions of all team members? (Annis et al., 2016)
- Is a patient-family-staff partnership video the most effective approach for preventing falls in hospitalized patients? (Silkworth et al., 2016)
- What is the impact of prompt nutrition care on patient outcomes and health care costs? (Meehan et al., 2016)

PCMH, Patient-centered medical home.

- The outcome addresses the effect of the treatment (e.g., intervention) for this patient or patient population in terms of quality and cost (e.g., decreased CAUTIs). It essentially answers whether the intervention makes a difference for the patient population.

The individual parts of the question are vital pieces of information to remember when it comes to searching for evidence in the literature. One of the easiest ways to do this is to use a table, as illustrated in Table 2.6. Examples of clinical questions are highlighted in Box 2.3. Chapter 3 provides examples of how to effectively search the literature to find answers to questions posed by researchers and research consumers.

QSEN EVIDENCE-BASED PRACTICE TIP

You should be formulating clinical questions that arise from your clinical practice. Once you have developed a focused clinical question using the PICO format, you will search the literature for the best available evidence to answer your clinical question.

APPRAISAL FOR EVIDENCE-BASED PRACTICE THE RESEARCH QUESTION AND HYPOTHESIS

When you begin to critically appraise a research study, consider the care the researcher takes when developing the research question or hypothesis; it is often representative of the overall conceptualization and design of the study. In a quantitative research study, the remainder of a study revolves around answering the research question or testing the hypothesis. In a qualitative research study, the objective is to answer the research question. Because this text focuses on you as a research consumer, the following sections will primarily pertain to the evaluation of research questions and hypotheses in published research reports.

Critiquing the Research Question and Hypothesis

The following Critical Appraisal Criteria box provides several criteria for evaluating the initial phase of the research process—the research question or hypothesis. Because the research question or hypothesis guides the study, it is usually introduced at the beginning of the research report to indicate the focus and direction of the study. You can then evaluate whether the rest of the study logically flows from its foundation—the research question or hypothesis. The author will often begin by identifying the background and significance of the issue that led to crystallizing development of the research question or hypothesis. The clinical and scientific background and/or significance will be summarized, and the purpose, aim, or objective of the study is then identified.

Often the research question or hypothesis will be proposed before or after the literature review. Sometimes you will find that the research question or hypothesis is not specifically stated. In some cases, it is only hinted at or is embedded in the purpose statement, and you are challenged to identify the research question or hypothesis. In other cases, the research question is embedded in the findings toward the end of the article. To some extent, this depends on the style of the journal.

Although a hypothesis can legitimately be nondirectional, it is preferable, and more common, for the researcher to indicate the direction of the relationship between the variables in the hypothesis. Quantifiable words such as "greater than," "less than," "decrease," "increase," and "positively," "negatively," or "related" convey the idea of objectivity and testability. You should immediately be suspicious of hypotheses or research questions that are not stated objectively. You will find that when there is a lack of data available for the literature review (i.e., the researcher has chosen to study a relatively undefined area of interest), a nondirectional hypothesis or research question may be appropriate.

You should recognize that how the proposed relationship of the hypothesis or research question is phrased suggests the type of research design that will be appropriate for the study, as well as the level of evidence to be derived from the findings. **Example:** ➤ If a hypothesis proposes that treatment $\mathbf{X_1}$ will have a greater effect on **Y** than treatment $\mathbf{X_2}$, an experimental (Level II evidence) or quasi-experimental design (Level III evidence) is suggested (see Chapter 9). If a research question asks if there will be a positive relationship between variables **X** and **Y**, a nonexperimental design (Level IV evidence) is suggested (see Chapter10).

Hypotheses and research questions are never proven beyond the shadow of a doubt. Researchers who claim that their data have "proven" the validity of their hypothesis or research question should be regarded with grave reservation. You should realize that, at best, findings that support a hypothesis or research question are considered tentative. If repeated replication of a study yields the same results, more confidence can be placed in the conclusions advanced by the researchers.

When critically appraising clinical questions, think about the fact that the clinical question should be focused and specify the patient population or clinical problem being addressed, the intervention, and the outcome for a particular patient population. There should be evidence that the clinical question guided the literature search and that appropriate types of research studies are retrieved in terms of the study design and level of evidence needed to answer the clinical question.

CRITICAL APPRAISAL CRITERIA

Developing Research Questions and Hypotheses

The Research Question

1. Does the research question express a relationship between two or more variables, or at least between an independent and a dependent variable, implying empirical testability?
2. How does the research question specify the nature of the population being studied?
3. How has the research question been supported with adequate experiential and scientific background material?
4. How has the research question been placed within the context of an appropriate theoretical framework?

Continued

5. How has the significance of the research question been identified?
6. Have pragmatic issues, such as feasibility, been addressed?
7. How have the purpose, aims, or goals of the study been identified?

The Hypothesis

1. Is the hypothesis concisely stated in a declarative form?
2. Are the independent and dependent variables identified in the statement of the hypothesis?
3. Is each hypothesis specific to one relationship so that each hypothesis can be either supported or not supported?
4. Is the hypothesis stated in such a way that it is testable?
5. Is the hypothesis stated objectively, without value-laden words?
6. Is the direction of the relationship in each hypothesis clearly stated?
7. How is each hypothesis consistent with the literature review?
8. How is the theoretical rationale for the hypothesis made explicit?
9. Given the level of evidence suggested by the research question, hypothesis, and design, what is the potential applicability to practice?

The Clinical Question

1. Does the clinical question specify the patient population, intervention, comparison intervention, and outcome?
2. Does the clinical question address an outcome applicable to practice?

KEY POINTS

- Developing the research question and stating the hypothesis are key preliminary steps in the research process.
- The research question is refined through a process that proceeds from the identification of a general idea of interest to the definition of a more specific and circumscribed topic.
- A preliminary literature review reveals related factors that appear critical to the research topic of interest and helps further define the research question.
- The significance of the research question must be identified in terms of its potential contribution to patients, nurses, the medical community in general, and society. Applicability of the question for nursing practice, as well as its theoretical relevance, must be established. The findings should also have the potential for formulating or altering nursing practices or policies.
- The final research question is a statement about the relationship of two or more variables. It clearly identifies the relationship between the independent and dependent variables, specifies the nature of the population being studied, and implies the possibility of empirical testing.
- Research questions that are nondirectional may be used in exploratory, descriptive, or qualitative research studies.
- Research questions can be directional, depending on the type of study design being used.
- Focused clinical questions arise from clinical practice and guide the literature search for the best available evidence to answer the clinical question.
- A hypothesis is a declarative statement about the relationship between two or more variables that predicts an expected outcome. Characteristics of a hypothesis include a relationship statement, implications regarding testability, and consistency with a defined theory base.

- Hypotheses can be formulated in a directional or a nondirectional manner and be further categorized as either research or statistical hypotheses.
- The purpose, research question, or hypothesis provides information about the intent of the research question and hypothesis and suggests the level of evidence to be obtained from the study findings.
- The interrelatedness of the research question or hypothesis and the literature review and the theoretical framework should be apparent.
- The appropriateness of the research design suggested by the research question or hypothesis is also evaluated.

CRITICAL THINKING CHALLENGES

- Discuss how the wording of a research question or hypothesis suggests the type of research design and level of evidence that will be provided.
- Using the study by Hawthorne, Youngblut, and Brooten (2016) (see Appendix B), describe how the background, significance, and purpose of the study are linked to the research questions.
- IPE The prevalence of catheter acquired urinary infections (CAUTIs) has increased on your hospital unit by 10% in the last two quarters. As a member of the Quality Improvement (QI) Committee on your unit, collaborate with your committee colleagues from other professions to develop an interprofessional action plan. Deliberate to develop a clinical question to guide the QI project.
- A nurse is in charge of discharge planning for frail older adults with congestive heart failure. The goal of the program is to promote self-care and prevent rehospitalizations. Using the PICO approach, the nurse wants to develop a clinical question for an evidence-based practice project to evaluate the effectiveness of discharge planning for this patient population. How can the nurse accomplish that objective?

REFERENCES

Angelhoff, C., Edell-Gustafason, L., & Morelius, E. (2015). Sleep of parents living with a child receiving hospital-based home care. *Nursing Research*, *64*(5), 372–380.

Annis, A. M., Harris, M., Robinson, C. H., & Krein, S. L. (2016). Do patient-centered medical home access and care coordination measures reflect the contributions of all team members? A systematic review. *Journal of Nursing Care Quality*, *31*(4), 357–366.

Bandura, A. (1997). *Self-efficacy: The Exercise of Control*. New York: Freeman.

Cullum, N. (2000). User's guides to the nursing literature: An introduction. *Evidence-Based Nursing*, *3*(2), 71–72.

Hawthorne, D. M., Youngblut, J. M., & Brooten, D. (2016). Patient spirituality, grief, and mental health at 1 and 3 months after their infant's/child's death in an intensive care unit. *Journal of Pediatric Nursing*, *31*, 73–80.

Johnson, M., Sanchez, P., & Zheng, C. (2016). Reducing patient clinical management errors using structured content and electronic nursing handover. *Journal of Nursing Care Quality*, *31*(3), 245–253.

Lazarus, R. L., & Folkman, S. (1984). *Stress, appraisal and coping*. New York, NY: Springer.

Lee, S. C., & Knobf, M. T. (2015). Primary breast cancer decision-making among Chinese American women. *Nursing Research*, *64*(5), 391–401.

Lewis, H. S., & Cunningham, C. J. L. (2016). Linking nurse leadership and work characteristics to nurse burnout and engagement. *Nursing Research*, *65*(1), 13–23.

Meehan, A., Loose, C., Bell, J., et al. (2016). Impact of prompt nutrition care on patient outcomes and health care costs. *Journal of Nursing Care Quality*, *31*(3), 217–223.

Morrison, J., Palumbo, M. V., & Rambur, B. (2016). Reducing preventable hospitalizations with two models of transitional care. *Journal of Nursing Scholarship*, *48*(3), 322–329.

Nyamathi, A., Salem, B. E., Zhang, S., et al. (2015). Nursing case management, peer coaching, and hepatitis A and B vaccine completion among homeless men recently released on parole: Randomized clinical trial. *Nursing Research*, *64*(3), 177–189.

NYU Langone Medical Center. (2016). *Personal Communication*. New York, NY.

Parry, M., Nielson, C. A., Muckle, F., et al. (2015). A novel noninvasive device to assess sympathetic nervous system function in patients with heart failure. *Nursing Research*, *64*(5), 351–360.

Rahn, D. (2016). Transformational teamwork: Exploring the impact of nursing teamwork on nurse-sensitive quality indicators. *Journal of Nursing Care Quality*, *31*(3), 262–268.

Rattanawiboon, C., Chaweewannakorn, C., Saisakphong, T., et al. (2016). Effective fluoride mouthwash delivery methods as an alternative to rinsing. *Nursing Research*, *65*(1), 68–75.

Richards, E. A., Ogata, N., & Cheng, C. (2016). Evaluation of the dogs, physical activity, and walking dogs (Dogs PAW) intervention. *Nursing Research*, *65*(3), 191–201.

Sackett, D., Straus, S. E., Richardson, W. S., et al. (2000). *Evidence-based medicine: How to practice and teach EBM*. London: Churchill Livingstone.

Schlotfeldt, R. (1981). Nursing in the future. *Nursing Outlook*, *29*, 295–301.

Shermont, H., Pignataro, S., Humphrey, K., & Bukoye, B. (2016). Reducing pediatric readmissions: Using a discharge bundle combined with teach-back methodology. *Journal of Nursing Care Quality*, *31*(3), 224–232.

Silkworth, A. I., Baker, J., Ferrara, J., et al. (2016). Nursing staff develop a video to prevent falls. A quality improvement project. *Journal of Nursing Care Quality*, *31*(1), 217–223.

Stoddard, S. A., Varela, J. J., & Zimmerman, M. (2015). Future expectations, attitude toward violence, and bullying perpetration during adolescence: A mediation evaluation. *Nursing Research*, *64*(6), 422–433.

Thabault, P. J., Burke, P. J., & Ades, P. A. (2015). Intensive behavioral treatment weight loss program in an adult primary care practice. *Journal of the American Association of Nurse Practitioners*, *28*, 249–257.

Thompson, C., Cullum, N., McCaughan, D., et al. (2004). Nurses, information use, and clinical decision-making: The real world potential for evidence-based decisions in nursing. *Evidence-Based Nursing*, *7*(3), 68–72.

Traeger, L., McDonnell, T. M., McCarty, C. E., et al. (2015). Nursing intervention to enhance outpatient chemotherapy symptom management: Patient-reported outcomes of a randomized controlled trial. *Cancer Nursing*, *121*(21), 3905–3913.

Turner-Sack, A. M., Menna, R., Setchell, S. R., et al. (2016). Psychological functioning, post-traumatic growth, and coping in parents and siblings of adolescent cancer survivors. *Oncology Nursing Forum*, *43*(1), 48–56.

Westbrook, A., Sherry, D., McDermott, M., et al. (2016). Examining IV insulin practice guidelines: Nurses evaluating quality outcomes. *Journal of Nursing Care Quality*, *31*(4), 344–349.

Go to Evolve at **http://evolve.elsevier.com/LoBiondo/** for review questions, critiquing exercises, and additional research articles for practice in reviewing and critiquing.

3

Gathering and Appraising the Literature

Barbara Krainovich-Miller

Go to Evolve at **http://evolve.elsevier.com/LoBiondo/** for review questions, critiquing exercises, and additional research articles for practice in reviewing and critiquing.

LEARNING OUTCOMES

After reading this chapter, you should be able to do the following:

- Discuss the purpose of a literature review in a research study.
- Discuss the purpose of reviewing the literature for an evidence-based and quality improvement (QI) project.
- Differentiate the purposes of a literature review from the evidence-based practice and the research perspective.
- Differentiate between primary and secondary sources.
- Differentiate between systematic reviews/meta-analyses and preappraised synopses.
- Discuss the purpose of reviewing the literature for developing evidence-based practice and QI projects.
- Use the PICO format to guide a search of the literature.
- Conduct an effective search of the literature.
- Apply critical appraisal criteria for the evaluation of literature reviews in research studies.

KEY TERMS

Boolean operator
citation management software
controlled vocabulary
electronic databases
electronic search
Grey literature
literature review
preappraised synopses
primary source
refereed, or peer-reviewed, journals
secondary source
web browser

You may wonder why an entire chapter of a research text is devoted to gathering and appraising the literature. The main reason is because searching for, retrieving, and critically appraising the literature is a key step for researchers and for practitioners who are basing their practice on evidence. Searching for, retrieving, critically appraising, and synthesizing research evidence is essential to support an evidence-based practice (EBP). A question you might ask is, "Will knowing more about how to search efficiently and critically appraise research really help me as a student and as a practicing nurse?" The answer is, "Yes, it most certainly will!" Your ability to locate, retrieve, critically appraise, and synthesize research articles will enable you to determine whether or not you have the best available evidence to inform your clinical practice (CP).

The critical appraisal of research studies is an organized, systematic approach to evaluating a research study or group of studies using a set of standardized critical appraisal criteria. The criteria are used to objectively determine the strength, quality, quantity, and consistency of evidence provided by the available literature to determine its applicability to practice, policy, and education (see Chapters 7, 11, and 18).

The purpose of this chapter is to introduce you to how to evaluate the literature review in a research study and how to critically appraise a group of studies for EBP and quality improvement (QI) projects. This chapter provides you with the tools to (1) locate, search, and retrieve individual research studies, systematic reviews/meta-analyses, and meta-syntheses (see Chapters 6, 9, 10, and 11), and other documents (e.g., CP guidelines); (2) differentiate between a research article and a theoretical/conceptual article or book; (3) critically appraise a research study or group of research studies; and (4) differentiate between a research article and a conceptual article or book. These tools will help you develop your competencies to develop EBP and develop QI projects.

REVIEW OF THE LITERATURE

The Literature Review: The Researcher's Perspective

The overall purpose of the literature review in a study is to present a systematic state of the science (i.e., what research exists) on a topic. In Box 3.1, Objectives 1 to 8 and 11 present the main purposes of a literature review found in a research article. In a published study, the literature review generally appears near the beginning of the report and may or may not be labeled. It provides an abbreviated version of the literature review conducted by a researcher and represents the building blocks, or framework, of the study. Keep in mind that researchers are constrained by page limitations and so do not expect to see a comprehensive literature review in an article. The researcher must present in a succinct manner an overview and critical appraisal of the literature on a topic in order to generate research

BOX 3.1 Overall Purposes of a Literature Review

Major Goal

To develop a strong knowledge base to conduct a research study or implement an evidence-based practice/QI project (1–3, 8–11) and carry out research (1–6, 11).

Objectives

A review of the literature supports the following:

1. Determine what is known and unknown about a subject, concept, or problem.
2. Determine gaps, consistencies, and inconsistencies in the literature about a subject, concept, or problem.
3. Synthesize the strengths and weaknesses of available studies to determine the state of the science on a topic/problem.
4. Describe the theoretical/conceptual frameworks that guide a study.
5. Determine the need for replication or refinement of a study.
6. Generate research questions and hypotheses.
7. Determine an appropriate research design, methodology, and analysis for a study.
8. Provide information to discuss the findings of a study, draw conclusions, and make recommendations for future research, practice, education, and/or policy changes.
9. Uncover a new practice intervention(s) or gain supporting evidence for revising, maintaining current intervention(s), protocols, and policies, or developing new ones.
10. Generate clinical questions that guide development of EBP/QI projects, policies, and protocols.
11. Identify recommendations from the conclusion for future research, practice, education, and/or policy actions.

QI, Quality improvement.

questions or hypotheses. A literature review is essential to all steps of the quantitative and qualitative research process, and is a broad, systematic critical review and evaluation of the literature in an area.

The following overview about use of the literature review in relation to the steps of the quantitative and qualitative research process will help you understand the researcher's focus. In quantitative studies, the literature review is at the beginning of the published research articles, and may or may not be titled *literature review* (see Appendix A, B, C, and D). As you read the selected research articles found in the appendices, you will see that none of these reports have a section titled *Literature Review*. But each has a literature review at the beginning of the article. **Example:** ➤ van Dijk and colleagues (2016) labeled this beginning section with the title *Introduction* (see Appendix C). Hawthorne and colleagues (2016), after a brief introduction about their topic, used sublevel headings for two major concepts of their review and then provided a sublevel heading to introduce their *Conceptual Framework* (see Appendix B). Appendix A's study by Nyamathi and colleagues (2015), after presenting their nonlabeled literature review, also provided a sublevel heading labeled "*Theoretical Framework.*"

A review of the relevant literature found in a quantitative study (Fig. 3.1) is valuable, as it provides the following:

- Theoretical or conceptual framework
    - Identifies concepts/theories used as a guide or map for developing research questions or hypotheses
    - Suggests the presumed relationship between the independent and dependent variables
    - Provides a rationale and definition for the variable(s) and concepts studied (see Chapters 1 and 2)
- Primary and secondary sources
    - Provides the researcher with a road map for designing the study
    - Includes **primary sources**, which are research articles, theoretical documents, or other documents used by the author(s) who is conducting the study, developing a theory, or writing an autobiography
    - Includes **secondary sources**, which are published articles or books written by persons other than the individual who conducted the research study or developed the theory. Table 3.1 provides definitions and examples of primary and secondary sources.

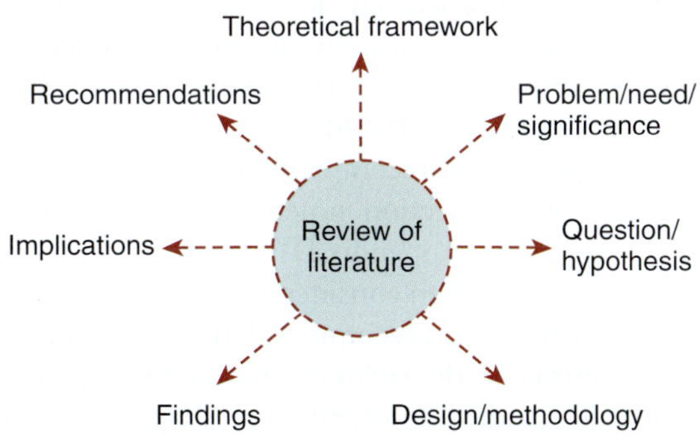

FIG 3.1 Relationship of the review of the literature to the steps of the quantitative research process.

TABLE 3.1 Examples of Primary and Secondary Sources

Primary: Essential	Secondary: Useful
Publications written by the person(s) who conducted the study or developed the theory/conceptual model.	Publications written by a person(s) other than the person who conducted the study or developed the theory or model. It usually appears as a summary/critique of another author's original work (research study, theory, or model); may appear in a study as the theoretical/conceptual framework, or paraphrased theory of the theorist.
Eyewitness accounts of historic events, autobiographies, oral histories, diaries, films, letters, artifacts, periodicals, and Internet communications on e-mail, Listservs, interviews, e-photographs, and audio/video recordings.	A biography or clinical article that cites original author's work.
Can be published or unpublished.	Can be published or unpublished.
A published research study (e.g., research articles in Appendices A–E).	An edited textbook (e.g., LoBiondo-Wood, G., & Haber, J. [2018]. *Nursing research: Methods and critical appraisal for evidence-based practice* [9th ed.], Elsevier).
Theory example: Dr. Jeffries in collaboration with the National League for Nursing developed and published a monograph entitled, *The NLN Jeffries Simulation Theory* (2015).	Theoretical framework example: Nyamathi and colleague's 2015 study used "comprehensive health seeking and coping paradigm" theoretical framework by Nyamathi (1989), which Nyamathi adopted from Lazarus and Folkman's (1984) "coping model" and Schlotfeldt's (1981) "health seeking and coping paradigm" (see study presented in Appendix A).
HINT: Critical appraisal of primary sources is essential to a thorough and relevant literature review.	HINT: Use secondary sources sparingly; however, secondary sources, especially a study's literature review that presents a critique of studies, are a valuable learning tool from an EBP perspective.

- Research question and hypothesis
  - Helps the researcher identify completed studies about the research topic of interest, including gaps or inconsistencies that suggest potential research questions or hypotheses about a subject, theory, or problem
- Design and method
  - Helps the researcher choose the appropriate design, sampling strategy, data collection methods, setting, measurement instruments, and data analysis method. Journal space guidelines limit researchers to include only abbreviated information about these areas
- Data analysis, discussion, conclusions, implications, recommendations
  - Helps the researcher interpret, discuss, and explain the study results/findings
  - Provides an opportunity for the researcher to return to the literature review and selects relevant studies to inform the discussion of the findings, conclusions, limitations, and recommendations. **Example:** ➤ Turner-Sack and colleagues' (2016) discussion section noted several times how their findings were similar to previous studies (Appendix D)
  - Useful when considering implications of research findings and making practice, education, and recommendations for practice, education, and research

In contrast to the styles of quantitative studies, literature reviews of qualitative studies are usually handled differently (see Chapters 5 to 7). In qualitative studies, often little is known about the topic under study, and thus the literature review may appear more abbreviated than in a quantitative study. However, qualitative researchers use the literature review in the same manner as quantitative researchers to interpret and discuss the study findings, draw conclusions, identify limitations, and suggest recommendations for future study.

Conducting a Literature Review: The EBP Perspective

The purpose of the literature review, from an EBP perspective, focuses on the critical appraisal of research studies, systematic reviews, CP guidelines, and other relevant documents. The literature review informs the development and/or refinement of the clinical question that will guide an EBP or QI project. When a clinical problem is identified, nurses and other team members collaborate to identify a clinical question using the PICO format (Yensen, 2013; see Chapter 2).

Once your clinical question is formulated, you will need to conduct a search in electronic database(s) (you may seek the help of a librarian) to gather and critically appraise relevant studies, and synthesize the strengths and weaknesses of the studies to determine if this is the "best available" evidence to answer your clinical question. Objectives 1 to 3 and 7 to 10 in Box 3.1 specifically reflect the purposes of a literature review for these projects.

A clear and precise articulation of a clinical question is critical to finding the best evidence. Clinical questions may sound like research questions, but they are questions used to search the literature for evidence-based answers, not to test research questions or hypotheses (see Chapter 2). The PICO format is as follows:

P Problem/patient population—What is the specifically defined group?
I Intervention—What intervention or event will be used to address the problem or population?
C Comparison—How does the intervention compare to current standards of care or another intervention?
O Outcome—What is the effect of the proposed or comparison intervention?

One group of students was interested in whether regular exercise prevented osteoporosis for postmenopausal women who had osteopenia. The PICO format for the clinical question that guided their search was as follows:

P Postmenopausal women with osteopenia (Age is part of the definition for this population.)
I Regular exercise program (How often is regular? Weekly? Twice a week?)
C No regular exercise program (comparing outcomes of regular exercise [I] and no regular exercise [C])
O Prevention of osteoporosis (How and when was this measured?)

These students' assignment to answer the PICO question requires the following:

- Search the literature using electronic databases (e.g., Cumulative Index to Nursing and Allied Health Literature [CINAHL via EBSCO], MEDLINE, and Cochrane Database of Systematic Reviews) for the information to identify the significance of osteopenia and osteoporosis as a women's health problem.
- Identify systematic reviews, practice guidelines, and research studies that provide the "best available evidence" related to the effectiveness of regular exercise programs for prevention of osteoporosis.
- Critically appraise information gathered using standardized critical appraisal criteria and tools (see Chapters 7, 11, 18, 19, and 20).
- Synthesize the overall strengths and weaknesses of the evidence provided by the literature.

- Draw a conclusion about the strength, quality, and consistency of the evidence.
- Make recommendations about applicability of evidence to CP to guide development of a health promotion project about osteoporosis risk reduction for postmenopausal women with osteopenia.

As a practicing nurse, you may be asked to work with colleagues to develop or create an EBP/QI project and/or to update current EBP protocols, CP standards/guidelines, or policies in your health care organization using the best available evidence. This will require that you know how to retrieve and critically appraise individual research articles, practice guidelines, and systematic reviews to determine each study's overall quality and then to determine if there is sufficient support (evidence) to change a current practice and/or policy or guideline.

HELPFUL HINT

Hunting for a quantitative study's literature review? Don't expect to find it labeled as *Literature Review*—many are not. Assume that the beginning paragraphs of the article comprise the literature review; the length and style will vary.

QSEN EVIDENCE-BASED PRACTICE TIPS

- Formulating a clinical question using the PICO format provides a focus that will guide an efficient electronic literature search.
- Remember, the findings of one study on a topic do not provide sufficient evidence to support a change in practice.
- The ability to critically appraise and synthesize the literature is essential to acquiring skills for making successful presentations, as well as participating in EBP/QI projects.

SEARCHING FOR EVIDENCE

Students often state, "I know how to do research; why I need to go see the librarian?" Perhaps you have thought the same thing because you too have "researched" a topic for many of your course requirements. However, it would be more accurate for you to say that you have "searched" the literature to uncover research studies and conceptual information to prepare an academic paper on a topic. During this process, you search for primary sources and secondary sources. It is best to use a primary source when available. Table 3.1 provides definitions and examples of primary and secondary sources, and Table 3.2 identifies the steps and strategies for conducting an efficient literature search. Table 3.3 indicates recommended databases. The top two, CINAHL Plus with full text and PubMed (MEDLINE), are always a must. There are multiple databases that health science libraries offer, and most offer online tutorials for how to use each database. Using the CINAHL Plus and PubMed databases and at least one additional resource database is recommended. **Example:** ➤ If your topic is about changing a patient's behavior, such as promoting smoking cessation or increasing weight-bearing exercises, you would use the top two as well as PsycINFO. Another recommendation if your clinical question focuses on interventions is to use the Cochrane Library (http://www.cochranelibrary.com), which has full text systematic reviews as well as an extensive list of randomized control trials (RCTs) and other sources of studies.

TABLE 3.2 **Steps and Strategies for Conducting a Literature Search: An EBP Perspective**

Steps of Literature Review	Strategy
Step I: Determine clinical question or research topic.	Focus on the types of patients (population) of interest. If the goal is to develop an EBP project, start with a PICO question. If the goal is to develop a research study, a researcher starts with a broad review of the literature to refine the research question or hypothesis (see Chapter 2).
Step II: Identify key variables/terms.	Review your library's online Help and Tutorial modules related to conducting a search, including the use of each databases' vocabulary, prior to meeting with your librarian for help. Make sure you have your PICO format completed so the librarian can help you limit the research articles that fit the parameters of your PICO question. If, after reviewing tutorials on Boolean connectors "AND, OR, and NOT" that connect your search terms when using a specific database, you don't understand the use of these connectors, clarify with a librarian.
Step III: Conduct electronic search using at least two, preferably three if needed for your topic, recognized electronic databases.	Conduct the search, and make a decision regarding which databases, in addition to CINAHL PLUS with Full Text via EBSCO and MEDLINE via Ovid, you should search; use key mesh terms and Boolean logic (AND, OR, NOT) to address your clinical question.
Step IV: Review abstracts online and weed out irrelevant articles.	Scan through your retrieved articles, read the abstracts, mark only those that fit the topic and are research; select "references" as well as "search history" and "full-text articles" if available, before printing and saving or e-mailing your search.
Step V: Retrieve relevant sources.	Organize by type or study design and year and reread the abstracts to determine if the articles chosen are relevant research to your topic and worth retrieving.
Step VI: Store or print relevant articles; if unable to print directly from the database, order through interlibrary loan.	Download the search to a web-based bibliography and database manager/writing and collaboration tool (e.g., RefWorks, EndNote); most academic institutions have "free" management tools, such as Zotero. Using a system will ensure that you have the information for each citation (e.g., journal name, year, volume number, pages), and it will format the reference list. Download PDF versions of articles as needed.
Step VII: Conduct preliminary reading; eliminate irrelevant sources.	First read each abstract to assess if the article is relevant.
Step VIII: Critically read each source (summarize and critique each source).	Use critical appraisal strategies (e.g., use an evidence table [see Chapter 20] or a standardized critiquing tool) to summarize and critique each articles; include references in APA format.
Step IX: Synthesize critical summaries of each article.	Decide how you will present the synthesis of overall strengths and weaknesses of the reviewed research articles (e.g., present chronologically or according to the designs); thus, the reader can review the evidence. Compare and contrast the studies in terms of the research process steps, so you conclude with the overall similarities and differences between and among studies. In the end, summarize the findings of the review—that is, determine if the strengths of the group of studies outweigh the limitations in order to determine confidence in the findings and draw a conclusion about the state of the science. Include the reference list.

CINAHL, Cumulative Index to Nursing and Allied Health Literature.

TABLE 3.3 **Databases for Nursing**

Database	Source
CINAHAL PLUS with FULL TEXT (EBSCO)	Full text database for nursing and allied health widely used by nursing and health care—a useful starting point (Source: https://health.ebsco.com/products/cinahl-plus-with-full-text)
PubMed (MEDLINE)	Provides free access to MEDLINE, NLM's database of citations and abstracts in medicine, nursing, dentistry, veterinary medicine, health care systems, and preclinical sciences, including full text (Source: https://www.nlm.nih.gov/bsd/pmresources.html)
PsycINFO	Centered on psychology, behavioral, and social sciences; interdisciplinary content, one of the most widely used databases (Source: http://www.apa.org/pubs/databases/psycinfo/)
Education Source with ERIC (EBSCO)	The largest and most complete collection of full-text education journals. This database provides research and information to meet needs of students, professionals, and policy makers, covers all levels of education—from early childhood to higher education—as well as all educational specialties such as multilingual education, health education, and testing. (Source: https://www.ebscohost.com/academic/education-source)

CINAHL, Cumulative Index to Nursing and Allied Health Literature.

Sources of Literature

Preappraised Literature

Preappraised literature is a secondary source of evidence, sometimes referred to as **preappraised synopses**, or simply *synopses*. Reading an expert's comment about another author's research can help develop your critical appraisal and synthesis skills. Some synopses include a commentary about the strength and applicability of the evidence to a patient population. It is important to keep in mind that there are limitations to using preappraised sources. These sources are useful for giving you a preview about the potential relevance of the publication to your clinical question and the strength of the evidence. You can then make a decision about whether to search for and critically appraise the primary source. Preappraised synopses can be found in journals such as *Evidence-Based Nursing* (http://ebn.bmj.com) and *Evidence-Based Medicine* (http://ebm.bmj.com) or the Joanna Briggs Institute (JBI) EBP Database (http://joannabriggs.org).

QSEN EVIDENCE-BASED PRACTICE TIP

If you find a preappraised commentary on an individual study related to your PICO question, read the preappraised commentary first. As a beginner, this strategy will make it easier for you to pick out the strengths and weaknesses in the primary source study.

Primary Sources

When searching the literature, primary sources should be a search strategy priority. Review Table 3.1 to identify the differences between primary and secondary sources. Then, as noted in Step VIII of Table 3.2, strategies to conduct a literature search, you need to apply your critiquing skills to determine the quality of the primary source publications. Review Chapters 7, 11, and 18 so you can apply the critical appraisal criteria outlined in these chapters to your retrieved studies. **Example:** ➤ For your PICO question, you searched for and found two types of primary source publications. One primary source was a rigorous systematic review related to your clinical question that provided strong evidence to support your PICO comparison intervention, the current standard of care; you also found two poorly designed RCTs that provided weak evidence supporting your proposed intervention. Which primary source would you recommend? You would need to make an evidence-based decision about the applicability of the primary source evidence supporting or not supporting the proposed or comparison intervention. The well-designed systematic review provided the highest level of evidence (Level I on the Fig. 1.1 evidence hierarchy). It also provided strong evidence that supported continuation of the current standard of care in comparison to the weak evidence supporting the proposed intervention provided by two poorly designed RCTs (Level II on the Fig. 1.1 evidence hierarchy). Your team would conclude that the primary source systematic review provided the strongest evidence supporting that the current standard of care be retained and recommended, and that there was insufficient evidence to recommend a practice change.

HELPFUL HINT

- If possible, consult a librarian before conducting your searches to determine which databases and keywords to use for your PICO question. Save your search history electronically.
- Learn how to use an online search management tool such as RefWorks, EndNote, or Zotero.

QSEN EVIDENCE-BASED PRACTICE TIP

- If you do not retrieve any studies from your search, review your PICO question and search strategies with a librarian.
- Every meta-analysis begins with a systematic review; however, not every systematic review results in a meta-analysis. Read Chapter 11 and find out why.

Performing an Electronic Search

Why Use an Electronic Database?

Perhaps you still are not convinced that electronic database searches are the best way to acquire information for a review of the literature. Maybe you have searched using Google or Yahoo! and found relevant information. This is an understandable temptation. Try to think about it from another perspective and ask yourself, "Is this the most appropriate and efficient way to find the latest and strongest research on a topic that affects patient care?" Yes, Google Scholar might retrieve some studies, but from an EBP perspective, you need to retrieve all the studies available on your topic/clinical question. The "I" and "C" of your PICO question require that you retrieve from your search all types of interventions, not just what you have proposed. To understand the literature in a specific area requires a review of all relevant studies. A way to decrease your frustration is to take the time to learn how to conduct an efficient database search by reviewing the steps presented in Table 3.2. Following these strategies and reviewing the Helpful Hints and EBP Tips provided in this chapter will help you gain the essential competencies needed for you to be successful in your search. The Critical Thinking Decision Path provides a means for locating evidence to support your clinical question (Kendall, 2008). Path shows a way to locate evidence to support your research or clinical question.

CRITICAL THINKING DECISION PATH

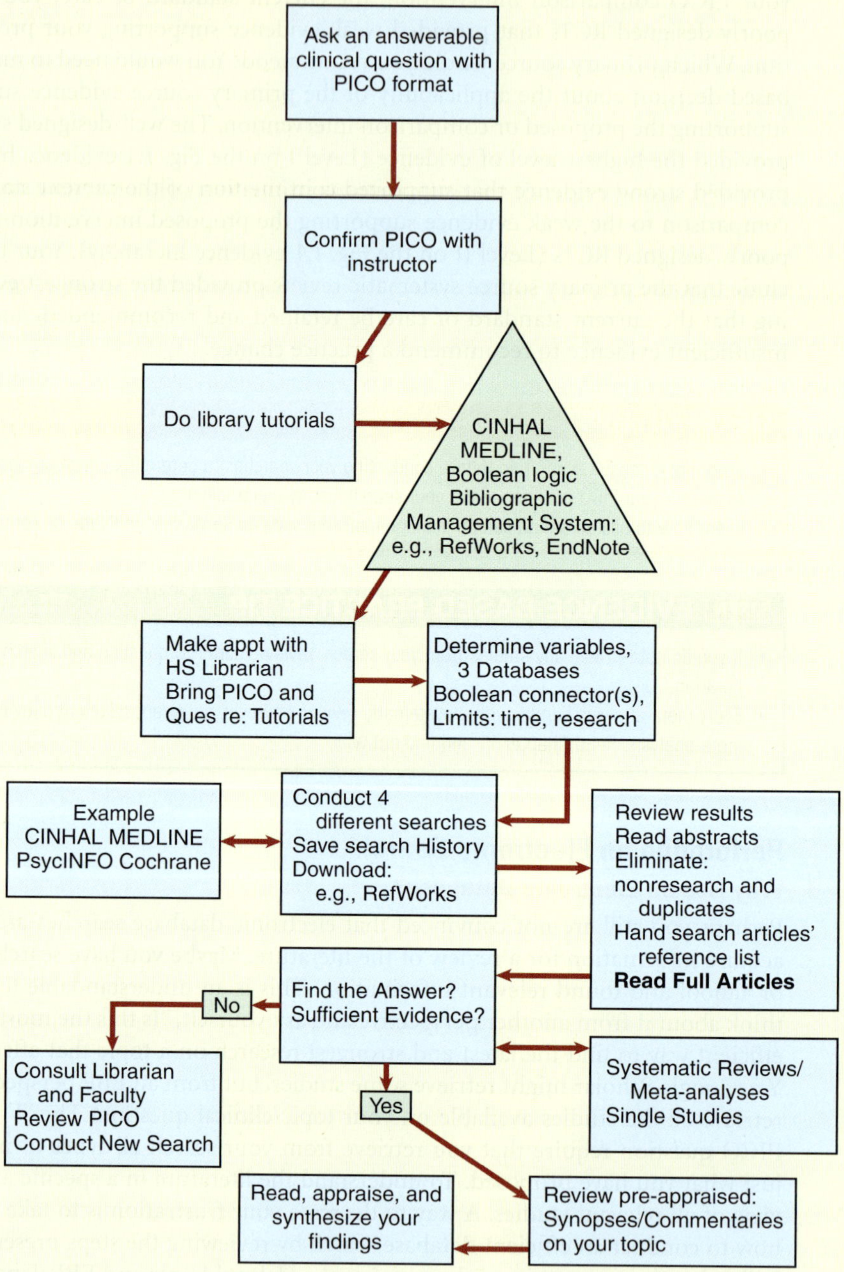

TYPES OF RESOURCES

Print and Electronic Indexes: Books and Journals

Most college/university libraries have management retrieval systems or databases to retrieve both print and online books, journals, videos, and other media items, scripts, monographs, conference proceedings, masters' theses, doctoral dissertations, archival materials, and **Grey literature** (e.g., information produced by government, industry, health care organizations, and professional organizations in the form of committee reports and policy documents; dissertations are included in the Grey literature). Print indexes are useful for finding sources that have not been entered into online databases. Print resources such as the Grey literature are still necessary if a search requires materials not entered into a database before a certain year. Also, another source is the citations/reference lists from the articles you retrieved; often they contain studies not captured with your search.

Refereed Journals

A major portion of most literature reviews consist of journal articles. Journals are published in print and online. In contrast to textbooks, which take much longer to publish, journals are a ready source of the latest information on almost any subject. Therefore, journals are the preferred mode of communicating the latest theory or study results. You should use **refereed or peer-reviewed journals** as your first choice when looking for primary sources of theoretical, clinical, or research articles. A refereed or peer-reviewed journal has a panel of internal and external reviewers who review submitted manuscripts for possible publication. The external reviewers are drawn from a pool of nurse scholars and scholars from related disciplines who are experts in various specialties. In most cases, the reviews are "blind"; that is, the manuscript to be reviewed does not include the name of the author(s). The reviewers use a set of criteria to judge whether a manuscript meets the publication journal's standards. These criteria are similar to what you will use to critically appraise the evidence you obtained in order to determine the strengths and weaknesses of a study (see Chapters 7 and 18). The credibility of a published research or theoretical/conceptual article is strengthened by the peer-review process.

Electronic: Bibliographic and Abstract Databases

Electronic databases are used to find research and theoretical/conceptual articles on a variety of topics, including doctoral dissertations. Electronic databases contain bibliographic citation information such as the author name, title, journal, and indexed terms for each record. Libraries have lists of electronic databases, including the ones indicated in Table 3.3 and Table 3.4. Usually these include the abstract, and some have the full text of the article or links to the full text. If the full text is not available, look for other options such as the abstract to learn more about the article before requesting an interlibrary loan of the article. Reading the abstract (see Chapter 1) is a critical step of the process to determine if you need to retrieve the full text article through another mechanism. Use both CINAHL and MEDLINE electronic databases as well as a third database; this will facilitate all steps of critically reviewing the literature, especially identifying the gaps. Your college/university most likely enables you to access such databases electronically whether on campus or not.

TABLE 3.4 Selected Examples of Websites for Evidence-Based Practice

Website	Scope	Notes
Virginia Henderson International Nursing Library (www.nursinglibrary.org)	Access to the *Registry of Nursing Research* database contains abstracts and the full text of research studies and conference papers	Offered without charge. Supported by Sigma Theta Tau International, Honor Society of Nursing.
National Guideline Clearinghouse (www.guidelines.gov)	Public resource for evidence-based CP guidelines	Offers a useful online feature of side-by-side comparison of guidelines and the ability to browse by disease/condition and treatment/intervention.
JBI (www.joannabriggs.org)	JBI is an international not-for-profit research and development center	Membership required for access. Recommended links worth reviewing, as well as descriptions on their levels of evidence and grading scale is provided.
TRIP (www.tripdatabase.com)	Content from free online resources, including synopses, guidelines, medical images, e-textbooks, and systematic reviews, organized under the TRIP search engine.	Site offers a wide sampling of available evidence and ability to filter by publication type—that is, evidence based synopses, systematic reviews, guidelines, textbooks, and research.
Agency for Health Research and Quality (www.ahrq.gov)	Evidence-based reports, statistical briefs, research findings and reports, and policy reports.	Free source of government documents, searchable via PubMed.
Cochrane Collaboration (www.cochrane.org)	Access to abstracts from Cochrane Database of Systematic Reviews. Full text of reviews and access to databases that are part of the Cochrane Library. Information is high quality and useful for health care decision making. It is a powerful tool for enhancing health care knowledge and decision making.	Abstracts are free and can be browsed or searched; uses many databases in its reviews, including CINAHL via EBSCO and MEDLINE; some are primary sources (e.g., systematic reviews/meta-analyses); others (if commentaries of single studies) are a secondary source; important source for clinical evidence.

CP, Clinical practice; *CINAHL,* Cumulative Index to Nursing and Allied Health Literature; *JBI,* Joanna Briggs Institute; *TRIP,* Turning Research into Practice.

Electronic: Secondary or Summary Databases

Some databases contain more than journal article information. These resources contain either summaries or synopses of studies, overviews of diseases or conditions, or a summary of the latest evidence to support a particular treatment. Table 3.4 provides a few examples.

Internet: Search Engines

You are probably familiar with accessing a **web browser** (e.g., Internet Explorer, Mozilla Firefox, Chrome, Safari) to conduct searches, and with using search engines such as Google or Google Scholar to find information. However, "surfing" the web is not a good use of your time when searching for scholarly literature. Table 3.4 indicates sources of online information; all are free except JBI. Most websites are not a primary source for research studies.

HELPFUL HINTS

Be sure to discuss with your instructor regarding the use of theoretical/conceptual articles and other Grey literature in your EBP/QI project or a review of the literature paper.

Less common and less used sources of scholarly material are audio, video, personal communications (e.g., letters, telephone or in-person interviews), unpublished doctoral dissertations, masters' theses, and conference proceedings.

QSEN EVIDENCE-BASED PRACTICE TIP

Reading systematic reviews, if available, on your clinical question/topic will enhance your ability to implement evidence-based nursing practice because they generally offer the strongest and most consistent level of evidence and can provide helpful search terms. A good first step for any question is to search the Cochrane Database of Systematic Reviews to see if someone has already completed a systematic review addressing your clinical question.

How Far Back Must the Search Go?

Students often ask questions such as, "How many articles do I need?"; "How much is enough?"; "How far back in the literature do I need to go?" When conducting a search, you should use a rigorous focused process or you may end up with hundreds or thousands of citations. Retrieving too many citations is usually a sign that there was something wrong with your search technique, or you may not have sufficiently narrowed your clinical question.

Each electronic database offers an explanation of its features; take the time and click on each icon and explore the explanations offered, because this will increase your confidence. Also, take advantages of tutorials offered to improve your search techniques. Keep in mind the types of articles you are retrieving. Many electronic resources allow you to limit your search to the article type (e.g., systematic reviews/meta-analyses, RCTs). Box 3.2 provides a number of features through which CINAHL Plus with Full Test allows you to choose and/or insert information so that your search can be targeted.

When conducting a literature review for any purpose, there is always a question of how far back one should search. There is no general time period. But if in your search you find a well-done meta-analysis that was published 6 years ago, you could continue your search, moving forward from that time period. Some research and EBP projects may warrant going back 10 or more years. Extensive literature reviews on particular topics or a concept clarification helps you limit the length of your search.

BOX 3.2 Tips: Using Cumulative Index to Nursing and Allied Health Literature via EBSCO

- Locate CINAHL from your library's home page. It may be located under databases, online resources, or nursing resources.
- In the Advanced Search, type in your keyword, subject heading, or phrase (e.g., maternal-fetal attachment, health behavior). Do not use complete sentences. (Ask your librarian for any tip sheets, or online tutorials or use the HELP feature in the database.)
- Before choosing "Search," make sure you mark "Research Articles" to ensure that you have retrieved articles that are actually research.
- In the "Limit Your Results" section, you can limit by year, age group, clinical queries, and so on.
- Using the Boolean connector "AND" between each of the words of your PICO variables narrows your search—that is, it will exclude an article that doesn't use both terms; using "OR" broadens your search.
- Once the search results appear, save them, review titles and abstracts online, export to your management system (e.g., RefWorks), and/or e-mail the results to yourself.

CINAHL, Cumulative Index to Nursing and Allied Health Literature.

As you scroll through and mark the citations you wish to include in your downloaded or printed search, make sure you include all relevant fields when you save or print. In addition to indicating which citations you want and choosing which fields, there is an opportunity to indicate if you want the "search history" included. It is always a good idea to include this information. It is especially helpful if you feel that some citations were missed; then you can replicate your search and determine which variable(s) you missed. This is also your opportunity to indicate if you want to e-mail the search to yourself. If you are writing a paper and need to develop a reference list, you can export your citations to **citation management software,** which formats and stores your citations so that they are available for electronic retrieval when they are needed for a paper. Quite a few of these software programs are available; some are free, such as Zotero, and others your institution has most likely purchased, including EndNote and RefWorks.

HELPFUL HINT

Ask your faculty for guidance if you are uncertain how far back you need to conduct your search. If you come across a systematic review/meta-analysis on your specific topic, review it to see what years the review covers; then begin your search from the last year of the studies included in the review and conduct your search from that year forward to the present to fill in the gap.

QSEN EVIDENCE-BASED PRACTICE TIP

You will be tempted to use Google, Google Scholar, or even Wikipedia instead of going through Steps I through III of Table 3.2 and using the databases suggested, but this will most likely result in thousands of citations that aren't classified as research and are not specific to your PICO question. Instead, use the specific parameters of your electronic database.

What Do I Need to Know?

Each database usually has a specific search guide that provides information on the organization of the entries and the terminology used. Academic and health science libraries continually update their websites in order to provide tutorials, guides, and tips for those who are using their databases. The strategies in Table 3.2 incorporate general search strategies, as well as those related to CINAHL and MEDLINE. Finding the right terms to "plug in" as keywords for a computer search is important for conducting an efficient search. In many electronic databases you can browse the **controlled vocabulary** terms and see how the terms of your question match up and then add them before you search. If you encounter a problem, ask your librarian for assistance.

HELPFUL HINT

One way to discover new terms for searching is to find a systematic review that includes the search strategy. Match your PICO words with the controlled vocabulary terms of each database.

In CINAHL the Full Text via EBSCO host provides you with the option of conducting a basic or advanced search using the controlled vocabulary of CINAHL headings. This user-friendly feature has a built-in tutorial that reviews how to use this option. You also can click on the "Help" feature at any time during your search. It is recommended that you conduct an Advanced Search with a Guided Style tutorial that outlines the steps for conducing your search. If you wanted to locate articles about maternal-fetal attachment as they relate to the health practices or health behaviors of low-income mothers, you would first want to construct your PICO:

P Maternal-fetal attachment in low-income mothers (specifically defined group)
I Health behaviors or health practices (event to be studied)
C None (comparison of intervention)
O Neonatal outcomes (outcome)

In this example, the two main concepts are maternal-fetal attachment and health practices and how these impact neonatal outcomes. Many times when conducting a search, you only enter in keywords or controlled vocabulary for the first two elements of your PICO—in this case, maternal-fetal attachment and health practices or behaviors. The other elements can be added if your list of results is overwhelming (review the Critical Thinking Decision Path).

Maternal-fetal attachment should be part of your keyword search; however, when you click the CINAHL heading, it indicates that you should use "prenatal bonding." To be comprehensive, you should use the **Boolean operator** of "OR" to link these terms together. The second concept, of health practices OR health behavior, is accomplished in a similar manner. The subject heading or controlled vocabulary assigned by the indexers could be added in for completeness. Boolean operators are "AND," "OR," and "NOT," and they dictate the relationship between words and concepts. Note that if you use "AND," then this would require that both concepts be located within the same article, while "OR" allows you to group together like terms or synonyms, and "NOT" eliminates terms from your search. It is suggested that you limit your search to "peer-reviewed" and "research" articles. Refine the publication range date to 10 years, or whatever the requirement is for your search, and save your search. Once these limits were chosen for the PICO search related to maternal-fetal attachment described previously, the search results decreased from an unmanageable 294 articles to 6 research articles. The key to understanding how to use this process is to try the search yourself using the terms just described. Developing search skills takes time, even if you complete the library tutorials and meet with a librarian to refine your PICO question, search terms, and limits. You should search several databases. Library database websites are continually being updated, so it is important to get to know your library database site.

HELPFUL HINT

When combining synonyms for a concept, use the Boolean operator "OR"—OR is more!

Review your library's tutorials on conducting a search for each type database (e.g., CINAHL and MEDLINE).

Use features in your database such as "limit search to" and choose peer review journal, research article, date range, age group, and country (e.g., United States).

How Do I Complete the Search?

Once you are confident about your search strategies for identifying key articles, it is time to critically read what you have found. Critically reading research articles requires several readings and the use of critical appraisal criteria (see Chapters 1, 7, and 18). Do not be discouraged if all of the retrieved articles are not as useful as you first thought, even though you limited your search to "research." This happens to even the most experienced searcher.

If most of the articles you retrieved were not useful, be prepared to do another search, but before you do, discuss the search terms with your librarian and faculty. You may also want to add a fourth database. It is a good practice to always save your search history when conducting a search. It is very helpful if you provide a printout of the search you have completed when consulting with your librarian or faculty. Most likely your library will have the feature that allows you to save your search, and it can be retrieved during your meeting. In the example of maternal-fetal bonding and health behaviors in low-income women, the third database of choice may be PsycINFO (see Table 3.3).

HELPFUL HINT

Read the abstract carefully to determine if it is a research article; you will usually see the use of headings such as "Methodology" and "Results" in research articles. It is also a good idea to review the reference list of the research articles you retrieved, as this strategy might uncover additional related articles you missed in your database search, and then you can retrieve them.

LITERATURE REVIEW FORMAT: WHAT TO EXPECT

Becoming familiar with the format of a literature review in the various types of review articles and the literature review section of a research article will help you use critical appraisal criteria to evaluate the review. To decide which style you will use so that your review is presented in a logical and organized manner, you must consider:

- The research or clinical question/topic
- The number of retrieved sources reviewed
- The number and type of research versus theoretical/conceptual materials and/or Grey literature

Some reviews are written according to the variables or concepts being studied and presented chronologically under each variable. Others present the material chronologically with subcategories or variables discussed within each time period. Still others present the variables and include subcategories related to the study's type or designs or related variables.

Hawthorne and colleagues (2016) (see Appendix B) stated that the purpose of their "longitudinal study was to test the relationships between spirituality/religious coping strategies and grief, mental health (depression and post-traumatic stress disorder), and mothers and fathers" at selected time periods after experiencing the death of an infant in the neonatal intensive care unit (NICU) or pediatric intensive care unit (PICU). At the beginning of their article, after some basic overall facts on infant deaths and parents' grieving, they logically presented the concepts they addressed in their quantitative study (see Appendix B). The researchers did not title the beginning of their article with a section labeled *Literature Review*. However, it is clear that the beginning of their article is a literature review. **Example:** ➤ After presenting general facts on infant deaths and parents grieving and related research, the authors title a section *Use of Spirituality/Religion as a Coping Strategy* and the next section *Parent Mental Health and Personal Growth*. In these sections they discuss studies related to each topic. Then, they present a section labeled *Conceptual Framework*, indicating that will use a specific grief framework to guide their study.

IPE HIGHLIGHT

Each member of your QI committee should be responsible for searching for one research study, using the agreed upon search terms and reviewing the abstract to determine its relevance to your QI project's clinical question.

HELPFUL HINT

The literature review for an EBP/QI project or another type of scholarly paper is different than one found in a research article.

Make an outline that will later become the level headings in your paper (i.e., title the concepts of your literature review). This is a good way to focus your writing and will let the reader know what to expect to read and demonstrate your logic and organization.

Include your search strategies so that a reader can re-create your search and come up with the same results. Include information on databases searched, time frame of studies chosen, search terms used, and any limits used to narrow the search.

Include any standardized tools used to critically appraise the retrieved literature.

APPRAISAL FOR EVIDENCE-BASED PRACTICE

When writing a literature review for an EBP/QI project, you need to critically appraise all research reports using appropriate criteria. Once you have conducted your search and obtained all your references, you need to evaluate the articles using standardized critical appraisal criteria (see Chapters 7, 11, and 18). Using the criteria, you will be able to identify the strengths and weaknesses of each study.

Critiquing research or theoretical/conceptual reports is a challenging task for seasoned consumers of research, so do not be surprised if you feel a little intimidated by the prospect of critiquing and synthesizing research. The important issue is to determine the overall value of the literature review, including both research and theoretical/conceptual materials. The purposes of a literature review (see Box 3.1) and the characteristics of a well-written literature review (Box 3.3) provide the framework for evaluating the literature.

The literature review should be presented in an organized manner. Theoretical/conceptual and research literature can be presented chronologically from earliest work of the theorist or first studies on a topic to most recent; sometimes the theoretical/conceptual

BOX 3.3 Characteristics of a Well-Written Review of the Literature—An EBP Perspective

Each reviewed source reflects critical thinking and writing and is relevant to the study/topic/project, and the content meets the following criteria:

- Uses mainly primary sources—that is, a sufficient number of research articles for answering a clinical question with a justification of the literature search dates and search terms used
- Organizes the literature review using a systematic approach
- Uses established critical appraisal criteria for specific study designs to evaluate strengths, weaknesses, conflicts, or gaps related to the PICO question
- Provides a synthesis and critique of the references indicating similarities, differences, strengths, and weaknesses between and among the studies
- Concludes with a summary that provides recommendations for practice and research
- In a table format, summarizes each article succinctly with references

literature that provided the foundation for the existing research will be presented first, followed by the research studies that were derived from this theoretical/conceptual base. Other times, the literature can be clustered by concepts, pro or con positions, or evidence that highlights differences in the theoretical/conceptual and/or research findings. The overall question to be answered from an EBP perspective is, "Does the review of the literature develop and present a knowledge base to provide sufficient evidence for an EBP/QI project?" Objectives 1 to 3, 5, 8, 10, and 11 in Box 3.1 specifically reflect the purposes of a literature review for EBP/QI project. Objectives 1 to 8 and 11 reflect the purposes of a literature review when conducting a research study.

Regardless of how the literature review is organized, it should provide a strong knowledge base for a CP or a research project. When a literature review ends with insufficient evidence, this provides a gap in knowledge and requires further research. The more you read published systematic and integrative reviews, as well as studies, the more competent you become at differentiating a well-organized literature review from one that has a limited organizing framework.

Another key to developing your competency in this area is to read both quantitative (meta-analyses) and qualitative (meta-syntheses) systematic reviews. A well-done meta-analysis adheres to the rigorous search, appraisal, and synthesis process for a group of like studies to answer a question and to meet the required guidelines, which include that it should be conducted by a team.

The systematic review on how nurses who lead clinics for patients with cardiovascular disease found in Appendix E is an example of a well-done quantitative systematic review that critically appraises and synthesizes the evidence from research studies related to the effect of the mortality and morbidity rates of patients with cardiovascular disease who are followed in nurse-led clinics.

The Critical Appraisal Criteria box summarizes general critical appraisal criteria for a review of the literature. Other sets of critical appraisal criteria may phrase these questions differently or more broadly. **Example:** ➤ "Does the literature search seem adequate?" "Does the report demonstrate scholarly writing?" These may seem to be difficult questions for you to answer; one place to begin, however, is by determining whether the source is a refereed journal. It is reasonable to assume that a refereed journal publishes manuscripts that are adequately searched, use mainly primary sources, and are written in a scholarly manner. This does not mean, however, that every study reported in a refereed journal will meet all of the critical appraisal criteria for a literature review and other components of the study in an equal manner. Because of style differences and space constraints, each citation summarized is often very brief, or related citations may be summarized as a group and lack a critique. You still must answer the critiquing questions. Consultation with a faculty advisor may be necessary to develop skill in answering these questions.

The key to a strong literature review is a careful search of published and unpublished literature. When critically appraising a literature review written for a published research study, it should reflect a synthesis or pulling together of the main points or value of all of the sources reviewed in relation to your research question, hypothesis, or clinical question (see Box 3.1). The relationship between and among these studies must be explained. The summary synthesis of a review of the literature in an area should appear at the end of a paper or article. When reading a research article, the summary of the literature appears before the methodology section and is referred to again when reviewing the results of the study.

CRITICAL APPRAISAL CRITERIA

Literature Review

1. Are all of the relevant concepts and variables included in the literature review?
2. Is the literature review presented in an organized format that flows logically (e.g., chronologically, clustered by concept or variables), enhancing the reader's ability to evaluate the need for the particular research study or evidence-based practice project?
3. Does the search strategy include an appropriate and adequate number of databases and other resources to identify key published and unpublished research and theoretical/conceptual sources?
4. Are both theoretical/conceptual and research sources used?
5. Are primary sources mainly used?
6. What gaps or inconsistencies in knowledge does the literature review uncover?
7. Does the literature review build on earlier studies?
8. Does the summary of each reviewed study reflect the essential components of the study design (e.g., type and size of sample, reliability and validity of instruments, consistency of data collection procedures, appropriate data analysis, identification of limitations)?
9. Does the critique of each reviewed study include strengths, weaknesses, or limitations of the design, conflicts, and gaps in information related to the area of interest?
10. Does the synthesis summary follow a logical sequence that presents the overall strengths and weaknesses of the reviewed studies and arrive at a logical conclusion on its topic?
11. Does the literature review for an evidence-based practice project answer a clinical question?
12. Is the literature review presented in an organized format that flows logically (e.g., chronologically, clustered by concepts or variables), enhancing the reader's ability to evaluate the need for the particular research study or evidence-based practice project?

HELPFUL HINT

- If you are doing an academic assignment, make sure you check with your instructor as to whether or not the following sources may be used: (1) unpublished material, (2) theoretical/conceptual articles, and (3) Grey literature.
- Use a standardized critical appraisal criteria appropriate to the study's design to evaluate research articles.
- Make a table of the studies found (see Chapter 20 for an example of a summary table).
- Synthesize the results of your analysis by comparing and contrasting the similarities and differences between the studies on your topic/clinical question and draw a conclusion.

KEY POINTS

- Review of the literature is defined as a broad, comprehensive, in-depth, systematic critique and synthesis of publications, unpublished print and online materials, audiovisual materials, and personal communication.
- Review of the literature is used for the development of EBP/QI clinical projects as well as research studies.
- There are differences between a review of the literature for research and for EBP/QI projects. For an EBP/QI project, your search should focus on the highest level of primary source literature available per the hierarchy of evidence, and it should relate to the specific clinical problem.

- The main objectives for conducting and writing a literature review are to acquire the ability to (1) conduct a comprehensive and efficient electronic research and/or print research search on a topic; (2) efficiently retrieve a sufficient amount of materials for a literature review in relation to the topic and scope of project; (3) critically appraise (i.e., critique) research and theoretical/conceptual material based on accepted critical appraisal criteria; (4) critically evaluate published reviews of the literature based on accepted standardized critical appraisal criteria; (5) synthesize the findings of the critique materials for relevance to the purpose of the selected scholarly project; and (6) determine applicability to answer your clinical question.
- Primary research and theoretical/conceptual resources are essential for literature reviews.
- Review the Grey literature for white papers and theoretical/conceptual materials not published in journals, and conduct "hand searches" of the reference list of your retrieved research articles as both provide background as well as uncover other studies.
- Secondary sources, such as commentaries on research articles from peer-reviewed journals, are part of a learning strategy for developing critical critiquing skills.
- It is more efficient to use electronic databases rather than print resources or general web search engines such as Google for retrieving materials.
- Strategies for efficiently retrieving literature for nursing include consulting the librarian and using at least three online sources (e.g., CINAHL, MEDLINE, and one that relates more specifically to your clinical question or topic).
- Literature reviews are usually organized according to variables, as well as chronologically.
- Critiquing and synthesizing a number of research articles, including systematic reviews, is essential to implementing evidence-based nursing practice.

CRITICAL THINKING CHALLENGES

- IPE Why is it important for your QI team colleagues to be able to challenge each other about the overall strength and quality of evidence provided by the group of studies retrieved from your search?
- For an EBP project, why is it necessary to critically appraise studies that are published in a refereed journal?
- How does reading preappraised commentaries of a study and systematic reviews/meta-analyses develop your critical appraisal skills?
- A general guideline for a literature search is to use a timeline of 5 years or more. Would your timeline possibly differ if you found a well-done systematic review?
- What is the relationship of the research article's literature review to the theoretical or conceptual framework?

REFERENCES

Hawthorne, D. M., Youngblut, J. M., & Brooten, D. (2016). Parent spirituality, grief, and mental health at 1 year and 3 months after their infants/child's death in an intensive care unit. *Journal of Pediatric Nursing*, *31*, 73–80.

Jeffries, P., & National League for Nursing (NLN). (2015). *The NLN Jeffries simulation theory*. Philadelphia, PA: Wolters Kluwer.

Kendall, S. (2008). Evidence-based resources simplified. *Canadian Family Physician*, *54*(2), 241–243.

Nyamathi, A., Salem, B. E., Zhang, S., et al. (2015). Nursing care management, peer coaching, and Hepatitis A and B vaccine completion among homeless men recently released on parole. *Nursing Research*, *64*(3), 177–189.

Turner-Sack, A. M., Menna, R., Setchell, S. R., et al. (2016). Psychological functioning, post traumatic growth, and coping in parent and siblings of adolescent cancer survivors. *Oncology Nursing Forum*, *43*, 48–56.

van Dijk, J. F., Vervoort, S. C., van Wijck, A. J., et al. (2016). Postoperative patients' perspective on rating pain: A qualitative study. *International Journal of Nursing Studies*, *53*, 260–269.

Yensen, J. (2013). PICO search strategies. *Online Journal of Nursing Informatics*, *17*(3). Retrieved from http://ojni.org/issues/?p=2860.

Go to Evolve at **http://evolve.elsevier.com/LoBiondo/** for review questions, critiquing exercises, and additional research articles for practice in reviewing and critiquing.

4

Theoretical Frameworks for Research

Melanie McEwen

Go to Evolve at **http://evolve.elsevier.com/LoBiondo/** for review questions, critiquing exercises, and additional research articles for practice in reviewing and critiquing.

LEARNING OUTCOMES

After reading this chapter, you should be able to do the following:

- Describe the relationship among theory, research, and practice.
- Identify the purpose of conceptual and theoretical frameworks for nursing research.
- Differentiate between conceptual and operational definitions.
- Identify the different types of theories used in nursing research.
- Describe how a theory or conceptual framework guides research.
- Explain the points of critical appraisal used to evaluate the appropriateness, cohesiveness, and consistency of a framework guiding research.

KEY TERMS

concept
conceptual definition
conceptual framework
construct
deductive
grand theory
inductive
middle range theory
model
operational definition
situation-specific theory
theoretical framework
theory

To introduce the discussion of the use of theoretical frameworks for nursing research, consider the example of Emily, a novice oncology nurse. From this case study, reflect on how nurses can understand the theoretical underpinnings of both nursing research and evidence-based nursing practice, and re-affirm how nurses should integrate research into practice.

The author would like to acknowledge the contribution of Patricia Liehr, who contributed this chapter in a previous edition.

Emily graduated with her bachelor of science in nursing (BSN) a little more than a year ago, and she recently changed positions to work on a pediatric oncology unit in a large hospital. She quickly learned that working with very ill and often dying children is tremendously rewarding, even though it is frequently heartbreaking.

One of Emily's first patients was Benny, a 14-year-old boy admitted with a recurrence of leukemia. When she first cared for Benny, he was extremely ill. Benny's oncologist implemented the protocols for cases such as his, but the team was careful to explain to Benny and his family that his prognosis was guarded. In the early days of his hospitalization, Emily cried with his mother when they received his daily lab values and there was no apparent improvement. She observed that Benny was growing increasingly fatigued and had little appetite. Despite his worsening condition, however, Benny and his parents were unfailingly positive, making plans for a vacation to the mountains and the upcoming school year.

At the end of her shift one night before several days off, Emily hugged Benny's parents, as she feared that Benny would die before her next scheduled workday. Several days later, when she listened to the report at the start of her shift, Emily was amazed to learn that Benny had been heartily eating a normal diet. He was ambulatory and had been cruising the halls with his baseball coach and playing video games with two of his cousins. When she entered Benny's room for her initial assessment, she saw the much-improved teenager dressed in shorts and a T-shirt, sitting up in bed using his iPad. A half-finished chocolate milkshake was on the table in easy reaching distance. He joked with Emily about *Angry Birds* as she performed her assessment. Benny steadily improved over the ensuing days and eventually went home with his leukemia again in remission.

As Emily became more comfortable in the role of oncology nurse, she continued to notice patterns among the children and adolescents on her unit. Many got better, even though their conditions were often critical. In contrast, some of the children who had better prognoses failed to improve as much, or as quickly, as anticipated. She realized that the kids who did better than expected seemed to have common attributes or characteristics, including positive attitudes, supportive family and friends, and strong determination to "beat" their cancer. Over lunch one day, Emily talked with her mentor, Marie, about her observations, commenting that on a number of occasions she had seen patients rebound when she thought that death was imminent.

Marie smiled. "Fortunately this is a pattern that we see quite frequently. Many of our kids are amazingly resilient." Marie told Emily about the work of several nurse researchers who studied the phenomenon of resilience and gave her a list of articles reporting on their findings. Emily followed up with Marie's prompting and learned about "psychosocial resilience in adolescents" (Tusaie et al., 2007) and "adolescent resilience" (Ahern, 2006; Ahern et al., 2008). These works led her to a "middle range theory of resilience" (Polk, 1997). Focusing her literature review even more, Emily was able to discover several recent research studies (Chen et al., 2014; Ishibashi et al., 2015; Wu et al., 2015) that examined aspects of resilience among adolescents with cancer, further piquing her interest in the subject.

From her readings, she gained insight into resilience, learning to recognize it in her patients. She also identified ways she might encourage and even promote resilience in children and teenagers. Eventually, she decided to enroll in a graduate nursing program to learn how to research different phenomena of concern to her patients and discover ways to apply the evidence-based findings to improve nursing care and patient outcomes.

PRACTICE-THEORY-RESEARCH LINKS

Several important aspects of how theory is used in nursing research are embedded in Emily's story. First, it is important to notice the links among practice, theory, and research. Each is intricately connected with the others to create the knowledge base for the discipline of nursing (Fig. 4.1). In her practice, Emily recognized a pattern of characteristics in some patients that appeared to enhance their recovery. Her mentor directed her to research that other nurses had published on the phenomenon of "resilience." Emily was then able to apply the information on resilience and related research findings as she planned and implemented care. Her goal was to enhance each child's resilience as much as possible and thereby improve their outcomes.

Another key message from the case study is the importance of reflecting on an observed phenomenon and discussing it with colleagues. This promotes questioning and collaboration, as nurses seek ways to improve practice. Finally, Emily was encouraged to go to the literature to search out what had been published related to the phenomenon she had observed. Reviewing the research led her to a middle range theory on resilience as well as current nursing research that examined its importance in caring for adolescents with cancer. This then challenged her to consider how she might ultimately conduct her own research.

OVERVIEW OF THEORY

Theory is a set of interrelated concepts that provides a systematic view of a phenomenon. A theory allows relationships to be proposed and predictions made, which in turn can suggest potential actions. Beginning with a theory gives a researcher a logical way of collecting data to describe, explain, and predict nursing practice, making it critical in research.

In nursing, science is the result of the interchange between research and theory. The purpose of research is to build knowledge through the generation or testing of theory that can then be applied in practice. To build knowledge, research should develop within a theoretical structure or blueprint that facilitates analysis and interpretation of findings. The use of theory provides structure and organization to nursing knowledge.

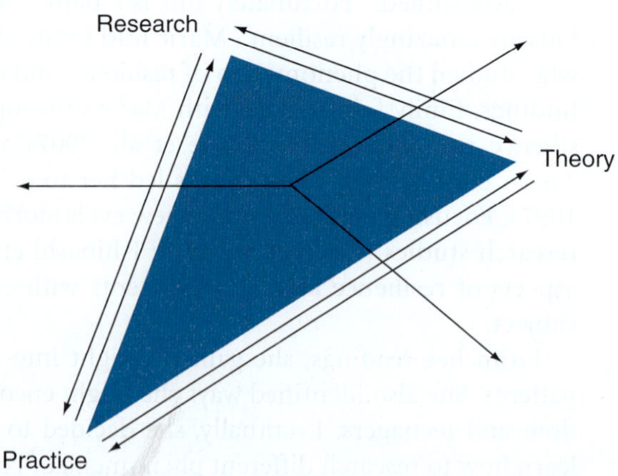

FIG 4.1 Discipline knowledge: Theory-practice-research connection.

It is important that nurses understand that nursing practice is based on the theories that are generated and validated through research (McEwen & Wills, 2014).

In an integrated, reciprocal manner, theory guides research and practice; practice enables testing of theory and generates research questions; and research contributes to theory building and establishing practice guidelines (see Fig. 4.1). Therefore, what is learned through practice, theory, and research interweaves to create the knowledge fabric of nursing. From this perspective, like Emily in the case study, each nurse should be involved in the process of contributing to the knowledge or evidence-based practice of nursing.

Several key terms are often used when discussing theory. It is necessary to understand these terms when considering how to apply theory in practice and research. They include **concept**, **conceptual definition**, **conceptual/theoretical framework**, **construct**, **model**, **operational definition**, and **theory**. Each term is defined and summarized in Box 4.1. Concepts and constructs are the major components of theories and convey the essential ideas or elements of a theory. When a nurse researcher decides to study a concept/construct, the researcher must precisely and explicitly describe and explain the concept, devise a mechanism to identify and confirm the presence of the concept of interest, and determine a method to measure or quantify it. To illustrate, Table 4.1 shows the key concepts and conceptual and operational definitions provided by Turner-Sack and colleagues (2016) in their study on psychological issues among parents and siblings of adolescent cancer survivors (see Appendix D).

BOX 4.1 Definitions

Concept

Image or symbolic representation of an abstract idea; the key identified element of a phenomenon that is necessary to understand it. Concept can be concrete or abstract. A concrete concept can be easily identified, quantified, and measured, whereas an abstract concept is more difficult to quantify or measure. For example, weight, blood pressure, and body temperature are concrete concepts. Hope, uncertainty, and spiritual pain are more abstract concepts. In a study, resilience is a relatively abstract concept.

Conceptual Definition

Much like a dictionary definition, a conceptual definition conveys the general meaning of the concept. However, the conceptual definition goes beyond the general language meaning found in the dictionary by defining or explaining the concept as it is rooted in theoretical literature.

Conceptual Framework/Theoretical Framework

A set of interrelated concepts that represents an image of a phenomenon. These two terms are often used interchangeably. The conceptual/theoretical framework refers to a structure that provides guidance for research or practice. The framework identifies the key concepts and describes their relationships to each other and to the phenomena (variables) of concern to nursing. It serves as the foundation on which a study can be developed or as a map to aid in the design of the study.

Construct

Complex concept; constructs usually comprise more than one concept and are built or "constructed" to fit a purpose. Health promotion, maternal-infant bonding, health-seeking behaviors, and health-related quality of life are examples of constructs.

Model

A graphic or symbolic representation of a phenomenon. A graphic model is empirical and can be readily represented. A model of an eye or a heart is an example. A symbolic or theoretical model depicts a phenomenon that is not directly observable and is expressed in language or symbols. Written music or Einstein's theory of relativity are examples of symbolic models. Theories used by nurses or developed by nurses frequently include symbolic models. Models are very helpful in allowing the reader to visualize key concepts/constructs and their identified interrelationships.

Operational Definition

Specifies how the concept will be measured. That is, the operational definition defines what instruments will be used to assess the presence of the concept and will be used to describe the amount or degree to which the concept exists.

Theory

Set of interrelated concepts that provides a systematic view of a phenomenon.

TABLE 4.1 Concepts and Variables: Conceptual and Operational Definitions

Concept	Conceptual Definition	Variable	Operational Definition
Post-traumatic growth (Turner-Sack et al., 2016)	Mastering a previously experienced trauma, perceiving benefits from it and developing beyond the original level of psychological functioning	PTG	Score on the post-traumatic growth inventory (a 21-item, Likert-type questionnaire)
Psychological distress (Turner-Sack et al., 2016)	Extent to which one experiences psychological symptoms (e.g., depression, anxiety, somatization)	Psychological distress (symptoms of somatization, depression, anxiety)	Scores on the brief symptom inventory (53 item, Likert-type questionnaire)
Coping strategies (Turner-Sack et al., 2016)	Methods or strategies used to respond to stressful events	Coping strategies (active coping, acceptance coping, avoidant coping, religious coping, social support)	Scores on COPE (60-item self-report questionnaire)
Life satisfaction (Turner-Sack et al., 2016)	Global life satisfaction with their lives	Life satisfaction	Responses to the "satisfaction with life scale" rating of 1 to 7 on five statements about their life

TYPES OF THEORIES USED BY NURSES

As stated previously, a theory is a set of interrelated concepts that provides a systematic view of a phenomenon. Theory provides a foundation and structure that may be used for the purpose of explaining or predicting another phenomenon. In this way, a theory is like a blueprint or a guide for modeling a structure. A blueprint depicts the elements of a structure and the relationships among the elements; similarly, a theory depicts the concepts that compose it and suggests how the concepts are related.

Nurses use a multitude of different theories as the foundation or structure for research and practice. Many have been developed by nurses and are explicitly related to nursing practice; others, however, come from other disciplines. Knowledge that draws upon both nursing and non-nursing theories is extremely important in order to provide excellent, evidence-based care.

Theories from Related Disciplines Used in Nursing Practice and Research

Like engineering, architecture, social work, and teaching, nursing is a practice discipline. That means that nurses use concepts, constructs, models, and theories from many disciplines in addition to nursing-specific theories. This is, to a large extent, the rationale for the "liberal arts" education that is required before entering a BSN program. Exposure to knowledge and theories of basic and natural sciences (e.g., mathematics, chemistry, biology) and social sciences (e.g., psychology, sociology, political science) provides a fundamental understanding of those disciplines and allows for application of key principles, concepts, and theories from each, as appropriate.

Likewise, BSN-prepared nurses use principles of administration and management and learning theories in patient-centered, holistic practices. Table 4.2 lists a few of the many theories and concepts from other disciplines that are commonly used by nurses in practice and research that become part of the foundational framework for nursing.

TABLE 4.2 **Theories Used in Nursing Practice and Research**

Discipline	Examples of Theories/Concepts Used by Nurses
Biomedical sciences	Germ theory (principles of infection), pain theories, immune function, genetics/genomics, pharmacotherapeutics
Sociologic sciences	Systems theory (e.g., VonBertalanffy), family theory (e.g., Bowen), role theory (e.g., Merton), critical social theory (e.g., Habermas), cultural diversity (e.g., Leininger)
Behavioral sciences	Developmental theories (e.g., Erikson), human needs theories (e.g., Maslow), personality theories (e.g., Freud), stress theories (e.g., Lazarus & Folkman), health belief model (e.g., Rosenstock)
Learning theories	Behavioral learning theories (e.g., Pavlov, Skinner), cognitive development/interaction theories (e.g., Piaget), adult learning theories (e.g., Knowles)
Leadership/management	Change theory (e.g., Lewin), conflict management (e.g., Rapaport), quality framework (e.g., Donabedian)

Nursing Theories Used in Practice and Research

In addition to the theories and concepts from disciplines other than nursing, the nursing literature presents a number of theories that were developed specifically by and for nurses. Typically, nursing theories reflect concepts, relationships, and processes that contribute to the development of a body of knowledge specific to nursing's concerns. Understanding these interactions and relationships among the concepts and phenomena is essential to evidence-based nursing care. Further, theories unique to nursing help define how it is different from other disciplines.

HELPFUL HINT

In research and practice, concepts often create descriptions or images that emerge from a conceptual definition. For instance, pain is a concept with different meanings based on the type or aspect of pain being referred to. As such, there are a number of methods and instruments to measure pain. So a nurse researching postoperative pain would conceptually define pain based on the patient's perceived discomfort associated with surgery, and then select a pain scale/instrument that allows the researcher to operationally define pain as the patient's score on that scale.

Nursing theories are often described based on their scope or degree of abstraction. Typically, these are reported as "grand," "middle range," or "situation specific" (also called "microrange") nursing theories. Each is described in this section.

Grand Nursing Theories

Grand nursing theories are sometimes referred to as nursing conceptual models and include the theories/models that were developed to describe the discipline of nursing as a whole. This comprises the works of nurse theorists such as Florence Nightingale, Virginia Henderson, Martha Rogers, Dorthea Orem, and Betty Neuman. Grand nursing theories/models are all-inclusive conceptual structures that tend to include views on persons, health, and environment to create a perspective of nursing. This most abstract level of theory has established a knowledge base for the discipline. These works are used as the conceptual basis for practice and research, and are tested in research studies.

One grand theory is not better than another with respect to research. Rather, these varying perspectives allow a researcher to select a framework for research that best depicts the concepts and relationships of interest, and decide where and how they can be measured as study variables. What is most important about the use of grand nursing theoretical frameworks for research is the logical connection of the theory to the research question and the study design. Nursing literature contains excellent examples of research studies that examine concepts and constructs from grand nursing theories. See Box 4.2 for an example.

Middle Range Nursing Theories

Beginning in the late 1980s, nurses recognized that grand theories were difficult to apply in research, and considerable attention moved to the development and research of "middle range" nursing theories. In contrast to grand theories, **middle range nursing theories** contain a limited number of concepts and are focused on a limited aspect of reality. As a result, they are more easily tested through research and more readily used as frameworks for research studies (McEwen & Wills, 2014).

A growing number of middle range nursing theories have been developed, tested through research, and/or are used as frameworks for nursing research. Examples are Pender's Health Promotion Model (Pender et al., 2015), the Theory of Uncertainty in Illness (Mishel, 1988, 1990, 2014), the Theory of Unpleasant Symptoms (Lenz, Pugh, et al., 1997; Lenz, Gift, et al., 2017), and the Theory of Holistic Comfort (Kolcaba, 1994, 2017).

Examples of development, use, and testing of middle range theories and models are becoming increasingly common in the nursing literature. The comprehensive health-seeking and coping paradigm (Nyamathi, 1989) is one example. Indeed, Nyamathi's model served as the conceptual framework of a recent research study that examined interventions to improve hepatitis A and B vaccine completion among homeless men (Nyamathi et al., 2015) (see Box 4.3 and Appendix A). In this study, the findings were interpreted according to the model. The researchers identified several predictors of vaccine completion and concluded that providers work to recognize factors that promote health-seeking and coping behaviors among high-risk populations.

Situation-Specific Nursing Theories: Microrange, Practice, or Prescriptive Theories

Situation-specific nursing theories are sometimes referred to as microrange, practice, or prescriptive theories. **Situation-specific theories** are more specific than middle range theories and are composed of a limited number of concepts. They are narrow in scope, explain a small aspect of phenomena and processes of interest to nurses, and are usually limited to specific populations or field of practice (Chinn & Kramer, 2015; Im, 2014; Peterson, 2017). Im and Chang (2012) observed that as nursing research began to require theoretical bases

BOX 4.2 Grand Theory Example

Wong and colleagues (2015) used Orem's self-care deficit nursing theory to examine the relationships among several factors such as parental educational levels, pain intensity, and self-medication on self-care behaviors among adolescent girls with dysmenorrhea. The researchers used a correlational study design that surveyed 531 high school–aged girls. Using constructs from Orem's theory, they determined health care providers should design interventions that promote self-care behaviors among adolescents with dysmenorrhea, specifically targeting those who are younger, those who report higher pain intensity, and those who do not routinely self-medicate for menstrual pain.

BOX 4.3 Middle Range Theory Exemplars

An integrative research review was undertaken to evaluate the connection between symptom experience and illness-related uncertainty among patients diagnosed with brain tumors. The Theory of Uncertainty in Illness (Mishel, 1988, 1990, 2014) was the conceptual framework for interpretation of the review's findings. The researchers concluded that somatic symptoms are antecedent to uncertainty among brain tumor patients, and that nursing strategies should attempt to understand and manage symptoms to reduce anxiety and distress by mitigating illness-related uncertainty (Cahill et al., 2012).

Bryer and colleagues (2013) conducted a study of health promotion behaviors of undergraduate nursing students. This study was based on Pender's HPM (Pender et al., 2015). Several variables for the study were operationalized and measured using the Health Promotion Lifestyle Profile II, a survey instrument that was developed to be used in studies that focus on HPM concepts.

HPM, Health Promotion Model.

that are easily operationalized into research, situation-specific theories provided closer links to research and practice. The idea and practice of identifying a work as a situation-specific theory is still fairly new. Often what is noted by an author as a middle range theory would more appropriately be termed situation specific. Most commonly, however, a theory is developed from a research study, and no designation (e.g., middle range, situation specific) is attached to it.

Examples of self-designated, situation-specific theories include the theory of men's healing from childhood maltreatment (Willis et al., 2015) and a situation-specific theory of health-related quality of life among Koreans with type 2 diabetes (Chang & Im, 2014). Increasingly, qualitative studies are being used by nurses to develop and support theories and models that can and should be expressly identified as situation specific. This will become progressively more common as more nurses seek graduate study and are involved in research, and increasing attention is given to the importance of evidence-based practice (Im & Chang, 2012; McEwen & Wills, 2014).

Im and Chang (2012) conducted a comprehensive research review that examined how theory has been described in nursing literature for the last decade. They reported a dramatic increase in the number of grounded theory research studies, along with increases in studies using both middle range and situation-specific theories. In contrast, the number and percentage directly dealing with grand nursing theories have fluctuated. Table 4.3 provides examples of grand, middle range, and situation-specific nursing theories used in nursing research.

HOW THEORY IS USED IN NURSING RESEARCH

Nursing research is concerned with the study of individuals in interaction with their environments. The intent is to discover interventions that promote optimal functioning and self-care across the life span; the goal is to foster maximum wellness (McEwen & Wills, 2014). In nursing research, theories are used in the research process in one of three ways:

- Theory is generated as the outcome of a research study (qualitative designs).
- Theory is used as a research framework, as the context for a study (qualitative or quantitative designs).
- Research is undertaken to test a theory (quantitative designs).

TABLE 4.3 Levels of Nursing Theory: Examples of Grand, Middle Range, and Situation-Specific Nursing Theories

Grand Nursing Theories	Middle Range Nursing Theories	Situation-Specific (or Micro) Nursing Theories
Florence Nightingale: Notes on Nursing (1860)	Health promotion model (Pender et al., 2015)	Theory of the peaceful end of life (Ruland & Moore, 1998)
Dorothy Johnson: The Behavioral Systems Model for Nursing (1990)	Uncertainty in illness theory (Mishel, 1988, 1990, 2014)	Theory of chronic sorrow (Eakes, 2017; Eakes et al., 1998)
Martha Rogers: Nursing: A Science of Unitary Human Beings (1970, 1990)	Theory of unpleasant symptoms (Lenz, Gift, et al., 2017)	Asian immigrant women's menopausal symptom experience in the United States (Im, 2012)
Betty Neuman: The Neuman Systems Model (2009)	Theory of holistic comfort/theory of comfort (Kolcaba, 1994, 2017)	Theory of Caucasians' cancer pain experience (Im, 2006)
Dorthea Orem: The Self Care Deficit Nursing Theory (2001)	Theory of resilience (Polk, 1997)	Becoming a mother (Mercer, 2004)
Callista Roy: Roy Adaptation Model (2009)	Theory of health promotion in preterm infants (Mefford, 2004)	
	Theory of flight nursing expertise (Reimer & Moore, 2010)	

Theory-Generating Nursing Research

When research is undertaken to create or generate theory, the idea is to examine a phenomenon within a particular context and identify and describe its major elements or events. Theory-generating research is focused on "What" and "How," but does not usually attempt to explain "Why." Theory-generating research is **inductive**; that is, it uses a process in which generalizations are developed from specific observations. Research methods used by nurses for theory generation include concept analysis, case studies, phenomenology, grounded theory, ethnography, and historical inquiry. Chapters 5, 6, and 7 describe these research methods. As you review qualitative methods and study examples in the literature, be attuned to the stated purpose(s) or outcomes of the research and note whether a situation-specific (practice or micro) theory or model or middle range theory is presented as a finding or outcome.

Theory as Framework for Nursing Research

In nursing research, theory is most commonly used as the conceptual framework, theoretical framework, or conceptual model for a study. Frequently, correlational research designs attempt to discover and specify relationships between characteristics of individuals, groups, situations, or events. Correlational research studies often focus on one or more concepts, frameworks, or theories to collect data to measure dimensions or characteristics of phenomena and explain why and the extent to which one phenomenon is related to another. Data is typically gathered by observation or self-report instruments (see Chapter 10 for nonexperimental designs).

HELPFUL HINT

When researchers use conceptual frameworks to guide their studies, you can expect to find a system of ideas synthesized for the purpose of organizing, thinking, and providing study direction. Whether the researcher is using a conceptual or a theoretical framework, conceptual and then operational definitions will emerge from the framework.

Often in correlational (nonexperimental/quantitative) research, one or more theories will be used as the conceptual/theoretical framework for the study. In these cases, a theory is used as the context for the study and basis for interpretation of the findings. The theory helps guide the study and enhances the value of its findings by setting the findings within the context of the theory and previous works, describing use of the theory in practice or research. When using a theory as a conceptual framework for research, the researcher will:

- Identify an existing theory (or theories) and designate and explain the study's theoretical framework.
- Develop research questions/hypotheses consistent with the framework.
- Provide conceptual definitions taken from the theory/framework.
- Use data collection instrument(s) (and operational definitions) appropriate to the framework.
- Interpret/explain findings based on the framework.
- Determine support for the theory/framework based on the study findings.
- Discuss implications for nursing and recommendations for future research to address the concepts and relationships designated by the framework.

Theory-Testing Nursing Research

Finally, nurses may use research to test a theory. Theory testing is **deductive**—that is, hypotheses are derived from theory and tested, employing experimental research methods. In experimental research, the intent is to move beyond explanation to prediction of relationships between characteristics or phenomena among different groups or in various situations. Experimental research designs require manipulation of one or more phenomena to determine how the manipulation affects or changes the dimension or characteristics of other phenomena. In these cases, theoretical statements are written as research questions or hypotheses. Experimental research requires quantifiable data, and statistical analyses are used to measure differences (see Chapter 9).

In theory-testing research, the researcher (1) chooses a theory of interest and selects a propositional statement to be examined; (2) develops hypotheses that have measurable variables; (3) conducts the study; (4) interprets the findings considering the predictive ability of the theory; and (5) determines if there are implications for further use of the theory in nursing practice and/or whether further research could be beneficial.

QSEN EVIDENCE-BASED PRACTICE TIP

In practice, you can use observation and analysis to consider the nuances of situations that matter to patient health. This process often generates questions that are cogent for improving patient care. In turn, following the observations and questions into the literature can lead to published research that can be applied in practice.

IPE HIGHLIGHT

When an interprofessional QI team launches a QI project to develop evidence-based behavior change self-management strategies for a targeted patient population, it may be helpful to think about the Transtheoretical Model of Change and health self-efficacy as an appropriate theoretical framework to guide the project.

APPLICATION TO RESEARCH AND EVIDENCE-BASED PRACTICE

To build knowledge that promotes evidence-based practice, research should develop within a theoretical structure that facilitates analysis and interpretation of findings. When a study is placed within a theoretical context, the theory guides the research process, forms the questions, and aids in design, analysis, and interpretation. In that regard, a theory, conceptual model, or conceptual framework provides parameters for the research and enables the researcher to weave the facts together.

As a consumer of research, you should know how to recognize the theoretical foundation of a study. Whether evaluating a qualitative or a quantitative study, it is essential to understand where and how the research can be integrated within nursing science and applied in evidence-based practice. As a result, it is important to identify whether the intent is to (1) generate a theory, (2) use the theory as the framework that guides the study, or (3) test a theory. This section provides examples that illustrate different types of theory used in nursing research (e.g., non-nursing theories, middle range nursing theories) and examples from the literature highlighting the different ways that nurses can use theory in research (e.g., theory-generating study, theory testing, theory as a conceptual framework).

Application of Theory in Qualitative Research

As discussed, in many instances, a theory, framework, or model is the outcome of nursing research. This is often the case in research employing qualitative methods such as grounded theory. From the study's findings, the researcher builds either an implicit or an explicit structure explaining or describing the findings of the research.

Example: ➤ van Dijk and colleagues (2016) (see Appendix C) reported findings from a study examining how postoperative patients rated their pain experiences. The researchers were interested in understanding potential differences in how postoperative patients interpret numeric pain rating scales. Using a qualitative approach to data collection, the team interviewed 27 patients 1 day after surgery. They discovered three themes (score-related factors, intrapersonal factors, and anticipated consequences of a pain score). The result of the research was a model that may be used by health providers to understand the factors that influence how pain scales may be interpreted by patients. Appropriate questions for calcification were also suggested.

Generally, when the researcher is using qualitative methods and inductive reasoning, you will find the framework or theory at the end of the manuscript in the discussion section (see Chapters 5 to 7). You should be aware that the framework may be implicitly suggested rather than explicitly diagrammed (Box 4.4).

The nursing literature is full of similar examples in which inductive, qualitative research methods were used to develop theory. **Example:** ➤ A team headed by Oneal and colleagues (2015) used grounded theory methods to conduct interviews with 10 low-income families who were involved in a program to reduce environmental risks to their children. Their findings were developed into the "theory of re-forming the risk message," which can be used by designing nursing interventions to reduce environmental risk. It was concluded that nurses working with low-income families should seek to discover how risk messages are heard and interpreted and develop interventions accordingly. Finally, a team led by Taplay and colleagues (2015) used grounded theory methods to develop a model to describe the process of adopting and incorporating simulation into nursing education. The

BOX 4.4 Research

Martz (2015) used grounded theory research methods to examine actions taken by hospice nurses to alleviate the feelings of guilt often experienced by caregivers. In this study, 16 hospice providers (most were nurses) were interviewed to identify interventions they used to reduce feelings of guilt among family caregivers during the transition from caring for their loved one at home to enlisting their loved one in an assisted living facility. The hospice nurses explained that the family caregivers worked through a five-stage process in their guilt experiences, moving from "feeling guilty" to "resolving their guilt" during the transition period. The actions of the hospice nurses varied based on the stage of the family caregiver's feelings of guilt. These actions included supporting, managing, navigating, negotiating, encouraging, monitoring, and coaching. A situation-specific model was proposed to explain the relationships among these processes and suggesting congruent hospice nursing interventions.

researchers interviewed 27 nursing faculty members from several schools to learn about their experiences incorporating simulation activities into their nursing programs. From the interviews, the researchers identified a seven-phase process of simulation adoption: securing resources, leaders working in tandem, "getting it out of the box," learning about simulation and its potential, trialing the equipment, finding a fit, and integrating simulation into the curriculum.

Examples of Theory as Research Framework

When the researcher uses quantitative methods, the framework is typically identified and explained at the beginning of the paper, before the discussion of study methods. **Example:** ➤ In their study examining the relationships among spirituality, coping strategies, grief, and mental health in bereaved parents, Hawthorne and colleagues (2016) (see Appendix B) indicated that their "conceptual framework" was derived from a Theory of Bereavement developed by Hogan and colleagues (1996). Specifically, Hawthorne's team used tools developed to measure variables from the Theory of Bereavement. In addition to grief, their research examined spiritual coping, mental health, and personal growth—all variables implicit or explicit in the bereavement theory. Their conclusions were interpreted with respect to the theory, suggesting that nurses and other health care providers promote coping strategies, including religious and spiritual activities, as these appear to be helpful for mental health and personal growth in many bereaved parents.

In another example, one of the works read by Emily from the case study dealt with resilience in adolescents (Tusaie et al., 2007). The researchers in this work used Lazarus and Folkman's (1984) theory of stress and coping as part of the theoretical framework, researching factors such as optimism, family support, age, and life events.

Examples of Theory-Testing Research

Although many nursing studies that are experimental and quasi-experimental (see Chapter 9) are frequently conducted to test interventions, examples of research expressly conducted to test a theory are relatively rare in nursing literature. One such work is a multisite, multimethods study examining women's perceptions of cesarean birth (Fawcett et al., 2012). This work tested multiple relationships within the Roy Adaptation Model as applied to the study population.

CRITICAL APPRAISAL CRITERIA

Critiquing Theoretical Framework

1. Is the framework for research clearly identified?
2. Is the framework consistent with a nursing perspective?
3. Is the framework appropriate to guide research on the subject of interest?
4. Are the concepts and variables clearly and appropriately defined?
5. Was sufficient literature presented to support study of the selected concepts?
6. Is there a logical, consistent link between the framework, the concepts being studied, and the methods of measurement?
7. Are the study findings examined in relationship to the framework?

Critiquing the Use of Theory in Nursing Research

It is beneficial to seek out, identify, and follow the theoretical framework or source of the background of a study. The framework for research provides guidance for the researcher as study questions are fine-tuned, methods for measuring variables are selected, and analyses are planned. Once data are collected and analyzed, the framework is used as a base of comparison. Ideally, the research should explain: Did the findings coincide with the framework? Did the findings support or refute findings of other researchers who used the framework? If there were discrepancies, is there a way to explain them using the framework? The reader of research needs to know how to critically appraise a framework for research (see the Critical Appraisal Criteria box).

The first question posed is whether a framework is presented. Sometimes a structure may be guiding the research, but a diagrammed model is not included in the manuscript. You must then look for the theoretical framework in the narrative description of the study concepts. When the framework is identified, it is important to consider its relevance for nursing. The framework does not have to be one created by a nurse, but the importance of its content for nursing should be clear. The question of how the framework depicts a structure congruent with nursing should be addressed. For instance, although the Lazarus Transaction Model of Stress and Coping was not created by a nurse, it is clearly related to nursing practice when working with people facing stress. Sometimes frameworks from different disciplines, such as physics or art, may be relevant. It is the responsibility of the author to clearly articulate the meaning of the framework for the study and to link the framework to nursing.

Once the meaning and applicability of the theory (if the objective of the research was theory development) or the theoretical framework to nursing are articulated, you will be able to determine whether the framework is appropriate to guide the research. As you critically appraise a study, you would identify a mismatch, for example, in which a researcher presents a study of students' responses to the stress of being in the clinical setting for the first time within a framework of stress related to recovery from chronic illness. You should look closely at the framework to determine if it is "on target" and the "best fit" for the research question and proposed study design.

Next, the reader should focus on the concepts being studied. Does the researcher clearly describe and explain concepts that are being studied and how they are defined and translated into measurable variables? Is there literature to support the choice of concepts? Concepts should clearly reflect the area of study. **Example:** ➤ Using the concept of "anger," when "incivility" or "hostility" is more appropriate to the research focus creates difficulties in defining variables and determining methods of measurement. These issues have to do with the logical consistency among the framework, the concepts being studied, and the methods of measurement.

Throughout the entire critiquing process, from worldview to operational definitions, the reader is evaluating the fit. Finally, the reader will expect to find a discussion of the findings as they relate to the theory or framework. This final point enables evaluation of the framework for use in further research. It may suggest necessary changes to enhance the relevance of the framework for continuing study, and thus serves to let others know where one will go from here.

Evaluating frameworks for research requires skills that must be acquired through repeated critique and discussion with others who have critiqued the same work. As with other abilities and skills, you must practice and use the skills to develop them further. With continuing education and a broader knowledge of potential frameworks, you will build a repertoire of knowledge to assess the foundation of a research study and the framework for research, and/or to evaluate findings where theory was generated as the outcome of the study.

KEY POINTS

- The interaction among theory, practice, and research is central to knowledge development in the discipline of nursing.
- The use of a framework for research is important as a guide to systematically identify concepts and to link appropriate study variables with each concept.
- Conceptual and operational definitions are critical to the evolution of a study.
- In developing or selecting a framework for research, knowledge may be acquired from other disciplines or directly from nursing. In either case, that knowledge is used to answer specific nursing questions.
- Theory is distinguished by its scope. Grand theories are broadest in scope and situation-specific theories are the narrowest in scope and at the lowest level of abstraction; middle range theories are in the middle.
- In critiquing a framework for research, it is important to examine the logical, consistent link among the framework, the concepts for study, and the methods of measurement.

CRITICAL THINKING CHALLENGES

- Search recent issues of a prominent nursing journal (e.g., *Nursing Research*, *Research in Nursing & Health*) for notations of conceptual frameworks of published studies. How many explicitly discussed the theoretical framework? How many did not mention any theoretical framework? What kinds of theories were mentioned (e.g., grand nursing theories, middle range nursing theories, non-nursing theories)? How many studies were theory generating? How many were theory testing?
- Identify a non-nursing theory that you would like to know more about. How could you find out information on its applicability to nursing research and nursing practice? How could you identify whether and how it has been used in nursing research?
- Select a nursing theory, concept, or phenomenon (e.g., resilience from the case study) that you are interested in and would like to know more about and consider: How could

you find studies that have used that theory in research and practice? How could you locate published instruments and tools that reportedly measure concepts and constructs of the theory?

- IPE You have just joined an interprofessional primary care QI Team focused on developing evidence-based self-management strategies to decrease hospital admissions for the practice's heart failure patients. Which theoretical framework could be used to guide your project?

REFERENCES

Ahern, N. R. (2006). Adolescent resilience: An evolutionary concept analysis. *Journal of Pediatric Nursing, 21*(3), 175–185.

Ahern, N. R., Ark, P., & Byers, J. (2008). Resilience and coping strategies in adolescents. *Pediatric Nursing, 20*(10), 32–36.

Bryer, J., Cherkis, F., & Raman, J. (2013). Health-promotion behaviors of undergraduate nursing students: A survey analysis. *Nursing Education Perspectives, 34*(6), 410–415.

Cahill, J., LoBiondo-Wood, G., Bergstrom, N., et al. (2012). Brain tumor symptoms as antecedents to uncertainty: An integrative review. *Journal of Nursing Scholarship, 44*(2), 145–155.

Chang, S. J., & Im, E. (2014). Development of a situation-specific theory for explaining health-related quality of life among older South Korean adults with type 2 diabetes. *Research and Theory for Nursing Practice: An International Journal, 28*(2), 113–126.

Chen, C. M., Chen, Y. C., & Wong, T. T. (2014). Comparison of resilience in adolescent survivors of brain tumors and health adolescents. *Cancer Nursing, 37*(5), 373–381.

Chinn, P. L., & Kramer, M. K. (2015). *Integrated theory and knowledge development in nursing* (9th ed.). St. Louis, MO: Elsevier.

Eakes, G. (2017). Chronic sorrow. In S. J. Peterson & T. S. Bredow (Eds.), *Middle range theories: Application to nursing research* (4th ed.). Philadelphia, PA: Wolters Kluwer.

Eakes, G., Burke, M. L., & Hainsworth, M. A. (1998). Middle rang theory of chronic sorrow. *Image: Journal of Nursing Scholarship, 30*(2), 179–185.

Fawcett, J., Abner, C., Haussler, S., et al. (2012). Women's perceptions of caesarean birth: A Roy international study. *Nursing Science Quarterly, 24*(40), 352–362.

Hawthorne, D. M., Youngblut, J. M., & Brooten, D. (2016). Parent spirituality, grief and mental health at 1 and 3 months after their infant's child's death in an intensive care unit. *Journal of Pediatric Nursing, 31*(1), 73–80.

Hogan, N. S., Morse, J. M., & Tason, M. C. (1996). Toward an experiential theory of bereavement. *Omega: Journal of Death and Dying, 33*, 43–65.

Im, E. (2006). A situation-specific theory of Caucasian cancer patients' pain experience. *Advances in Nursing Science, 28*(2), 137–151.

Im, E. (2014). The status quo of situation-specific theories. *Research and Theory for Nursing Practice: An International Journal, 28*(4), 278–298.

Im, E., & Chang, S. J. (2012). Current trends in nursing theories. *Journal of Nursing Scholarship, 44*(2), 156–164.

Ishibashi, A., Okamura, J., Ueda, R., et al. (2016). Psychological strength enhancing resilience in adolescents and young adults with cancer. *Journal of Pediatric Oncology Nursing, 33*(1), 45–54.

Johnson, D. E. (1990). The behavioral system model for nursing. In M. E. Parker (Ed.), *Nursing theories in practice* (pp. 23–32). New York, NY: National League for Nursing Press.

Kolcaba, K. Y. (1994). A theory of holistic comfort for nursing. *Journal of Advanced Nursing, 19*(6), 1178–1184.

Kolcaba, K. Y. (2017). Comfort. In S. J. Peterson & T. S. Bredow (Eds.), *Middle range theories: Application to nursing research* (4th ed., pp. 254–272). Philadelphia, PA: Wolters Kluwer.

Lazarus, R. S., & Folkman, S. (1984). *Stress, appraisal and coping*. New York, NY: Springer.
Lenz, E. R., Gift, A., Pugh, L. C. & Milligan, R.A. (2017). Unpleasant symptoms. In S. J. Peterson & T. S. Bredow (Eds.), *Middle range theories: Application to nursing research* (4th ed.). Philadelphia, PA: Wolters Kluwer.
Lenz, E. R., Pugh, L. C., Miligan, R. A., et al. (1997). The middle range theory of unpleasant symptoms: An update. *Advances in Nursing Science, 19*(3), 14–27.
Martz, K. (2015). Actions of hospice nurses to alleviate guilt in family caregiver during residential care transitions. *Journal of Hospice and Palliative Nursing, 17*(1), 48–55.
McEwen, M., & Wills, E. (2014). *Theoretical basis for nursing* (4th ed.). Philadelphia, PA: Lippincott.
Mefford, L. C. (2004). A theory of health promotion for preterm infants based on Levine's conservation model of nursing. *Nursing Science Quarterly, 17*(3), 260–266.
Mercer, R. T. (2004). Becoming a mother versus maternal role attainment. *Journal of Nursing Scholarship, 36*(3), 226–232.
Mishel, M. H. (1988). Uncertainty in illness. *Journal of Nursing Scholarship, 20*(4), 225–232.
Mishel, M. H. (1990). Reconceptualization of the uncertainty in illness theory. *Image: Journal of Nursing Scholarship, 22*(4), 256–262.
Mishel, M. H. (2014). Theories of uncertainty in illness. In M. J. Smith & P. R. Liehr (Eds.), *Middle range theory for nursing* (3rd ed., pp. 53–86). New York, NY: Springer Publishing Co.
Neuman, B., & Fawcett, J. (2009). *The Neuman systems model* (5th ed.). Upper Saddle River, NJ: Pearson Education.
Nightingale, F. (1969). *Notes on nursing: What it is and what it is not*. New York, NY: Dover Publications (Original work published 1860).
Nyamathi, A. (1989). Comprehensive health seeking and coping paradigm. *Journal of Advanced Nursing, 14*(4), 281–290.
Nyamathi, A., Salem, B. E., Zhang, S., et al. (2015). Nursing case management, peer coaching, and hepatitis A and B vaccine completion among homeless men recently released on parole. *Nursing Research, 64*(3), 177–189.
Oneal, G. A., Eide, P., Hamilton, R., et al. (2015). Rural families' process of re-forming environmental health risk messages. *Journal of Nursing Scholarship, 47*(4), 354–362.
Orem, D. E. (2001). *Nursing: Concepts of practice* (6th ed.). St Louis, MO: Mosby.
Pender, N. J., Murdaugh, C., & Parsons, M. (2015). *Health promotion in nursing practice* (7th ed.). Upper Saddle River, NJ: Pearson Education.
Peterson, S. J. (2017). Introduction to the nature of nursing knowledge. In S. J. Peterson & T. S. Bredow (Eds.), *Middle range theories: Application to nursing research* (4th ed., pp. 3–41). Philadelphia, PA: Wolters Kluwer.
Polk, L. V. (1997). Toward a middle range theory of resilience. *Advances in Nursing Science, 19*(3), 1–13.
Reimer, A. P., & Moore, S. M. (2010). Flight nursing expertise: towards a middle-range theory. *Journal of Advanced Nursing, 66*(5), 1183–1192.
Rogers, M. E. (1970). *An introduction to the theoretical basis of nursing*. Philadelphia, PA: Davis.
Rogers, M. E. (1990). Nursing: the science of unitary, irreducible, human beings: Update: 1990. In E. A. M. Barrett (Ed.), *Visions of Rogers' science-based nursing* (pp. 5–11). New York, NY: National League for Nursing Press.
Roy, C. (2009). *The Roy adaptation model* (3rd ed.). Upper Saddle River, NJ: Pearson.
Ruland, C. M., & Moore, S. M. (1998). Theory construction based on standards of care: A proposed theory of the peaceful end of life. *Nursing Outlook, 46*(4), 169–175.
Taplay, K., Jack, S. M., Baxter, P., et al. (2015). The process of adopting and incorporating simulation into undergraduate nursing curricula: A grounded theory study. *Journal of Professional Nursing, 31*(1), 26–36.
Turner-Sack, A. M., Menna, R., Setchell, S. R., et al. (2016). Psychological functioning, post-traumatic growth and coping in parents and sibling of adolescent cancer survivors. *Oncology Nursing Forum, 43*(10), 48–56.

Tusaie, K., Puskar, K., & Sereika, S. M. (2007). A predictive and moderating model of psychosocial resilience in adolescents. *Journal of Nursing Scholarship*, *39*(1), 54–60.

van Dijk, J. F. M., Vervoort, S. C. J. M., van Wijck, A. J. M., et al. (2016). Postoperative patients' perspectives on rating pain: A qualitative study. *International Journal of Nursing Studies*, *53*, 260–269.

Willis, D. G., DeSanto-Madeya, S., & Fawcett, J. (2015). Moving beyond dwelling in suffering: A situation-specific theory of men's healing form childhood maltreatment. *Nursing Science Quarterly*, *28*(1), 57–63.

Wong, C. L., Ip, W. Y., Choi, K. C., & Lam, L.W. (2015). Examining self-care behaviors and their associated factors among adolescent girls with dysmenorrhea: An application of Orem's Self-care Deficit Nursing Theory. *Journal of Nursing Scholarship*, *47*(3), 219–227.

Wu, W. W., Tsai, S. Y., Liang, S. Y., et al. (2015). The mediating role of resilience on quality of life and cancer symptom distress in adolescent patients with cancer. *Journal of Pediatric Oncology Nursing*, *32*(5), 304–313.

Go to Evolve at **http://evolve.elsevier.com/LoBiondo/** for review questions, critiquing exercises, and additional research articles for practice in reviewing and critiquing.

PART II

Processes and Evidence Related to Qualitative Research

Research Vignette: Gail D'Eramo Melkus

RESEARCH VIGNETTE

TYPE 2 DIABETES: JOURNEY FROM DESCRIPTION TO BIOBEHAVIORAL INTERVENTION

Gail D'Eramo Melkus, EdD, ANP, FAAN
Florence and William Downs Professor in Nursing Research
Director, Muriel and Virginia Pless Center for Nursing Research
Associate Dean for Research
New York University Rory Meyers College of Nursing

My nursing career began at a time when there was an emphasis on health promotion, disease prevention, and active participation of patients and families in health care decision making and interactions. This emphasis was consistent with an ever-increasing incidence and prevalence of chronic conditions, particularly diabetes and cardiovascular disease. It became apparent in time through epidemiological studies that certain populations had a disproportionate burden of these chronic conditions that resulted in premature morbidity and mortality. It also became apparent that the health care workforce was not prepared to deal with the changing paradigm of chronic disease management that necessitated active patient involvement. Thus I came to understand the best way to enhance diabetes care for all persons was to improve clinical practice through research and professional education.

Diabetes is a prevalent chronic illness affecting approximately 29 million individuals in the United States and 485 million globally. Thus the dissemination and translation of research findings to clinical practice is necessary to decrease the personal and economic burden of disease. In order to contribute to the improvement of diabetes care and outcomes, my role as a direct care provider extended to and encompassed clinical research and education and served as a model for my mentees. My integrated scholarship addresses the quality and effectiveness of diabetes behavioral interventions and care in the context of the patient and culture, primary care, and professional practice while also serving as a training ground for clinical practice and clinical research. This work has extended to collaborations with colleagues nationally and internationally. My research collectively demonstrated the beneficial effects of behavioral self-management interventions combined with diabetes care in primary care.

My program of research has contributed to the body of literature that has demonstrated the effectiveness of behavioral interventions in improving metabolic control (hemoglobin A1c [HbA1c], BP, lipids, and weight) and diabetes-related emotional distress. One of my early studies tested a comprehensive intervention for obese men and women with type 2 diabetes that demonstrated efficacy in significantly improving diabetes control and weight loss compared to a control group that received a customary intervention of diabetes patient education (D'Eramo-Melkus et al., 1992). Post-hoc analysis of study participants with equal weight loss yet disparate HbA1c levels revealed that persons with elevated HbA1c levels had decreased insulin secretion capacity that was associated with a 10 years or greater duration of type 2 diabetes. This study contributed to clinical practice recommendations that called for assessment of insulin secretion capacity to direct therapeutic interventions such that persons with low insulin secretory reserve should be started on insulin rather than continued weight loss intervention alone. It became apparent during the implementation of the intervention study that the majority of participants received diabetes care in primary care settings where diabetes care and self-management resources were scarce or nonexistent. In an effort to better understand the delivery of diabetes care within primary care settings so that we could best develop effective patient centered interventions, my research turned to assessing nurse practitioner (NP) and physician diabetes care practice patterns in a large urban primary care center. This study showed that both primary NPs and physicians were not providing diabetes care according to the American Diabetes Association clinical care guidelines. In fact, screening for diabetes complications occurred in fewer than 50% of cases, and NPs performed foot exams less often than physicians (Fain & D'Eramo-Melkus, 1994). These findings along with other studies that found similar results provided an impetus to develop and implement a model program of advanced practice nursing education and subspecialty training in diabetes care (D'Eramo-Melkus & Fain, 1995). Graduates of this program (over 300 to date) have assumed leadership roles in facilitating diabetes care in generalist and specialty settings throughout the United States, Canada, and various international sites. During this education and training program, many of the students participated in my program of research and contributed to a growing body of literature on diabetes care.

Epidemiological studies in the early 1990s showed that increasingly ethnic minorities suffered a disproportionate burden of type 2 diabetes and related complications. In particular, black women had and continue to have the highest rate of disease and diabetes-related complications, with the poorest health outcomes, and a 40% greater mortality compared to black men and white men and women. Therefore my program of research came to focus on this group, beginning with descriptive studies that described the context of type 2 diabetes for black women. The first study of a small convenience sample of volunteers from an urban center revealed a group of midlife black women, the majority of whom were employed and customary utilizers of primary care. Despite their poor glycemic control (average HbA1c 12.8%), only 68% received diabetes medications, and less than 50% of the time were they screened for diabetes complications. In order to better understand factors contributing to such findings, we conducted focus groups to elicit information on diabetes beliefs and practices of black women with type 2 diabetes. Key themes that emerged were a need for diabetes education and health care provider rapport, importance of culturally appropriate diabetes education materials, and the importance of family support (Maillet et al., 1996; Melkus et al., 2002).

Based on an informant survey and focus group data, using social learning theory and cognitive behavioral methods that incorporated the context of culture for black women with type 2 diabetes and input from a community advisory board, we developed and tested a culturally relevant intervention of group diabetes self-management education and skills training (DSME/T), along with nurse practitioner care. This intervention was first tested for feasibility using a one group repeated measures pretest, posttest design that demonstrated participant acceptability based on high rates of attendance at both group sessions and NP care visits, and feasibility of methods based on formative and summative process and fidelity measures. Further glycemic control was significantly improved baseline to 3 months and maintained at 6 months ($p = .008$), and the psychosocial outcome of diabetes-related emotional distress was also greatly reduced ($p = .06$) (Melkus et al., 2004). Given these promising results, we went on to test the efficacy of the DSME/T intervention using a two-group repeated measures design with a comparison group (control) that received customary group diabetes education; time and attention were controlled for in both groups. The primary outcome of glycemic control as measured by HbA1c was significantly improved from baseline to 3 and 6 months ($p = .01$, $F = 6.15$). The gold standard for glycemic control is HbA1c. HbA1c, when maintained in a normal range (≥7.0%), has been shown to prevent or slow the progression of diabetes-related complications (The Diabetes Control and Complications Trial Research Group, 1993).

One of the salient findings in all of the work-up to this point was that the women reported high levels of diabetes-related emotional distress, given the demands of diabetes self-management and complex lives that often included multigenerational family caregiving and work. The majority were grandmothers responsible for some extent of child care, which for many negatively affected their diabetes control (Balukonis et al., 2008). Recognizing the need to address this concern, we added a coping skills training component that followed DSME/T when we conducted a prospective randomized clinical trial (RCT) to test intervention effectiveness. The control/comparison group received a customary diabetes education program followed by drop-in question and answer sessions equivalent in time so to control for a potential attention effect. The experimental ($n = 52$) and control group ($n = 57$) participants were in active intervention for 12 months, consisting of assigned group sessions and monthly NP visits for the first 2 months and quarterly thereafter; they were followed for a total of 24 months. As with any prospective behavioral intervention, trial attrition occurred resulting in a sample of 77 study completers. An intention to treat analysis that included all participants as randomly assigned showed that the primary outcome of HbA1c was significantly improved over time for both groups ($p < .0001$) up to 12 months, after which time control group levels showed an increase from 12 to 24 months while the intervention group remained stable (Melkus et al., 2010). This finding demonstrates the importance of active intervention that includes numerous contacts and feedback in order to facilitate optimal diabetes self-management and glycemic control. When data of completers ($n = 77$) were analyzed, the same significant finding resulted over time for HbA1c at 12 and 24 months. Low-density and high-density lipoprotein cholesterol levels also significantly improved over time for both groups. Quality of life (MOS-36) vitality domain, social support, and diabetes-related emotional distress were all significantly changed in the intervention group at 24 months compared to the control group. The results showed that we reached the intended target group of black women with suboptimal glycemic control, cardiovascular risk factors, poor quality of life, and high levels of emotional distress, in need of social support. Moreover, it is important to note that both groups received intervention beyond standard "real world" primary care. Thus patients with type 2 diabetes cared for in primary care settings when given the opportunity to participate in DSME/T may improve in both physiological and psychosocial outcomes. Further evidence is needed to promote the need for chronic disease self-management programs and psychosocial care beyond the medical visit that focuses on physiological parameters and prescribing of therapeutic regimens.

REFERENCES

Balukonis, J., Melkus, G. D., & Chyun, D. (2008). Grandparenthood status and health outcomes in midlife African American women with type 2 diabetes. *Ethnicity and Disease*, *18*(2), 141–146.

D'Eramo Melkus, G., & Fain, J. A. (1995). Diabetes care concentration: a program of study for advanced practice nurses. *Clinical Nurse Specialist*, *9*(6), 313–316.

D'Eramo-Melkus, G., Wylie-Rosett, J., & Hagan, J. (1992). Metabolic impact of education on NIDDM. *Diabetes Care, 15*(7), 864–869.

The Diabetes Control and Complications Trial Research Group. (1993). The effect of intensive treatment of diabetes on the development and progression of long-term complications in insulin-dependent diabetes mellitus. *New England Journal of Medicine, 329*, 977–986.

Fain, J. A., & D'Eramo-Melkus, G. (1994). Nurse practitioner practice patterns based on standards of medical care for patients with diabetes. *Diabetes Care, 17*(8), 879–881.

Maillet, N. A., D'Eramo Melkus, G., & Spollett, G. (1996). Using focus groups to characterize beliefs and practices of African American women with NIDDM. *The Diabetes Educator, 22*(1), 39–45.

Melkus, G. D., Chyun, D., Newlin, K., et al. (2010). Effectiveness of a diabetes self-management intervention on physiological and psychosocial outcomes. *Biological Research in Nursing, 12*(1), 7–19.

Melkus, G. D., Maillet, N., Novak, J., et al. (2002). Primary care cancer screening and diabetes complications screening for black women with type 2 diabetes. *Journal of the American Academy of Nurse Practitioners, 4*(1), 43–48.

Melkus, G. D., Spollett, G., Jefferson, V., et al. (2004). Feasibility testing of a culturally competent intervention of education and care for black women with type 2 diabetes. *Applied Nursing Research, 17*(1), 10–20.

5

Introduction to Qualitative Research

Mark Toles and Julie Barroso

Go to Evolve at **http://evolve.elsevier.com/LoBiondo/** for review questions, critiquing exercises, and additional research articles for practice in reviewing and critiquing.

LEARNING OUTCOMES

After reading this chapter, the student should be able to do the following:

- Describe the components of a qualitative research report.
- Describe the beliefs generally held by qualitative researchers.
- Identify four ways qualitative findings can be used in evidence-based practice.

KEY TERMS

context dependent
data saturation
grand tour question
inclusion and exclusion criteria
inductive
naturalistic setting
paradigm
qualitative research
theme

Let's say that you are reading an article that reports findings that HIV-infected men are more adherent to their antiretroviral regimens than HIV-infected women. You wonder, "Why is that? Why would women be less adherent in taking their medications? Certainly, it is not solely due to the fact that they are women." Or say you are working in a postpartum unit and have just discharged a new mother who has debilitating rheumatoid arthritis. You wonder, "What is the process by which disabled women decide to have children? How do they go about making that decision?" These, like so many other questions we have as nurses, can be best answered through research conducted using qualitative methods. Qualitative research gives us the answers to those difficult "why?" questions. Although qualitative research can be used at many different places in a program of research, you will most often find it answering questions that we have when we understand very little about some phenomenon in nursing.

WHAT IS QUALITATIVE RESEARCH?

Qualitative research is a broad term that encompasses several different methodologies that share many similarities. Qualitative studies help us formulate an understanding of a phenomenon. Nurse scholars who are trained in qualitative methods use these methods to best answer discovery-oriented research questions.

Qualitative research is explanatory, descriptive, and **inductive** in nature. It uses words, as opposed to numbers, to explain a phenomenon. Qualitative research lets us see the world through the eyes of another—the woman who struggles to take her antiretroviral medication, or the woman who has carefully thought through what it might be like to have a baby despite a debilitating illness. Qualitative researchers assume that we can only understand these things if we consider the context in which they take place, and this is why most qualitative research takes place in naturalistic settings. Qualitative studies make the world of an individual visible to the rest of us. Qualitative research involves an "interpretative, naturalistic approach to the world; meaning that qualitative researchers study things in their natural settings, attempting to make sense of or interpret phenomena in terms of the meaning people bring to them" (Denzin & Lincoln, 2011, p. 3).

WHAT DO QUALITATIVE RESEARCHERS BELIEVE?

Qualitative researchers believe that there are multiple realities that can be understood by carefully studying what people can tell us or what we can observe as we spend time with them. **Example:** ➤ The experience of having a baby, while it has some shared characteristics, is not the same for any two women, and it is definitely different for a disabled mother. Thus qualitative researchers believe that reality is socially constructed and **context dependent**. Even the experience of reading this book is different for any two students; one may be completely engrossed by the content, while another is reading but at the same time worrying about whether or not her financial aid will be approved soon.

Because qualitative researchers believe that the discovery of meaning is the basis for knowledge, their research questions, approaches, and activities are often quite different from quantitative researchers (see the Critical Thinking Decision Path). Qualitative researchers seek to understand the "lived experience" of the research participants. They might use interviews or observations to gather new data, and use new data to create narratives about research phenomena. Thus qualitative researchers know that there is a very strong imperative to clearly describe the phenomenon under study. Ideally, the reader of a qualitative research report, if even slightly acquainted with the phenomenon, would have an "aha!" moment in reading a well-written qualitative report.

So, you may now be saying, "Wow! This sounds great! Qualitative research is for me!" Many nurses feel very comfortable with this approach because we are educated with regard to how to speak with people about the health issues concerning them; we are used to listening, and listening well. But the most important consideration for any research study is whether or not the methodology fits the question. This means that qualitative researchers must select an approach for exploring phenomena that will actually answer their research questions. Thus, as you read studies and are considering them as evidence on which to base your practice, you should ask yourself, "Does the methodology fit with the research question under study?"

HELPFUL HINT

All research is based on a paradigm, but this is seldom specifically stated in a research report.

DOES THE METHODOLOGY FIT WITH THE RESEARCH QUESTION BEING ASKED?

As we said before, qualitative methods are often best for helping us determine the nature of a phenomenon and the meaning of experience. Sometimes authors will state that they are using qualitative methods because little is known about a phenomenon, but that alone is not a good reason for conducting a study. Little may be known about a phenomenon because it does not matter! When researchers ask people to participate in a study, to open themselves and their lives for analysis, they should be asking about things that will help make a difference in people's lives or help provide more effective nursing care. You should be able to articulate a valid reason for conducting a study, beyond "little is known about this topic."

Considering the examples at the start of this chapter, we may want to know why HIV-infected women are less adherent to their medication regimens, so we can work to change these barriers and anticipate them when our patients are ready to start taking these pills. Similarly, we need to understand the decision-making processes women use to decide whether or not to have a child when they are disabled, so we can guide or advise the next woman who is going through this process. To summarize, a qualitative approach "fits" a research question when the researchers seek to understand the nature or experience of phenomena by attending to personal accounts of those with direct experiences related to the phenomena. Keeping in mind the purpose of qualitative research, let's discuss the parts of a qualitative research study.

COMPONENTS OF A QUALITATIVE RESEARCH STUDY

The components of a qualitative research study include the review of literature, study design, study setting and sample, approaches for data collection and analysis, study findings, and conclusions with implications for practice and research. As we reflect on these parts of qualitative studies, we will see how nurses use the qualitative research process to develop new knowledge for practice (Box 5.1).

Review of the Literature

When researchers are clear that a qualitative approach is the best way to answer the research question, their first step is to review the relevant literature and describe what is already

BOX 5.1 Steps in the Research Process

- Review of the literature
- Study design
- Sample
- Setting: Recruitment and data collection
- Data collection
- Data analysis
- Findings
- Conclusions

CRITICAL THINKING DECISION PATH

Selecting a Research Process

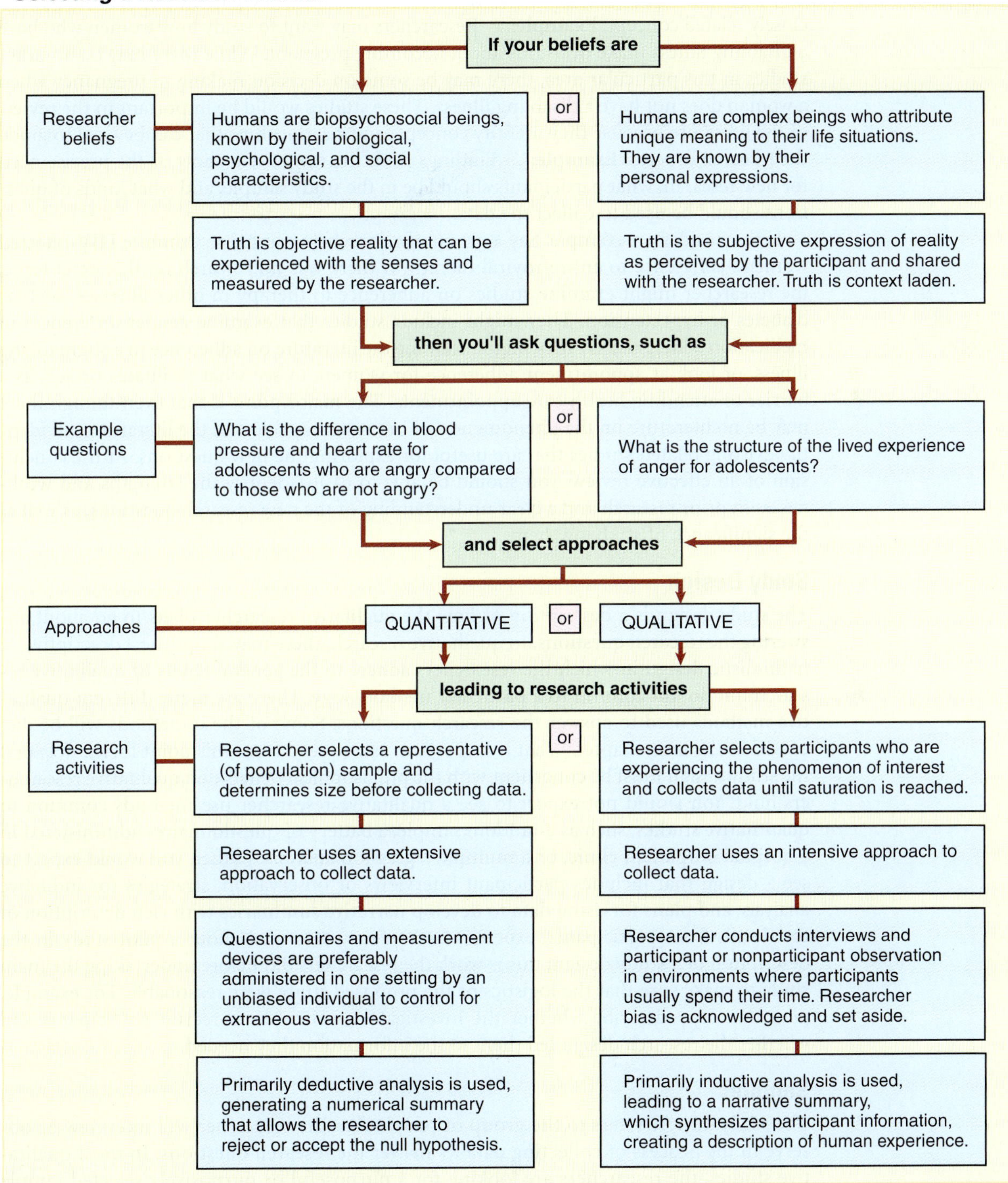

known about the phenomena of interest. This may require creativity on the researcher's part, because there may not be any published research on the phenomenon in question. Usually there are studies on similar subjects, or with the same patient population, or on a closely related concept. **Example:** ➤ Researchers may want to study how women who have a disabling illness make decisions about becoming pregnant. While there may be no other studies in this particular area, there may be some on decision making in pregnancy when a woman does not have a disabling illness. These studies would be important in the review of the literature because they identify concepts and relationships that can be used to guide the research process. **Example:** ➤ Findings from the review can show us the precise need for new research, what participants should be in the study sample, and what kinds of questions should be used to collect the data.

Let's consider an example. Say a group of researchers wanted to examine HIV-infected women's adherence to antiretroviral therapy. If there was no research on this exact topic, the researcher might examine studies on adherence to therapy in other illnesses, such as diabetes or hypertension. They might include studies that examine gender differences in medication adherence. Or they might examine the literature on adherence in a stigmatizing illness, or look at appointment adherence for women, to see what facilitates or acts as a barrier to attending health care appointments. The major point is that even though there may be no literature on the phenomenon of interest, the review of the literature will identify existing related studies that are useful for exploring the new questions. At the conclusion of an effective review, you should be able to easily identify the strengths and weaknesses in prior research and a clear understanding of the new research questions, as well as the significance of studying them.

Study Design

The study design is a description of how the qualitative researcher plans to go about answering the research questions. In qualitative research, there may simply be a descriptive or naturalistic design in which the researchers adhere to the general tenets of qualitative research but do not commit to a particular methodology. There are many different qualitative methods used to answer the research questions. Some of these methods will be discussed in the next chapter. What is important, as you read from this point forward, is that the study design must be congruent with the philosophical beliefs that qualitative researchers hold. You would not expect to see a qualitative researcher use methods common to quantitative studies, such as a random sample, a battery of questionnaires administered in a hospital outpatient clinic, or a multiple regression analysis. Rather, you would expect to see a design that includes participant interviews or observation, strategies for inductive analysis, and plans for using data to develop narrative summaries with rich description of the details from participants' experiences. You may also read about a pilot study in the description of a study design; this is work the researchers did before undertaking the main study to make sure that the logistics of the proposed study were reasonable. For example, pilot data may describe whether the investigators were able to recruit participants and whether the research design led them to the information they needed.

Sample

The study sample refers to the group of people that the researcher will interview or observe in the process of collecting data to answer the research questions. In most qualitative studies, the researchers are looking for a purposeful or purposively selected sample (see Chapter 10). This means that they are searching for a particular kind of person who can illuminate the phenomenon they want to study. **Example:** ➤ The researchers may want to interview women with multiple sclerosis or rheumatoid arthritis. There may be other parameters—called **inclusion** and **exclusion criteria**—that the researchers impose as well, such as requiring that participants be older than 18 years, not under the influence of illicit drugs, or experiencing a first pregnancy (as opposed to subsequent pregnancies). When researchers are clear about these criteria, they are able to identify and recruit participants with the experiences needed to shed light on the phenomenon in question. Often the researchers make decisions such as determining who might be a "long-term survivor" of a certain illness. In this case, they must clearly describe why and how they decided who would fit into this category. Is a long-term survivor someone who has had an illness for 5 years or 10 years? What is the median survival time for people with this diagnosis? Thus, as a reader of nursing research, you are looking for evidence of sound scientific reasoning behind the sampling plan.

When the researchers have identified the type of person to include in the research sample, the next step is to develop a strategy for recruiting participants, which means locating and engaging them in the research. Recruitment materials are usually very specific. **Example:** ➤ If the researchers want to talk to HIV-infected women about adherence to their medication regimen, they may distribute flyers or advertise their interest in recruiting women who consistently take their medication as indicated, as well as those who do not. Or, they may want to talk to women who fit into only one of those categories. Similarly, the researchers who are examining decision making in pregnancy among women with disabling conditions would develop recruitment strategies that identify subjects with the conditions or characteristics they want to study.

In a research report, the researcher may include a description of the study sample in the findings. (This can also be reported in the description of the sample.) In any event, besides a demographic description of the study participants, a qualitative researcher should also report on key axes of difference in the sample. **Example:** ➤ In a sample of HIV-infected women, there should be information about the stage of illness, what kind/how many pills they must take, how many children they have, and so on. This information helps you place the findings into a context.

Setting: Recruitment and Data Collection

The study setting refers to the places where participants are recruited and the data are collected. Settings for recruitment are usually a point of contact for people of common social, medical, or other individual traits. In the example of HIV-infected women who are having difficulties adhering to their antiretroviral regimens, researchers might distribute flyers describing the study at AIDS service organizations, support groups for HIV-infected women, clinics, online support groups, and other places people with HIV may seek services. The settings for data collection are another critical area of difference between quantitative and qualitative studies. Data collection in a qualitative study is usually done in a **naturalistic setting**, such as someone's home, not in a clinic interview room or researcher's office. This is important in qualitative research because the researcher's observations can inform the data collection. To be in someone else's home is a great advantage, as it helps the researcher to understand what that participant values. An entire wall in a participant's living room might contain many pictures of a loved one, so anyone who enters the home would immediately understand the centrality of that person in the participant's life. In the home of someone who is ill, many household objects may be clustered around a favorite chair: perhaps an oxygen tank, a glass of water, medications, a telephone, tissues, and so on. A good qualitative researcher will use clues like these in the study setting to complete the complex, rich drawing that is being rendered in the study.

> **IPE HIGHLIGHT**
>
> Reading and critically appraising qualitative research studies may be the best way for interprofessional teams to understand the experience of living with a chronic illness so they can provide more effective whole person care.

Data Collection

The procedures for data collection differ significantly in qualitative and quantitative studies. Where quantitative researchers focus on statistics and numbers, qualitative researchers are usually concerned with words: what people can tell them and the narratives about meaning or experience. Qualitative researchers interview participants; they may interview an individual or a group of people in what is called a focus group. They may observe individuals as they go about daily tasks, such as sorting medications into a pill minder or caring for a child. But in all cases, the data collected are expressed in words. Most qualitative researchers use voice recorders so that they can be sure that they have captured what the participant says. This reduces the need to write things down and frees researchers to listen fully. Interview recordings are usually transcribed verbatim and then listened to for accuracy. In a research report, investigators describe their procedures for collecting the data, such as obtaining informed consent, the steps from initial contact to the end of the study visit, and how long each interview or focus group lasted or how much time the researcher spent "in the field" collecting data.

A very important consideration in qualitative data collection is the researcher's decision that they have a sufficient sample and that data collection is complete. Researchers generally continue to recruit participants until they have reached redundancy or **data saturation**, which means that nothing new is emerging from the interviews. There usually is *not* a predetermined number of participants to be selected as there is in quantitative studies; rather, the researcher keeps recruiting until she or he has all of the data needed. One important exception to this is if the researcher is very interested in getting different types of people in the study. **Example:** ➤ In the study of HIV-infected women and medication adherence, the researchers may want some women who were very adherent in the beginning but then became less so over time, or they may want women who were not adherent in the beginning but then became adherent; alternately, they may want to interview women with children and women without children to determine the influence of having children on adherence. Whatever the specific questions may be, sample sizes tend to be fairly small (fewer than 30 participants) because of the enormous amounts of written text that will need to be analyzed by the researcher.

Investigators use great care to design the interview questions because they must be crafted to help study participants describe their personal experiences and perceptions. Interview questions are different from research questions. Research questions are typically broad, encompassing, and written in scientific language. The interview questions may also be broad, like the overview or **grand tour question** that seeks the "big picture." **Example:** ➤ Researchers might ask, "Tell me about taking your medications—the things that make it easier, and the things that make it harder," or "Tell me what you were thinking about when you decided to get pregnant." Along with overview questions, there are usually a series of prompts (additional questions) that were derived from the literature. These are areas that the researcher believes are important to cover (and that the participant will likely cover), but the prompts are there to remind the researcher in case the material is not mentioned. **Example:** ➤ With regard to medication adherence, the researcher may have read in other studies that motherhood can influence adherence in two very different ways: children can become a reason to live, which would facilitate taking antiretroviral medication; and children can be all-demanding, leaving the mother with little to no time to take care of herself. Thus, a neutrally worded question about the influence of children would be a prompt if the participants do not mention it spontaneously. In a research report, you should expect to find the primary interview questions identified verbatim; without them, it is impossible to know how the data were collected and how the researcher shaped what was discovered in the interviews.

QSEN EVIDENCE-BASED PRACTICE TIP

Qualitative researchers use more flexible procedures than quantitative researchers. While collecting data for a project, they consider all of the experiences that may occur.

Data Analysis

Next is the description of data analysis. Here, researchers tell you how they handled the raw data, which, in a qualitative study, are usually transcripts of recorded interviews. The goal of qualitative analysis is to find commonalities and differences in the interviews, and then to group these into broader, more abstract, overarching categories of meaning, sometimes called **themes**, that capture much of the data. In the example we have been using about decision making regarding pregnancy for disabled women, one woman might talk about discussing the need for assistance with her friends if she became pregnant, and finding out that they were willing and able to help her with the baby. Another woman might talk about how she discussed the decision with her parents and siblings, and found them to be a ready source of aid. And yet a third woman may say that she talked about this with her church study group, and they told her that they could arrange to bring meals and help with housework during the pregnancy and afterward. On a more abstract level, these women are all talking about social support. So an effective analysis would be one that identifies this pattern in social support and, perhaps, goes further by also describing how social support influences some other concept in the data. **Example:** ➤ Consider women's decision making about having a baby. In an ideal situation, written reports about the data will give you an example like the one you just read, but the page limitations of most journals limit the level of detail that researchers can present.

Many qualitative researchers use computer-assisted qualitative data analysis programs to find patterns in the interviews and field notes, which, in many studies, can seem overwhelming due to the sheer quantity of data to be dealt with. With a computer-assisted data analysis program, researchers from multiple sites can simultaneously code and analyze data from hundreds of files without using a single piece of paper. The software is a tool for managing and remembering steps in analysis; however, it does not replace the thoughtful work of the researcher who must apply the program to guide the analysis of the data. In research reports, you should see a description of the way data were managed and analyzed, and whether the researchers used software or other paper-based approaches, such as using index cards with handwritten notes.

Findings

At last, we come to the results. Findings in qualitative reports, as we have suggested already, are words—the findings are patterns of any kind in the data, such as the ways that participants talked, the things that they talked about, even their behaviors associated with where the researcher spent time with them. When researchers describe patterns in the data, they may describe a process (such as the way decision making occurs); they may identify a list of things that are functioning in some way (such as a list of barriers and facilitators to taking medications for HIV-infected women); they may specify a set of conditions that must be present for something to occur (such as what parents state they need to care for a ventilator-dependent child at home); or they may describe what it is like to go through some health-related transition (such as what it is like to become the caregiver for a parent with dementia). This is by no means an all-inclusive list; rather, it is a range of examples to help you recognize what types of findings might be possible. It may help to think of the findings as discoveries. The qualitative researcher has explored a phenomenon, and the findings are a report on what he or she "found"—that is, what was discovered in the interviews and observations.

When researchers describe their results, they usually break the data down into units of meaning that help the data cohere and tell a story. Effective research reports will describe the logic that was used for breaking down the units of data. **Example:** ➤ Are the themes—a means of describing a large quantity of data in a condensed format—identified from the most prevalent to the least prevalent? Are the researchers describing a process in temporal (time ordered) terms? Are they starting with things that were most important to the subject, then moving to less important items? As a report on the findings unfolds, the researcher should proceed with a thorough description of the phenomenon, defining each of the themes and fleshing out each of the themes with a thorough explanation of the role that it plays in the question under study. The researcher should also provide quotations that support their themes. Ideally, they will stage the quote, giving you some information about the subject from whom it came. For example, was the subject a newly diagnosed HIV-infected African American woman without children? Or was it a disabled woman who has chosen to become pregnant, but who has suffered two miscarriages? The staging of quotes is important because it allows you to put the information into some social context.

In a well-written report of qualitative research, some of the quotes will give you an "aha!" feeling. You will have a sense that the researcher has done an excellent job of getting to the core of the problem. Quotes are as critical to qualitative reports as numbers are to a quantitative study; you would not have a great deal of confidence in a quantitative or qualitative report in which the author asks you to believe the conclusion without also giving concrete, verifiable findings to back it up.

HELPFUL HINT

Values are involved in all research. It is important, however, that they not influence the results of the research.

DISCUSSION OF THE RESULTS AND IMPLICATIONS FOR EVIDENCE-BASED PRACTICE

When the researchers are satisfied that their findings answer the research questions, they should summarize the results for you and should compare their findings to the existing literature. Researchers usually explain how these findings are similar to or different from the existing literature. This is one of the great contributions of qualitative research—using findings to open up new venues of discovery that were not anticipated when the study was designed. **Example:** ➤ The researchers can use findings to develop new concepts or new conceptual models to explain broader phenomena. The conceptual work also identifies implications for how findings can be used in practice and can direct future research. Another alternative is for researchers to use their findings to extend or refine existing theoretical models. For example, a researcher may learn something new about stigma that has not been described in the literature, and in writing about these findings, the researcher may refer to an existing stigma theory, pointing out how his or her work extends that theory.

Nursing is a practice discipline, and the goal of nursing research is to use research findings to improve patient care. Qualitative methods are the best way to start to answer clinical and research questions that have not been addressed or when a new perspective is needed in practice. The qualitative answers to these questions provide important evidence that offers the first systematic insights into phenomena previously not well understood and often lead to new perspectives in nursing practice and improved patient care outcomes.

Kearney (2001) developed a typology of levels and applications of qualitative research evidence that helps us see how new evidence can be applied to practice (Table 5.1). She described five categories of qualitative findings that are distinguished from one another in their levels of complexity and discovery: those restricted by a priori frameworks, descriptive categories, shared pathway or meaning, depiction of experiential variation, and dense explanatory description. She argued that the greater the complexity and discovery within qualitative findings, the stronger the potential for clinical application.

Findings developed with only a priori frameworks provide little or no evidence for changing practice, because the researchers have prematurely limited what they are able to learn from participants or describe in their analysis. Findings that identify descriptive categories portray a higher level of discovery when a phenomenon is vividly portrayed from a new perspective. For nursing practice, these findings serve as maps of previously uncharted territory in human experience. Findings in Kearney's third category, shared pathway or meaning, are more complex. In this type of finding, there is an integration of concepts or themes that results in a synthesis of a shared process or experience that leads to a logical, complex portrayal of the phenomenon. The researcher's ideas at this level reveal how discrete bits of data come together in a meaningful whole. For nursing practice, this allows us to reflect on the bigger picture and what it means for the human experience (Kearney, 2001). Findings that depict experiential variation describe the essence of an experience and how this experience varies, depending on the individual or context. For nursing practice, this type of finding helps us see a variety of viewpoints, realizations of a human experience, and the contextual sources of that variety. In nursing practice, these findings explain how different variables can produce different consequences in different people or settings. Finally, findings that are presented as a dense explanatory description are at the highest level of complexity and discovery. They provide a rich, situated understanding of a multifaceted and varied human phenomenon in a unique situation. These

TABLE 5.1 Kearney's Categories of Qualitative Findings, from Least to Most Complex

Category	Definition	Example
Restricted by a priori frameworks	Discovery aborted because researcher has obscured the findings with an existing theory	Use of the theory of "relatedness" to describe women's relationships without substantiation in the data, or when there may be an alternative explanation to describe how women exist in relationship to others; the data seem to point to an explanation other than "relatedness"
Descriptive categories	Phenomenon is vividly portrayed from a new perspective; provides a map into previously uncharted territory in the human experience of health and illness	Children's descriptions of pain, including descriptors, attributed causes, and what constitutes good care during a painful episode
Shared pathway or meaning	Synthesis of a shared experience or process; integration of concepts that provides a complex picture of a phenomenon	Description of women's process of recovery from depression; each category was fully described, and the conditions for progression were laid out; able to see the origins of a phase in the previous phase
Depiction of experiential variation	Describes the main essence of an experience, but also shows how the experience varies, depending on the individual or context	Description of how pregnant women recovering from cocaine addiction might or might not move forward to create a new life, depending on the amount of structure they imposed on their behavior and their desire to give up drugs and change their lives
Dense explanatory description	Rich, situated understanding of a multifaceted and varied human phenomenon in a unique situation; portray the full range and depth of complex influences; densely woven structure to findings	Unique cultural conditions and familial breakdown and hopelessness led young people to deliberately expose themselves to HIV infection in order to find meaning and purpose in life; describes loss of social structure and demands of adolescents caring for their diseased or drugged parents who were unable to function as adults

types of findings portray the full depth and range of complex influences that propel people to make decisions. Physical and social contexts are fully accounted for. There is a densely woven structure of findings in these studies that provide a rich fund of clinically and theoretically useful information for nursing practice. The layers of detail work together in the findings to increase understanding of human choices and responses in particular contexts (Kearney, 2001).

QSEN EVIDENCE-BASED PRACTICE TIP

Qualitative research findings can be used in many ways, including improving ways clinicians communicate with patients and with each other.

So how can we further use qualitative evidence in nursing? The evidence provided by qualitative studies is used conceptually by the nurse: qualitative studies let nurses gain access to the experiences of patients and help nurses expand their ability to understand their patients, which should lead to more helpful approaches to care (Table 5.2).

Kearney (2001) proposed four modes of clinical application: insight or empathy, assessment of status or progress, anticipatory guidance, and coaching. The simplest mode, according to Kearney, is to use the information to better understand the experiences of our

TABLE 5.2 Kearney's Modes of Clinical Application for Qualitative Research

Mode of Clinical Application	Example
Insight or empathy: Better understanding our patients and offering more sensitive support	Nurse is better able to understand the behaviors of a woman recovering from depression
Assessment of status or progress: Descriptions of trajectories of illness	Nurse is able to describe trajectory of recovery from depression and can assess how the patient is moving through this trajectory
Anticipatory guidance: Sharing of qualitative findings with the patient	Nurse is able to explain the phases of recovery from depression to the patient and to reassure her that she is not alone, that others have made it through a similar experience
Coaching: Advising patients of steps they can take to reduce distress or improve adjustment to an illness, according to the evidence in the study	Nurse describes the six stages of recovery from depression to the patient, and in ongoing contact, points out how the patient is moving through the stages, coaching her to recognize signs that she is improving and moving through the stages

patients, which in turn helps us to offer more sensitive support. Qualitative findings can also help us assess the patient's status or progress through descriptions of trajectories of illness or by offering a different perspective on a health condition. They allow us to consider a range of possible responses from patients. We can then determine the fit of a category to a particular client, or try to locate them on an illness trajectory. Anticipatory guidance includes sharing of qualitative findings directly with patients. The patient can learn about others with a similar condition and can learn what to anticipate. This allows them to better garner resources for what might lie ahead or look for markers of improvement. Anticipatory guidance can also be tremendously comforting in that the sharing of research results can help patients realize they are not alone, that there are others who have been through a similar experience with an illness. Finally, coaching is a way of using qualitative findings; in this instance, nurses can advise patients of steps they can take to reduce distress, improve symptoms, or monitor trajectories of illness (Kearney, 2001).

Unfortunately, qualitative research studies do not fare well in the typical systematic reviews upon which evidence-based practice recommendations are based. Randomized clinical trials and other types of intervention studies traditionally have been the major focus of evidence-based practice. Typically, the selection of studies to be included in systematic reviews is guided by levels of evidence models that focus on the effectiveness of interventions according to their strength and consistency of their predictive power. Given that the levels of evidence models are hierarchical in nature and they perpetuate intervention studies as the "gold standard" of research design, the value of qualitative studies and the evidence offered by their results have remained unclear. Qualitative studies historically have been ranked lower in a hierarchy of evidence, as a "weaker" form of research design.

Remember, however, that qualitative research is not designed to test hypotheses or make predictions about causal effects. As we use qualitative methods, these findings become more and more valuable as they help us discover unmet patient needs, entire groups of patients that have been neglected, and new processes for delivering care to a population. Though qualitative research uses different methodologies and has different goals, it is important to explore how and when to use the evidence provided by findings of qualitative studies in practice.

APPRAISAL FOR EVIDENCE-BASED PRACTICE FOUNDATION OF QUALITATIVE RESEARCH

A final example illustrates the differences in the methods discussed in this chapter and provides you with the beginning skills of how to critique qualitative research. The information in this chapter, coupled with information presented in Chapter 7, provides the underpinnings of critical appraisal of qualitative research (see the Critical Appraisal Criteria box, Chapter 7). Consider the question of nursing students learning how to conduct research. The empirical analytical approach (quantitative research) might be used in an experiment to see if one teaching method led to better learning outcomes than another. The students' knowledge might be tested with a pretest, the teaching conducted, and then a posttest of knowledge obtained. Scores on these tests would be analyzed statistically to see if the different methods produced a difference in the results.

In contrast, a qualitative researcher may be interested in the process of learning research. The researcher might attend the class to see what occurs and then interview students to ask them to describe how their learning changed over time. They might be asked to describe the experience of becoming researchers or becoming more knowledgeable about research. The goal would be to describe the stages or process of this learning. Alternately, a qualitative researcher might consider the class as a culture and could join to observe and interview students. Questions would be directed at the students' values, behaviors, and beliefs in learning research. The goal would be to understand and describe the group members' shared meanings. Either of these examples are ways of viewing a question with a qualitative perspective. The specific qualitative methodologies are described in Chapter 6.

Many other research methods exist. Although it is important to be aware of the qualitative research method used, it is most important that the method chosen is the one that will provide the best approach to answering the question being asked. One research method does not rank higher than another; rather, a variety of methods based on different paradigms are essential for the development of a well informed and comprehensive approach to evidence-based nursing practice.

KEY POINTS

- All research is based on philosophical beliefs, a worldview, or a paradigm.
- Qualitative research encompasses different methodologies.
- Qualitative researchers believe that reality is socially constructed and is context dependent.
- Values should be acknowledged and examined as influences on the conduct of research.
- Qualitative research follows a process, but the components of the process vary.
- Qualitative research contributes to evidence-based practice.

CRITICAL THINKING CHALLENGES

- Discuss how a researcher's values could influence the results of a study. Include an example in your answer.
- Can the expression, "We do not always get closer to the truth as we slice and homogenize and isolate [it]" be applied to both qualitative and quantitative methods? Justify your answer.

- What is the value of qualitative research in evidence-based practice? Give an example.
- IPE Discuss how your interprofessional team could apply the findings of a qualitative study about coping with a diagnosis of multiple sclerosis.

REFERENCES

Denzin, N. K., & Lincoln, Y. S. (2011). *The SAGE handbook of qualitative research* (4th ed.). Thousand Oaks, CA: Sage.

Kearney, M. H. (2001). Levels and applications of qualitative research evidence. *Research in Nursing and Health*, *24*, 145–153.

Go to Evolve at **http://evolve.elsevier.com/LoBiondo/** for review questions, critiquing exercises, and additional research articles for practice in reviewing and critiquing.

6

Qualitative Approaches to Research

Mark Toles and Julie Barroso

Go to Evolve at **http://evolve.elsevier.com/LoBiondo/** for review questions, critiquing exercises, and additional research articles for practice in reviewing and critiquing.

LEARNING OUTCOMES

After reading this chapter, you should be able to do the following:

- Identify the processes of phenomenological, grounded theory, ethnographic, and case study methods.
- Recognize appropriate use of community-based participatory research (CBPR) methods.
- Discuss significant issues that arise in conducting qualitative research in relation to such topics as ethics, criteria for judging scientific rigor, and combination of research methods.
- Apply critical appraisal criteria to evaluate a report of qualitative research.

KEY TERMS

auditability
bracketing
case study method
community-based participatory research
constant comparative method
credibility
culture
data saturation
domains
emic view
ethnographic method
etic view
fittingness
grounded theory method
instrumental case study
intrinsic case study
key informants
lived experience
meta-summary
meta-synthesis
mixed methods
phenomenological method
theoretical sampling

Qualitative research combines the science and art of nursing to enhance understanding of the human health experience. This chapter focuses on four commonly used qualitative research methods: phenomenology, grounded theory, ethnography, and case study. Community-based participatory research (CBPR) is also presented. Each of these methods, although distinct from the others, shares characteristics that identify it as a method within the qualitative research tradition.

Traditional hierarchies of research evaluation and how they categorize evidence from strongest to weakest, with emphasis on support for the effectiveness of interventions, are presented in Chapter 1. This perspective is limited because it does not take into account the ways that qualitative research can support practice, as discussed in Chapter 5. There is no doubt about the merit of qualitative studies; the problem is that no one has developed a satisfactory method for including them in current evidence hierarchies. In addition, qualitative studies can answer the critical *why* questions that emerge in many evidence-based practice summaries. Such summaries may report the answer to a research question, but they do not explain *how* it occurs in the landscape of caring for people.

As a research consumer, you should know that qualitative methods are the best way to start to answer clinical and research questions when little is known or a new perspective is needed for practice. The very fact that qualitative research studies have increased exponentially in nursing and other social sciences speaks to the urgent need of clinicians to answer these *why* questions and to deepen our understanding of experiences of illness. Thousands of reports of well-conducted qualitative studies exist on topics such as the following:

- Personal and cultural constructions of disease, prevention, treatment, and risk
- Living with disease and managing the physical, psychological, and social effects of multiple diseases and their treatment
- Decision-making experiences at the beginning and end of life, as well as assistive and life-extending, technological interventions
- Contextual factors favoring and mitigating against quality care, health promotion, prevention of disease, and reduction of health disparities (Sandelowski, 2004; Sandelowski & Barroso, 2007)

Findings from qualitative studies provide valuable insights about unique phenomena, patient populations, or clinical situations. In doing so, they provide nurses with the data needed to guide and change practice.

In this chapter, you are invited to look through the lens of human experience to learn about phenomenological, grounded theory, ethnographic, CBPR, and case study methods. You are encouraged to put yourself in the researcher's shoes and imagine how it would be to study an issue of interest from the perspective of each of these methods. No matter which method a researcher uses, there is a focus on the human experience in natural settings.

The researcher using these methods believes that each unique human being attributes meaning to their experience and that experience evolves from one's social and historical context. Thus one person's experience of pain is distinct from another's and can be elucidated by the individual's subjective description of it. **Example:** ➤ Researchers interested in studying the lived experience of pain for the adolescent with rheumatoid arthritis will spend time in the adolescents' natural settings, perhaps in their homes and schools (see Chapter 5). Research efforts will focus on uncovering the meaning of pain as it extends beyond the number of medications taken or a rating on a pain scale. Qualitative methods are grounded in the belief that objective data do not capture the whole of the human experience. Rather, the meaning of the adolescent's pain emerges within the context of personal history, current relationships, and future plans, as the adolescent lives daily life in dynamic interaction with the environment.

QUALITATIVE APPROACH AND NURSING SCIENCE

The evidence provided by qualitative studies that consider the unique perspectives, concerns, preferences, and expectations each patient brings to a clinical encounter offers

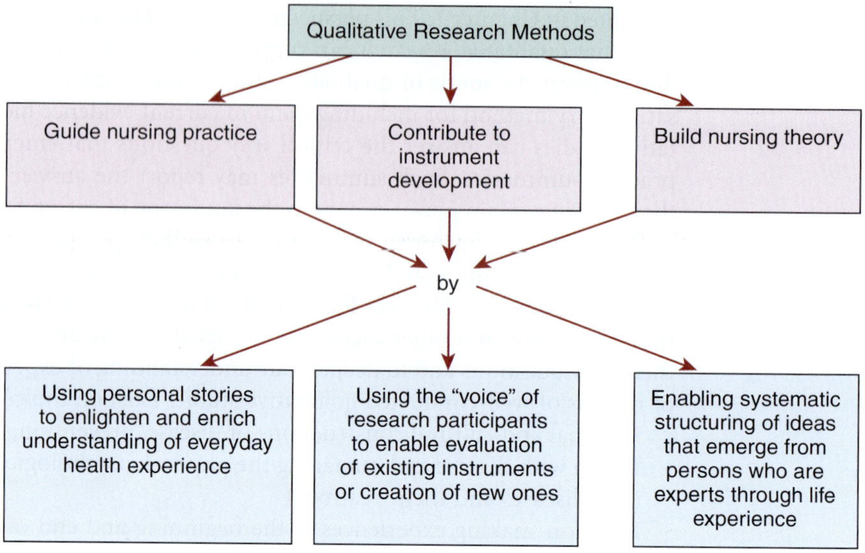

FIG 6.1 Qualitative approach and nursing science.

in-depth understanding of human experience and the contexts in which they occur. Thus findings in qualitative research often guide nursing practice, contribute to instrument development (see Chapter 15), and develop nursing theory (Fig. 6.1).

QUALITATIVE RESEARCH METHODS

Thus far you have studied an overview of the qualitative research approach (see Chapter 5). Recognizing how the choice to use a qualitative approach reflects one's worldview and the nature of some research questions, you have the necessary foundation for exploring selected qualitative methodologies. Now, as you review the Critical Thinking Decision Path and study the remainder of Chapter 6, note how different qualitative methods are appropriate for distinct areas of interest. Also note how unique research questions might be studied with each qualitative research method. In this chapter, we will explore five qualitative research methods in depth, including phenomenological, grounded theory, ethnographic, case study, and CBPR methods.

Phenomenological Method

The **phenomenological method** is a process of learning and constructing the meaning of human experience through intensive dialogue with persons who are living the experience. It rests on the assumption that there is a structure and essence to shared experiences that can be narrated (Marshall & Rossman, 2011). The researcher's goal is to understand the meaning of the experience as it is lived by the participant. Phenomenological studies usually incorporate data about the lived space, or spatiality; the lived body, or corporeality; lived time, or temporality; and lived human relations, or relationality. Meaning is pursued through a process of dialog, which extends beyond a simple interview and requires

CRITICAL THINKING DECISION PATH

Selecting a Qualitative Research Method

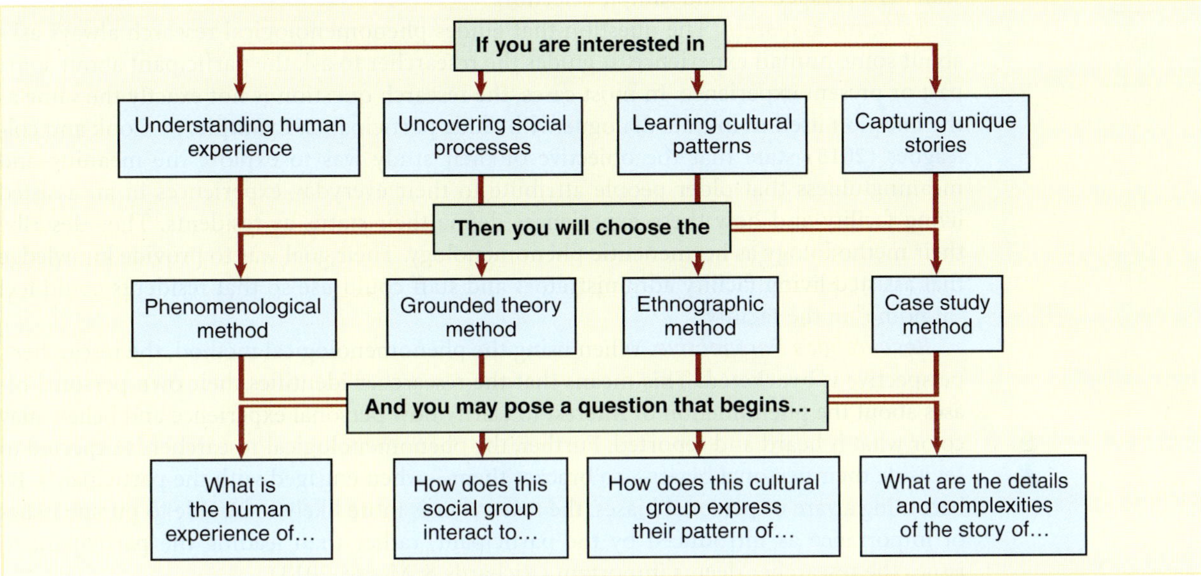

thoughtful presence on the part of the researcher. There are many schools of phenomenological research, and each school of thought uses slight differences in research methods. **Example:** ➤ Husserl belonged to the group of transcendental phenomenologists, who saw phenomenology as an interpretive, as opposed to an objective, mode of description. Using vivid and detailed attentiveness to description, researchers in this school explore the ways knowledge comes into being. They seek to understand knowledge that is based on insights rather than objective characteristics (Richards & Morse, 2013). In contrast, Heidegger was an existential phenomenologist who believed that the observer cannot separate him/herself from the lived world. Researchers in this school of thought study how being in the world is a reality that is perceived; they study a reciprocal relationship between observers and the phenomenon of interest (Richards & Morse, 2013). In all forms of phenomenological research, you will find researchers asking a question about the lived experience and using methods that explore phenomena as they are embedded in people's lives and environments.

Identifying the Phenomenon

Because the focus of the phenomenological method is the lived experience, the researcher is likely to choose this method when studying a dimension of day-to-day existence for a particular group of people. An example of this is provided later in this chapter, in which Cook and colleagues (2015) studied the complex issues surrounding the residential status of assisted living residents in terms of fundamental human needs.

Structuring the Study

When thinking about methods, we say the methodological approach "structures the study." This phrase means that the method shapes the way we think about the phenomenon of interest and the way we would go about answering a research question. For the purpose of describing structuring, the following topics are addressed: the research question, the researcher's perspective, and sample selection.

Research Question. The question that guides phenomenological research always asks about some human experience. It guides the researcher to ask the participant about some past or present experience. In most cases, the research question is not exactly the same as the question used to initiate dialogue with study participants. **Example:** ➤ Cook and colleagues (2015) state that the objective of their study was to explore the meaning and meaningfulness that older people attribute to their everyday experiences in an assisted living facility and how these experiences define their status as residents. They describe their methodology as hermeneutic phenomenology. Their goal was to provide knowledge that assisted living facility administrators and staff could use so that residents could feel "at home" in the facility.

Researcher's Perspective. When using the phenomenological method, the researcher's perspective is **bracketed**. This means that the researcher identifies their own personal biases about the phenomenon of interest to clarify how personal experience and beliefs may color what is heard and reported. Further, the phenomenological researcher is expected to set aside their personal biases—to bracket them—when engaged with the participants. By becoming aware of personal biases, the researcher is more likely to be able to pursue issues of importance as introduced by the participant, rather than leading the participant to issues the researcher deems important (Richards & Morse, 2013).

IPE HIGHLIGHT

Discuss with your interprofessional QI team why searching for qualitative studies might be most appropriate for understanding about living with Hepatitis C and managing the physical, psychological, and social effects of multiple treatments and their effects.

Using phenomenological methods, researchers strive to identify personal biases and hold them in abeyance while querying the participant. Readers of phenomenological articles may find it difficult to identify bracketing strategies because they are seldom explicitly identified in a research manuscript. Sometimes a researcher's worldview or assumptions provide insight into biases that have been considered and bracketed.

Sample Selection. As you read a phenomenological study, you will find that the participants were selected purposively (selecting subjects who are considered typical of the population) and that members of the sample either are living the experience the researcher studies or have lived the experience in their past. Because phenomenologists believe that each individual's history is a dimension of the present, a past experience exists in the present moment. For the phenomenologist, it is a matter of asking the right questions and listening. Even when a participant is describing a past experience, remembered information is being gathered in the present at the time of the interview.

HELPFUL HINT

Qualitative studies often use purposive sampling (see Chapter 12).

Data Gathering

Written or oral data may be collected when using the phenomenological method. The researcher may pose the query in writing and ask for a written response, or may schedule a time to interview the participant and record the interaction. In either case, the researcher may return to ask for clarification of written or recorded transcripts. To some extent, the particular data collection procedure is guided by the choice of a specific analysis technique. Different analysis techniques require different numbers of interviews. A concept known as *data saturation* usually guides decisions regarding how many interviews are enough. **Data saturation** is the situation of obtaining the full range of themes from the participants, so that in interviewing additional participants, no new data emerge (Marshall & Rossman, 2011).

Data Analysis

Several techniques are available for data analysis when using the phenomenological method. Although the techniques are slightly different from each other, there is a general pattern of moving from the participant's description to the researcher's synthesis of all participants' descriptions. Colaizzi (1978) suggests a series of seven steps:

1. Read the participants' narratives to acquire a feeling for their ideas in order to understand them fully.
2. Extract significant statements to identify keywords and sentences relating to the phenomenon being studied.
3. Formulate meanings for each of these significant statements.
4. Repeat this process across participants' stories and cluster recurrent meaningful themes. Validate these themes by returning to the informants to check interpretation.
5. Integrate the resulting themes into a rich description of the phenomenon under study.
6. Reduce these themes to an essential structure that offers an explanation of the behavior.
7. Return to the participants to conduct further interviews or elicit their opinions on the analysis in order to cross-check interpretation.

Cook and colleagues (2015) do not cite a reference for data analysis; they describe using narrative analysis to interpret how participants viewed their experiences and environment over a series of up to eight interviews with each resident over 6 months.

It is important to note that giving verbatim transcripts to participants can have unanticipated consequences. It is not unusual for people to deny that they said something in a certain way, or that they said it at all. Even when the actual recording is played for them, they may have difficulty believing it. This is one of the more challenging aspects of any qualitative method: every time a story is told, it changes for the participant. The participant may sincerely feel that the story as it was recorded is not the story as it is now.

QSEN EVIDENCE-BASED PRACTICE TIP

Phenomenological research is an important approach for accumulating evidence when studying a new topic about which little is known.

Describing the Findings

When using the phenomenological method, the nurse researcher provides you with a path of information leading from the research question, through samples of participants' words and the researcher's interpretation, to the final synthesis that elaborates the lived experience as a narrative. When reading the report of a phenomenological study, the reader should find that detailed descriptive language is used to convey the complex meaning of the lived experience that offers the evidence for this qualitative method (Richards & Morse, 2013). Cook and colleagues (2015) described five themes that emerged from the narratives that collectively demonstrate that residents wanted their residential status to involve "living with care" rather than "existing in care."

1. Caring for oneself/being cared for
2. Being in control/losing control
3. Relating to others/putting up with others
4. Active choosers and users of space/occupying space
5. Engaging in meaningful activity/lacking meaningful activity

The themes in their phenomenological report describe the need for assisted living facility staff to be more focused on recognizing, acknowledging, and supporting residents' aspirations regarding their future lives and their status as residents. By using direct participant quotes, researchers enable readers to evaluate the connections between what individual participants said and how the researcher labeled or interpreted what they said.

Grounded Theory Method

The **grounded theory method** is an inductive approach involving a systematic set of procedures to arrive at a theory about basic social processes (Silverman & Marvasti, 2008). The emergent theory is based on observations and perceptions of the social scene and evolves during data collection and analysis (Corbin & Strauss, 2015). Grounded theory describes a research approach to construct theory where no theory exists, or in situations where existing theory fails to provide evidence to explain a set of circumstances.

Developed originally as a sociologist's tool to investigate interactions in social settings (Glaser & Strauss, 1967), the grounded theory method is used in many disciplines; in fact, investigators from different disciplines use grounded theory to study the same phenomenon from their varying perspectives (Corbin & Strauss, 2015; Denzin & Lincoln, 2003; Marshall & Rossman, 2011; Strauss & Corbin, 1994, 1997). **Example:** ➤ In an area of study such as chronic illness, a nurse might be interested in coping patterns within families, a psychologist might be interested in personal adjustment, and a sociologist might focus on group behavior in health care settings. In grounded theory, the usefulness of the study stems from the transferability of theories; that is, a theory derived from one study is applicable to another. Thus the key objective of grounded theory is the development of theories spanning many disciplines that accurately reflect the cases from which they were derived (Sandelowski, 2004).

Identifying the Phenomenon

Researchers typically use the grounded theory method when interested in social processes from the perspective of human interactions or patterns of action and interaction between and among various types of social units (Denzin & Lincoln, 2003). The basic social process is sometimes expressed in the form of a gerund (i.e., the -ing form of a verb when functioning as a noun), which is designed to indicate change occurring over time as individuals negotiate social reality. **Example:** ➤ Hyatt and colleagues (2015) explore soldiers and their family reintegration experiences, as described by married dyads, following a combat-related mild traumatic brain injury.

Structuring the Study

Research Question. Research questions for the grounded theory method are those that address basic social processes that shape human behavior. In a grounded theory study, the research question can be a statement or a broad question that permits in-depth explanation of the phenomenon. For example, Hyatt and colleagues (2015) examined the following research question: "How do soldiers and their spouses identify the special challenges, sources of support, and overall rehabilitation process of post–mild traumatic brain injury family reintegration?"

Researcher's Perspective. In a grounded theory study, the researcher brings some knowledge of the literature to the study, but an exhaustive literature review may not be done. This allows theory to emerge directly from data and to reflect the contextual values that are integral to the social processes being studied. In this way, the new theory that emerges from the research is "grounded in" the data (Richards & Morse, 2013).

Sample Selection. Sample selection involves choosing participants who are experiencing the circumstance and selecting events and incidents related to the social process under investigation. Hyatt and colleagues (2015) obtained their purposive (see Chapter 12) sample through self-referral from flyers posted in military health care clinics, health care provider referrals, and directly approaching potential participants while in the traumatic brain injury clinic of a military health care system; it is important to note that Hyatt was an active military member herself at the time of data collection.

Data Gathering

In the grounded theory method, data are collected through interviews and skilled observations of individuals interacting in a social setting. Interviews are recorded and transcribed, and observations are recorded as field notes. Open-ended questions are used initially to identify concepts for further focus. At their first data collection point, Hyatt and colleagues (2015) interviewed couples (soldiers and their spouses) together; then they interviewed each of them separately, to probe the themes that emerged in the joint interviews.

Data Analysis

A unique and important feature of the grounded theory method is that data collection and analysis occur simultaneously. The process requires systematic data collection and documentation using field notes and transcribed interviews. Hunches about emerging patterns in the data are noted in memos that the researcher uses to direct activities in fieldwork. This technique, called **theoretical sampling**, is used to select experiences that will help the researcher to test hunches and ideas and to gather complete information about developing concepts. The researcher begins by noting indicators or actual events, actions, or words in the data. As data are concurrently collected and analyzed, new concepts, or abstractions, are developed from the indicators (Charmaz, 2003; Strauss, 1987).

The initial analytical process is called *open coding* (Strauss, 1987). Data are examined carefully line by line, broken down into discrete parts, then compared for similarities and differences (Corbin & Strauss, 2015). Coded data are continuously compared with new data as they are acquired during research. This is a process called the **constant comparative method**. When data collection is complete, codes in the data are clustered to form categories. The categories are expanded and developed, or they are collapsed into one another, and relationships between the categories are used to develop new "grounded" theories. As a result, data collection, analysis, and theory generation have a direct, reciprocal relationship which grounds new theory in the perspectives of the research participants (Charmaz, 2003; Richards & Morse, 2013; Strauss & Corbin, 1990).

HELPFUL HINT

In a report of research using the grounded theory method, you can expect to find a diagrammed model of a theory that synthesizes the researcher's findings in a systematic way.

Describing the Findings

Grounded theory studies are reported in detail, permitting readers to follow the exact steps in the research process. Descriptive language and diagrams of the research process are used as evidence to document the researchers' procedures for moving from the raw data to the new theory. Hyatt and colleagues (2015) found the basic social process of family reintegration after mild traumatic brain injury to be "finding a new normal." The couples described this new normal as the phenomenon of finding or adjusting to changes in their new, post-mild traumatic brain injury family roles or routines. The following were the core categories:

1. Facing the unexpected—"Homecoming"— and adjusting to having the soldier back home; noticing changes in the soldier
2. Managing unexpected change—Assuming a caregiver role, managing the post-mild traumatic brain injury changes within the context of the married relationship
3. Experiencing mismatched expectations—Coping with the shifting state of the relationship, losing a career, or a shifting future
4. Adjusting to new expectations—Accepting changes, building a new family life
5. Learning to live with new expectations—Accepting the new normal

QSEN EVIDENCE-BASED PRACTICE TIP

When thinking about the evidence generated by the grounded theory method, consider whether the theory is useful in explaining, interpreting, or predicting the study phenomenon of interest.

Ethnographic Method

Derived from the Greek term *ethnos*, meaning people, race, or cultural group, the **ethnographic method** focuses on scientific description and interpretation of cultural or social groups and systems (Creswell, 2013). The goal of the ethnographer is to understand the research participants' views of their world, or the emic view. The **emic view** (insiders' view) is contrasted with the **etic view** (outsiders' view), which is obtained when the researcher uses quantitative analyses of behavior. The ethnographic approach requires that the researcher enter the world of the study participants to watch what happens, listen to what is said, ask questions, and collect whatever data are available. It is important to note that the term *ethnography* is used to mean both the research technique and the product of that technique—that is, the study itself (Creswell, 2013; Richards & Morse, 2013; Tedlock, 2003). Vidick and Lyman (1998) trace the history of ethnography, with roots in the disciplines of sociology and anthropology, as a method born out of the need to understand "other" and "self." Nurses use the method to study cultural variations in health and patient groups as subcultures within larger social contexts.

Identifying the Phenomenon

The phenomenon under investigation in an ethnographic study varies in scope from a long-term study of a very complex culture, such as that of the Aborigines (Mead, 1949), to a short-term study of a phenomenon within subunits of cultures. Kleinman (1992) notes the clinical utility of ethnography in describing the "local world" of groups of patients who are experiencing a particular phenomenon, such as suffering. The local worlds of patients have cultural, political, economic, institutional, and social-relational dimensions in much the same way as larger complex societies. An example of ethnography is found in Grassley and colleagues' (2015) study of nurses' support of breastfeeding on the night shift. Grassley and colleagues used institutional ethnography, which has as its goal to explore how social experiences and processes, in particular those of everyday work, are organized. Institutional ethnography also considers the institutional processes and interactions that mediate the context of nurses' everyday work (Grassley et al., 2015).

Structuring the Study

Research Question. In ethnographic studies, questions are asked about "lifeways" or particular patterns of behavior within the social context of a culture or subculture. In this type of research, **culture** is viewed as the system of knowledge and linguistic expressions used by social groups that allows the researcher to interpret or make sense of the world (Aamodt, 1991; Richards & Morse, 2013). Thus ethnographic nursing studies address questions that concern how cultural knowledge, norms, values, and other contextual variables influence people's health experiences. **Example:** ➤ Grassley and colleagues' (2015) research question is implied in their purpose statement: "To describe nurses' support of breastfeeding on the night shift and to identify the interpersonal interactions and institutional structures that affect their ability to offer breastfeeding support and to promote exclusive breastfeeding on the night shift." Remember that ethnographers have a broader definition of culture, where a particular social context is conceptualized as a culture. In this case, nurses who provide care on a mother/baby unit to mother/infant dyads in the immediate postpartum period are seen as a cultural entity that is appropriate for ethnographic study.

Researcher's Perspective. When using the ethnographic method, the researcher's perspective is that of an interpreter entering an alien world and attempting to make sense of that world from the insider's point of view (Richards & Morse, 2013). Like phenomenologists and grounded theorists, ethnographers make their own beliefs explicit and bracket, or set aside, their personal biases as they seek to understand the worldview of others.

Sample Selection. The ethnographer selects a cultural group that is living the phenomenon under investigation. The researcher gathers information from general informants and from key informants. **Key informants** are individuals who have special knowledge, status, or communication skills, and who are willing to teach the ethnographer about the phenomenon (Richards & Morse, 2013). **Example:** ➤ Grassley and colleagues' (2015) research took place in a tertiary care hospital with 4200 births per year (20% of the state's total births) and an exclusive breastfeeding rate of 75% on discharge. They described the setting and its employees in detail.

HELPFUL HINT

Managing personal bias is an expectation of researchers using all of the methods discussed in this chapter.

Data Gathering

Ethnographic data gathering involves immersion in the study setting and the use of participant observation, interviews of informants, and interpretation by the researcher of cultural patterns (Richards & Morse, 2013). Ethnographic research involves face-to-face interviewing with data collection and analysis taking place in the natural setting. Thus fieldwork is a major focus of the method. Other techniques may include obtaining life histories and collecting material items reflective of the culture. **Example:** ➤ Photographs and films of the informants in their world can be used as data sources. In their study, Grassley and colleagues (2015) collected data using focus groups, individual and group interviews, and mother/baby unit observations.

Data Analysis

Like the grounded theory method, ethnographic data are collected and analyzed simultaneously. Data analysis proceeds through several levels as the researcher looks for the meaning of cultural symbols in the informant's language. Analysis begins with a search for **domains** or symbolic categories that include smaller categories. Language is analyzed for semantic relationships, and structural questions are formulated to expand and verify data. Analysis proceeds through increasing levels of complexity until the data, grounded in the informant's reality, are synthesized by the researcher (Richards & Morse, 2013). Grassley and colleagues (2015) described analysis of data as beginning with interview transcripts using content analysis, with subsequent team meetings to discuss findings and agree on categories. The observation notes were used to substantiate the themes.

Describing the Findings

Ethnographic studies yield large quantities of data that reflect a wide array of evidence amassed as field notes of observations, interview transcriptions, and sometimes other artifacts such as photographs. The first level description is the description of the scene, the parameters or boundaries of the research group, and the overt characteristics of group members (Richards & Morse, 2013). Strategies that enhance first level description include maps and floor plans of the setting, organizational charts, and documents. Researchers may report item-level analysis, followed by pattern and structure level of analysis. Ethnographic research articles usually provide examples from data, thorough descriptions of the analytical process, and statements of the hypothetical propositions and their relationship to the ethnographer's frame of reference, which can be rather detailed and lengthy. Grassley and colleagues (2015) identified three main themes that described nurses' support of breastfeeding on the night shift: competing priorities, incongruent expectations, and influential institutional structure; these described the interpersonal interactions and institutional structures that affected the nurses. Competing priorities included maternal rest, the newborn night feeding pattern, the presence of visitors, support of the breastfeeding dyad, and other patients' care needs. Incongruent expectations included the breastfeeding expectations of parents, the newborn's breastfeeding behaviors, parental night feeding expectations, the newborn's nocturnal sleep pattern, the nurses' expectations about support, and challenging breastfeeding dyads. Finally, influential institutional structures included hospital practices, staffing (including the nurse/patient ratio, RN experience, and lactation of RNs), and feeding policies.

QSEN EVIDENCE-BASED PRACTICE TIP

Evidence generated by ethnographic studies will answer questions about how cultural knowledge, norms, values, and other contextual variables influence the health experience of a particular patient population in a specific setting.

Case Study

Case study research, which is rooted in sociology, has a complex history and many definitions (Aita & McIlvain, 1999). As noted by Stake (2000), a case study design is not a methodological choice; rather, it is a choice of what to study. Thus the **case study method** is about studying the peculiarities and the commonalities of a specific case, irrespective of the actual strategies for data collection and analysis that are used to explore research questions. Case studies include quantitative and/or qualitative data but are defined by their focus on uncovering an individual case and, in some instances, identifying patterns in variables that are consistent across a set of cases. Stake (2000) distinguishes intrinsic from instrumental case studies. **Intrinsic case study** is undertaken to have a better understanding of the case—for example, one child with chickenpox, as opposed to a group or all children with chickenpox. The researcher at least temporarily subordinates other curiosities so that the stories of those "living the case" will be teased out (Stake, 2000). **Instrumental case study** is used when researchers are pursuing insight into an issue or want to challenge some generalization—for example, the qualities of sleep and restfulness in a set of four children with chickenpox. Very often, in case studies, there is an emphasis on holism, which means that researchers are searching for global understanding of a case within a spatially or temporally defined context.

Identifying the Phenomenon

Although some definitions of case study demand that the focus of research be contemporary, Stake's (1995, 2000) defining criterion of attention to the single case broadens the scope of phenomenon for study. By a single case, Stake is designating a focus on an individual, a family, a community, an organization—some complex phenomenon that demands close scrutiny for understanding. Walker and colleagues (2015) used a case study design to examine how older, early-stage breast and prostate cancer patients managed the transition from active treatment of cancer to recovery when treatment was completed. To explore the strategies that cancer patients used, Walker and colleagues used a purposive sampling strategy to select a sample of 11 patient and caregiver dyads from a larger group of dyads enrolled in a randomized clinical trial of a new cancer treatment.

Structuring the Study

Research Question. Stake (2000) suggests that research questions be developed around issues that serve as a foundation to uncover complexity and pursue understanding. Although researchers pose questions to begin discussion, the initial questions are never all-inclusive; rather, the researcher uses an iterative process of "growing questions" in the field. That is, as data are collected to address these questions, it is expected that other questions will emerge and serve as guides to the researcher to untangle the complex, context-laden story within the case. **Example:** ➤ In Walker and colleagues' (2015) study, data were collected from patients' daily written journals, patient interview transcripts, and researcher notes from telephone calls with patients and caregivers. By using multiple ways of identifying how patients recovered after treatment, the researchers were able to describe a central theme about cancer recovery—with the return of a sense of "normalcy," patients experienced less anxiety and greater quality of life. Using rich description in the case study data, the researchers were also able to describe resources, such as conversations with family members and health care workers, which promote a sense of normalcy and well-being after treatment.

Researcher's Perspective. When the researcher begins with questions developed around suspected *issues* of importance, they are said to have an "etic" focus, which means the research is focused on the perspective of the researcher. As case study researchers engage the phenomenon of interest in individual cases, the uniqueness of individual stories unfold and shift from an etic (researcher orientation) to an "emic" (participant orientation) focus (Stake, 2000). Ideally, the case study researcher will develop an insider view that permits narration of the way things happen in the case. **Example:** ➤ In the study by Walker and colleagues (2015), the etic focus on the abstract concept of "recovery" shifted to the emic focus on the precise details about the way patients returned to a sense of normalcy after treatment.

Sample Selection. This is one of the areas where scholars in the field present differing views, ranging from only choosing the most common cases to only choosing the most unusual cases (Aita & McIlvain, 1999). Stake (2000) advocates selecting cases that may offer the best opportunities for learning. In some instances, the convenience of studying the case may even be a factor. For instance, if there are several patients who have undergone heart transplantation and are willing to participate in the study, practical factors may influence which patient offers the best opportunity for learning. Persons who live in the area and can be easily visited at home or in the medical center might be better choices than those living much farther away (where multiple contacts over time might be impossible). Similarly, the researcher may choose to study a case in which a potential participant has an actively involved family, because understanding the family context of transplant patients may shed important new light on their healing. It can safely be said that no choice is perfect when selecting a case; however, selecting cases for their contextual features fosters the strength of data that can be learned at the level of the individual case. **Example:** ➤ In the Walker and colleagues' (2015) study, the selection of 11 patient and caregiver dyads permitted the detailed data collection necessary to describe the actual process of returning to normalcy and how factors in the environment contributed to this process.

Data Gathering

Case study data are gathered using interviews, field observations, document reviews, and any other methods that accumulate evidence for describing or explaining the complexity of the case. Stake (1995) advocates development of a data gathering plan to guide the progress of the study from definition of the case through decisions regarding data collection involving multiple methods, at multiple time points, and sometimes with multiple participants within the case. In the Walker and colleagues' (2015) study, multiple methods for collecting data were used, including daily written diaries, interview transcripts, and notes from phone calls. Using data from multiple sources, the researchers used data from different times and points of view to describe the step-by-step process of returning to normal after cancer treatment.

Data Analysis/Describing Findings

Data analysis is often concurrent with data gathering and description of findings as the narrative in the case develops. Qualitative case study is characterized by researchers spending extended time on site, personally in contact with activities and operations of the case, and reflecting and revising meanings of what transpires (Stake, 2000). Reflecting and revising meanings are the work of the case study researcher, who records data, searches for patterns, links data from multiple sources, and develops preliminary thoughts regarding the meaning of collected data. This reflective and iterative process for writing the case narrative produces a unique form of evidence. Many times case study research reports do not list all of the research activities. However, reported findings are usually embedded in the following: (1) a chronological development of the case; (2) the researcher's story of coming to know the case; (3) the one-by-one description of case dimensions; and (4) vignettes that highlight case qualities (Stake, 1995). **Example:** ➤ As Walker and colleagues (2015) analyzed "cases" of patient recovery after treatment, the diversity of cases in the study permitted the researchers to identify behaviors, such as conversations with trusted health care workers, which patients used to reassess their wellness and realize they were healing after treatment. Analysis consisted of the search for patterns in raw data, variation in the patterns within and between cases, and identification of themes that described common patterns within and between the cases. In the study by Walker and colleagues (2015), the researchers ultimately used patterns in the case data to develop a theory about the process of working toward normalcy after cancer treatment; this was significant because the new theory is focused on patient experiences and will be a guide for assisting cancer patients in the future.

QSEN EVIDENCE-BASED PRACTICE TIP

Case studies are a way of providing in-depth evidence-based discussion of clinical topics that can be used to guide practice.

Community-Based Participatory Research

Community-based participatory research is a research method that systematically accesses the voice of a community to plan context-appropriate action. CBPR provides an alternative to traditional research approaches that assume a phenomenon may be separated from its context for purposes of study. Investigators who use CBPR recognize that engaging members of a study population as active and equal participants, in all phases of the research, is crucial for the research process to be a means of facilitating change (Holkup et al., 2004). Change or action is the intended end product of CBPR, and "action research" is a term related to CBPR. Many scholars consider CBPR to be a type of action research and group this within the tradition of critical science (Fontana, 2004).

In his book *Action Research,* Stringer (1999) distilled the research process into three phases: look, think, and act. In the look phase Stringer (1999) describes "building the picture" by getting to know stakeholders so that the problem is defined in their terms and the problem definition is reflective of the community context. He characterizes the think phase as interpretation and analysis of what was learned in the look phase. As investigators "think," the researcher is charged with connecting the ideas of the stakeholders so that they provide evidence that is understandable to the larger community group (Stringer, 1999). Finally, in the act phase, Stringer (1999) advocates planning, implementation, and evaluation based on information collected and interpreted in the other phases of research.

Bisung and colleagues (2015) used photovoice as a CBPR tool to understand water, sanitation, and hygiene behaviors and to catalyze community-led solutions to change behaviors among women in Western Kenya. Changing these behaviors is essential for reducing waterborne and water-related diseases. Photovoice is a CBPR tool that can be used to foster trust and capacity building for community-led solutions to environment and health issues. Through photography, participants, who take the pictures themselves, are able to identify, represent, discuss, and find solutions to their everyday environment and health problems. In the first part of their study, photovoice one-on-one interviews were used to explore local perceptions and practices around water-health linkages and how the ecological and sociopolitical environment shapes these perceptions and practices. The second component consisted of using photovoice group discussions to explore participants' experiences with and reactions to the photographs and the photovoice project. From the group discussions, three major themes emerged: awareness, immediate reactions, and planned actions. Awareness involved the photos serving as prompts to certain behaviors and practices in the community and the influence of these practices on their health. Immediate reactions involved spontaneous decisions to educate people and stop children from certain negative practices and having discussions on how to find solutions to common negative behaviors and practices. Planned actions involved working with village leaders and the whole community.

Mixed Methods Research

Mixed methods research is basically the use of both qualitative and quantitative methods in one study. Mixed methods research has evolved over the past decade. There are several types of mixed methods designs (Creswell & Plano Clark, 2011). Researchers who choose a mixed methods study choose on the basis of the question. (See Chapter 10 for further information.)

Data from different sources can be used to corroborate, elaborate, or illuminate the phenomenon in question. **Example:** ➤ Bhandari and Kim (2016) conducted a mixed methods study. The study aimed to develop an exploratory model for self-care in type 2 diabetic adults and enhance the model's interpretation through qualitative input. For the qualitative component, the researchers conducted semistructured interviews with a subset ($N = 13$) of the total sample ($N = 230$). For the quantitative component, the subjects responded to several questionnaires related to self-care behaviors. As you read research, you will quickly discover that approaches and methods, such as mixed methods, are being combined to contribute to theory building, guide practice, and facilitate instrument development.

Although certain questions may be answered effectively by combining qualitative and quantitative methods in a single study, this does not necessarily make the findings and related evidence stronger. In fact, if a researcher inappropriately combines methods in a single study, the findings could be weaker and less credible.

SYNTHESIZING QUALITATIVE EVIDENCE: META-SYNTHESIS

The depth and breadth of qualitative research has grown over the years, and it has become important to qualitative researchers to synthesize critical masses of qualitative findings.

The terms most commonly used to describe this activity are qualitative meta-summary and qualitative meta-synthesis. Qualitative **meta-summary** is a quantitatively oriented aggregation of qualitative findings that are topical or thematic summaries or surveys of data. Meta-summaries are integrations that are approximately equal to the sum of parts, or the sum of findings across reports in a target domain of research. They address the manifest content in findings and reflect a quantitative logic: to discern the frequency of each finding and to find in higher frequency the evidence of replication foundational to validity in most quantitative research. Qualitative meta-summary involves the extraction and further abstraction of findings, and the calculation of manifest frequency effect sizes (Sandelowski & Barroso, 2003a). Qualitative **meta-synthesis** is an interpretive integration of qualitative findings that are interpretive syntheses of data, including the phenomenologies, ethnographies, grounded theories, and other integrated and coherent descriptions or explanations of phenomena, events, or cases that are the hallmarks of qualitative research. Meta-syntheses are integrations that are more than the sum of parts in that they offer novel interpretations of findings. These interpretations will not be found in any one research report; rather, they are inferences derived from taking all of the reports in a sample as a whole. Meta-syntheses offer a description or explanation of a target event or experience, instead of a summary view of unlinked features of that event or experience. Such interpretive integrations require researchers to piece the individual syntheses constituting the findings in individual research reports together to craft one or more meta-syntheses. Their validity does not reside in a replication logic, but in an inclusive logic whereby all findings are accommodated and the accumulative analysis displayed in the final product. Meta-synthesis methods include constant comparison, taxonomic analysis, the reciprocal translation of in vivo concepts, and the use of imported concepts to frame data (Sandelowski & Barroso, 2003b). Meta-synthesis integrates qualitative research findings on a topic and is based on comparative analysis and interpretative synthesis of qualitative research findings that seek to retain the essence and unique contribution of each study (Sandelowski & Barroso, 2007).

Fleming and colleagues (2015) published a meta-synthesis of qualitative studies related to antibiotic prescribing in long-term care facilities. The synthesis of qualitative research was used to facilitate determination of antibiotic prescribing in long-term care settings. This meta-synthesis provided a way to describe findings across a set of qualitative studies and create knowledge that is relevant to clinical practice. Sandelowski (2004) cautions that the use of qualitative meta-synthesis is laudable and necessary, but requires careful application of qualitative meta-synthesis methods. There are a number of meta-synthesis studies being conducted by nurse scientists. It will be interesting for research consumers to follow the progress of researchers who seek to develop criteria for appraising a set of qualitative studies and use those criteria to guide the incorporation of these studies into systematic literature reviews.

QSEN EVIDENCE-BASED PRACTICE TIP

Although qualitative in its approach to research, community-based participatory research leads to an action component in which a nursing intervention is implemented and evaluated for its effectiveness in a specific patient population.

ISSUES IN QUALITATIVE RESEARCH

Ethics

Protection of human subjects is a critical aspect of all scientific investigation. This demand exists for both quantitative and qualitative research approaches. Protection of human subjects in quantitative approaches is discussed in Chapter 13. These basic tenets hold true for the qualitative approach. However, several characteristics of the qualitative methodologies outlined in Table 6.1 generate unique concerns and require an expanded view of protecting human subjects.

Naturalistic Setting

The central concern that arises when research is conducted in naturalistic settings focuses on the need to gain informed consent. The need to obtain informed consent is a basic researcher responsibility but is not always easy to obtain in naturalistic settings. For instance, when research methods include observing groups of people interacting over time, the complexity of gaining consent becomes apparent: Have all parties consented for all periods of time? Have all parties been consented? What have all parties consented to doing? These complexities generate controversy and debate among qualitative researchers. The balance between respect for human participants and efforts to collect meaningful data must be continuously negotiated. The reader should look for information indicating that the researcher has addressed this issue of balance by recording attention to human participant protection.

Emergent Nature of Design

The emergent nature of the research design in qualitative research underscores the need for ongoing negotiation of consent with participants. In the course of a study, situations change, and what was agreeable at the beginning may become intrusive. Sometimes, as data collection proceeds and new information emerges, the study shifts direction in a way that is not acceptable to participants. For instance, if the researcher were present in a family's home during a time when marital discord arose, the family may choose to renegotiate the consent. From another perspective, Morse (1998) discussed the increasing involvement of participants in the research process, sometimes resulting in their request to have their names published in the findings or be included as a coauthor. If the participant originally signed a consent form and then chose an active identified role, Morse (1998) suggests that the participant then sign a "release for publication" form to address this request. The emergent qualitative research process demands ongoing negotiation of researcher-participant relationships, including the consent relationship. The opportunity

TABLE 6.1 Characteristics of Qualitative Research Generating Ethical Concerns

Characteristics	Ethical Concerns
Naturalistic setting	Some researchers using participant observation methods may believe that consent is not always possible or necessary.
Emergent nature of design	Planning for questioning and observation emerges over the time of the study. Thus it is difficult to inform the participant precisely of all potential threats before he or she agrees to participate.
Researcher-participant interaction	Relationships developed between the researcher and participant may blur the focus of the interaction.
Researcher as instrument	The researcher is the study instrument, collecting data and interpreting the participant's reality.

to renegotiate consent establishes a relationship of trust and respect characteristic of the ethical conduct of research.

Researcher-Participant Interaction

The nature of the researcher-participant interaction over time introduces the possibility that the research experience will become a therapeutic one. It is a case of research becoming practice. It is important to recognize that there are basic differences between the intent of nurses when engaging in practice and when conducting research (Smith & Liehr, 2003). In practice, the nurse has caring-healing intentions. In research, the nurse intends to "get the picture" from the perspective of the participant. The process of "getting the picture" may be a therapeutic experience for the participant. When a research participant talks to a caring listener about things that matter, the conversation may promote healing, even though it was not intended. From an ethical perspective, the qualitative researcher is promising only to listen and encourage the other's story. If this experience is therapeutic for the participant, it becomes an unplanned benefit of the research. If it becomes harmful, the ethics of continuing the research becomes an issue and the study design will require revision.

Researcher as Instrument

The responsibility to establish rigor in data collection and analysis requires that the researcher acknowledge any personal bias and strive to interpret data in a way that accurately reflects the participant's point of view. This serious ethical obligation may require that researchers return to the subjects at critical interpretive points and ask for clarification or validation.

Credibility, Auditability, and Fittingness

Quantitative studies are concerned with reliability and validity of instruments, as well as internal and external validity criteria as measures of scientific rigor (see the Critical Thinking Decision Path), but these are not appropriate for qualitative work. The rigor of qualitative methodology is judged by unique criteria appropriate to the research approach. Credibility, auditability, and fittingness were scientific criteria proposed for qualitative research studies by Guba and Lincoln (1981). Although these criteria were proposed decades ago, they still capture the rigorous spirit of qualitative inquiry and persist as reasonable criteria for appraisal of scientific rigor in the research. The meanings of **credibility**, **auditability**, and **fittingness** are briefly explained in Table 6.2.

TABLE 6.2 **Criteria for Judging Scientific Rigor: Credibility, Auditability, Fittingness**

Criteria	Criteria Characteristics
Credibility	Truth of findings as judged by participants and others within the discipline. For instance, you may find the researcher returning to the participants to share interpretation of findings and query accuracy from the perspective of the persons living the experience.
Auditability	Accountability as judged by the adequacy of information leading the reader from the research question and raw data through various steps of analysis to the interpretation of findings. For instance, you should be able to follow the reasoning of the researcher step by step through explicit examples of data, interpretations, and syntheses.
Fittingness	Faithfulness to participants' everyday reality, described in enough detail so that others can evaluate importance for practice, research, and theory development. For instance, you will know enough about the human experience being reported that you can decide whether it "rings true" and is useful for guiding your practice.

QSEN EVIDENCE-BASED PRACTICE TIPS

- Mixed methods research offers an opportunity for researchers to increase the strength and consistency of evidence provided by the use of both qualitative and quantitative research methods.
- The combination of stories with numbers (qualitative and quantitative research approaches) through use of mixed methods may provide the most complete picture of the phenomenon being studied and, therefore, the best evidence for guiding practice.

APPRAISAL FOR EVIDENCE-BASED PRACTICE QUALITATIVE RESEARCH

General criteria for critiquing qualitative research are proposed in the following Critical Appraisal Criteria box. Each qualitative method has unique characteristics that influence what the research consumer may expect in the published research report, and journals often have page restrictions that penalize qualitative research. The criteria for critiquing are formatted to evaluate the selection of the phenomenon, the structure of the study, data collection, data analysis, and description of the findings. Each question of the criteria focuses on factors discussed throughout the chapter. Appraising qualitative research is a useful activity for learning the nuances of this research approach. You are encouraged to identify a qualitative study of interest and apply the criteria for critiquing. Keep in mind that qualitative methods are the best way to start to answer clinical and/or research questions that previously have not been addressed in research studies or that do not lend themselves to a quantitative approach. The answers provided by qualitative data reflect important evidence that may provide the first insights about a patient population or clinical phenomenon.

CRITICAL APPRAISAL CRITERIA

Qualitative Approaches

Identifying the Phenomenon

1. Is the phenomenon focused on human experience within a natural setting?
2. Is the phenomenon relevant to nursing and/or health?

Structuring the Study

Research Question

3. Does the question specify a distinct process to be studied?
4. Does the question identify the context (participant group/place) of the process that will be studied?
5. Does the choice of a specific qualitative method fit with the research question?

Researcher's Perspective

6. Are the biases of the researcher reported?
7. Do the researchers provide a structure of ideas that reflect their beliefs?

Sample Selection

8. Is it clear that the selected sample is living the phenomenon of interest?

Data Collection

9. Are data sources and methods for gathering data specified?
10. Is there evidence that participant consent is an integral part of the data-gathering process?

Data Analysis

11. Can the dimensions of data analysis be identified and logically followed?
12. Does the researcher paint a clear picture of the participant's reality?
13. Is there evidence that the researcher's interpretation captured the participant's meaning?
14. Have other professionals confirmed the researcher's interpretation?

Describing the Findings

15. Are examples provided to guide the reader from the raw data to the researcher's synthesis?
16. Does the researcher link the findings to existing theory or literature, or is a new theory generated?

In summary, the term *qualitative research* is an overriding description of multiple methods with distinct origins and procedures. In spite of distinctions, each method shares a common nature that guides data collection from the perspective of the participants to create a story that synthesizes disparate pieces of data into a comprehensible whole that provides evidence and promises direction for building nursing knowledge.

KEY POINTS

- Qualitative research is the investigation of human experiences in naturalistic settings, pursuing meanings that inform theory, practice, instrument development, and further research.
- Qualitative research studies are guided by research questions.
- Data saturation occurs when the information being shared with the researcher becomes repetitive.
- Qualitative research methods include five basic elements: identifying the phenomenon, structuring the study, gathering the data, analyzing the data, and describing the findings.
- The phenomenological method is a process of learning and constructing the meaning of human experience through intensive dialogue with persons who are living the experience.
- The grounded theory method is an inductive approach that implements a systematic set of procedures to arrive at theory about basic social processes.
- The ethnographic method focuses on scientific descriptions of cultural groups.
- The case study method focuses on a selected phenomenon over a short or long time period to provide an in-depth description of its essential dimensions and processes.
- CBPR is a method that systematically accesses the voice of a community to plan context-appropriate action.
- Ethical issues in qualitative research involve issues related to the naturalistic setting, emergent nature of the design, researcher-participant interaction, and researcher as instrument.
- Credibility, auditability, and fittingness are criteria for judging the scientific rigor of a qualitative research study.
- Mix methods approaches to research are promising.

CRITICAL THINKING CHALLENGES

- How can mixed methods increase the effectiveness of qualitative research?
- How can a nurse researcher select a qualitative research method when he or she is attempting to accumulate evidence regarding a new topic about which little is known?
- How can the case study approach to research be applied to evidence-based practice?
- Describe characteristics of qualitative research that can generate ethical concerns.
- IPE Your interprofessional team is asked to provide a rationale about why they are searching for a meta-synthesis rather than individual qualitative studies to answer their clinical question.

REFERENCES

Aamodt, A. A. (1991). Ethnography and epistemology: Generating nursing knowledge. In J. M. Morse (Ed.), *Qualitative nursing research: A contemporary dialogue*. Newbury Park, CA: Sage.

Aita, V. A., & McIlvain, H. E. (1999). An armchair adventure in case study research. In B. Crabtree & W. L. Miller (Eds.), *Doing qualitative research*. Thousand Oaks, CA: Sage.

Bhandari, P., & Kim, M. (2016). Self-care behaviors of Nepalese adults with Type 2 diabetes. *Nursing Research*, *65*(3), 202–241.

Bisung, E., Elliott, S. J., Abudho, B., et al. (2015). Using photovoice as a community based participatory research tool for changing water, sanitation, and hygiene behaviours in Usoma, Kenya. *BioMed Research International*, *2015*, 903025. doi:1155/2015/903025.

Charmaz, K. (2003). Grounded theory: Objectivist and constructivist methods. In N. K. Denzin & Y. S. Lincoln (Eds.), *Handbook of qualitative research*. Thousand Oaks, CA: Sage.

Colaizzi, P. (1978). Psychological research as a phenomenologist views it. In R. S. Valle & M. King (Eds.), *Existential phenomenological alternatives for psychology*. New York, NY: Oxford University Press.

Cook, G., Thompson, J., & Reed, J. (2015). Reconceptualising the status of residents in a care home: Older people wanting to "live with care." *Ageing and Society*, *35*, 1587–1613.

Corbin, J., & Strauss, A. (2015). *Basics of qualitative research*. Los Angeles, CA: Sage.

Creswell, J. W. (2013). *Qualitative inquiry and research design: Choosing among five traditions*. Thousand Oaks, CA: Sage.

Creswell, J. W., & Plano-Clark, V. L. (2011). *Designing and conducting mixed methods research* (2nd ed.). Thousand Oakes, CA: Sage.

Denzin, N. K., & Lincoln, Y. S. (2003). *The landscape of qualitative research*. Thousand Oaks, CA: Sage.

Fleming, A., Bradley, C., Cullinan, S., et al. (2015). Antibiotic prescribing in long-term care facilities: A meta-synthesis of qualitative research. *Drugs & Aging*, *32*(4), 295–303. doi:10.1007/s40266-015-0252-2.

Fontana, J. S. (2004). A methodology for critical science in nursing. *Advances in Nursing Science*, *27*(2), 93–101.

Glaser, B. G., & Strauss, A. L. (1967). *The discovery of grounded theory: Strategies for qualitative research*. Chicago, IL: Aldine.

Grassley, J. S., Clark, M., & Schleis, J. (2015). An institutional ethnography of nurses' support of breastfeeding on the night shift. *Journal of Obstetric, Gynecologic & Neonatal Nursing*, *44*, 567–577.

Guba, E., & Lincoln, Y. (1981). *Effective evaluation*. San Francisco, CA: Jossey-Bass.

Holkup, P. A., Tripp-Reimer, T., Salois, E. M., et al. (2004). Community-based participatory research: An approach to intervention research with a Native American community. *ANS Advance in Nursing Science*, *27*(3), 162–175.

Hyatt, K. S., Davis, L. L., & Barroso, J. (2015). Finding the new normal: Accepting changes after combat-related mild traumatic brain injury. *Journal of Nursing Scholarship*, *47*, 300–309.
Kleinman, A. (1992). Local worlds of suffering: An interpersonal focus for ethnographies of illness experience. *Qualitative Health Research*, *2*(2), 127–134.
Marshall, C., & Rossman, G. B. (2011). *Designing qualitative research* (5th ed.). Los Angeles, CA: Sage.
Mead, M. (1949). *Coming of age in Samoa*. New York, NY: New American Library, Mentor Books.
Morse, J. M. (1998). The contracted relationship: Ensuring protection of anonymity and confidentiality. *Qualitative Health Research*, *8*(3), 301–303.
Richards, L., & Morse, J. M. (2013). *Read me first for a user's guide to qualitative methods* (2nd ed.). Los Angeles, CA: Sage.
Sandelowski, M. (2004). Using qualitative research. *Qualitative Health Research*, *14*(10), 1366–1386.
Sandelowski, M., & Barroso, J. (2003a). Creating metasummaries of qualitative findings. *Nursing Research*, *52*, 226–233.
Sandelowski, M., & Barroso, J. (2003b). Toward a metasynthesis of qualitative findings on motherhood in HIV-positive women. *Research in Nursing & Health*, *26*, 153–170.
Sandelowski, M., & Barroso, J. (2005). The travesty of choosing after positive prenatal diagnosis. *Journal of Obstetric, Gynecologic, and Neonatal Nursing*, *34*(4), 307–318.
Sandelowski, M., & Barroso, J. (2007). *Handbook for synthesizing qualitative research*. Philadelphia, PA: Springer.
Silverman, D., & Marvasti, A. (2008). *Doing qualitative research*. Los Angeles, CA: Sage.
Smith, M. J., & Liehr, P. (2003). The theory of attentively embracing story. In M. J. Smith & P. Liehr (Eds.), *Middle range theory for nursing*. New York, NY: Springer.
Stake, R. E. (1995). *The art of case study research*. Thousand Oaks, CA: Sage.
Stake, R. E. (2000). Case studies. In N. K. Denzin & Y. S. Lincoln (Eds.), *Handbook of qualitative research* (2nd ed.). Thousand Oaks, CA: Sage.
Strauss, A. L. (1987). *Qualitative analysis for social scientists*. New York, NY: Cambridge University Press.
Strauss, A., & Corbin, J. (1990). *Basics of qualitative research: Grounded theory procedures and techniques*. Newbury Park, CA: Sage.
Strauss, A., & Corbin, J. (1994). Grounded theory methodology. In N. K. Denzin & Y. S. Lincoln (Eds.), *Handbook of qualitative research*. Thousand Oaks, CA: Sage.
Strauss, A., & Corbin, J. (Eds.), (1997). *Grounded theory in practice*. Thousand Oaks, CA: Sage.
Stringer, E. T. (1999). *Action research* (2nd ed.). Thousand Oaks, CA: Sage.
Tedlock, B. (2003). Ethnography and ethnographic representation. In N. K. Denzin & Y. S. Lincoln (Eds.), *Handbook of qualitative research*. Thousand Oaks, CA: Sage.
Vidick, A. J., & Lyman, S. M. (1998). Qualitative methods: their history in sociology and anthropology. In N. K. Denzin & Y. S. Lincoln (Eds.), *The landscape of qualitative research: Theories and issues*. Thousand Oaks, CA: Sage.
Walker, R., Szanton, S. L., & Wenzel, J. (2015). Working toward normalcy post-treatment: A qualitative study of older adult breast and prostate cancer survivors. *Oncology Nursing Forum*, *42*(6), 358–367.

Go to Evolve at **http://evolve.elsevier.com/LoBiondo/** for review questions, critiquing exercises, and additional research articles for practice in reviewing and critiquing.

7

Appraising Qualitative Research

Dona Rinaldi Carpenter

Go to Evolve at **http://evolve.elsevier.com/LoBiondo/** for review questions, critiquing exercises, and additional research articles for practice in reviewing and critiquing.

LEARNING OUTCOMES

After reading this chapter, you should be able to do the following:

- Understand the role of critical appraisal in research and evidence-based practice.
- Identify the criteria for critiquing a qualitative research study.
- Identify the stylistic considerations in a qualitative study.
- Apply critical reading skills to the appraisal of qualitative research.
- Evaluate the strengths and weaknesses of a qualitative study.
- Describe applicability of the findings of a qualitative study.
- Construct a written critique of a qualitative study.

KEY TERMS

bracketing	auditability	phenomena	theme
phenomenology	credibility	saturation	trustworthiness

Qualitative and quantitative research methods vary in terms of purpose, approach, analysis, and conclusions. Therefore, the use of each requires an understanding of the traditions on which the methods are based. This chapter aims to provide a set of criteria that can be used to critique qualitative research studies through a process of critical analysis and evaluation.

The critical appraisal of qualitative research continues to be discussed in nursing and related health care professions, providing a framework that includes key concepts for evaluation (Beck, 2009; Bigby, 2015; Flannery, 2016; Horsburgh, 2003; Ingham-Broomfield, 2015; Pearson et al., 2015; Russell & Gregory, 2003; Sandelowski, 2015; Williams, 2015).

CRITICAL APPRAISAL AND QUALITATIVE RESEARCH CONSIDERATIONS

Qualitative research represents a basic level of inquiry that seeks to discover and understand concepts, phenomena, or cultures. In a qualitative study, you should not expect to find hypotheses; theoretical frameworks; dependent and independent variables; large, random samples; complex statistical procedures; scaled instruments; or definitive conclusions about how to use the findings. A primary reason for conducting a qualitative study is to develop a theory or to discover knowledge about a phenomenon. Sample size is expected to be small. This type of research is not generalizable, nor should it be. Findings are presented in a narrative format with raw data used to illustrate identified **themes**. Thick, rich data are essential in order to document the rigor of the research, which is called **trustworthiness** in a qualitative research study. Ensuring trustworthiness in qualitative inquiry is critical, as qualitative researchers seek to have their work recognized in an evidence-driven world (Beck, 2009; Bigby, 2015).

APPLICATION OF QUALITATIVE RESEARCH FINDINGS

The purpose of qualitative research is to describe, understand, or explain phenomenon important to nursing. **Phenomena** are those things that are perceived by our senses. For example, pain and losing a loved one are considered phenomena. In a qualitative study, the researcher gathers narrative data that uses the participants' voices and experiences to describe the phenomenon under investigation. Barbour and Barbour (2003) offer that qualitative research can provide the opportunity to give voice to those who have been disenfranchised and have no history. Therefore, the application of qualitative findings will necessarily be context-bound (Russell & Gregory, 2003).

Qualitative research also has the ability to contribute to evidenced-based practice literature (Anthony & Jack, 2009; Cesario et al., 2002; Donnelly & Wiechula, 2013; Walsh & Downe, 2005). Describing the lived human experience of patients can contribute to the improvement of care, adding a dimension of understanding to our work as it is described by those who live it on a day-to-day basis. Fundamentally, principles for evaluating qualitative research are the same. Reviewers are concerned with the plausibility and trustworthiness of the researcher's account of the findings and its potential and/or actual relevance to current or future theory and practice (Horsburgh, 2003; Ingham-Bloomfield, 2015; Pearson et al., 2015; Sandelowski, 2015; Williams, 2015). As a framework for understanding how the appraisal of qualitative research can support evidence-based practice, a published research report and critical appraisal criteria follow (Table 7.1). The critical appraisal

TABLE 7.1 Critical Appraisal of Qualitative Research

Elements of style	1. Was there sufficient detail to enable critical appraisal? 2. Is there evidence that the researcher has the qualifications, knowledge, and expertise to conduct the research? 3. Does the abstract give a clear summary of the study, including the research problem, sample, methodology, findings, and recommendations? 4. Is the title clear, accurate, and reflective of the topic and method?
Statement of the phenomenon of interest	1. Was the title clear, accurate, and related to the research question? 2. What is the phenomenon of interest and is it clearly stated for the reader? 3. What is the justification for using a qualitative method? 4. What are the philosophical underpinnings of the research method?
Purpose	1. What is the purpose of the study? 2. What is the projected significance of the work to nursing?

Continued

TABLE 7.1 Critical Appraisal of Qualitative Research—cont'd

Ethical considerations	1. Is protection of human participants addressed? 2. Did the author address IRB approval? 3. Were the participants fully informed about the nature of the research? 4. Did the researcher address participant autonomy and confidentiality?
Method	1. Is the method used to collect data compatible with the purpose of the research? 2. Is the method adequate to address the phenomenon of interest? 3. If a particular approach is used to guide the inquiry, does the researcher complete the study according to the processes described?
Sampling	1. What type of sampling is used? Is it appropriate, given the particular method? 2. Are the informants who were chosen appropriate to inform the research? 3. Were the participants and setting adequately described and appropriate for informing the research? 4. Was saturation achieved?
Data collection	1. Is data collection focused on human experience? 2. Does the researcher describe data collection strategies (i.e., interview, observation, field notes)? 3. Were the data gathered of sufficient depth and richness? 4. Were the questions asked and observations made and recorded in an appropriate way? 5. Is saturation of the data described? 6. What are the procedures for collecting data?
Data analysis	1. What strategies are used to analyze the data? 2. Has the researcher remained true to the data? 3. Is there a logical connection between raw data and themes? 4. Does the reader follow the steps described for data analysis?
Authenticity and trustworthiness of data	1. Does the researcher address the credibility, auditability, and transferability of the data? Credibility • Were the study purpose and method clearly described? • Do the participants recognize the experience as their own? • Has adequate time been allowed to fully understand the phenomenon? Auditability • Can the reader follow the researcher's thinking? • Does the researcher document the research process? • Is there a logical connection between data and themes? • Is there a clear description of findings? • Is there agreement between the findings of the study and the conclusions? Transferability • Are the findings applicable outside of the study situation? • Was the selection of participants described? • Did participants fit the context of the study? • Are the results meaningful to individuals not involved in the research? • Is the strategy used for analysis compatible with the purpose of the study?
Findings	1. Are the findings presented within a context? 2. Is the reader able to apprehend the essence of the experience from the report of the findings? 3. Are the researcher's conceptualizations true to the data? 4. Does the researcher place the report in the context of what is already known about the phenomenon? Was the existing literature on the topic related to the findings?
Conclusions, implications, and recommendations	1. Do the conclusions, implications, and recommendations give the reader a context in which to use the findings? 2. How do the conclusions reflect the study findings? 3. What are the recommendations for future study? Do they reflect the findings? 4. How has the researcher made explicit the significance of the study to nursing theory, research, or practice?

criteria will be used to demonstrate the process of appraising a qualitative research report. For information on specific guidelines for appraisal of phenomenology, ethnography, grounded theory, and action research, see Chapters 5 and 6 and Streubert and Carpenter (2011).

CRITICAL APPRAISAL CRITERIA

Qualitative Research Study

As evidenced by published works, **phenomenology** is one approach to qualitative research. From a nursing perspective, qualitative research allows caregivers to understand the life experience of the patients they care for. Excerpts from "A Woman's Experience: Living With an Implantable Cardioverter Defibrillator" by Jaclyn Conelius are provided throughout this chapter as examples of phenomenological research. The article was published in *Applied Nursing Research* in 2015. The following sections critique Conelius's study. The primary purpose of this critique is to carefully examine how each step of the research process has been articulated in the study and to examine how the research has contributed to nursing knowledge. The article by Conelius (2015) provides an example of a phenomenological study true to qualitative methods.

CRITIQUE OF A QUALITATIVE RESEARCH STUDY

THE RESEARCH STUDY

The study "A Woman's Experience: Living With an Implantable Cardioverter Defibrillator" by Jaclyn Conelius, published in *Applied Nursing Research,* is critiqued. The article is presented in its entirety and followed by the critique.

A Woman's Experience: Living with an Implantable Cardioverter Defibrillator

Jaclyn Conelius, PhD, FNP-BC

Abstract

The implantable cardioverter defibrillators (ICD) have decreased mortality rates from those who are at risk for sudden cardiac death or who have survived sudden cardiac death and has been shown to be superior to antiarrhythmic medications (Greenburg et al., 2004). This advance in technology may improve physical health but can impose some challenges to patients, such as depression, anxiety, fear, and unpredictability. Published research on how ICD affects a woman's life experience using phenomenology is limited. Therefore, the purpose of this article is to describe the experiences of women who have an ICD using Colaizzi's method of phenomenology since their implant. Analysis of the three interviews resulted in five themes that described the essence of this experience. The results of this study could not only help clinicians understand what their patients are experiencing but also it can be used as an education tool.

Introduction

Implantable cardioverter defibrillators (ICDs) have decreased mortality rates from those who are at risk for sudden cardiac death or who have survived sudden cardiac death and has been shown to be superior to anti-arrhythmic medications (Greenburg et al., 2004). ICDs have been supported by many clinical trials and it is now the treatment of choice in primary and secondary prevention for these patients (Bardy et al., 2005; Bristow et al., 2004; Moss et al., 2002). This mainstay of treatment has increased steadily from 486,025 implants from 2006 to 2009 to 850,068 from 2010 to 2011 (Hammill et al., 2010; Kremers et al., 2013). Of these implants approximately 28% were female only.

This advance in technology may improve physical health but can impose some challenges to patients. They include the adjustments to the device in their everyday living, such as; quality of life issues as well as psychological issues. Through quantitative research the following have been reported; a fear of physical activity and a fear of shock from the device to prevent the sudden cardiac arrest (Lampert et al., 2002; Wallace et al., 2002; Whang et al., 2005). Other studies have reported anxiety, fear, and depression in these patients. Some specific fears included; malfunctioning, unpredictability, and the inability to control events (Dickerson, 2005; Dunbar, 2005; Eckert & Jones, 2002; Kamphuis et al., 2004; Lemon, Edelman, & Kirkness, 2004). These quality of life and psychological issues reported in the studies are not reported as gender specific; therefore, female specific challenges are not well studied. Furthermore, there have been few qualitative studies based on a patient's experience of living with an ICD. Previous studies reported themes such as the feeling of gratitude, safety, belief in the future, adjustment to the device, lifesaving yet changing, fear of receiving a shock, physical/mental deterioration, confrontation with mortality and conditional acceptance (Dickerson, 2002; Fridlund et al., 2000; Kamphuis et al., 2004; Morken, Severinsson, & Karlsen, 2009; Tagney, James, & Alberran, 2003).

Based on the available research studies, there is very little reported data specific to females and specifically how an ICD affects a woman's lived experience. A lived experience is how a person immediately experiences the world (Husserl, 1970). In order to understand a woman's lived experience living with an ICD, phenomenology was used. Phenomenology is a philosophy and a research method used to understand everyday lived experiences. Therefore, the purpose of this study was to describe what those experiences were, specifically, to describe their thoughts, feelings, and perceptions that they have experienced since their implant. It is important to gain an understanding and formulate a description of what life is for a woman who had received an implantable cardioverter defibrillator in order to describe the universal essence of that experience. Descriptive phenomenology emphasizes describing universal essences, viewing the person as one representative of the world in which she lives, an assumption of self-reflection, a belief that the consciousness is what people share and a belief that stripping of previous knowledge (bracketing) helps prevent investigator bias and interpretation bias (Wojnar & Swanson, 2007). Specifically, Colaizzi's (1978) descriptive phenomenological method uses seven steps as a method of analyzing data so that by the end of the study a description of the lived experience could be reported.

Method

Descriptive phenomenology originated from the philosopher Husserl (1970), who believed that the meaning of a lived experience may be discovered though one to one interaction between the researcher and the subject. It assumes that for any human experience, there are distinct structures that make up the phenomenon. Studying the individual experiences highlights these essential structures. It is an inductive method that describes a phenomenon as it is experienced by an individual rather than by transforming it into an operationally defined behavior. An important aspect of descriptive phenomenology, according to

Husserl, is the process of bracketing in which he describes as separating the phenomenon from the world and having the researcher suspend all preconceptions (Wojnar & Swanson, 2007). The goal of descriptive phenomenology is to provide a universal description of the lived experience as described by the participants of the phenomenon. Colaizzi's (1978) method of descriptive phenomenology is the method used for this study. In his method, interviewing is the selected strategy for collecting data, which is necessary for describing an experience. This method works well with a small sample size.

Sample. Ten women were asked to participate, of these, three women agreed to participate from a private cardiology office in the United States. This convenient sample of women were all Caucasian and their ages ranged from 34 to 50 years old. All three women had college degrees and have had the device over one year. None of the women were previously diagnosed with any psychiatric disease.

Procedure. After receiving approval from the university's institutional review board (IRB), women were recruited from a private cardiology office in the United States for 4 months. The participant population only included women that had an implantable cardioverter defibrillator (ICD). Women needed to be 18 years or older, and speak English. Women of all ethnic backgrounds were eligible to participate. There was no cost to the participant and no compensation provided. Once the informed consent was signed, they were asked to stay for an interview that day. All women were interviewed privately in the office and each interview lasted approximately 45 minutes to an hour. They were asked to "describe their experiences after having received an ICD, specifically, to describe their thoughts, feelings, and perceptions that they had experienced since their implant?" They were then asked to share as much of those experiences to the point that they did not have anything else to contribute. The interviews were recorded and then transcribed. The researcher conducted all of the interviews since the researcher in trained in the method. Interviews were conducted until an accurate description of the phenomenon had occurred, repetition of data and no new themes where described. This saturation of data did occurs after the three interviews. After each interview, follow up questions were asked in order to clarify any points the participant described. The researcher kept a journal to write down any notes needed during the interview.

In order for the description to be pure, the researcher's prior knowledge was bracketed to capture the essence of the description without bias (Wojnar & Swanson, 2007). Husserl (1970) introduced the term, and it means to set aside one's own assumption and preunderstanding. In order to be true to the method, the researcher reflected and kept a journal of all assumptions, clinical experiences, understandings and biases to reference during the entire study.

Significant statements and phrases pertaining to a woman's experience living with an ICD were extracted from each transcript. These statements were written on separate sheets and coded. Meanings were formulated from the significant statements. Accordingly, each underlying meaning was coded into a specific category as it reflected an exhaustive description. Then the significant statements with the formulated meanings where grouped into themes.

To ensure confidentiality, the signed informed consent forms were kept separate from the transcripts. The recorded tapes and hard copy were in a locked cabinet. Identifying information was deleted and names were never used in any research reports. Audiotapes were destroyed once the pilot study was completed.

Data Analysis. Each transcript was analyzed using Colaizzi's (1978) method. The method of data analysis consisted of the following steps; (1) read all the participants' descriptions of the phenomenon, (2) extract significant statements that pertain directly to the phenomenon, (3) formulate meanings for each significant statement, (4) categorizing into clusters of themes and validation with the original transcript, (5) describing, (6) validate the description by returning to the participant to ask them how it compares with their experience, and (7) incorporate any changes offered by the participant into the final description of the essence of the phenomenon.

Rigor. There were efforts made to limit any potential bias of the researcher. One such effort was to bracket any of the researcher's prior perspective and knowledge of the subject (Aher, 1999). To ensure the credibility of the data collected, two of the women in the study reviewed the description of the lived experiences as suggested by Lincoln and Guba (1985). This was performed as a validity check of the data. In order to address for auditability, a tape recorder was used and the researcher reviewed the transcripts and cross-referenced the field noted (Beck, 1993).

Additionally, the transcripts were transcribed verbatim by a secretary in order to ensure they were free of bias. Also, the data analysis and description of the lived experience were reviewed by an independent judge with phenomenological experience to ensure intersubjective agreement. All of the themes reported were agreed upon by the judge.

Finally, the researcher validated the description by returning to the participants to ask them how it compared with their experience and incorporated any changes offered by the participants into the final description of the essence of the phenomenon. This final description was reviewed by other women with ICDs who were not a part of the study to ensure fittingness.

Results

At the conclusion of verifying and reviewing the transcripts, there were 46 significant statements extracted that pertained directly to the phenomenon. From each significant statement formulated meanings were created. These statements were then formed into five themes (Table 1) that described the essence of these experiences.

Theme 1: Security Blanket: If it Keeps me Alive it's Worth it. Women who had an ICD felt a sense of security with the device. They felt that this device acted as a security blanket. Prior to their device they had a constant worry about how soon they could get medical treatment and now that they had the device, that worry was lifted. The feeling of worry was no longer apparent for them. One woman said:

> *Now I just think this will keep me alive long enough for somebody to make a decision, at least it will give me a chance. I do not have anything to worry about anymore. I used to worry that if something happened, how soon I could get to a hospital or what could they do to try to save me.*

The women also described how their worry decreased should they require medical treatment while they were with their family also was decreased. "Now I do not have to worry if I am with my family, I have ICD in my chest to give me treatment right away."

Another woman felt that the device just being there saved her life. "If the device can save her life it's worth it." The device prevents the heart from having sustained lethal arrhythmias. She explained: "I feel like it saved my life, I feel like it keeps my heart beating nice and smooth."

There was an overall feeling that the device improved their lives. Based on their past medical history, the device was needed since it is the next step in their medical

TABLE 1 Selected Examples of Significant Statements and their Formulated Meaning for Five Themes

Theme Number	Significant Statement	Formulated Meaning
1 Security blanket: If it keeps me alive It's worth it.	"I do not have anything to worry about anymore. I used to worry that if something happened, how soon I can get to a hospital or what could they do to try to save me."	The women did not have to worry anymore about medical emergencies.
2 A piece of cake: I do more than before.	"Actually, I probably do a little more than before. But I can do everything that I did before. I have not eased up on anything."	She felt as if nothing has changed. She does everything she did prior.
3 A constant reminder: I know it's there.	"The children sometimes bump into that side and I am literally guarding that side all the time."	She is aware of it and guards it when others come in contact with it.
4 Living on the edge: I do not want it to go off.	"I do have a little fear of that but so far, it hasn't happened."	She has an extreme fear of the device shocking her.
5 Catch 22: I'd rather not have it.	"I would rather not personally have it but I know medically, I need to have it, which is a good thing."	She would rather not have to have it, but she knows she needs it.

treatment. All the women were glad they were able to receive the device. One woman explained:

It could be both ways. I mean, I feel knowing what my family history is, yeah, I am glad I have it. I needed it. It made me feel that I can go anywhere and do anything because it acts like my insurance policy.

Theme 2: A Piece of Cake: I do more than before. The women did not have a decrease in physical functioning or quality of life. Their quality of life remained stable or improved once the post operative period was over.

One woman explained:

Actually, I probably do a little more than before. But I can do everything that I did before. I have not eased up on anything. I felt like after the surgery, I was tired for 2 days then I could go on and do everything I used to do; now I do not even think about it. I just go about my day as usual and even do more because I know I have this to protect me.

The women felt that the whole process of receiving an ICD was easy. Nothing much changed in their everyday lives. They live and do everything that they did before with no restrictions.

Another woman shared,

After that, I really have had no change in lifestyle. My life has been as normal as it was before. Physically, I see no change, or even see an improvement.

Theme 3: A Constant Reminder. I know it's there. The women felt as if they had a constant reminder of the ICD. Their family was aware of the device in their body since they can see the scar. Some family members would comment on the device if they could feel it when given a hug. This in turn would remind the women that it was there. The device did affect their body image; it made them more conscious of the device in their chest.

One woman with school aged children explained:

> *And it is hard when the kids cuddle up to me and I have to say I can't have you on my left side anymore. With four kids, you know the pile up, at least the two youngest ones, they want to lie next to me while watching TV or when we are praying or reading books or doing anything. I have to remind them that you can't put your head up there. The children sometimes bump into that side and I am literally guarding that side all the time.*

The most amount of pain that women had experienced was postoperative. After that, it varied when the pain decreased. The actual incision is "hardly noticeable" in all of the women although the knowledge that the device is in fact in their chest is a "constant reminder." The degree at which it reminds them varies depending on body type.

One woman stated: "I am reminded of this all the time, I can feel it, I know it is there. Everyday activities like opening a jar, it pops and moves. Anytime I use my pectoral muscle, I know it is there, which is a lot of what I do during the day, like laundry."

Another woman stated: "The only thing that bothers me a little bit sometimes, it feels like it moves in my chest when I am in bed. When I lay a certain way it sometimes feels like it is popping out or something."

> *Yeah, I mean just being that it is there and it should not be there and it shows itself all the time. I especially know it's there in the summer when you were fewer clothes, especially bathing suits. To me it is constant reminder that I may feel fine, but I am technically sick.*

Theme 4: Living on the Edge. I do not want it to go off. All of the women had a common fear that was constantly in their thoughts. They feared that the device would have to do its job; it would have to "fire." They did not want this fear to become a reality. They feared that they would be somewhere in public and the device would have to administer therapy or shock them. The women stated such things as:

> *I do have a little fear of that but so far, it hasn't happened. Oh! I don't want it to go off!*
> *I am completely scared it will go off and no one will know what the heck happened.*

The fear of the device firing has a significant impact on these women. The most concerning part, is the wonder on what it will actually feel like, the uncertainty. These women could not possibly know how it would feel like since none of them have ever received a shock. They have been told that it feels like an "animal kicking you in the chest." None of them to date have yet to experience it. To them that is unimaginable until it becomes a reality.

> *I am scared. I am afraid it is going to kick off and I was told it would feel like a pair of boots kicking you in the chest. And I am afraid, but it has never gone off. You know, I am wondering what it would feel like. The doctor explained it almost like getting kicked in the chest by a horse. Well, that would be a jolt, I guess? I am afraid that I will be doing something, not feel anything, then all of a sudden boom!*

Theme 5: Catch 22: I'd Rather Not Have It. The women received these ICDs because it was medically necessary for them to have it based on the current guidelines. They have various cardiac medical conditions that require an implant of a defibrillator. The women understood that it was essential and yet they would rather not have had to go through it. They would rather not have the heart disease that comes with needing the device.

> *I would rather not personally have it but I know it is medically, I need to have it, which is a good thing that I have it. Mentally it bothers me, mentally; I know I cannot avoid it.*

The women felt that the experience was depressing. They were mostly depressed immediately preceding the implantation. Although, it had decreased over time, there was a constant reminder of the device still there. They needed to adjust to the device, which was hard for them. They felt as if they had no choice to adjust to this new situation.

One woman explained:

> *Well, I have adjusted to it, I had no choice. But in another aspect, no, I would rather not be going through this. Interestingly, no one has ever asked me how I feel about having one before. I just got it and the doctor does not even ask me about it. I mean it comes and goes, because a lot of things I know are happening are like, it could get depressing. I do feel anxious at times, then I feel depressed at times, then I am fine at times. So, I guess it depends on what is going on.*

Discussion

Aspects of the five themes that describe the essence of a woman's experience living with an ICD have been reported in previous studies, but nowhere is there a study that is an exact comparison to this study. For instance, theme 1 (security blanket: if it keeps me alive it's worth it) is similar to the concept in Fridlund et al. (2000), a feeling of gratitude, and a feeling of safety. The women in this study expressed a feeling of safety and appreciation since they received their ICDs. This sense of safety and trust in the device is consistent with other studies (Bilge et al., 2006; Dickerson, 2002; Morken et al., 2009).

Contrary to what is found in the literature, the women in this study reported how they have more energy than before and noticed an actual increase in physical functioning. Previous studies have identified decreased physical functioning (Dickerson, 2005; Kamphuis et al., 2004; Williams, Young, Nikoletti, & McRae, 2007) and a decrease in activity levels in their day-to-day lives (Bolse, Hamilton, Flanangan, Caroll, & Fridlund, 2005; Eckert & Jones, 2002). This contradiction can be related to the types of studies conducted. Previous studies have used questionnaires while this study focused on actual descriptions experienced by participants who had undergone the device implant.

Theme 3 (a constant reminder: I know it's there) described the women "knowing that the device was in their chest," and it was a reminder of their condition. They also described how it affected their body image. There were two other studies that had mentioned this as a concern for women. One study by Walker et al. (2004) reported body image concerns of women. The women in that study were more concerned on how the device appeared in their chest (i.e. the scar) than any other aspect. A second study by Tagney et al. (2003), also reported body image concerns in women since it can be seen in their chest which makes them aware of the device. There were similarities with respect to body image only. They were not concerned with the constant reminder aspect of the cardiac disease, only a constant reminder of their mortality (Dickerson, 2002).

The common concern as described in theme 4 (Living on the Edge: I do not want my device going off) was the fear of the device having to shock them as well as the uncertainty of when, where, and who would be around for support. This was foremost in their thoughts. There have been common themes of fear of the device going off or shocking them in the literature reviewed. Dickerson (2002, 2005) reported that uncertainty of when and where shocks can be triggered was a prevailing concern of the male and female participants. Also, participants in Albarran, Tagney, and James (2004) study reported a feeling of uncertainty regarding the device firing.

The prevailing concern in theme 5 (catch 22: I'd rather not have it.) is the conflict women have after receiving a device. These women knew that they medically needed the device yet would have rather not have gone through with it. Dickerson (2005) reported the theme of conditional acceptance that touches on the same concept. Also, a greater acceptance of the new situation was reported in previous studies (Carroll & Hamilton, 2005; Kamphuis et al., 2004).

The women in this study offered specific experiences of living with an ICD which is not completely seen in any previous study as stated previously. Moreover, there were some similar aspects identified in other studies such as receiving a shock and feeling of safety but most were not specific to women (Bilge et al., 2006; Dickerson, 2002, 2005; Morken et al., 2009). This study was able to describe the essence of women who are living with an ICD. As stated previously, the majority of the patients who receive ICD s are male and all of the samples in previous studies have been predominantly male. This study is specific to women and allows special insight to women who are living with cardiac disease and more specifically cardiac disease requiring a medical device.

Clinical Implications and Future Research

This study can have an impact on clinical practice as a whole by helping clinicians understand what their patients are experiencing. The women in this study stated that they experienced a lot of uncertainty regarding the need for the device and its functionality. This uncertainty can be reduced or eliminated by educating the patients with respect to how the device operates. An increase in education pre and post operatively on device functionality would benefit patients by relieving some of that uncertainty. These concerns are not being addressed properly in the healthcare system. This study can help clinicians gain the understanding of the experience these women are having and perhaps pay closer attention to these issues when they are seen in outpatient settings.

Furthermore, this study can also advocate for support groups for women. Support groups would allow these patients to converse with other women with the same health condition. There are multiple studies in the literature regarding the use of support groups in heart failure patients, however, there are very few studies involving patients with ICDs. Support groups can expose women to different types of resources in order to cope better, decrease anxiety and answer any questions that arise (Myers & James, 2008). Also, it would give them a security knowing that they would be able to have each other as a support system.

The women in this study were similar in that they were Caucasian from affluent areas with numerous resources available to them (Smeulders et al., 2010). An additional study involving women of various ethnical backgrounds and ages would allow capture of a wider range of experiences. Also, since the women have an outstanding fear of the device firing/shocking them, a noteworthy follow-up study would be to describe their experience post firing/shock. These studies would help clinicians understand what their patients are experiencing. It would allow them to be more empathetic and identify the gaps in knowledge. The results would become a valuable teaching tool to help educate patients regarding their device function.

REFERENCES

Aher, K. (1999). Pearls, pith, and provocation: Ten tips forreflexive bracketing. *Qualitative Health Research, 9*, 407–411.

Albarran, J. W., Tagney, J., & James, J. (2004). Partners of ICD patients—An exploratory study of their experiences. *European Journal of Cardiovascular Nursing, 3*(3), 201–210.

Bardy, G. H., Lee, K. L., Mark, D. B., Poole, J. E., Packer, D. L., Boineau, R., et al. (2005). Sudden Cardiac Death in Heart Failure (SCD-HeFT). *The New England Journal of Medicine, 352*(3), 225–237.

Beck, C. T. (1993). Qualitative research: Evaluation of its credibility, auditability, and fittingness. *Western Journal of NursingResearch, 15*, 263–26.

Bilge, A. K., Ozben, B., Demircan, S., Cinar, M., Yilmaz, E., & Adalet, K. (2006). Depression and anxiety status of patients with implantable cardioverter defibrillators and precipitating factors. *Pacing and Clinical Electrophysiology, 29*, 619–626.

Bolse, K., Hamilton, G., Flanangan, J., Caroll, D. L, & Fridlund, B. (2005). Ways of experiencing the life situation among United States patients with an implantable cardioverter defibrillator: A qualitative study. *Progress in CardiovascularNursing, 20*, 4–10.

Bristow, M. R., Saxon, L. A., Boechmer, J., Krueger, S., Kass, D. A., DeMarco, T., et al. (2004). Cardiac-resynchronization therapy with or without an implantable cardioverter in advanced chronic heart failure. *The New England Journal of Medicine, 250*, 2140–2150.

Carroll, D. L., & Hamilton, G. A. (2005). Long-term effects of implanted cardioverter- defibrillators on health status, quality of life, and psychological state. *American Journal of Critical Care, 17*, 222–230.

Colaizzi, P. (1978). Psychological research as the phenomenologist view it. In R. Valle, & M. King (Eds.), *Existential phenomenological alternatives for psychology* (pp. 48–71). New York: Oxford University Press.

Dickerson, S. (2002). Redefining life while forestalling death: Living an implantable cardioverter defibrillator after a sudden cardiac death experience. *Qualitative Health Research, 12*, 360–372.

Dickerson, S. (2005). Technology-patient interactions: Internet use for gaining a healthy context for living with an implantable cardioverter defibrillator. *Heart & Lung, 34*(3), 157–168.

Dunbar, S. B. (2005). Psychological signs of patients with implantable cardioverter defibrillators. *American Journal of Critical Care, 14*(4), 294–303.

Eckert, M., & Jones, T. (2002). How does an implantable cardioverter defibrillator (ICD) affect the lives of patients and their families? *International Journal of Nursing Practice, 8*(3), 152–157.

Fridlund, B., Lindgren, E., Ivarson, A., Jinhage, B. B., Bolse, K., Flemme, I., et al. (2000). Patients with implantable cardioverter defibrillators and their conceptions of the life situation: A qualitative analysis. *Journal of Clinical Nursing, 9*, 37–45.

Greenburg, H., Case, R. B., Moss, A. J., Brown, N. M., Carroll, E. R., Andrews, M. L., et al. (2004). Analysis of mortality events in the Multicenter Automatic Defibrillator Implantation Trial (MADIT-II). *Journal of the American College of Cardiology, 43*, 1429–1465.

Hammill, S. C, Kremers, M. S., Stevenson, L W., Heidenreich, P. A., Lang, C. M., Curtis, J. P., et al. (2010). Review of the Registry's fourth year, incorporating lead data and pediatric ICD procedures, and use as a national performance measure. *Heart Rhythm, 7*(9), 1340–1345.

Husserl, E. (1970). *Crisis of European sciences and transcendentalphenomenology*. Evanston: Northwestern University Press.

Kamphuis, H., Verhoeven, N., Leeuw, R., Derksen, R., Hauer, R., & Winnubst, J. A. (2004). ICD: A qualitative study of patient experience the first year after implantation. *Journal of Clinical Nursing, 13*(8), 1008–l031.

Kremers, M. S., Hammill, S. C., Berul, C. I., Koutras, C., Curtis, J. S., Wang, Y., et al. (2013). The National Registry Report: Version 2.1 including leads and pediatrics for years 2010 and 2011. *Heart Rhythm, 10*(4), 59–65.

Lampert, R., Joska, T., Burg, M. M., Batsford, W. P., McPherson, C. A., &Jain, D. (2002). Emotional and physical precipitants of ventricular arrhythmias. *Circulation, 106*, 1800–1805.

Lemon, J., Edelman, S., & Kirkness, A. (2004). Avoidance behaviors in patients with implantable cardioverter defibrillators. *Heart &Lung, 33*, 176–182.
Lincoln, Y., & Guba, E. (1985). *Naturalistic Inquiry*. Newbury Park: Sage Publications.
Morken, I., Severinsson, E., & Karlsen, B. (2009). Reconstructing unpredictability: Experiences of living with an implantable cardioverter defibrillator over time. *Journal of Clinical Nursing, 19*, 537–546.
Moss, A., Zareba, W., Hall, J., Klein, H., Wilbur, D., Cannom, D., et al. (2002). Prophylactic implantation of a defibrillator in patients with myocardial infarction and reduced ejection fraction. *The New England Journal of Medicine, 346*, 877–883.
Myers, G. M., & James, G. D. (2008). Social support, anxiety, and support group participation in patients with an implantable cardioverter defibrillator. *Progress in Cardiovascular Nursing, 23*, 160–167.
Smeulders, J., van Haastregt, T., Ambergen, T., Uszko-Lencer, N. H., Janssen-Boyne, J. J., Gorgeis, P., et al. (2010). Nurse-led self-management group programme for patients with congestive heart failure: Randomized control trial. *Journal of Advanced Nursing, 66*, 1487–1499.
Tagney, J., James, J., & Alberran, J. (2003). Exploring the patient's experiences of learning to live with an implantable cardioverter defibrillator (ICD) from one UK centre: A qualitative study. *European Journal of Cardiovascular Nursing, 2*, 195–203.
Walker, R., Campell, K., Sears, S., Glenn, B., Sotile, R., Curtis, A., et al. (2004). Women and the implantable cardioverter defibrillator: A lifespan perspective on key psychological issues. *Clinical Cardiology, 27*, 543–546.
Wallace, B., Sears, S., Lewis, T., Griffis, J., Curtis, A., & Conti, J. (2002). Predictors of quality of life in long-term recipients of implantable cardioverter defibrillators. *Journal of Cardiopulmonary Rehabilitation, 22*, 278–281.
Whang, W., Albert, C. M., Sears, S. F., Lampert, R., Conti, J. B., Wang, P. J., et al. (2005). Depression as a predictor for appropriate shocks among patients with implantable cardioverter defibrillators: Results from the Triggers of Ventricular Arrhythmias (TOVA) study. *Journal of the American College of Cardiology, 45*, 1090–1095.
Williams, A. M., Young, J., Nikoletti, S., & McRae, S. (2007). Getting on with life; Accepting the permanency of an implantable cardioverter defibrillator. *International Journal of Nursing Practice, 13*, 166–172.
Wojnar, D. M., & Swanson, K. M. (2007). Phenomenology: An exploration. *Journal of Holistic Nursing, 25*, 172–180.

THE CRITIQUE

This is a critical appraisal of the article, "A Woman's Experience: Living With an Implantable Cardioverter Defibrillator" (Conelius, 2015) to determine its usefulness and applicability for nursing practice.

Abstract

The purpose of the abstract is to provide a clear overview of the study and summarize the main features of the findings and recommendations. The abstract should accurately represent the remainder of the article. Conelius (2015) summarized the research in the following narrative:

The implantable cardioverter defibrillators (ICD) have decreased mortality rates from those who are at risk for sudden cardiac death or who have survived sudden cardiac death and has been shown to be superior to antiarrhythmic medications (Greenburg et al., 2004). This advance in technology may improve physical health but can impose some challenges to patients, such as depression, anxiety, fear, and unpredictability. Published research on how an ICD affects a woman's life experience using phenomenology is limited. Therefore, the purpose of this article is to describe the experiences of women who have an ICD using Colaizzi's method of phenomenology since their implant. Analysis of the three interviews resulted in five themes that described the essence of this experience. The results of this study could not only help clinicians understand what their patients are experiencing but also it can be used as an education tool.

Introduction/Review of Literature

All research requires the investigator to review the literature. This is the point at which gaps are identified with regard to what is known about a particular topic and what is not known.

In qualitative research, the literature review is generally brief, because there is not a great deal known about the topic; nor is there an existing body of research studies. This essentially means that the researcher needs to have an understanding of the substantive body of knowledge on the topic and a clear perspective of what areas still need to be explored. A clear rationale for why the research is needed should be established. The researcher must be clear that a gap in nursing knowledge was identified, there is a clear need for the study, and the selected research method is appropriate. **Bracketing** what is known about the phenomenon is one way to prevent bias and keep what is known about the topic separate, prior to data collection and analysis (see Chapter 6). Conelius (2015) discusses bracketing in the data collection section of her research on women and implantable cardiac defibrillators. The background information provided in her introduction establishes a need for a qualitative study. Conelius (2015) emphasizes the fact that to date much of the research has been quantitative. She further notes that qualitative studies to date have not been gender specific, emphasizing the need for a study related to women's experiences.

Implantable cardioverter defibrillators (ICDs) have decreased mortality rates from those who are at risk for sudden cardiac death or who have survived sudden cardiac death and has been shown to be superior to anti-arrhythmic medications (Greenburg et al., 2004). ICDs have been supported by many clinical trials and it is now the treatment of choice in primary and secondary prevention for these patients (Bardy et al., 2005; Bristow et al., 2004; Moss et al., 2002). This mainstay of treatment has increased steadily from 486,025 implants from 2006 to 2009 to 850,068 from 2010 to 2011 (Hammill et al., 2010; Kremers et al., 2013). Of these implants approximately 28% were female only. (Conelius, 2015)

This advance in technology may improve physical health but can impose some challenges to patients. They include the adjustments to the device in their everyday living, such as; quality of life issues as well as psychological issues. Through quantitative research the following have been reported; a fear of physical activity and a fear of shock from the device to prevent the sudden cardiac arrest (Lampert et al., 2002; Wallace et al., 2002; Whang et al., 2005). Other studies have reported anxiety, fear, and depression in these patients. Some specific fears included; malfunctioning, unpredictability, and the inability to control events (Dickerson, 2005; Dunbar, 2005; Eckert & Jones, 2002; Kamphuis et al., 2004; Lemon, Edelman, & Kirkness, 2004). These quality of life and psychological issues reported in the studies are not reported as gender specific; therefore, female specific challenges are not well studied. Furthermore, there have been few qualitative studies based on a patient's experience of living with an ICD. Previous studies reported themes such as the feeling of gratitude, safety, belief in the future, adjustment to the device, lifesaving yet changing, fear of receiving a shock, physical/mental deterioration, confrontation with mortality and conditional acceptance (Dickerson, 2002; Fridlund et al., 2000; Kamphuis et al., 2004; Morken, Severinsson, & Karlsen, 2009; Tagney, James, & Alberran, 2003). Based on the available research studies, there is very little reported data specific to females and specifically how an ICD affects a woman's lived experience. (Conelius, 2015)

Phenomenology is a philosophy and a research method used to understand everyday lived experiences and is an appropriate methodology for the phenomena of interest. The subjective experience of women with an ICD is central to study and key to developing interventions to help these women cope. Conelius (2015) clearly articulates the focus of the study and makes a clear case for why a qualitative design is appropriate.

When critiquing the literature review of a qualitative study, it is important to remember that this component of the study must be critiqued within the context of the qualitative methodology selected. In phenomenological studies, the literature review may be delayed until the data analysis is complete in order to minimize bias. Conelius (2015) does not indicate that the review was delayed.

Philosophical Underpinnings

In addition to making a case for the study and qualitative approach, it is also important to give the reader perspective on the philosophical traditions of the method selected. Conelius (2015) describes the philosophical underpinnings of phenomenology and then relates the traditions to the method used in the study. In most published studies, the author is most concerned about sharing the findings of the study. This limits the space for in-depth literature reviews or discussion of the method used. Conelius (2015) discusses the work of Husserl (1970) as being an integral component of her philosophical grounding of phenomenology as method. She then connects this fundamental work to the method developed by Colaizzi (1978).

A lived experience is how a person immediately experiences the world (Husserl, 1970). In order to understand a woman's lived experience living with an ICD, phenomenology was used. Phenomenology is a philosophy and a research method used to understand everyday lived experiences. Descriptive phenomenology emphasizes describing universal essences, viewing the person as one representative of the world in which she lives, an assumption of self-reflection, a belief that the consciousness is what people share and a belief that stripping of previous knowledge (bracketing) helps prevent investigator bias and interpretation bias (Wojnar & Swanson, 2007). Specifically, Colaizzi's (1978) descriptive phenomenological method uses seven steps as a method of analyzing data so that by the end of the study a description of the lived experience could be reported. (Conelius, 2015)

The specific qualitative research approach selected helps determine the focus of the research and the manner in which sampling, data collection, and analysis are undertaken. The qualitative research example provided here used phenomenology as method. Research studies using a qualitative approach other than phenomenology should be critiqued relative to the philosophical underpinnings of the method.

Purpose

The author explained why the study was important and the significant contribution the study would make to nursing's body of knowledge. The background information justified the use of a qualitative approach as well as why phenomenology was used.

The researcher states that "The purpose of this study was to describe a woman's experience living with an ICD. More specifically to describe their thoughts, feelings and perceptions that they have experienced since their implant" (Conelius, 2015). The purpose is clearly articulated, first in the abstract and then in the introduction of the study. Conelius (2015) makes it clear that there is a gap in nursing knowledge related to ICDs and the experience of women living with an ICD.

Ethical Considerations

Addressing the ethical aspect of a research report involves being able to know whether participants were told what the research entailed, how their autonomy and confidentiality were protected, and what arrangements were made to avoid harm. In qualitative research the data collection tools generally include interview and participant observation, making anonymity impossible. Because the interviews are open-ended, the possibility of disclosing personal information or uncomfortable experiences related to the topic may occur. Consent must be a process of continuous negotiation (Oye et al., 2016).

The study by Conelius (2015) was approved by the Institutional Review Board. The author clearly states how the participants were protected. "To ensure confidentiality the signed informed consent forms were kept separate from the transcripts. The recorded tapes and hard copy were in a locked cabinet. Identifying information was deleted and names were never used in any research reports. Audiotapes were destroyed once the pilot study was completed" (Conelius, 2015). Participants were fully informed about the nature of the research and were protected from harm; their autonomy and confidentiality were protected.

Conelius (2015) also made clear to the participants that they had the right to withdraw from the research at any time. This is true for any research; however, in a qualitative investigation, ethical issues may arise at any point in the study (Hegney & Chan, 2010). Conelius (2015) clearly articulated the ethical rigor of this study.

Sample

In qualitative research, participants are recruited because of their life experience with the phenomena of interest. This is referred to as purposeful sampling. The goal is to ensure rich, thick data about the phenomenon of interest. Data are generally collected until no new material is emerging and data **saturation** has been reached. Cleary and colleagues (2014) discuss sampling in qualitative research in relationship to sample size. Qualitative studies generally have a small sample. Following the steps for sampling in qualitative research, Conelius (2015) offers the following information related to participant selection:

> *After receiving approval from the university's institutional review board (IRB), women were recruited from a private cardiology office in the United States for 4 months. The participant population only included women that had an implantable cardioverter defibrillator (ICD). Women needed to be 18 years or older, and speak English. Women of all ethnic backgrounds were eligible to participate. There was no cost to the participant and no compensation provided. Once the informed consent was signed, they were asked to stay for an interview that day. (Conelius, 2015)*

In qualitative research, purposive sampling is the approach of choice. Participants must have experience with the phenomenon of interest and be appropriate to inform the research. In this case, Conelius (2015) needed women with an ICD. Her selection process supports a qualitative sampling paradigm that is appropriate for phenomenology.

Data Generation

The data generation approach should be sufficiently described so that it is clear to the reader why a particular strategy was selected.

Conelius (2015) clearly articulates that the data generation method supports a qualitative paradigm and allows for discovery, description, and understanding of the participants' lived experience. The researcher uses open-ended questioning and asks each individual to exhaust their ideas and describe their experiences. She also completes three in-depth interviews with each participant, allowing for clarification of responses as well as an opportunity for the participants to add experiences that may have been omitted at the first interview. Recording and transcribing the interview verbatim helps maintain authenticity of the data. The following excerpts from the article illustrate these points:

> *All women were interviewed privately in the office and each interview lasted approximately 45 minutes to an hour. They were asked to "describe their experiences after having received an ICD, specifically, to describe their thoughts, feelings, and perceptions that they had experienced since their implant?" They were then asked to share as much of those experiences to the point that they did not have anything else to contribute. The interviews were recorded and then transcribed. The researcher conducted the interviews since the researcher was trained in the method. Interviews were conducted until an accurate description of the phenomenon had occurred, repetition of data and no new themes where described. This saturation of data did occur after the three interviews. (Conelius, 2015)*
>
> *The researcher kept a journal to write down any notes needed during the interview. "In order for the description to be pure, the researcher's prior knowledge was **bracketed** to capture the essence of the description without bias (Wojnar & Swanson, 2007). Husserl (1970) introduced the term, and it means to set aside one's own assumption and preunderstanding. In order to be true to the method, the researcher reflected and kept a journal of all assumptions, clinical experiences, understandings and biases to reference during the entire study. Significant statements and phrases pertaining to a woman's experience living with an ICD were extracted from each transcript. These statements were written on separate sheets and coded. Meanings were formulated from the significant statements. Accordingly, each underlying meaning was coded into a specific category as it reflected an exhaustive description. Then the significant statements with the formulated meanings where grouped into themes." (Conelius, 2015)*

Data generation was appropriate for this study and followed the steps described by Colaizzi (1978).

Data Analysis

The process of data analysis is fundamental to determining the credibility of qualitative research findings. Data analysis involves the transformation of raw data into a final description or narrative, identifying common thematic elements found in the raw data. The description should enable a reviewer to confirm the processes of concurrent data collection and analysis as well as steps in coding and identifying themes.

Data analysis followed the method described by Colaizzi (1978). The author developed a table to allow the reader to follow the line of thinking and establish thematic elements. The reader can clearly follow the researcher's stated processes. Further, Conelius (2015) followed clear processes to establish authenticity and trustworthiness of the data. The findings reported demonstrate the participants' realities. During data analysis the researcher made every effort to eliminate potential bias. Bracketing, verbatim transcription of taped interviews, and an independent reviewer were used to establish intersubjective agreement.

Authenticity and Trustworthiness

Critical to the meaning of the findings is the researcher's ability to demonstrate that the data were authentic and trustworthy or valid. Rigor ensures there is a correlation between the steps of the research process and the actual study. Procedural rigor relates to accuracy of data collection and analysis. Rigor or trustworthiness is a means of demonstrating the credibility and integrity of the qualitative research process (Cope, 2014). A study's rigor may be established if the reviewer is able to audit the actions and development of the researcher. It is at this point that the review of literature becomes critical and should be systematically related to the findings. This was addressed by the author, and every effort was clearly employed to reduce any bias or misinterpretation of findings.

Conelius (2015) was able to demonstrate rigor with regard to data analysis in multiple ways. She stated:

> *There were efforts made to limit any potential bias of the researcher. One such effort was to* **bracket** *any of the researcher's prior perspective and knowledge of the subject (Aher, 1999). To ensure the credibility of the data collected,* **two of the women in the study reviewed the description** *of the lived experiences as suggested by Lincoln and Guba (1985).*
>
> *This was performed as a validity check of the data. In order to address for* **auditability**, *a tape recorder was used and the research was reviewed the transcripts and cross-referenced the field noted (Beck, 1993). Additionally, the* **transcripts were transcribed verbatim** *by a secretary in order to ensure they were free of bias. The data analysis and description of the lived experience were reviewed by an independent judge with phenomenological experience to ensure* **intersubjective agreement**. *All of the themes reported were agreed upon by the judge. Finally, the researcher* **validated the description by returning to the participants** *to ask them how it compared with their experience and incorporated any changes offered by the participants into the final description of the essence of the phenomenon were created.*

Conelius (2015) provided clear evidence of rigor for the reader. Bracketing, having participants read the final description and thematic elements, taping and transcribing interviews verbatim, and using an independent judge to establish intersubjective agreement are key elements in a well done qualitative study. The author also left an audit trail illustrated in table format. This table establishes the researcher's line of thinking. Examples of how raw data lead to the identification of thematic elements were provided and further establish rigor for this study.

Findings, Conclusions, Implications, and Recommendations

Findings from a qualitative study generally are discussed in a narrative format that tells the story of the experience through an exhaustive description and thematic elements. Conelius

(2015) summarized conclusions, implications, and recommendations from the study. The findings were also compared to prior research studies. In qualitative research, this is the area that must include a comprehensive incorporation of current research on the topic. According to Conelius (2015):

*Aspects of the five themes that describe the essence of a woman's experience living with an ICD have been reported in previous studies, but nowhere is there a study that is an exact comparison to this study. For instance, theme 1 (***security blanket:** *if it keeps me alive it's worth It) is similar to the concept in Fridlund et al. (2000), a feeling of gratitude, and a feeling of safety. The women in this study expressed a feeling of safety and appreciation since they received their ICDs. This* **sense of safety and trust** *in the device is consistent with other studies. (Bilge et al., 2006; Dickerson, 2002; Morken et al., 2009)*

Contrary to what is found in the literature, the women in this study reported how they have **more energy** *than before and noticed an actual* **increase in physical functioning.** *Previous studies have identified decreased physical functioning (Dickerson, 2005; Kamphuis et al., 2004; Williams, Young, Nikoletti, & McRae, 2007) and a decrease in activity levels in their day-to-day lives (Bolse, Hamilton, Flanangan, Caroll, & Fridlund, 2005; Eckert & Jones, 2002). This contradiction can be related to the types of studies conducted. Previous studies have used questionnaires while this study focused on actual descriptions experienced by participants who had undergone the device implant. Theme 3 (a constant reminder: I know it's there) described the women "knowing that the device was in their chest," and it was a reminder of their condition. They also described how it affected their* **body image.** *There were two other studies that had mentioned this as a concern for women. One study by Walker et al. (2004) reported body image concerns of women. The women in that study were more concerned on how the device appeared in their chest (i.e., the scar) than any other aspect. A second study by Tangney et al. (2003), also reported body image concerns in women since it can be seen in their chest which makes them aware of the device. There were similarities with respect to body image only. They were not concerned with the constant reminder aspect of the cardiac disease, only a constant reminder of their mortality. (Dickerson, 2002)*

The common concern as described in theme 4 (Living on the Edge: I do not want my device going off) was the fear of the device having to shock them as well as the uncertainty of when, where, and who would be around for support. This was foremost in their thoughts. There have been common themes of fear of the device going off or shocking them in the literature reviewed. Dickerson (2002, 2005) reported that uncertainty of when and where shocks can be triggered was a prevailing concern of the male and female participants. Also, participants in Albarran, Tagney, and James' (2004) study reported a feeling of uncertainty regarding the device firing. The prevailing concern in theme 5 (catch 22: I'd rather not have it.) Is the conflict women have after receiving a device. These women knew that they medically needed the device yet would have rather not have gone through with it. Dickerson (2005) reported the theme of conditional acceptance that touches on the same concept. Also, a greater acceptance of the new situation was reported in previous studies. (Carroll & Hamilton, 2005; Kamphuis et al., 2004)

The women in this study offered specific experiences of living with an ICD which is not completely seen in any previous study. Moreover, there were some similar aspects identified in other studies such as receiving a shock and feeling of safety but most were not specific to women. (Bilge et al., 2006; Dickerson, 2002, 2005; Morken et al., 2009)

This study was able to describe the essence of women who are living with an ICD. The study remained true to qualitative research design. The focus on women was important, as there have been no gender specific studies to date. Capturing the fear and uncertainty for women with an ICD can have an impact on clinical practice and patient education. The author emphasized that these concerns are not being addressed properly in the healthcare system. This study can help clinicians gain an understanding of the experience these women are having and perhaps pay closer attention to these issues when they are seen in outpatient settings (Conelius, 2015).

The research may also be helpful in the establishment of support groups for women with ICDs. "Support groups can expose women to different types of resources in order to cope better, decrease anxiety, and answer any questions that arise" (Myers & James, 2008). "Since the women have an outstanding fear of the device firing/shocking them, a noteworthy follow-up study would be to describe their experience post firing/shock" (Conelius, 2015). By capturing the experiences of women with ICDs, the potential for better sensitivity toward the patient experience exists. This may be critical to overall quality of life and extends beyond the actual purpose and operation of the device. Conelius (2015) has made an important contribution to the understanding of women's experiences with an ICD.

The critical appraisal of a qualitative study involves an in-depth review of each step of the research process. The example of a qualitative critique in this chapter provides a foundation for the development of critiquing skills in qualitative research.

REFERENCES

Anthony, S., & Jack, S. (2009). Qualitative case study methodology in nursing research: An integrative review. *Journal of Advanced Nursing*, *65*(6), 1171–1181. doi:10.1111/j.1365-2648.2009.04998.x.

Barbour, R. S., & Barbour, M. (2003). Evaluating and synthesizing qualitative research: The need to develop a distinctive approach. *Journal of Evaluation in Clinical Practice*, *9*(2), 179–186.

Beck, C. (2009). Critiquing qualitative research. *AORN Journal*, *90*(4), 543–554. doi:10.1016/j.aorn.2008.12.023.

Bigby, C. (2015). Preparing manuscripts that report qualitative research: Avoiding common pitfalls and illegitimate questions. *Australian Social Work*, *68*(3), 384–391. doi:10.1080/0312407X.2015.1035663.

Cesario, S., Morin, K., & Santa-Donato, A. (2002). Evaluating the level of evidence of qualitative research. *Journal of Obstetric, Gynecologic and Neonatal Nursing*, *31*(6), 708–714.

Cleary, M., Escott, P., Horsfall, J., et al. (2014). Qualitative research: The optimal scholarly means of understanding the patient experience. *Issues in Mental Health Nursing*, *35*(11), 902–904. doi:10.3109/01612840.2014.965619.

Cleary, M., Horsfall, J., & Hayter, M. (2014). Data collection and sampling in qualitative research: Does size matter? *Journal of Advanced Nursing*, *70*(3), 473–475. doi:10.1111.

Colaizzi, P. (1978). Psychological research as the phenomenologist view it. In R. Valle & M. King (Eds.), *Existential phenomenological alternatives for psychology* (pp. 48–71). New York: Oxford University Press.

Cope, D. G. (2014). Methods and meanings: Credibility and trustworthiness of qualitative Research. *Oncology Nursing Forum*, *41*(1), 89–91. doi:10.1188/14.ONF.

Donnelly, F., & Wiechula, R. (2013). An example of qualitative comparative analysis in nursing research. *Nurse Researcher*, *20*(6), 6–11.

Flannery, M. (2016). Common perspectives in qualitative research. *Oncology Nursing Forum*, *43*(4), 517–518. doi:10.1188/16.ONF.

Hegney, D., & Chan, T. W. (2010). Ethical challenges in the conduct of qualitative research. *Nurse Researcher*, *18*(1), 4–7.

Horsburgh, D. (2003). Evaluation of qualitative research. *Journal of Clinical Nursing*, *12*, 307–312.

Ingham-Broomfield, R. (2015). A nurses' guide to qualitative research. *Australian Journal of Advanced Nursing*, *32*(3), 34–40.

Oye, C., Sørensen, N. O., & Glasdam, S. (2016). Qualitative research ethics on the spot. *Nursing Ethics*, *23*(4), 455–464. doi:10.1177/0969733014567023.

Pearson, A., Jordan, Z., Lockwood, C., et al. (2015). Notions of quality and standards for qualitative research reporting. *International Journal of Nursing Practice*, *21*(5), 670–676. doi:10.1111/ijn.12331.

Russell, C. K., & Gregory, D. M. (2003). Evaluation of qualitative research studies. *Evidence-Based Nursing*, *6*(2), 36–40.

Sandelowski, M. (2015). A matter of taste: Evaluating the quality of qualitative research. *Nursing Inquiry*, *22*(2), 86–94. doi:10.1111/nin.12080.

Streubert, H. J., & Carpenter, D. R. (2011). *Qualitative nursing research: Advancing the humanistic imperative*. Philadelphia, PA: Wolters Klower Health.

Walsh, D., & Downe, S. (2005). Meta-synthesis method of qualitative research: A literature review. *Journal of Advanced Nursing*, *50*(2), 204–211.

Williams, B. (2015). How to evaluate qualitative research. *American Nurse Today*, *10*(11), 31–38.

Go to Evolve at **http://evolve.elsevier.com/LoBiondo/** for review questions, critiquing exercises, and additional research articles for practice in reviewing and critiquing.

PART III

Processes and Evidence Related to Quantitative Research

RESEARCH VIGNETTE

SOMETIMES THE *SIMPLEST* THINGS ARE THE MOST COMPLICATED

Elaine Larson, PhD, RN, FAAN, CIC
Professor of Epidemiology
Associate Dean of Scholarship & Research
Columbia University
School of Nursing
New York, New York

Every nurse researcher has a story, which usually emanates from clinical experiences. I had several such experiences that instilled in me a passion for research. In the year following my graduation decades ago from a BSN program, I was working on a medical unit and a young patient of mine with mitral valve disease called me to her bedside to tell me that she did not feel well, was having trouble breathing, and that something was terribly wrong. I took her vital signs, did not detect anything serious, and set her up with a pillow on the bedside stand so she could breathe more easily. Within a few minutes she was in acute pulmonary edema, and within the hour she was dead. Of course, this would not happen today because of more sophisticated monitoring, but as a novice nurse I was devastated and promised myself that I would do everything in my power to keep this from happening again. So I learned what I could about acute pulmonary edema and submitted a paper to the *American Journal of Nursing* about the case (Larson, 1986). The paper would never be published now, as it was primarily a summary of information from medical textbooks, but putting my thoughts down on paper was a helpful way for me to deal with my feelings of failure and wanting to be a better nurse. The editor of the journal wrote me a letter to say that she hoped more clinical nurses would submit articles addressing relevant practice issues. So I was hooked on publishing!

The second clinical experience that cinched my passion for research and dissemination of findings happened when I was a clinical nurse specialist in a surgical intensive care unit. At that time, the unit was designed with a central nursing station surrounded by five patient beds in a semicircle so that they could all be observed. The ICU had several sinks adjacent to the patient beds, but at least one of them was usually unavailable because it was hooked up to a dialysis machine. When plans were made for a new, updated unit with many more beds in separate rooms (for the stated purposes of improving patients' privacy and ability to sleep and preventing transmission of infections), a colleague and I decided to formally evaluate the impact of this architectural change on rates of infection. We wrote a protocol, collected data before and after the ICU design change, did air sampling, monitored numbers of interactions between staff and patients and hand hygiene, and obtained cultures from patients for six surveillance organisms every 4 days. Rates of infection did not change after the ICU was redesigned, nor did staff infection prevention or hand hygiene practices, despite the fact that there was a sink available at the entrance to every patient room (Preston et al., 1981). It was clear from that project that just changing the physical environs of the ICU was insufficient to reduce the risk of infections; in fact, the problem seemed to be more behavioral than structural.

As a result of the ICU project, completed while I was working fulltime as a clinician, I returned to school for a PhD. With a small grant from the American Nurses Foundation (http://www.anfonline.org/), I studied the hand flora of patient care staff and found that 21% of nosocomial infections over a 7-month period were caused by species found on personnel hands and that such organisms were much more prevalent on normal skin than generally thought (Larson, 1981). Ironically, I had to provide a strong rationale for choosing to study such a *simple* topic as hand hygiene, because the doctoral faculty of epidemiology at the time felt that there was really little to study about the issue that was not already known. Since that time, however, hand hygiene has become a major topic of interdisciplinary research and has resulted in the publication in this decade of two international evidence-based guidelines citing hundreds of publications (Boyce & Pittet, 2002; Pittet et al., 2009). The point is that our research must go full circle, from clinical observation, to scholarly and rigorous data collection, and then back to evidence-based practice. Sometimes nurse researchers stop at the second step, but evidence-based practice is the raison d'être for pursuing a research career in nursing.

Conducting a well-designed, rigorous study is a primary responsibility of the nurse researcher, but only one responsibility among many. Evidence-based practice and the increasing adoption of practice guidelines (similar to what was previously referred to as research utilization) help ensure that important research findings are translated into clinical practice and public policy (Melnyk & Gallagher-Ford, 2014; Melnyk et al., 2014). It is often at the translational gap between publishing findings, even in influential, peer-reviewed journals, and communicating these findings in meaningful ways that the potential impact of nursing research is lost. In reality, research matters only to the extent that it is communicated and that it results in improved practice and policy—in the work environment, in the quality of life of our individual patients, and in the general health of the public. For that reason, the dissemination of research is essential in all appropriate media and to all appropriate audiences, not just to other researchers.

For me, the *simple* research related to hand hygiene and infections has become increasingly complex over the years. Despite multiple, intensive interventions, international dissemination of practice guidelines, and changes in national policy and mandates from The Joint Commission and the Centers for Disease Control and Prevention, hand hygiene remains stubbornly resistant to change, requiring more sophisticated interventions and conceptual underpinnings (Carter et al., 2016; Haas & Larson, 2007; Srigley et al., 2015). It is clearer now than it has been for several decades that new, emerging, and re-emerging infectious diseases will be a constant. While my research contributions have been primarily in one small field—that of the prevention and control of infectious diseases—the cumulative contributions of each of us to the broader scholarly community in our respective areas of concentration together make up the building blocks of a healthier world. That's my fundamental belief and commitment—nursing research as part of a global collective to improve health. Sounds simple, but it's not!

REFERENCES

Boyce, J. M., & Pittet, D. (2002). Guideline for hand hygiene in health-care settings. Recommendations of the Healthcare Infection Control Practices Advisory Committee and the HIPAC/SHEA/APIC/IDSA Hand Hygiene Task Force. *American Journal of Infection Control, 30*(8), S1–S46.

Carter, E. J., Wyer, P., Giglio, J., et al. (2016). Environmental factors and their association with emergency department hand hygiene compliance: an observational study. *BMJ Quality and Safety, 25*(5), 372–378.

Haas, J. P., & Larson, E. L. (2007). Measurement of compliance with hand hygiene. *Journal of Hospital Infection, 66*(1), 6–14.

Larson, E. (1986). The patient with acute pulmonary edema. *American Journal of Nursing, 68*, 1019–1022.

Larson, E. L. (1981). Persistent carriage of gram-negative bacteria on hands. *American Journal of Infection Control, 9*(4), 112–119.

Melnyk, B. M., & Gallagher-Ford, L. (2014). Evidence-based practice as mission critical for healthcare quality and safety: a disconnect for many nurse executives. *Worldviews on Evidence-Based Nursing/Sigma Theta Tau International, Honor Society of Nursing, 11*(3), 145–146.

Melnyk, B. M., Gallagher-Ford, L., Long, L. E., & Fineout-Overholt, E. (2014). The establishment of evidence-based practice competencies for practicing registered nurses and advanced practice nurses in real-world clinical settings: proficiencies to improve healthcare quality, reliability, patient outcomes, and costs. *Worldviews on Evidence-Based Nursing/Sigma Theta Tau International, Honor Society of Nursing, 11*(1), 5–15.

Pittet, D., Allegranzi, B., & Boyce, J. (2009). World Health Organization World Alliance for Patient Safety First Global Patient Safety Challenge Core Group of E. The World Health Organization Guidelines on Hand Hygiene in Health Care and their consensus recommendations. *Infection Control and Hospital Epidemiology, 30*(7), 611–622.

Preston, G.A., Larson, E.L., & Stamm, W.E. (1981). The effect of private isolation rooms on patient care practices, Colonization and infection in an intensive care unit. *American Journal of Medicine, 70*(3), 641–645.

Srigley, J.A., Corace, K., Hargadon, D.P., et al. (2015). Applying psychological frameworks of behaviour change to improve healthcare worker hand hygiene: a systematic review. *Journal of Hospital Infection, 91*(3), 202–210.

8

Introduction to Quantitative Research

Geri LoBiondo-Wood

Go to Evolve at **http://evolve.elsevier.com/LoBiondo/** for review questions, critiquing exercises, and additional research articles for practice in reviewing and critiquing.

LEARNING OUTCOMES

After reading this chapter, you should be able to do the following:

- Define research design.
- Identify the purpose of a research design.
- Define control and fidelity as it affects research design and the outcomes of a study.
- Compare and contrast the elements that affect fidelity and control.
- Begin to evaluate what degree of control should be exercised in a study.
- Define internal validity.
- Identify the threats to internal validity.
- Define external validity.
- Identify the conditions that affect external validity.
- Identify the links between study design and evidence-based practice.
- Evaluate research design using critiquing questions.

KEY TERMS

bias
constancy
control
control group
dependent variable
experimental group
external validity
extraneous or mediating variable
generalizability
history
homogeneity
independent variable
instrumentation
internal validity
intervening variable
intervention fidelity
maturation
measurement effects
mortality
pilot study
randomization
reactivity
selection
selection bias
testing

The word *design* implies the organization of elements into a masterful work of art. In the world of art and fashion, design conjures up images that are used to express a total concept. When an individual creates a structure such as a dress pattern or blueprints for a house, the type of structure depends on the aims of the creator. The same can be said of the research process. The framework that the researcher creates is the design. When reading a study, you should be able to recognize that the literature review, theoretical framework, and research question or hypothesis all interrelate with, complement, and assist in the operationalization

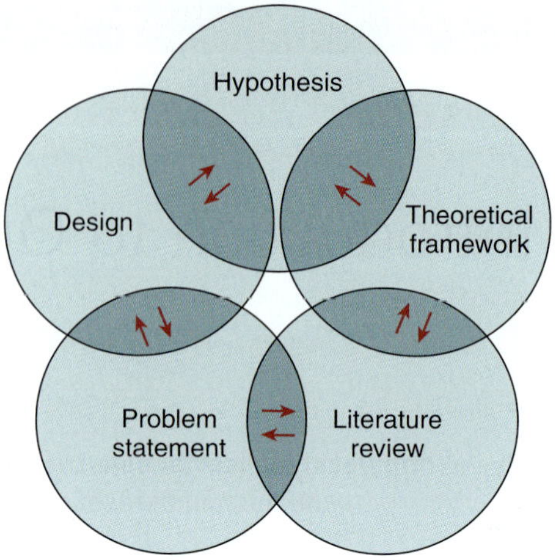

FIG 8.1 Interrelationships of design, problem statement, literature review, theoretical framework, and hypothesis.

of the design (Fig. 8.1). The degree to which there is a fit between these elements and the steps of the research process strengthens the study and also your confidence in the evidence's potential for applicability to practice.

How a researcher structures, implements, or designs a study affects the results of a study and ultimately its application to practice. For you to understand the implications and usefulness of a study for evidence-based practice, the key issues of research design must be understood. This chapter provides an overview of the meaning, purpose, and issues related to quantitative research design, and Chapters 9 and 10 present specific types of quantitative designs.

RESEARCH DESIGN—PURPOSE

Researchers choose from different design types. But the design choice must be consistent with the research question/hypotheses. Quantitative research designs include:

- A plan or blueprint
- Vehicle for systematically testing research questions and hypotheses
- Structure for maintaining control in the study

The design coupled with the methods and analysis provides control for the study. **Control** is defined as the measures that the researcher uses to hold the conditions of the study consistent and avoid possible potential of **bias** or error in the measurement of the **dependent variable** (outcome variable). Control measures help control threats to the validity of the study.

An example that demonstrates how the design can aid in the solution of a research question and maintain control is illustrated in the study by Nyamathi and colleagues (2015; Appendix A), whose aim was to evaluate the effectiveness of peer coaching, and hepatitis A and B vaccine completion in subjects who met the study's inclusion criteria were randomly assigned to one of the three groups. The interventions were clearly defined. The authors also discuss how they maintained **intervention fidelity** or constancy of interventionists, data-collector training and supervision, and follow-up throughout the study. By establishing the

TABLE 8.1 Pragmatic Considerations in Determining the Feasibility of a Research Question

Factor	Pragmatic Considerations
Time	A question must be one that can be studied within a realistic time period.
Subject availability	A researcher must determine if a sufficient number of subjects will be available and willing to participate. If one has a captive audience (e.g., students in a classroom), it may be relatively easy to enlist subjects. If a study involves subjects' independent time and effort, they may be unwilling to participate when there is no apparent reward. Potential subjects may have fears about harm and confidentiality and be suspicious of research. Subjects with unusual characteristics may be difficult to locate. Dependent on the design, a researcher may consider enlisting more subjects than needed to prepare for subject attrition. At times, a research report may note how the inclusion criteria were liberalized or the number of subjects altered, as a result of some unforeseen recruitment or attrition consideration.
Facility and equipment availability	All research requires equipment such as questionnaires or computers. Most research requires availability of a facility for data collection (e.g., a hospital unit or laboratory space).
Money	Research requires expenditure of money. Before starting a study, the researcher itemizes expenses and develops a budget. Study costs can include postage, printing, equipment, computer charges, and salaries. Expenses can range from about $1000 for a small study to hundreds of thousands of dollars for a large federally funded project.
Ethics	Research that places unethical demands on subjects is not feasible for study. Ethical considerations affect the design and methodology choice.

sample criteria and subject eligibility (inclusion criteria; see Chapter 12) and by clearly describing and designing the experimental intervention, the researchers demonstrated that they had a well-developed plan and were able to consistently maintain the study's conditions. A variety of considerations, including the type of design chosen, affect a study's successful completion and utility for evidence-based practice. These considerations include the following:

- Objectivity in conceptualizing the research question or hypothesis
- Accuracy
- Feasibility (Table 8.1)
- Control and intervention fidelity
- Validity—internal
- Validity—external

There are statistical principles associated with the mechanisms of control, but it is more important that you have a clear conceptual understanding of these mechanisms.

The next two chapters present experimental, quasi-experimental, and nonexperimental designs. As you will recall from Chapter 1, a study's type of design is linked to the level of evidence. As you appraise the design, you must also take into account other aspects of a study's design and conduct. These aspects are reviewed in this chapter. How they are applied depends on the type of design (see Chapters 9 and 10).

OBJECTIVITY IN THE RESEARCH QUESTION CONCEPTUALIZATION

Objectivity in the conceptualization of the research question is derived from a review of the literature and development of a theoretical framework (see Fig. 8.1). Using the literature, the researcher assesses the depth and breadth of available knowledge on the question (see Chapters 3 and 4), which in turn affects the design chosen. **Example:** ➤ A research question about the length of a breastfeeding teaching program in relation to adherence to breastfeeding may suggest either a correlational or an experimental design (see Chapters 9 and 10), whereas a question related to coping of parents and siblings of adolescent cancer survivors may suggest a survey or correlational study (see Chapter 10).

> **IPE HIGHLIGHT**
>
> There is usually more than one threat to internal and external validity in a research study. It is helpful to have a team discussion to summarize specific threats that affect the overall strength and quality of evidence provided by the studies your team is critically appraising.

ACCURACY

Accuracy in determining the appropriate design is aided by a thoughtful theoretical framework and literature review (see Chapters 3 and 4). Accuracy means that all aspects of a study systematically and logically follow from the research question or hypothesis. The simplicity of a research study does not render it useless or of less value. You should feel that the researcher chose a design that was consistent with the research question or hypothesis and offered the maximum amount of control. Issues of control are discussed later in this chapter.

Many research questions have not yet been researched. Therefore, a preliminary or **pilot study** is also a wise approach. A pilot study can be thought of as a beginning study in an area conducted to test and refine a study's data collection methods, and it helps to determine the sample size needed for a larger study. **Example:** ➤ Patterson (2016) published a report of a pilot study that tested the effect of an emotional freedom technique on stress and anxiety in nursing students. The key is the accuracy, validity, and objectivity used by the researcher in attempting to answer the question. Accordingly, when consulting research, you should read various types of studies and assess how and if the criteria for each step of the research process were followed.

CONTROL AND INTERVENTION FIDELITY

A researcher chooses a design to maximize the degree of **control**, fidelity, or uniformity of the study methods. Control is maximized by a well-planned study that considers each step of the research process and the potential threats to internal and external validity. In a study that tests interventions (randomized controlled trial; see Chapter 9), **intervention fidelity** (also referred to as **treatment fidelity**) is a key concept. *Fidelity* means trustworthiness or faithfulness. In a study, intervention fidelity means that the researcher standardized the intervention and planned how to administer the intervention to each subject in the same manner under the same conditions. A study designed to address issues related to fidelity maximizes results, decreases bias, and controls preexisting conditions that may affect outcomes. The elements of control and fidelity differ based on the design type. Thus, when various research designs are critiqued, the issue of control is always raised but with varying levels of flexibility. The issues discussed here will become clearer as you review the various designs types discussed in later chapters (see Chapters 9 and 10).

Control is accomplished by ruling out mediating or intervening variables that compete with the independent variables as an explanation for a study's outcome. An **extraneous**, **mediating**, or **intervening variable** is one that occurs in between the independent and dependent variable and interferes with interpretation of the dependent variable. An example would be the effect of the stage of cancer and depression during different phases of cancer treatment. Means of controlling mediating variables include the following:

- Use of a homogeneous sample
- Use of consistent data-collection procedures
- Training and supervision of data collectors and interventionists
- Manipulation of the independent variable
- Randomization

> **QSEN EVIDENCE-BASED PRACTICE TIP**
>
> As you read studies, assess if the study includes an intervention and whether there is a clear description of the intervention and how it was controlled. If the details are not clear, it should make you think that the intervention may have been administered differently among the subjects, therefore affecting bias and the interpretation of the results.

Homogeneous Sampling

In a smoking cessation study, extraneous variables may affect the dependent variable. The characteristics of a study's subjects are common extraneous variables. Age, gender, length of time smoked, amount smoked, and even smoking rules may affect the outcome in a smoking cessation study. These variables may therefore affect the outcome. As a control for these and other similar problems, the researcher's subjects should demonstrate **homogeneity**, or similarity, with respect to the extraneous variables relevant to the particular study (see Chapter 12). Extraneous variables are not fixed but must be reviewed and decided on, based on the study's purpose and theoretical base. By using a sample of homogeneous subjects, based on inclusion and exclusion criteria, the researcher has implemented a straightforward method of control.

Example: ➤ In the study by Nyamathi and colleagues (2015; see Appendix A), the researchers ensured homogeneity of the sample based on age, history of drug use, homelessness, and participation in a drug treatment unit. This step limits the **generalizability** or application of the findings to similar populations when discussing the outcomes (see Chapter 17). As you read studies, you will often see the researchers limit the generalizability of the findings to similar samples.

> **HELPFUL HINT**
>
> When critiquing studies, it is better to have a "clean" study with clearly identified controls that enhance generalizability from the sample to the specific population than a "messy" one from which you can generalize little or nothing.

If the researcher feels that an extraneous variable is important, it may be included in the design. In the smoking example, if individuals are working in an area where smoking is not allowed and this is considered to be important, the researcher could establish a control for it. This can be done by comparing two different work areas: one where smoking is allowed and one where it is not. The important idea to keep in mind is that before data are collected, the researcher should have identified, planned for, or controlled the important extraneous variables.

Constancy in Data Collection

A critical component of control is constancy in data collection. **Constancy** refers to the notion that the data-collection procedures should reflect a cookbook-like recipe of how the researcher controlled the study's conditions. This means that environmental conditions, timing of data collection, data-collection instruments, and data-collection procedures are the same for each subject (see Chapter 14). Constancy in data collection is also referred to as **intervention fidelity.** The elements of intervention fidelity (Breitstein et al., 2012; Gearing et al., 2011; Preyde & Burnham, 2011) are as follows:

- *Design:* The study is designed to allow an adequate testing of the hypothesis (or hypotheses) in relation to the underlying theory and clinical processes
- *Training:* Training and supervision of the data collectors and/or interventionists to ensure that the intervention is being delivered as planned and in a similar manner with all the subjects
- *Delivery:* Assessing that the intervention is delivered as intended, including that the "dose" (as measured by the number, frequency, and length of contact) is well described for all subjects and that the dose is the same in each group, and that there is a plan for possible problems
- *Receipt:* Ensuring that the treatment has been received and understood by the subject
- *Enactment:* Assessing that the intervention skills of the subject are enlisted as intended

The study by Nyamathi and colleagues (Appendix A; see the "Interventions" section) is an example of how intervention fidelity was maintained. A review of this study shows that data were collected from each subject in the same manner and under the same conditions by trained data collectors. This type of control aided the investigators' ability to draw conclusions, discuss limitations, and cite the need for further research. When interventions are implemented, researchers will often describe the training of and supervision of interventionists and/or data collectors that took place to ensure constancy. All study designs should demonstrate constancy (fidelity) of data collection, but studies that test an intervention require the highest level of intervention fidelity.

Manipulation of Independent Variable

A third means of control is manipulation of the **independent variable**. This refers to the administration of a program, treatment, or intervention to one group within the study and not to the other subjects in the study. The first group is known as the **experimental group** or **intervention group,** and the other group is known as the **control group**. In a control group, the variables under study are held at a constant or comparison level. **Example:** ➤ Nyamathi and colleagues (2015; see Appendix A) manipulated the provision of three levels of peer coaching and nurse-delivered interventions.

Experimental and quasi-experimental designs are used to test whether a treatment or intervention affects patient outcomes. Nonexperimental designs do not manipulate the independent variable and thus do not have a control group. The use of a control group in an experimental or quasi-experimental design is related to the aim of the study (see Chapter 9).

HELPFUL HINT

The lack of manipulation of the independent variable does not mean a weaker study. The type of question, amount of theoretical development, and the research that has preceded the study affects the researcher's design choice. If the question is amenable to a design that manipulates the independent variable, it increases the power of a researcher to draw conclusions—that is, if all of the considerations of control are equally addressed.

Randomization

Researchers may also choose other forms of control, such as randomization. **Randomization of subjects** is used when the required number and type of subjects from the population are obtained in such a manner that each potential subject has an equal chance of being assigned to a treatment group. Randomization eliminates bias, aids in the attainment of a representative sample, and can be used in various designs (see Chapter 12). Nyamathi and colleagues (2015; see Appendix A) randomized subjects to intervention and control groups.

Randomization can also be accomplished with questionnaires. By randomly ordering items on the questionnaires, the investigator can assess if there is a difference in responses that can be related to the order of the items. This may be especially important in longitudinal studies where bias from giving the same questionnaire to the same subjects on a number of occasions can be a problem.

QUANTITATIVE CONTROL AND FLEXIBILITY

The same level of control or elimination of bias *cannot* be exercised equally in all design types. When a researcher wants to explore an area in which little or no literature and/or research on the concept exists, the researcher may use a qualitative method or a nonexperimental design (see Chapters 5 through 7 and 10). In these types of studies, the researcher is interested in describing a phenomenon in a group of individuals.

Control must be exercised as strictly as possible in quantitative research. All studies should be evaluated for potential variables that may affect the outcomes; however, all studies, based on their design, exercise different levels of control. You should be able to locate in the research report how the researcher maintained control in accordance with its design.

QSEN EVIDENCE-BASED PRACTICE TIP

Remember that establishing evidence for practice is determined by assessing the validity of each step of the study, assessing if the evidence assists in planning patient care, and assessing if patients respond to the evidence-based care.

INTERNAL AND EXTERNAL VALIDITY

When reading research, you must be convinced that the results of a study are valid, are obtained with precision, and remain faithful to what the researcher wanted to measure. For the findings of a study to be applicable to practice and provide the foundation for further research, the study should indicate how the researcher avoided bias. Bias can occur at any step of the research process. Bias can be a result of which research questions are asked (see Chapter 2), which hypotheses are tested (see Chapter 2), how data are collected or observations made (see Chapter 14), the number of subjects and how subjects are recruited and

BOX 8.1 Threats to Validity

Internal Validity
- History
- Maturation
- Testing
- Instrumentation
- Mortality
- Selection bias

External Validity
- Selection effects
- Reactive effects
- Measurement effects

included (see Chapter 12), how subjects are randomly assigned in an experimental study (see Chapter 9), and how data are analyzed (see Chapter 16). There are two important criteria for evaluating bias, credibility, and dependability of the results: internal validity and external validity. An understanding of the threats to internal validity and external validity is necessary for critiquing research and considering its applicability to practice. Threats to validity are listed in Box 8.1, and discussion follows.

Internal Validity

Internal validity asks whether the *independent variable* really made the difference or the change in the *dependent variable.* To establish internal validity, the researcher rules out other factors or threats as rival explanations of the relationship between the variables—essentially sources of bias. There are a number of threats to internal validity. These are considered by researchers in planning a study and by clinicians before implementing the results in practice (Campbell & Stanley, 1966). You should note that threats to internal validity can compromise outcomes for all studies, and thereby the overall strength and quality of evidence of a study's findings should be considered to some degree in all quantitative designs. How these threats may affect specific designs are addressed in Chapters 9 and 10. Threats to internal validity include history, maturation, testing, instrumentation, mortality, and selection bias. Table 8.2 provides examples of the threats to internal validity. Generally, researchers will note the threats to validity that they encountered in the discussion and/or limitations section of a research article.

History

In addition to the independent variable, another specific event that may have an effect on the dependent variable may occur either inside or outside the experimental setting; this is referred to as **history**. An example may be that of an investigator testing the effects of a research program aimed at young adults to increase bone marrow donations in the community. During the course of the educational program, an ad featuring a known television figure is released on television and Facebook about the importance of bone marrow donation. The release of this information on social media with a television figure engenders a great deal of media and press attention. In the course of the media attention, medical experts are interviewed widely, and awareness is raised regarding the importance of bone marrow donation. If the researcher finds an increase in the number of young adults who donate bone marrow in their area, the researcher may not be able to conclude that the change in behavior is the result of the teaching program, as the change may have been influenced by the result of the information on social media and the resultant media coverage. See Table 8.2 for another example.

TABLE 8.2 **Examples of Internal Validity Threats**

Threat	Example
History	A study tested an exercise program intervention in a cardiac care rehabilitation center at one center and compared outcomes to those of another center in which usual care was given. During the final months of data collection, the control hospital implemented an e-health physical activity intervention; as a result data from the control hospital (cohort) was not included in the analysis.
Maturation	Hernandez-Martinez and colleagues (2016) evaluated the effects of prenatal nicotine exposure on infants' cognitive development at 6, 12, and 30 months. They noted that cognitive development and intelligence are clearly influenced by environment and genetics and not just by nicotine exposure.
Testing	Nyamathi and colleagues (2015) discussed the lack of treatment differences found in terms of vaccine completion rates possibly due to the bundled nature of the program (see Appendix A).
Instrumentation	Lee and colleagues (in press) acknowledged in a study of obesity and disability in young adults that "our measures of disability are not directly comparable to more traditional measures of disability used in studies of older adults."
Mortality	Nyamathi and colleagues (2015) noted that more than one-quarter (27%) did not complete the vaccine series, despite being informed of their risk for HBV infection (see Appendix A).
Selection bias	Nyamathi and colleagues (2015) controlled for selection bias by establishing inclusion and exclusion participation criteria for participation. Subjects were also stratified using a specific procedure that ensured balance across the three groups (see Nyamathi et al., 2015, Appendix A, Fig. 1).

Maturation

Maturation refers to the developmental, biological, or psychological processes that operate within an individual as a function of time and are external to the events of the study. **Example:** ➤ Suppose one wishes to evaluate the effect of a teaching method on baccalaureate students' achievement on a skills test. The investigator would record the students' abilities before and after the teaching method. Between the pretest and posttest, the students have grown older and wiser. The growth or change is unrelated to the study and may explain the differences between the two testing periods rather than the experimental treatment. It is important to remember that maturation is more than change resulting from an age-related developmental process, but could be related to physical changes as well. **Example:** ➤ In a study of new products to stimulate wound healing, one might ask whether the healing that occurred was related to the product or to the natural occurrence of wound healing. See Table 8.2 for another example.

Testing

Taking the same test repeatedly could influence subjects' responses the next time the test is completed. **Example:** ➤ The effect of taking a pretest on the subject's posttest score is known as **testing**. The effect of taking a pretest may sensitize an individual and improve the score of the posttest. Individuals generally score higher when they take a test a second time, regardless of the treatment. The differences between posttest and pretest scores may not be a result of the independent variable but rather of the experience gained through the testing. Table 8.2 provides an example.

Instrumentation

Instrumentation threats are changes in the measurement of the variables or observational techniques that may account for changes in the obtained measurement. **Example:** ➤ A researcher may wish to study types of thermometers (e.g., tympanic, oral, infrared) to compare the accuracy of using a digital thermometer to other temperature-taking methods. To prevent instrumentation threat, a researcher must check the calibration of the thermometers according to the manufacturer's specifications before and after data collection.

Another example that fits into this area is related to techniques of observation or data collection. If a researcher has several raters collecting observational data, all must be trained in a similar manner so that they collect data using a standardized approach, thereby ensuring interrater reliability (see Chapter 13) and intervention fidelity (see Table 8.2). At times, even though the researcher takes steps to prevent instrumentation problems, this threat may still occur and should be evaluated within the total context of the study.

Mortality

Mortality is the loss of study subjects from the first data-collection point (pretest) to the second data-collection point (posttest). If the subjects who remain in the study are not similar to those who dropped out, the results could be affected. The loss of subjects may be from the sample as a whole or, in a study that has both an experimental and a control group, there may be differential loss of subjects. A differential loss of subjects means that more of the subjects in one group dropped out than the other group. See Table 8.2 for an example.

Selection Bias

If the precautions are not used to gain a representative sample, **selection bias** could result from how the subjects were chosen. Suppose an investigator wishes to assess if a new exercise program contributes to weight reduction. If the new program is offered to all, chances are only individuals who are more motivated to exercise will take part in the program. Assessment of the effectiveness of the program is problematic, because the investigator cannot be sure if the new program encouraged exercise behaviors or if only highly motivated individuals joined the program. To avoid selection bias, the researcher could randomly assign subjects to groups. In a nonexperimental study, even with clearly defined inclusion and exclusion criteria, selection bias is difficult to avoid completely. See Table 8.2 for an example.

HELPFUL HINT

More than one threat can be found in a study, depending on the type of study design. Finding a threat to internal validity in a study does not invalidate the results and is usually acknowledged by the investigator in the "Results" or "Discussion" or "Limitations" section of the study.

QSEN EVIDENCE-BASED PRACTICE TIP

Avoiding threats to internal validity can be quite difficult at times. Yet this reality does not render studies that have threats useless. Take them into consideration and weigh the total evidence of a study for not only its statistical meaningfulness but also its clinical meaningfulness.

External Validity

External validity concerns the generalizability of the findings of one study to additional populations and other environmental conditions. External validity questions under what conditions and with what types of subjects the same results can be expected to occur.

The factors that may affect external validity are related to selection of subjects, study conditions, and type of observations. These factors are termed *selection effects, reactive effects,* and *testing effects.* You will notice the similarity in the names of the factors of selection and testing to those of the threats to internal validity. When considering internal validity threats factors as internal threats, you should assess them as they relate to the testing of *independent* and *dependent* variables within the study. When assessing external validity threats, you should consider them in terms of the *generalizability* or use outside of the study to other populations and settings. The internal validity threats ask if the independent variable changed or was related to the dependent variable or if was affected by something else. The Critical Thinking Decision Path for threats to validity displays the way threats to internal and external validity can interact with each other. It is important to remember that this decision path is not exhaustive of the type of threats and their interaction. Problems of internal validity are generally easier to control. Generalizability issues are more difficult to deal with because they indicate that the researcher is assuming that other populations are similar to the one being tested.

CRITICAL THINKING DECISION PATH

Potential Threats to a Study's Validity

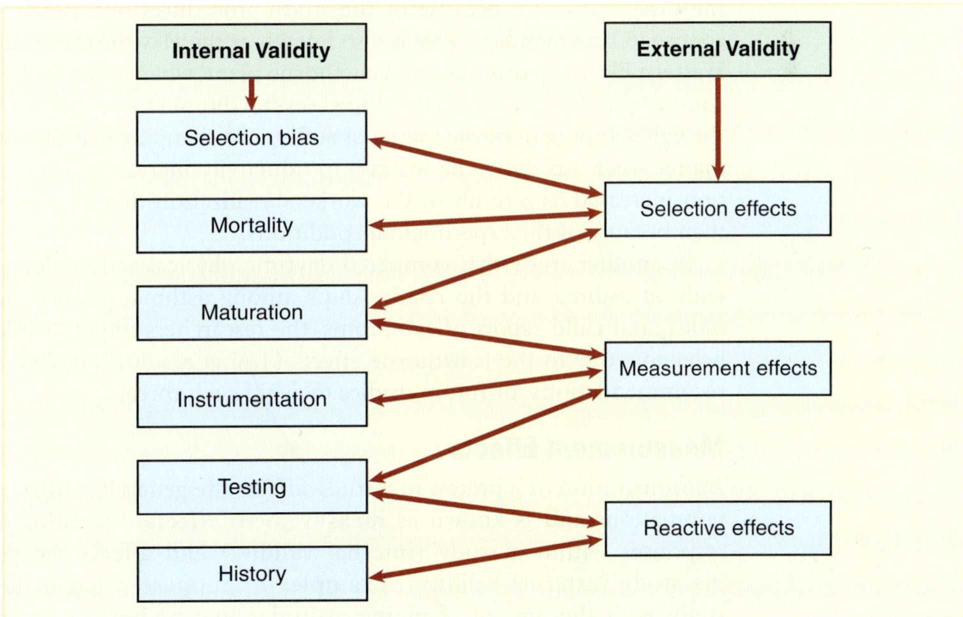

QSEN EVIDENCE-BASED PRACTICE TIP

Generalizability depends on who actually participates in a study. Not everyone who is approached actually participates, and not everyone who agrees to participate completes a study. As you review studies, think about how well the subjects represent the population of interest.

Selection Effects

Selection refers to the generalizability of the results to other populations. An example of selection effects occurs when the researcher cannot attain the ideal sample. At times, the numbers of available subjects may be low or not accessible (see Chapter 12). Therefore, the type of sampling method used and how subjects are assigned to research conditions affect the generalizability to other groups, the external validity.

Examples of selection effects are reported when researchers note any of the following:

- "There are several limitations to the study. At 1 and 3 months' post-death, parents were in early stages of grieving. Thus these findings may not be applicable to parents who are later in their grieving process" (Hawthorne et al., 2016, Appendix B).
- "The sample size was small, which could have limited the power and obscured significant effects that may have been revealed with a larger sample" (Turner-Sack et al., 2016, Appendix D).

These remarks caution you about potentially generalizing beyond the type of sample in a study, but also point out the usefulness of the findings for practice and future research aimed at building the research in these areas.

Reactive Effects

Reactivity is defined as the subjects' responses to being studied. Subjects may respond to the investigator not because of the study procedures but merely as an independent response to being studied. This is also known as the Hawthorne effect, which is named after Western Electric Corporation's Hawthorne plant, where a study of working conditions was conducted. The researchers developed several different working conditions (i.e., turning up the lights, piping in music loudly or softly, and changing work hours). They found that no matter what was done, the workers' productivity increased. They concluded that production increased as a result of the workers' realization that they were being studied rather than because of the experimental conditions.

In another study that compared daytime physical activity levels in children with and without asthma and the relationships among asthma, physical activity and body mass index, and child report of symptoms, the researchers noted, "Children may change their behaviors due to the Hawthorne effect" (Tsai et al., 2012, p. 258). The researchers made recommendations for future studies to avoid such threats.

Measurement Effects

Administration of a pretest in a study affects the generalizability of the findings to other populations and is known as **measurement effects**. Pretesting can affect the posttest responses within a study (internal validity) and affects the generalizability outside the study (external validity). **Example:** ➤ Suppose a researcher wants to conduct a study with the aim of changing attitudes toward breast cancer screening behaviors.

To accomplish this, an education program on the risk factors for breast cancer is incorporated. To test whether the education program changes attitudes toward screening behaviors, tests are given before and after the teaching intervention. The pretest on attitudes allows the subjects to examine their attitudes regarding cancer screening. The subjects' responses on follow-up testing may differ from those of individuals who were given the education program and did not see the pretest. Therefore, when a study is conducted and a pretest is given, it may "prime" the subjects and affect the researcher's ability to generalize to other situations.

HELPFUL HINT

When reviewing a study, be aware of the internal and external validity threats. These threats do not make a study useless—but actually more useful—to you. Recognition of the threats allows researchers to build on data, and allows you to think through what part of the study can be applied to practice. Specific threats to validity depend on the design type.

There are other threats to external validity that depend on the type of design and methods of sampling used by the researcher, but these are beyond the scope of this text. Campbell and Stanley (1966) offer detailed coverage of the issues related to internal and external validity.

APPRAISAL FOR EVIDENCE-BASED PRACTICE QUANTITATIVE RESEARCH

Critiquing a study's design requires you to first have knowledge of the overall implications that the choice of a design may have for the study as a whole (see the Critical Appraisal Criteria box). When researchers ask a question they design a study, decide how the data will be collected, what instruments will be used, what the sample's inclusion and exclusion criteria will be, and how large the sample will be, to diminish threats to the study's validity. These choices are based on the nature of the research question or hypothesis. Minimizing threats to internal and external validity of a study enhances the strength of evidence. In this chapter, the meaning, purpose, and important factors of design choice, as well as the vocabulary that accompanies these factors, have been introduced.

Several criteria for evaluating the design related to maximizing control and minimizing threats to internal/external validity and, as a result, sources of bias can be drawn from this chapter. Remember that the criteria are applied differently with various designs (see Chapters 9 and 10). The following discussion pertains to the overall appraisal of a quantitative design.

The research design should reflect that an objective review of the literature and establishment of a theoretical framework guided the development of the hypothesis and the design choice. When reading a study, there may be no explicit statement regarding how the design was chosen, but the literature reviewed will provide clues as to why the researcher chose the study's design. You can evaluate this by critiquing the study's theoretical framework and literature review (see Chapters 3 and 4). Is the question new and not extensively researched? Has a great deal of research been done on the question, or is it a new or different way of looking at an old question? Depending on the level of the question, the investigators make certain choices. **Example:** ➤ In the study by Nyamathi and colleagues (2015), the researchers wanted to test a controlled intervention; thus they developed a randomized controlled trial (Level II design). However, the purpose of the study by Turner-Sack and colleagues (2016) was much different. The Turner-Sack study examined the relationship between and among variables. The study did not test an intervention but explored how variables related to each other in a specific population (Level IV design).

CRITICAL APPRAISAL CRITERIA

Quantitative Research

1. Is the type of design used appropriate?
2. Are the various concepts of control consistent with the type of design chosen?
3. Does the design used seem to reflect consideration of feasibility issues?
4. Does the design used seem to flow from the proposed research question, theoretical framework, literature review, and hypothesis?
5. What are the threats to internal validity or sources of bias?
6. What are the controls for the threats to internal validity?
7. What are the threats to external validity or generalizability?
8. What are the controls for the threats to external validity?
9. Is the design appropriately linked to the evidence hierarchy?

You should be alert for the means investigators use to maintain control (i.e., homogeneity in the sample, consistent data-collection procedures, how or if the independent variable was manipulated, and whether randomization was used). Once it has been established whether the necessary control or uniformity of conditions has been maintained, you must determine whether the findings are valid. To assess this aspect, the threats to internal validity should be reviewed. If the investigator's study was systematic, well grounded in theory, and followed the criteria for each step of the research process, you will probably conclude that the study is internally valid. No study is perfect; there is always the potential for bias or threats to validity. This is not because the research was poorly conducted or the researcher did not think through the process completely; rather, it is that when conducting research with human subjects there is always some potential for error. Subjects can drop out of studies, and data collectors can make errors and be inconsistent. Sometimes errors cannot be controlled by the researcher. If there are policy changes during a study, an intervention can be affected. As you read studies, note how each facet of the study was conducted, what potential errors could have arisen, and how the researcher addressed the sources of bias in the limitations section of the study.

Additionally, you must know whether a study has external validity or generalizability to other populations or environmental conditions. External validity can be claimed only after internal validity has been established. If the credibility of a study (internal validity) has not been established, a study cannot be generalized (external validity) to other populations. Determination of external validity of the findings goes hand in hand with sampling issues (see Chapter 12). If the study is not representative of any one group or one event of interest, external validity may be limited or not present at all. The issues of internal and external validity and applications for specific designs (see Chapters 9 and 10) provide the remaining knowledge to fully critique the aspects of a study's design.

KEY POINTS

- The purpose of the design is to provide the master plan for a study.
- There are many types of designs.
- You should be able to locate within the study the question that the researcher wished to answer. The question should be proposed with a plan for the accomplishment of the study. Depending on the question, you should be able to recognize the steps taken by the investigator to ensure control, eliminate bias, and increase generalizability.
- The choice of a design depends on the question. The research question and design chosen should reflect the investigator's attempts to maintain objectivity, accuracy, and, most important, control.
- Control affects not only the outcome of a study but also its future use. The design should reflect how the investigator attempted to control both internal and external validity threats.
- Internal validity must be established before external validity can be established.
- The design, literature review, theoretical framework, and hypothesis should all interrelate.
- The choice of the design is affected by pragmatic issues. At times, two different designs may be equally valid for the same question.
- The choice of design affects the study's level of evidence.

CRITICAL THINKING CHALLENGES

- How do the three criteria for an experimental design, manipulation, randomization, and control, minimize bias and decrease threats to internal validity?
- Argue your case for supporting or not supporting the following claim: "A study that does not use an experimental design does not decrease the value of the study even though it may influence the applicability of the findings in practice." Include examples to support your rationale.
- IPE Have your interprofessional team provide rationale for why evidence of selection bias and mortality are important sources of bias in research studies. As you critically appraise a study that uses an experimental or quasi-experimental design, why is it important for you to look for evidence of intervention fidelity? How does intervention fidelity increase the strength and quality of the evidence provided by the findings of a study using these types of designs?

REFERENCES

Breitstein, S., Robbins, L., & Cowell, M. (2012). Attention to fidelity: Why is it important? *Journal of School Nursing*, *28*(6), 407–408. doi:1186/1748-5908-1-1.

Campbell, D., & Stanley, J. (1966). *Experimental and quasi-experimental designs for research*. Chicago, IL: Rand-McNally.

Gearing, R. E., El-Bassel, N., Ghesquiere, A., et al. (2011). Major ingredients of fidelity: A review and scientific guide to improving quality of intervention research implementation. *Clinical Psychology Review*, *31*, 79–88. doi:10.1016/jcpr.2010.09.007.

Hawthorne, D. M., Youngblut, J. M., & Brooten, D. (2016). Parent spirituality, grief, and mental health at 1 and 3 months after their infant/child's death in an intensive care unit. *Journal of Pediatric Nursing*, *31*, 73–80.

Hernandez-Martinez, Moreso, N. V., Serra, B. R., Val, V. A., et al. (2016). *Maternal Child Health Journal*. Epub ahead of print.

Lee, H., Pantazis, A., Cheng, P., et al. (2016). The association between adolescent obesity and disability incidence in young adulthood. *Journal of Adolescent Health*, *59*(4), 472–478.

Nyamathi, A., Salem, B., Zhang, S., et al. (2015). Nursing case management, peer coaching, and Hepatitis A and B vaccine completion among homeless men recently released on parole: A randomized trial. *Nursing Research*, *64*(3), 177–189.

Patterson, S. L. (2016). The effect of emotional freedom technique on stress and anxiety in nursing students. *Nurse Education Today*, *5*(40), 104–111.

Preyde, M., & Burnham, P. V. (2011). Intervention fidelity in psychosocial oncology. *Journal of Evidence-Based Social Work*, *8*, 379–396. doi:10.1080/15433714.2011.54234.

Tsai, S. Y., Ward, T., Lentz, M., & Kieckhefer, G. M. (2012). Daytime physical activity levels in school-age children with and without asthma. *Nursing Research*, *61*(4), 252–159.

Turner-Sack, A. M., Menna, R., Setchell, S. R., et al. (2016). Psychological functioning, post traumatic growth, and coping in parent and siblings of adolescent cancer survivors. *Oncology Nursing Forum*, *43*(1), 48–56.

Go to Evolve at **http://evolve.elsevier.com/LoBiondo/** for review questions, critiquing exercises, and additional research articles for practice in reviewing and critiquing.

9

Experimental and Quasi-Experimental Designs

Susan Sullivan-Bolyai and Carol Bova

Go to Evolve at **http://evolve.elsevier.com/LoBiondo/** for review questions, critiquing exercises, and additional research articles for practice in reviewing and critiquing.

LEARNING OUTCOMES

After reading this chapter, you should be able to do the following:

- Describe the purpose of experimental and quasi-experimental research.
- Describe the characteristics of experimental and quasi-experimental designs.
- Distinguish between experimental and quasi-experimental designs.
- List the strengths and weaknesses of experimental and quasi-experimental designs.
- Identify the types of experimental and quasi-experimental designs.
- Identify potential internal and external validity issues associated with experimental and quasi-experimental designs.
- Critically evaluate the findings of experimental and quasi-experimental studies.
- Identify the contribution of experimental and quasi-experimental designs to evidence-based practice.

KEY TERMS

after-only design
after-only nonequivalent control group design
antecedent variable
classic experiment
control
dependent variable
design
effect size
experimental design
extraneous variable
independent variable
intervening variable
intervention fidelity
manipulation
mortality
nonequivalent control group design
one-group (pretest-posttest) design
power analysis
quasi-experimental design
randomization (random assignment)
randomized controlled trial
Solomon four-group design
testing
time series design
treatment effect

RESEARCH PROCESS

One purpose of research is to determine cause-and-effect relationships. In nursing practice, we are concerned with identifying interventions to maintain or improve patient outcomes, and base practice on evidence. We test the effectiveness of nursing interventions by using **experimental** and **quasi-experimental designs**. These **designs** differ from nonexperimental designs in one important way: the researcher does not observe behaviors and actions, but actively intervenes by manipulating study variables to bring about a desired effect. By manipulating an independent variable, the researcher can measure a change in behavior(s) or action(s), which is the dependent variable. Experimental and quasi-experimental studies provide the two highest levels of evidence, Level II and Level III, for a single study (see Chapter 1).

Experimental designs are particularly suitable for testing cause-and-effect relationships because they are structured to minimize potential threats to internal validity (see Chapter 8). To infer causality requires that these three criteria be met:

- The causal (independent) and effect (dependent) variables must be associated with each other.
- The cause must precede the effect.
- The relationship must not be explainable by another variable.

When critiquing experimental and/or quasi-experimental designs, the primary focus is on to what extent the experimental treatment, or **independent variable**, caused the desired effect on the outcome, the **dependent variable**. The strength of the conclusion depends on how well other extraneous study variables may have influenced or contributed to the findings.

The purpose of this chapter is to acquaint you with the issues involved in interpreting and applying to practice the findings of studies that use experimental and quasi-experimental designs (Box 9.1). The Critical Thinking Decision Path shows an algorithm that influences a researcher's choice of experimental or quasi-experimental design. In the literature, these types of studies are often referred to as *therapy* or *intervention* articles.

CRITICAL THINKING DECISION PATH

Experimental and Quasi-Experimental Designs

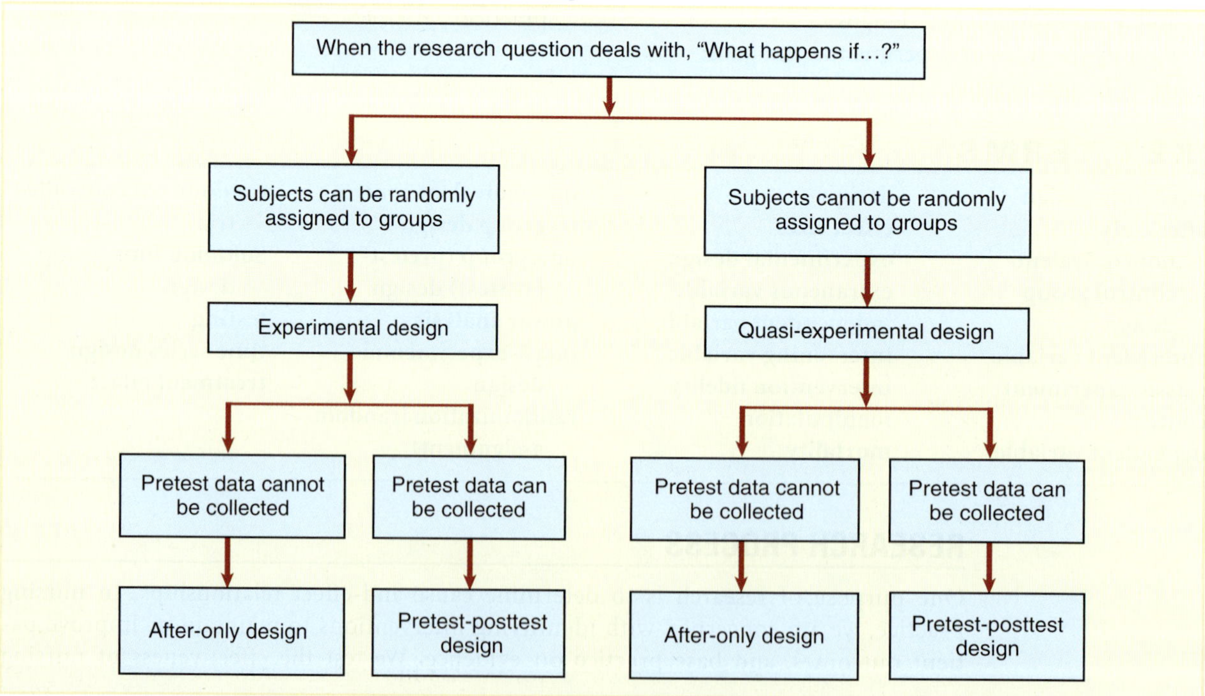

BOX 9.1 Summary of Experimental and Quasi-Experimental Research Designs

Experimental Designs
- True experiment (pretest-posttest control group) design
- Solomon four-group design
- After-only design

Quasi-Experimental Designs
- Nonequivalent control group design
- After-only nonequivalent control group design
- One group (pretest-posttest) design
- Time series design

EXPERIMENTAL DESIGN

An **experimental design** has three identifying properties:

- **Randomization**
- **Control**
- **Manipulation**

A study using an experimental design is commonly called a **randomized controlled trial (RCT)**. In clinical settings, it may be referred to as a *clinical trial* and is commonly used in drug trials. An RCT is considered the "gold standard" for providing information about cause-and-effect relationships. An RCT generates Level II evidence (see Chapter 1) because randomization, control, and manipulation minimize bias or error. A well-controlled RCT using these properties provides more confidence that the intervention is effective and will produce the same results over time (see Chapters 1 and 8). Box 9.2 shows examples of how these properties were used in the study in Appendix A.

Randomization

Randomization, or **random assignment**, is required for a study to be considered an experimental design with the distribution of subjects to either the experimental or the control group on a random basis. As shown in Box 9.2, each subject has an equal chance of being assigned to one of the three groups. This ensures that other variables that could affect change in the dependent variable will be equally distributed among the groups, reducing systematic bias. It also decreases selection bias (see Chapter 8). Randomization may be done individually or by groups. Several procedures are used to randomize subjects to groups, such as a table of random numbers or computer-generated number sequences (Suresh, 2011). Note that random assignment to groups is different from random sampling as discussed in Chapter 12.

Control

Control refers to the process by which the investigator holds conditions constant to limit bias that could influence the dependent variable(s). Control is acquired by manipulating the independent variable, randomly assigning subjects to a group, using a control group, and preparing intervention and data collection protocols that are consistent for all study participants (intervention fidelity) (see Chapters 8 and 14). Box 9.2 illustrates how a control group was used by Nyamathi and colleagues (2015; see Appendix A). In an experimental study, the control group (or in Nyamathi's study, referred to as *Usual Care* group) receives the usual treatment or a placebo (an inert pill in drug trials).

Manipulation

Manipulation is the process of "doing something," a different dose of "something," or comparing different types of treatment by manipulating the independent variable for at

BOX 9.2 Experimental Design Exemplar: Nursing Case Management, Peer Coaching, and Hepatitis A and B Vaccine Completion among Homeless Men Recently Released on Parole, Randomized Clinical Trial

- This study reports specifically on whether seronegative parolees involved and randomized in the original education and support intervention study were more likely to complete the hepatitis A and B vaccination series and variable predictors of their adherence for completion. The study consisted of parolee participants randomization to one of three groups:
  - Peer coaching–nurse case management over 6 months whereby a combination of a peer coach who provided weekly (~45 minutes) interactions focused on using coping and communication skills, self-management, and access to community resources; and interactions with a nurse case manager (~20 minutes over 8 consecutive weeks) focused on health promotion, completion of drug treatment, vaccination adherence, and reduction of risky drug and sexual behaviors
  - Peer coaching alone as described in group 1 along with a one-time nurse interaction (20 minutes) focused on hepatitis and HIV risk reduction
  - Usual care that consisted of encouragement by a nurse to complete the three-series HAV/HBV vaccine and a one-time 20-minute peer counselor session on health promotion. A detailed power analysis for sample size was reported.
- Fig. 2 in Appendix A: The CONSORT diagram illustrates how $N = 669$ study participants were approached, of which 69 were excluded, and why; followed by the *N* of 600 participants who were randomized to one of the three study arms to control for confounding variables and to ensure balance across groups: $n = 195$ in peer coaching–nurse care manager group; $n = 120$ in peer coaching group; and $n = 209$ in usual care group.
- The researchers also statistically assessed whether random assignment produced groups that were similar; Table 1 illustrates that except for personal health status there were no differences in the baseline characteristics (each group had similar distribution of study participants) across the three intervention arms for demographics, social, situational, coping, and personal characteristics. Fair/poor health was more commonly reported for the usual care group (37.2%). Thus, we would want to consider the fact that randomization did not work for that variable. Subanalyses might be necessary (controlling for that variable) to determine if perception of health affected that group's adherence for completion of the vaccination series.
- There is no report within this article of **attention-control** (all groups receiving same amount of *attention time*), so we do not know the average amount of time each study arm received. Thus time alone could explain adherence improvement (spending more time teaching/interacting with group members).
- Of the 345 study participants, the vaccination completion rate for three or more doses was 73% across all three groups with no differences across groups. In other words, there was not a higher rate of vaccination completion for the study participants who were in arm 1 or 2 compared to usual care.
- The authors identify several limitations that could have attributed to the findings, such as the fact that self-report has the potential for bias.

least some of the involved subjects (typically those randomly assigned to the experimental group). The independent variable might be a treatment, a teaching plan, or a medication. The effect of this manipulation is measured to determine the result of the experimental treatment on the dependent variable compared with those who did not receive the treatment.

Box 9.2 provides an illustration of how the properties of experimental designs, randomization, control, and manipulation are used in an intervention study and how the researchers ruled out other potential explanations or bias (threats to internal validity) influencing the results. The description in Box 9.2 is also an example of how the researchers used control to minimize bias and its effect on the intervention (Nyamathi et al., 2015). This control helped rule out the following potential internal validity threats:

- *Selection effect:* Bias in the sample contributed to the results versus the intervention.
- *History:* External events may have contributed to the results versus the intervention.

- *Maturation:* Developmental processes that occur and potentially alter the results versus the intervention.

Researchers also tested statistically for differences among the groups and found that there were none, reassuring the reader that the randomization process worked. We have briefly discussed RCTs and how they precisely use control, manipulation, and randomization to test the effectiveness of an intervention.

- RCTs use an experimental and control group, sometimes referred to as experimental and control arms.
- Have a specific sampling plan, using clear-cut *inclusion* and *exclusion* criteria (see Chapter 12).
- Administer the intervention in a consistent way, called *intervention fidelity.*
- Perform statistical comparisons to determine any baseline and/or postintervention differences between groups.
- Calculate the sample size needed to detect a treatment effect.

It is important that researchers establish a large enough sample size to ensure that there are enough subjects in each study group to statistically detect differences among those who receive the intervention and those who do not. This is called the ability to statistically detect the **treatment effect** or **effect size**—that is, the impact of the independent variable/intervention on the dependent variable (see Chapter 12). The mathematical procedure to determine the number for each arm (group) needed to test the study's variables is called a **power analysis** (see Chapter 12). You will usually find power analysis information in the sample section of the research article. **Example:** ➤ You will know there was an appropriate plan for an adequate sample size when a statement like the following is included: "With at least 114 men in each intervention condition there was 80% power to detect differences of 15-20 percentage points (e.g., 50% vs. 70%, 75% vs. 90%) for vaccine completion between either of the two intervention conditions and the UC intervention condition at $p = .05$" (Nyamathi et al., 2015). This information demonstrates that the researchers sought an adequate sample size. This information is critical to assess because with a small sample size, differences may not be statistically evident, thus creating the potential for a *type II error*—that is, acceptance of the null hypothesis when it is false (see Chapter 16). Carefully read the intervention and control group section of an article to see exactly what each group received and what the differences were between groups either at baseline or following the intervention.

In Appendix A, Nyamathi and colleagues (2015) provide a detailed description and illustration of the intervention. The discussion section reports that the patients' self-report (they may report doing better than they really did) may have posed an accuracy bias in reporting health behaviors. When reviewing RCTs, you also want to assess how well the study incorporates intervention fidelity measures. Fidelity covers several elements of an experimental study (Gearing et al., 2011; Preyde & Burnham, 2011; Wickersham et al., 2011) that must be evaluated and that can enhance a study's internal validity. These elements are as follows:

1. Well-defined intervention, sampling strategy, and data collection procedures
2. Well-described characteristics of study participants and environment
3. Clearly described protocol for delivering the intervention systematically to all subjects in the intervention group
4. Discussion of threats to internal and *external validity*

Types of Experimental Designs

There are numerous experimental designs (Campbell & Stanley, 1966). Each is based on the **classic experimental design** called the RCT (Fig. 9.1A). The classic RCT is conducted as follows:

1. The researcher recruits a sample from the accessible population.
2. Baseline measurements are taken of preintervention demographics, personal characteristics.
3. Baseline measurement is taken of the dependent variable(s).
4. Subjects are randomized to either the intervention or the control group.
5. Each group receives the experimental intervention *or* comparison/control intervention (usual care or standard treatment, or placebo).
6. Both groups complete postintervention measures to see which, if any, changes have occurred in the dependent variables (determining the differential effects of the treatment).
7. Reliability and validity data are clearly described for measurement instruments.

QSEN EVIDENCE-BASED PRACTICE TIP

The term *RCT* is often used to refer to an experimental design in health care research and is frequently used in nursing research as the gold standard design because it minimizes bias or threats to study validity. Because of ethical issues, rarely is "no treatment" acceptable. Typically, either "standard treatment" or another version or dose of "something" is provided to the control group. Only when there is no standard or comparable treatment available is a no-treatment control group appropriate.

The degree of difference between the groups at the end of the study indicates the confidence the researcher has in a causal link (i.e., the intervention caused the difference) between the independent and dependent variables. Because random assignment and control minimizes the effects of many threats to internal validity or bias (see Chapter 8), it is a strong design for testing cause-and-effect relationships. However, the design is not perfect. Some threats to internal validity cannot be controlled in RCTs, including but not limited to:

- **Mortality**: People tend to drop out of studies, especially those that require participation over an extended period of time. When reading RCTs, examine the sample and the results carefully to see if excessive dropouts or deaths occurred, or one group had more dropouts than the other, which can affect the study findings.
- **Testing**: When the same measurement is given twice, subjects tend to score better the second time just by remembering the test items. Researchers can avoid this problem in one of two ways: They might use different or equivalent forms of the same test for the two measurements (see Chapter 15), or they might use a more complex experimental design called the Solomon four-group design.

Solomon Four-Group Design. The **Solomon four-group design**, shown in Fig. 9.1B, has two groups that are identical to those used in the classic experimental design, plus two additional groups: an experimental after-group and a control after-group. As the diagram shows, subjects are randomly assigned to one of four groups before baseline data are collected. This design results in two groups that receive only a posttest (rather than pretest and posttest), which provides an opportunity to rule out testing biases that may have occurred because of exposure to the pretest (also called pretest sensitization). In other words, pretest

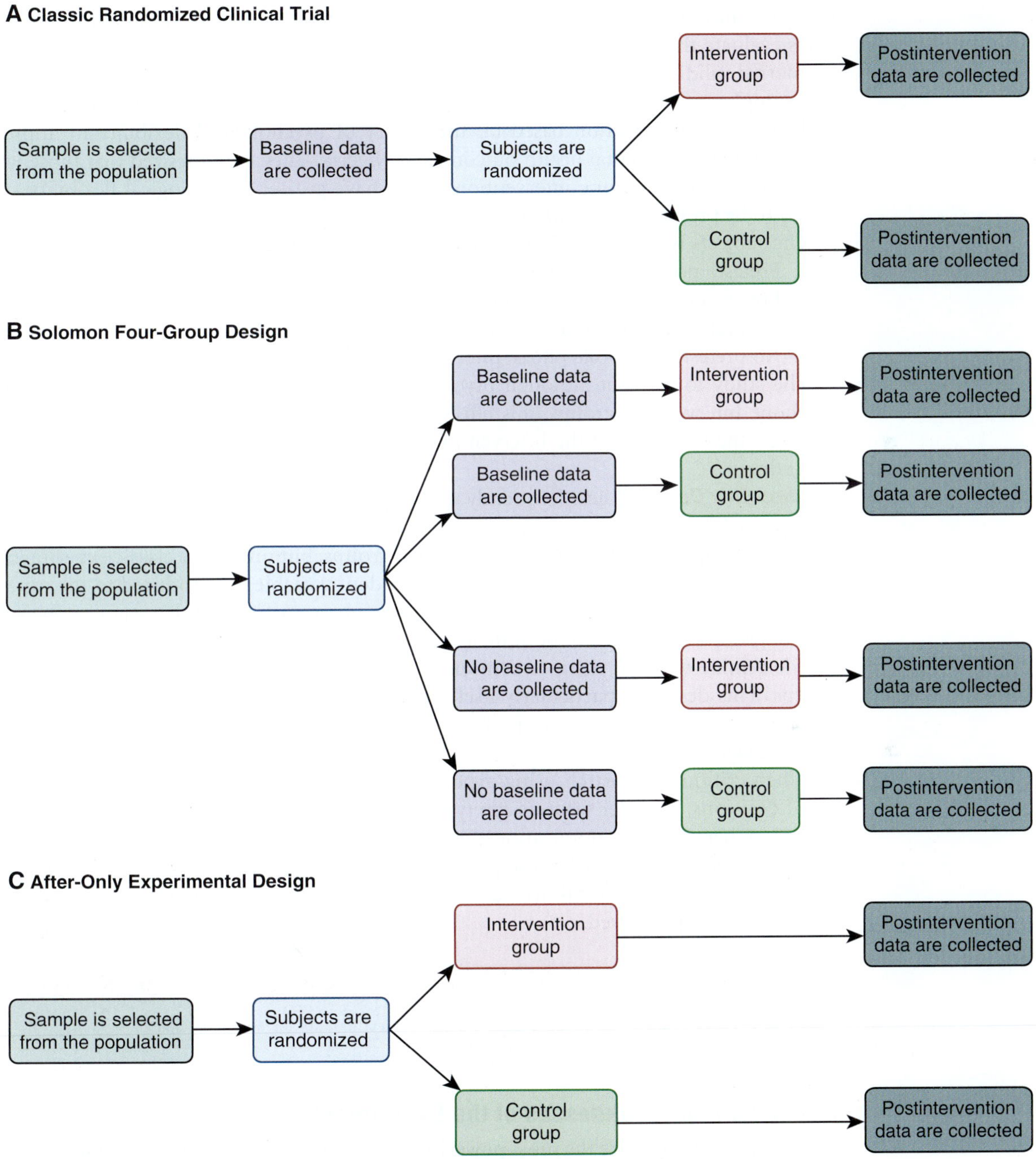

FIG 9.1 Experimental Designs. **A,** Classic randomized clinical trial. **B,** Solomon four-group design. **C,** After-only experimental design.

sensitization suggests that those who take the pretest learn what to concentrate on during the study and may score higher after the intervention is completed. Although this design helps evaluate the effects of testing, the threat of mortality (dropout) is a potential threat to internal validity.

Example: ➤ Ishola and Chipps (2015) used the Solomon four-group design to test a mobile phone intervention based on the theory of psychological flexibility to improve pregnant women's mental health outcomes in Nigeria. They hypothesized that those who received the mobile phone intervention would have greater psychological flexibility (the ability to be present and act when necessary).

- The subjects were randomly assigned to one of four groups:
  1. Pretest, mobile phone intervention, immediate posttest
  2. Pretest, no mobile phone intervention, immediate posttest
  3. No pretest, mobile phone intervention, posttest only
  4. No pretest, no mobile phone intervention, posttest only
- The study found that although psychological flexibility was improved in the mobile phone intervention groups, this effect was influenced by a significant interaction between the pretests and the intervention; thus, pretest sensitization was present in this study.

After-Only Design. A less frequently used experimental design is the **after-only design** (see Fig. 9.1C). This design, which is sometimes called the posttest-only control group design, is composed of two randomly assigned groups, but unlike the classic experimental design, neither group is pretested. The independent variable is introduced to the experimental group and not to the control group. The process of randomly assigning the subjects to groups is assumed to be sufficient to ensure lack of bias so that the researcher can still determine whether the intervention created significant differences between the two groups. This design is particularly useful when testing effects that are expected to be a major problem, or when outcomes cannot be measured beforehand (e.g., postoperative pain management).

When critiquing research using experimental designs, to help inform your evidence-based decisions, consider what design type was used; how the groups were formed (i.e., if the researchers used randomization); whether the groups were equivalent at baseline; if they were not equivalent, what the possible threats to internal validity were; what kind of manipulation (i.e., intervention) was administered to the experimental group; and what the control group received.

HELPFUL HINT

Look for evidence of pre-established inclusion and exclusion criteria for the study participants.

Strengths and Weaknesses of the Experimental Design

Experimental designs are the most powerful for testing cause-and-effect relationships due to the control, manipulation, and randomization components. Therefore, the design offers a better chance of measuring if the intervention caused the change or difference in the two groups. **Example:** ➤ Nyamathi and colleagues (2015) tested several types of interventions (peer coaching with nurse case management, peer coaching alone, and usual care) with paroled men to examine hepatitis A and B vaccine completion rates and found no significant differences between the groups. If you were working in a clinic caring for this population, you would consider this evidence as a starting point for putting research findings into clinical practice.

Experimental designs have weaknesses as well. They are complicated to design and can be costly to implement. **Example:** ➤ There may not be an adequate number of potential study participants in the accessible population. These studies may be difficult or impractical to carry out in a clinical setting. An example might be trying to randomly assign patients from one hospital unit to different groups when nurses might talk to each other about the different treatments. Experimental procedures also may be disruptive to the setting's usual routine. If several nurses are involved in administering the experimental program, it may be impossible to ensure that the program is administered in the same way with each subject. Another problem is that many important variables that are related to patient care outcomes are not amenable to manipulation for ethical reasons. **Example:** ➤ Cigarette smoking is known to be related to lung cancer, but you cannot randomly assign people to smoking or nonsmoking groups. Health status varies with age and socioeconomic status. No matter how careful a researcher is, no one can assign subjects randomly by age or by a certain income level. Because of these problems in carrying out experimental designs, researchers frequently turn to another type of research design to evaluate cause-and-effect relationships. Such designs, which look like experiments but lack some of the control of the true experimental design, are called quasi-experimental designs.

QUASI-EXPERIMENTAL DESIGNS

Quasi-experimental designs also test cause-and-effect relationships. However, in quasi-experimental designs, random assignment or the presence of a control group is lacking. The characteristics of an experimental study may not be possible to include because of the nature of the independent variable or the available subjects.

Without all the characteristics associated with an experimental study, internal validity may be compromised. Therefore, the basic problem with the quasi-experimental approach is a weakened confidence in making causal assertions that the results occurred because of the intervention. Instead, the findings may be a result of other extraneous variables. As a result, quasi-experimental studies provide Level III evidence. **Example:** ➤ Letourneau and colleagues (2015) used a quasi-experimental design to evaluate the effect of telephone peer support on maternal depression and social support with mothers diagnosed with postpartum depression. This one-group pretest-posttest design, where peer volunteers were trained and delivered phone social support, resulted in promising improvement in lower depression and higher perception of social support scores among the participants. However, there was a small group (11%) of mothers who had a "relapse" of depressive symptoms despite peer phone support. In this study there was no comparison group to see if the peer support was more effective than a comparison group and if the 11% of relapse to depression was a common occurrence among women with postpartum depression.

HELPFUL HINT

Remember that researchers often make trade-offs and sometimes use a quasi-experimental design instead of an experimental design because it may be impossible to randomly assign subjects to groups. Not using the "purest" design does not decrease the value of the study even though it may decrease the strength of the findings.

Types of Quasi-Experimental Designs

There are many different quasi-experimental designs, but we will limit the discussion to only those most commonly used in nursing research. Refer back to the experimental design shown in Fig. 9.1A, and compare it with the **nonequivalent control group design** shown in Fig. 9.2A. Note that this design looks exactly like the true experiment, except that subjects are not randomly assigned to groups. Suppose a researcher is interested in the effects of a new diabetes education program on the physical and psychosocial outcomes of patients newly diagnosed with diabetes. Under certain conditions, the researcher might be able to randomly assign subjects to either the group receiving the new program or the group receiving the usual program, but for any number of reasons, that might not be possible.

- For example, nurses on the unit where patients are admitted might be so excited about the new program that they cannot help but include the new information for all patients.
- The researcher has two choices: to abandon the study or to conduct a quasi-experiment.
- To conduct a quasi-experiment, the researcher might use one unit as the intervention group for the new program, find a similar unit that has not been introduced to the new

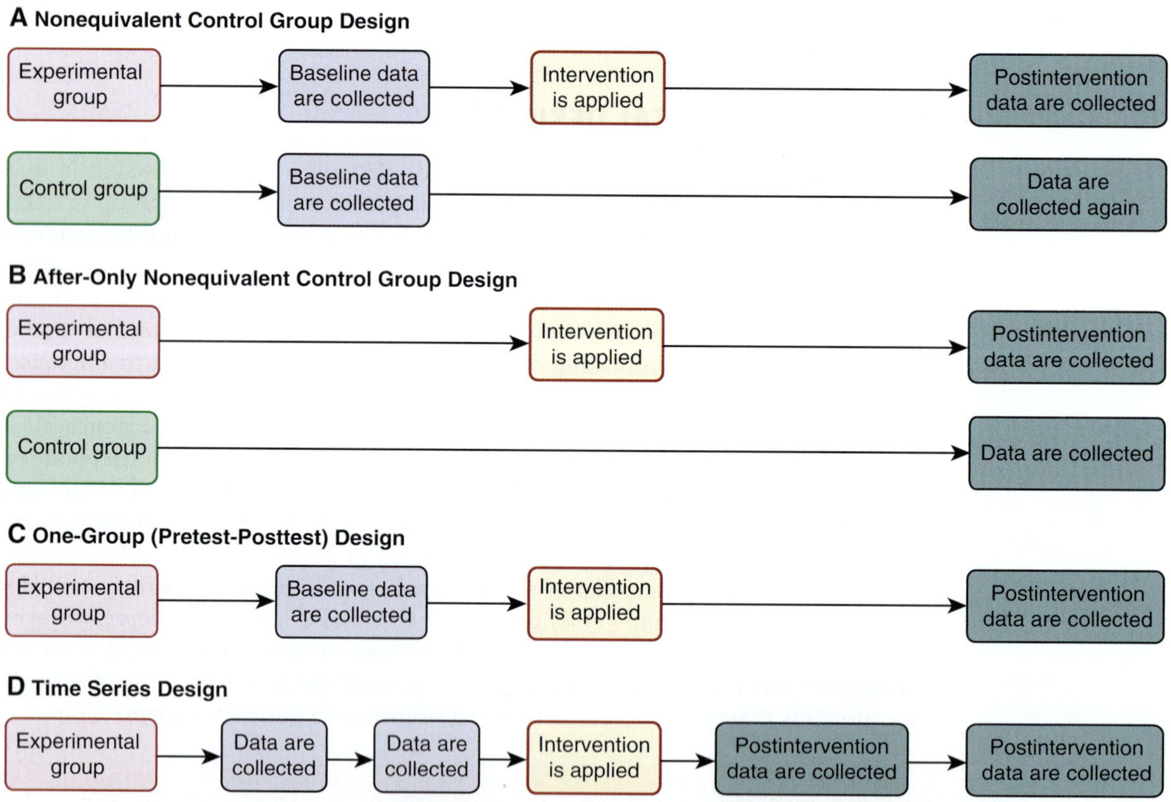

FIG 9.2 Quasi-experimental designs. **A,** Nonequivalent control group design. **B,** After-only nonequivalent control group design. **C,** One-group (pretest-posttest) design. **D,** Time series design.

program, and study the newly diagnosed patients with diabetes who are admitted to that unit as a comparison group. The study would then involve a quasi-experimental design.

Nonequivalent Control Group. The **nonequivalent control group design** is commonly used in nursing studies conducted in clinical settings. The basic problem with this design is the weakened confidence the researcher can have in assuming that the experimental and comparison groups are similar at the beginning of the study. Threats to internal validity, such as *selection effect, maturation, testing,* and *mortality,* are possible. However, the design is relatively strong because by gathering pretest data, the researcher can compare the equivalence of the two groups on important antecedent variables before the independent variable is introduced. **Antecedent variables** are variables that occur within the subjects prior to the study, such as in the previous example, where the patients' motivation to learn about their medical condition might be important in determining the effect of the diabetes education program. At the outset of the study, the researcher could include a measure of motivation to learn. Thus, differences between the two groups on this variable could be tested, and if significant differences existed, they could be controlled statistically in the analysis.

After-Only Nonequivalent Control Group. Sometimes the outcomes simply cannot be measured before the intervention, as with prenatal interventions that are expected to affect birth outcomes. The study that could be conducted would look like the **after-only nonequivalent control group design** shown in Fig. 9.2B. This design is similar to the after-only experimental design, but randomization is not used to assign subjects to groups and makes the assumption that the two groups are equivalent and comparable before the introduction of the independent variable. The soundness of the design and the confidence that we can put in the findings depend on the soundness of this assumption of preintervention comparability. Often it is difficult to support the assertion that the two nonrandomly assigned groups are comparable at the outset of the study, because there is no way of assessing its validity.

One-Group (Pretest-Posttest). Another quasi-experimental design is a **one-group (pretest-posttest) design** (see Fig. 9.2C), such as the Letourneau and colleagues (2015) example described earlier. This is used when only one group is available for study. Data are collected before and after an experimental treatment on one group of subjects. In this design, there is no control group and no randomization, which are important characteristics that enhance internal validity. Therefore, it becomes important that the evidence generated by the findings of this type of quasi-experimental design is interpreted with careful consideration of the design limitations.

Time Series. Another quasi-experimental approach used by researchers when only one group is available to study over a longer period of time is called a **time series design** (see Fig. 9.2D). Time series designs are useful for determining trends over time. Data are collected multiple times before the introduction of the treatment to establish a baseline point of reference on outcomes. The experimental treatment is introduced, and data are collected on multiple occasions to determine a change from baseline. The broad range and number of data collection points help rule out alternative explanations, such as history effects. However, the internal validity of testing is always present because of multiple data collection points. Without a control group, the internal validity threats of selection and maturation cannot be ruled out (see Chapter 8).

IPE HIGHLIGHT

When your team is critically appraising studies that use experimental and quasi-experimental designs, it is important to make sure that your team members understand the difference between random selection and random assignment (randomization).

Strengths and Weaknesses of Quasi-Experimental Designs

Quasi-experimental designs are used frequently because they are practical, less costly, and feasible, with potentially generalizable findings. These designs are more adaptable to the real-world practice setting than the controlled experimental designs. For some research questions and hypotheses, these designs may be the only way to evaluate the effect of the independent variable.

The weaknesses of the quasi-experimental approach involve the inability to make clear cause-and-effect statements.

QSEN EVIDENCE-BASED PRACTICE TIP

Experimental designs provide Level II evidence, and quasi-experimental designs provide Level III evidence. Quasi-experimental designs are lower on the evidence hierarchy because of lack of control, which limits the ability to make confident cause-and-effect statements that influence applicability to practice and clinical decision making.

EVIDENCE-BASED PRACTICE

As nursing science expands, and accountability for cost-effective quality clinical outcomes increases, nurses must become more cognizant of what constitutes best practice for their patient population. An understanding of the value of intervention studies that use an experimental or quasi-experimental design is critical for improving clinical outcomes. These study designs provide the strongest evidence for making informed clinical decisions. These designs are those most commonly included in systematic reviews (see Chapter 11).

One cannot assume that because an intervention study has been published that the findings apply to your practice population. When conducting an evidence-based practice project, the clinical question provides a guide for you and your team to collect the strongest, most relevant evidence related to your problem. If your search of the literature reveals experimental and quasi-experimental studies, you will need to evaluate them to determine which studies provide the best available evidence. The likelihood of changing practice based on one study is low, unless it is a large clinical RCT based on prior research evidence.

Key points for evaluating the evidence and whether bias has been minimized in experimental and quasi-experimental designs include:

- Random group assignment (experimental or intervention and control or comparison)
- Inclusion and exclusion criteria that are relevant to the clinical problem studied
- Equivalence of groups at baseline on key demographic variables
- Adequate sample size recruitment of a homogeneous sample
- Intervention fidelity and consistent data collection procedures
- Control of antecedent, **intervening**, or **extraneous variables**

CRITICAL APPRAISAL CRITERIA

Experimental and Quasi-Experimental Designs

1. Is the design used appropriate to the research question or hypothesis?
2. Is there a detailed description of the intervention?
3. Is there a clear description of the intervention group treatment in comparison to the control group? How is intervention fidelity maintained?
4. Is power analysis used to calculate the appropriate sample size for the study?

Experimental Designs

1. What experimental design is used in the study?
2. How are randomization, control, and manipulation implemented?
3. Are the findings generalizable to the larger population of interest?

Quasi-Experimental Designs

1. What quasi-experimental design is used in the study, and is it appropriate?
2. What are the most common threats to internal and external validity of the findings of this design?
3. What does the author say about the limitations of the study?
4. To what extent are the study findings generalizable?

APPRAISAL FOR EVIDENCE-BASED PRACTICE EXPERIMENTAL AND QUASI-EXPERIMENTAL DESIGNS

Research designs differ in the amount of control the researcher has over the antecedent and intervening variables that may affect the study's results. Experimental designs, which provide Level II evidence, provide the most possibility for control. Quasi-experimental designs, which provide Level III evidence, provide less control. When conducting an evidence-based practice or quality improvement project, you must always look for studies that provide the highest level of evidence (see Chapter 1). For some PICO questions (see Chapter 2), you will find both Level II and Level III evidence. You will want to determine if the choice of design, experimental or quasi-experimental, is appropriate to the purpose of the study and can answer the research question or hypotheses.

HELPFUL HINT

When reviewing the experimental and quasi-experimental literature, do not limit your search only to your patient population. For example, it is possible that if you are working with adult caregivers, related parent caregiver intervention studies may provide you with strategies as well. Many times, with some adaptation, interventions used with one sample may be applicable for other populations.

Questions that you should pose when reading studies that test cause-and-effect relationships are listed in the Critical Appraisal Criteria box. These questions should help you judge whether a causal relationship exists.

For studies in which either experimental or quasi-experimental designs are used, first try to determine the type of design that was used. Often a statement describing the design of the study appears in the abstract and in the methods section of the article. If such a statement is not present, you should examine the article for evidence of control, randomization, and manipulation. If all are discussed, the design is probably experimental. On the other hand, if the study involves the administration of an experimental treatment but does not involve the random assignment of subjects to groups, the design is quasi-experimental. Next, try to identify which of the experimental and quasi-experimental designs was used. Determining the answer to these questions gives you a head start, because each design has its inherent threats to internal and external validity. This step makes it a bit easier to critically evaluate the study. It is important that the author provide adequate accounts of how the procedures for randomization, control, and manipulation were carried out. The report should include a description of the procedures for random assignment to such a degree that the reader could determine just how likely it was for any one subject to be assigned to a particular group. The description of the intervention that each group received provides important information about what intervention fidelity strategies were implemented.

The inclusion of this information helps determine if the intervention group and control group received different treatments that were consistently carried out by trained interventionists and data collectors. The question of threats to internal validity, such as testing and mortality, is even more important to consider when critically evaluating a quasi-experimental study, because quasi-experimental designs cannot possibly feature as much control; there may be a lack of randomization or a control group. A well-written report of a quasi-experimental study systematically reviews potential threats to the internal and external validity of the findings. Your work is to decide if the author's explanations make sense. For either experimental or quasi-experimental studies, you should also check for a reported power analysis that assures you that an appropriate sample size for detecting a treatment effect was planned.

KEY POINTS

- Experimental designs or RCTs provide the strongest evidence (Level II) for a single study that tests whether an intervention or treatment affects patient outcomes.
- Experimental designs are characterized by the ability of the researcher to control extraneous variation, to manipulate the independent variable, and to randomly assign subjects to intervention groups.
- Experimental studies conducted either in clinical settings or in the laboratory provide the best evidence in support of a causal relationship because the following three criteria can be met: (1) the independent and dependent variables are related to each other; (2) the independent variable chronologically precedes the dependent variable; and (3) the relationship cannot be explained by the presence of a third variable.
- Researchers turn to quasi-experimental designs to test cause-and-effect relationships because experimental designs may be impractical or unethical.
- Quasi-experiments may lack the randomization and/or the comparison group characteristics of true experiments. The usefulness of quasi-experiments for studying causal relationships depends on the ability of the researcher to rule out plausible threats to the validity of the findings, such as history, selection, maturation, and testing effects.

CRITICAL THINKING CHALLENGES

- Describe the ethical issues included in a true experimental research design used by a nurse researcher.

- Describe how a true experimental design could be used in a hospital setting with patients.
- How should a nurse go about critiquing experimental research articles in the research literature so that his or her evidence-based practice is enhanced?
- IPE Discuss whether your QI team would use an experimental or quasi-experimental design for a quality improvement project.
- Identify a clinical quality indicator that is a problem on your unit (e.g., falls, ventilator-acquired pneumonia, catheter-acquired urinary tract infection), and consider how a search for studies using experimental or quasi-experimental designs could provide the foundation for a quality improvement project.

REFERENCES

Campbell, D., & Stanley, J. (1966). *Experimental and quasi-experimental designs for research.* Chicago, IL: Rand-McNally.

Gearing, R. E., El-Bassel, N., Ghesquiere, A., et al. (2011). Major ingredients of fidelity: A review and scientific guide to improving quality of intervention research implementation. *Clinical Psychology Review*, *31*, 79–88. doi:10.1016/jcpr.2010.09.007.

Ishola, A. G., & Chipps, J. (2015). The use of mobile phones to deliver acceptance and commitment therapy in the prevention of mother-child HIV transmission in Nigeria. *Journal of Telemedicine and Telecare*, *21*, 423–426. doi:10.1177/1357633X15605408.

Letourneau, N., Secco, L., Colpitts, J., et al. (2015). Quasi-experimental evaluation of a telephone-based peer support intervention for maternal depression. *Journal of Advanced Nursing*, *71*, 1587–1599. doi:10.1111/jan.12622.

Nyamathi, A., Salem, B. E., Zhang, S., et al. (2015). Nursing care management, peer coaching, and hepatitis A and B vaccine completion among homeless men recently released on parole. *Nursing Research*, *64*(3), 177–189.

Preyde, M., & Burnham, P. V. (2011). Intervention fidelity in psychosocial oncology. *Journal of Evidence-Based Social Work*, *8*, 379–396. doi:10.1080/15433714.2011.54234.

Suresh, K. P. (2011). An overview of randomization techniques: An unbiased assessment of outcome in clinical research. *Journal of Human Reproductive Science*, *4*, 8–11.

Wickersham, K., Colbert, A., Caruthers, D., et al. (2011). Assessing fidelity to an intervention in a randomized controlled trial to improve medication adherence. *Nursing Research*, *60*, 264–269.

Go to Evolve at **http://evolve.elsevier.com/LoBiondo/** for review questions, critiquing exercises, and additional research articles for practice in reviewing and critiquing.

10

Nonexperimental Designs

Geri LoBiondo-Wood and Judith Haber

Go to Evolve at **http://evolve.elsevier.com/LoBiondo/** for review questions, critiquing exercises, and additional research articles for practice in reviewing and critiquing.

LEARNING OUTCOMES

After reading this chapter, you should be able to do the following:

- Describe the purpose of nonexperimental designs.
- Describe the characteristics of nonexperimental designs.
- Define the differences between nonexperimental designs.
- List the advantages and disadvantages of nonexperimental designs.
- Identify the purpose and methods of methodological, secondary analysis, and mixed method designs.
- Identify the critical appraisal criteria used to critique nonexperimental research designs.
- Evaluate the strength and quality of evidence by nonexperimental designs.

KEY TERMS

case control study
cohort study
correlational study
cross-sectional study
developmental study
ex post facto study
longitudinal study
methodological research
mixed methods
prospective study
psychometrics
repeated measures studies
retrospective study
secondary analysis
survey studies

Many phenomena relevant to nursing do not lend themselves to an experimental design. For example, nurses studying cancer-related fatigue may be interested in the amount of fatigue, variations in fatigue, and patient fatigue in response to chemotherapy. The investigator would not design an experimental study and implement an intervention that would potentially intensify an aspect of a patient's fatigue just to study the fatigue experience. Instead, the researcher would examine the factors that contribute to the variability in a patient's cancer-related fatigue experience using a nonexperimental design. Nonexperimental designs are used when a researcher wishes to explore events, people, or situations as they occur; or test relationships and differences among variables. Nonexperimental designs construct a picture of variables at one point or over a period of time.

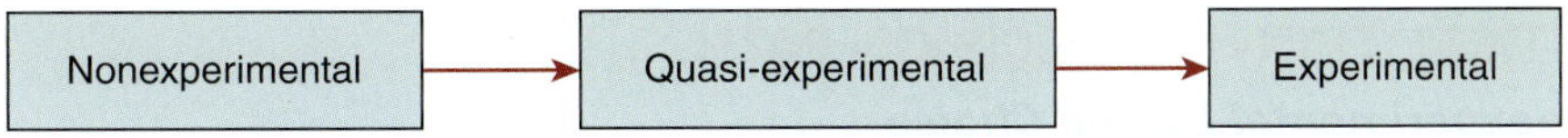

FIG 10.1 Continuum of quantitative research design.

In nonexperimental research the independent variables have naturally occurred, so to speak, and the investigator cannot directly control them by manipulation. As the researcher does not actively manipulate the variables, the concepts of control and potential sources of bias (see Chapter 8) should be considered. Nonexperimental designs provide Level IV evidence. The information yielded by these types of designs is critical to developing an evidence base for practice and may represent the best evidence available to answer research or clinical questions.

Researchers are not in agreement on how to classify nonexperimental studies. A continuum of quantitative research design is presented in Fig. 10.1. Nonexperimental studies explore the relationships or the differences between variables. This chapter divides nonexperimental designs into survey studies and relationship/difference studies as illustrated in Box 10.1. These categories are somewhat flexible, and other sources may classify nonexperimental studies differently. Some studies fall exclusively within one of these categories, whereas other studies have characteristics of more than one category (Table 10.1). As you

BOX 10.1 Summary of Nonexperimental Research Designs

I. Survey Studies
- A. Descriptive
- B. Exploratory
- C. Comparative

II. Relationship/Difference Studies
- A. Correlational studies
- B. Developmental studies
  1. Cross-sectional
  2. Cohort, longitudinal, and prospective
  3. Case control, retrospective, and ex post facto

TABLE 10.1 Examples of Studies With More Than One Design Label

Design Type	Study's Purpose
Retrospective, predictive correlation	To identify predictors of initial and repeated unplanned hospitalizations and potential financial impact among Medicare patients with early stage (Stages I–III) colorectal cancer receiving outpatient chemotherapy using the SEER Medicare database (Fessele et al., 2016)
Descriptive, exploratory, secondary analysis of a randomized controlled trial	To describe drug use and sexual behavior (sex with multiple partners) prior to incarceration and 6 and 12 months after study enrollment using data obtained as part of a randomized controlled trial designed to study the effects of intensive peer coaching and nurse case management, intensive peer coaching, and brief nurse counseling on hepatitis A and B vaccination adherence (Nyamathi et al., 2015, 2016; see Appendix A)
Longitudinal, descriptive	This longitudinal, single group study was conducted to determine whether empirically selected and social cognitive theory-based factors, including baseline characteristics and modifiable behavioral and psychosocial factors, were determinants of PA maintenance in breast cancer survivors after a physical activity intervention (Lee, Von, et al., 2016).

PA, Physical activity; *SEER,* Surveillance, Epidemiology, and End Results.

CRITICAL THINKING DECISION PATH

Nonexperimental Design Choice

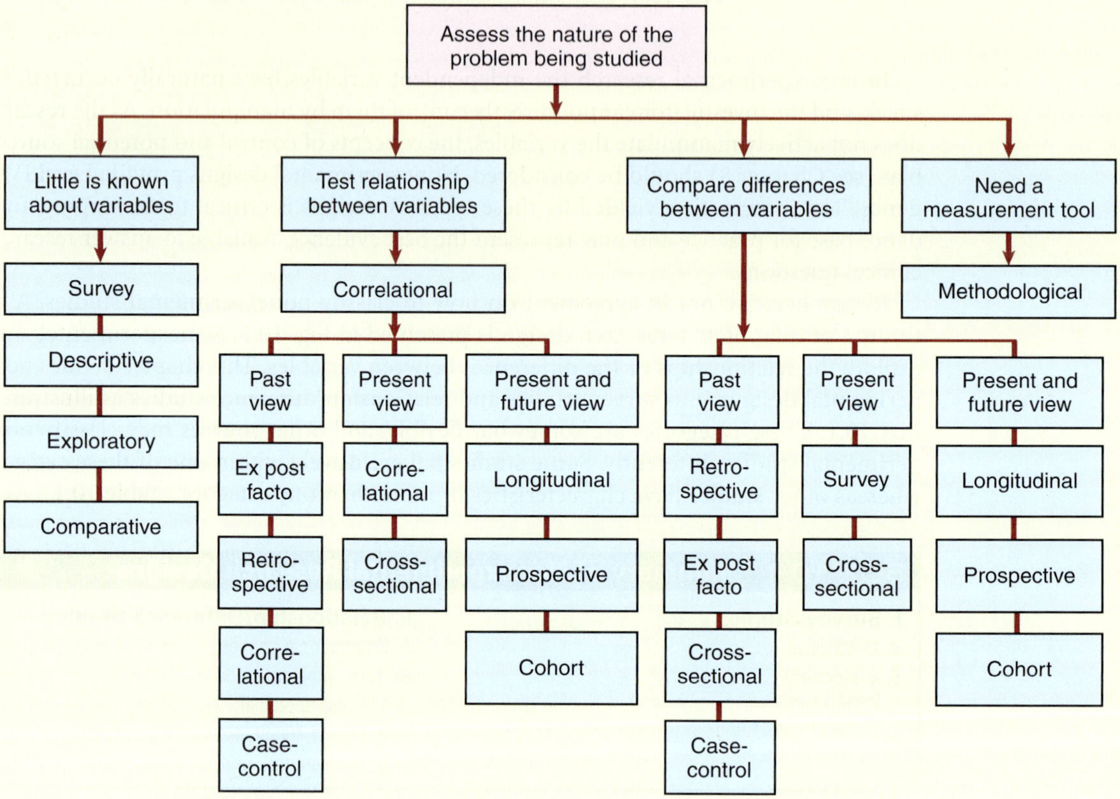

read the research literature, you will often find that researchers use several design classifications for one study. This chapter introduces the types of nonexperimental designs and discusses their advantages and disadvantages, the use of nonexperimental research, the issues of causality, and the critiquing process as it relates to nonexperimental research. The Critical Thinking Decision Path outlines the path to the choice of a nonexperimental design.

QSEN EVIDENCE-BASED PRACTICE TIPS

When critically appraising nonexperimental studies, you need to be aware of possible sources of bias that can be introduced at any point in the study.

SURVEY STUDIES

The broadest category of nonexperimental designs is the survey study. **Survey studies** are further classified as *descriptive*, *exploratory*, or *comparative*. *Surveys* collect detailed descriptions of variables and use the data to justify and assess conditions and practices or to make

BOX 10.2 Survey Design Examples

- Bender and colleagues (2016) developed and administered a survey to a nationwide sample ($n = 585$) of certified clinical nurse leaders (CNLs) and managers, leaders, educators, clinicians, and change agents involved in planning and integrating CNLs into a health system's nursing care delivery model. Items addressed organizational and implementation characteristics and perceived level of CNL initiative success.
- Lee, Fan, and colleagues (2016) conducted a survey to investigate the differences between perceptions of injured patients and their caregivers. Participants completed the Chinese Illness Perception Questionnaire Revised–Trauma. Exploring the differences in illness perceptions between injured patients and their caregivers can help clinicians provide individualized care and design interventions that meets patients' and caregivers' needs.

plans for improving health care practices. You will find that the terms *exploratory, descriptive, comparative,* and *survey* are used either alone, interchangeably, or together to describe this type of study's design (see Table 10.1).

- A survey is used to search for information about the characteristics of particular subjects, groups, institutions, or situations, or about the frequency of a variable's occurrence, particularly when little is known about the variable. Box 10.2 provides examples of survey studies.
- Variables can be classified as opinions, attitudes, or facts.
- Fact variables include gender, income level, political and religious affiliations, ethnicity, occupation, and educational level.
- Surveys provide the basis for the development of intervention studies.
- Surveys are described as comparative when used to determine differences between variables.
- Survey data can be collected with a questionnaire or an interview (see Chapter 14).
- Surveys have small or large samples of subjects drawn from defined populations, can be either broad or narrow, and can be made up of people or institutions.
- Surveys relate one variable to another or assess differences between variables, but do not determine causation.

The advantages of surveys are that a great deal of information can be obtained from a large population in a fairly economical manner, and that survey research information can be surprisingly accurate. If a sample is representative of the population (see Chapter 12), even a relatively small number of subjects can provide an accurate picture of the population.

Survey studies do have disadvantages. The information obtained in a survey tends to be superficial. The breadth rather than the depth of the information is emphasized.

QSEN EVIDENCE-BASED PRACTICE TIPS

Evidence gained from a survey may be coupled with clinical expertise and applied to a similar population to develop an educational program, to enhance knowledge and skills in a particular clinical area (e.g., a survey designed to measure the nursing staff's knowledge and attitudes about evidence-based practice where the data are used to develop an evidence-based practice staff development course).

HELPFUL HINT

You should recognize that a well-constructed survey can provide a wealth of data about a particular phenomenon of interest, even though causation is not being examined.

RELATIONSHIP AND DIFFERENCE STUDIES

Investigators also try to assess the relationships or differences between variables that can provide insight into a phenomenon. These studies can be classified as relationship or difference studies. The following types of **relationship/difference studies** are discussed: correlational studies and developmental studies.

Correlational Studies

In a **correlational study** the *relationship* between two or more variables is examined. The researcher does not test whether one variable causes another variable. Rather, the researcher is:

- Testing whether the variables co-vary (i.e., As one variable changes, does a related change occur in another variable?)
- Interested in quantifying the strength of the relationship between variables, or in testing a hypothesis or research question about a specific relationship

The direction of the relationship is important (see Chapter 16 for an explanation of the correlation coefficient). For example, in their correlational study, Turner-Sack and colleagues (2016) examined psychological functioning, post-traumatic growth (PTG), and coping and cancer–related characteristics of adolescent cancer survivors' parents and siblings (see Appendix D). This study tested multiple variables to assess the relationship and differences among the sample. One finding was that parents' psychological distress was negatively correlated with their survivor child's active coping ($r = -0.53, p < .001$). The study findings revealed that younger age, higher life satisfaction, and less avoidant coping were strong predictors of lower psychological distress in parents of adolescent cancer survivors. Thus the variables were related to (not causal of) outcomes. Each step of this study was consistent with the aims of exploring relationships among variables.

When reviewing a correlational study, remember what relationship the researcher tested and notice whether the researcher implied a relationship that is consistent with the theoretical framework and research question(s) or hypotheses being tested. Correlational studies offer the following advantages:

- An efficient and effective method of collecting a large amount of data about a problem
- A potential for evidence-based application in clinical settings
- A potential foundation for future experimental research studies
- A framework for exploring the relationship between variables that cannot be manipulated

The following are disadvantages of correlational studies:

- Variables are not manipulated.
- Randomization is not used because the groups are preexisting, and therefore generalizability is decreased.
- The researcher is unable to determine a causal relationship between the variables because of the lack of manipulation, control, and randomization.
- The strength and quality of evidence is limited by the associative nature of the relationship between the variables.

Correlational studies may be further labeled as *descriptive correlational* or *predictive correlational.* In terms of evidence for practice, the researchers based on the literature review and findings, frame the utility of the results in light of previous research and therefore help establish the "best available" evidence that, combined with clinical expertise, informs clinical decisions regarding the study's applicability to a specific patient population. A correlational design is a very useful design for clinical studies because many of the phenomena of clinical interest are beyond the researcher's ability to manipulate, control, and randomize.

> **IPE HIGHLIGHT**
>
> When your QI team's search of the literature for intervention studies reporting evidence-based strategies for preventing ventilator acquired pneumonia (VAP) yields only studies using nonexperimental designs, your team members should debate whether the evidence is of sufficient quality to be applied to answering your clinical question.

Developmental Studies

There are also classifications of nonexperimental designs that use a time perspective. Investigators who use **developmental studies** are concerned not only with the existing status and the relationship and differences among phenomena at one point in time, but also with changes that result from elapsed time. The following types of designs are discussed: cross-sectional, cohort/longitudinal/prospective, and case control/retrospective/ex post facto. In the literature, studies may be designated by more than one design name. This practice is accepted because many studies have elements of several designs. Table 10.1 provides examples of studies classified with more than one design label.

> **QSEN EVIDENCE-BASED PRACTICE TIPS**
>
> Replication of significant findings in nonexperimental studies with similar and/or different populations increases your confidence in the conclusions offered by the researcher and the strength of evidence generated by consistent findings from more than one study.

Cross-Sectional Studies

A **cross-sectional study** examines data at one point in time; that is, data are collected on only one occasion with the same subjects rather than with the same subjects at several time points. For example, a cross-sectional study was conducted by Koc and Cinarli (2015) to determine knowledge, awareness, and practices of Turkish hospital nurses in relation to cervical cancer, human papillomavirus (HPV), and HPV vaccination. The researchers aimed to answer several research questions:

- What is the level of knowledge about cancer risk factors?
- What is the level of knowledge about early diagnosis?
- What are the awareness, knowledge, information sources, and practices regarding HPV infection and HPV vaccine administration?
- What are the relationships between the sociodemographic (age, willingness to receive HPV vaccination, willingness for their children to receive HPV vaccination) and professional characteristics (education, belief that cervical cancer can be prevented by HPV vaccination), and overall level of knowledge about cervical cancer, HPV, and HPV vaccines?

As you can see, the variables were related to, not causal of, outcomes. Each step of this study was consistent with the aims of exploring the relationship and differences among variables in a cross-sectional design.

In this study the sample subjects participated on one occasion; that is, data were collected on only one occasion from each subject and represented a cross section of 464 Turkish nurses working in hospital settings, rather than the researchers following a group of nurses over time. The purpose of this study was not to test causality, but to explore the potential relationships between and among variables that can be related to knowledge about HPV, belief in the effectiveness of early cervical cancer screening, and HPV vaccination. The authors concluded that higher levels of knowledge among nurses may increase their willingness to recommend the HPV vaccine to patients. Cross-sectional studies can explore relationships and correlations, or differences and comparisons, or both. Advantages and disadvantages of cross-sectional studies are as follows:

- Cross-sectional studies, when compared to longitudinal/cohort/prospective studies are less time-consuming, less expensive, and thus more manageable.
- Large amounts of data can be collected at one point, making the results more readily available.
- The confounding variable of maturation, resulting from the elapsed time, is not present.
- The investigator's ability to establish an in-depth developmental assessment of the relationships of the variables being studied is lessened. The researcher is unable to determine whether the change that occurred is related to the change that was predicted because the same subjects were not followed over a period of time. In other words, the subjects are unable to serve as their own controls (see Chapter 8).

Cohort/Prospective/Longitudinal/Repeated Measures Studies

In contrast to the cross-sectional design, cohort studies collect data from the same group at different points in time. **Cohort studies** are also referred to as **longitudinal, prospective,** and **repeated measures studies**. These terms are interchangeable. Like cross-sectional studies, cohort studies explore differences and relationships among variables. An example of a longitudinal (cohort) study is found in the study by Hawthorne and colleagues (2016; see Appendix B). This study tested the relationships between spiritual/religious coping strategies and grief, mental health (depression and post-traumatic stress disorder), and personal growth for mothers and fathers at 1 and 3 months after their infant/child's death in the NICU/PICU with and without control for race/ethnicity and religion. They concluded that spiritual strategies and activities were associated with lower symptoms of grief and depression in parents and post-traumatic stress in mothers but not post-traumatic stress in fathers.

Cohort designs have advantages and disadvantages. When assessing the appropriateness of a cross-sectional study versus a cohort study, first assess the nature of the research question or hypothesis: Cohort studies allow clinicians to assess the incidence of a problem over time and potential reasons for changes in the study's variables. However, the disadvantages inherent in a cohort study also must be considered. Data collection may be of long duration; therefore, subject loss or mortality can be high due to the time it takes for the subjects to progress to each data collection point. The internal validity threat of testing is also present and may be unavoidable in a cohort study. Subject loss to follow-up or attrition, may lead to unintended sample bias affecting both the internal validity and external validity of the study.

These realities make a cohort study costly in terms of time, effort, and money. There is also a chance of confounding variables that could affect the interpretation of the results.

Subjects in such a study may respond in a socially desirable way that they believe is congruent with the investigator's expectations (Hawthorne effect). Advantages of a cohort study are as follows:

- Each subject is followed separately and thereby serves as his or her own control.
- Increased depth of responses can be obtained and early trends in the data can be analyzed.
- The researcher can assess changes in the variables of interest over time, and both relationships and differences can be explored between variables.

In summary, cohort studies begin in the present and end in the future, and cross-sectional studies look at a broader perspective of a population at a specific point in time.

Case Control/Retrospective/Ex Post Facto Studies

A **case control study** is essentially the same as an **ex post facto study** and a **retrospective study**. In these studies, the dependent variable already has been affected by the independent variable, and the investigator attempts to link present events to events that occurred in the past. When researchers wish to explain causality or the factors that determine the occurrence of events or conditions, they prefer to use an experimental design. However, they cannot always manipulate the independent variable, or use random assignments. When experimental designs that test the effect of an intervention or condition cannot be employed, case control (ex post facto or retrospective) studies may be used. Ex post facto literally means "from after the fact." Case control, ex post facto, retrospective, or case control studies also are known as *causal-comparative* studies or *comparative* studies. As we discuss this design further, you will see that many elements of this category are similar to quasi-experimental designs because they explore differences between variables (Campbell & Stanley, 1963).

In case control studies, a researcher hypothesizes, for instance:

- That X (cigarette smoking) is related to and a determinant of Y (lung cancer).
- But X, the presumed cause, is not manipulated and subjects are not randomly assigned to groups.
- Rather, a group of subjects who have experienced X (cigarette smoking) in a normal situation is located and a control group of subjects who have not experienced X is chosen.
- The behavior, performance, or condition (lung tissue) of the two groups is compared to determine whether the exposure to X had the effect predicted by the hypothesis.

Table 10.2 illustrates this example. Examination of Table 10.2 reveals that although cigarette smoking appears to be a determinant of lung cancer, the researcher is still not able to conclude that a causal relationship exists between the variables, because the independent variable has not been manipulated and subjects were not randomly assigned to groups.

TABLE 10.2 Paradigm for the Ex Post Facto Design

Groups (Not Randomly Assigned)	Independent Variable (Not Manipulated by Investigator)	Dependent Variable
Exposed group: Cigarette smokers	X	Y_e
	Cigarette smoking	Lung cancer
Control group: Nonsmokers	—	Y_c
	—	No lung cancer

Kousha and Castner (2016) conducted a case control study to explore novel multipollutant exposure assessments using the Air Quality Health Index in relation to emergency department (ED) visits over a 6-year period for otitis media (OM). They used information from ED visits (n = 4815 children from 3 years of age and younger) for OM, air pollution, and weather databases. The findings indicate that there was an increase in ED visits with OM diagnoses 6 to 7 days after exposure to increased ozone and 3 to 4 days after exposure to particulate matter. These findings confirm that there is an association between changes in the Air Quality Index and ED visits for OM. These findings can be used to inform risk communication, patient education, and policy.

QSEN EVIDENCE-BASED PRACTICE TIPS

The quality of evidence provided by a cohort/longitudinal/prospective study is stronger than that from other nonexperimental designs because the researcher can determine the incidence of a problem and its possible causes.

The advantages of the case control/retrospective/ex post facto design are similar to those of the correlational design. The additional benefit is that it offers a higher level of control than a correlational study, thereby increasing the confidence the research consumer would have in the evidence provided by the findings. For example, in the cigarette smoking study, a group of nonsmokers' lung tissue samples are compared with samples of smokers' lung tissue. This comparison enables the researcher to establish the existence of a differential effect of cigarette smoking on lung tissue. However, the researcher remains unable to draw a causal linkage between the two variables, and this inability is the major disadvantage of the case control/retrospective/ex post facto/case control design.

Another disadvantage is the problem of an alternative hypothesis being the reason for the documented relationship. If the researcher obtains data from two existing groups of subjects, such as one that has been exposed to X and one that has not, and the data support the hypothesis that X is related to Y, the researcher cannot be sure whether X or some extraneous variable is the real cause of the occurrence of Y. As such, the impact or effect of the relationship cannot be estimated accurately. Finding naturally occurring groups of subjects who are similar in all respects except for their exposure to the variable of interest is very difficult. There is always the possibility that the groups differ in some other way, such as exposure to other lung irritants (e.g., asbestos), that can affect the findings of the study and produce spurious or unreliable results. Consequently, you need to cautiously evaluate the conclusions drawn by the investigator.

HELPFUL HINT

When reading research reports, you will note that at times researchers classify a study's design with more than one design type label. This is correct because research studies often reflect aspects of more than one design label.

Cohort/longitudinal/prospective studies are considered to be stronger than case control/retrospective studies because of the degree of control that can be imposed on extraneous variables that might confound the data and lead to bias.

HELPFUL HINT

Remember that nonexperimental designs can test relationships, differences, comparisons, or predictions, depending on the purpose of the study.

PREDICTION AND CAUSALITY IN NONEXPERIMENTAL RESEARCH

A concern of researchers and research consumers is the issues of prediction and causality. Researchers are interested in explaining cause-and-effect relationships—that is, estimating the effect of one phenomenon on another without bias. Historically, researchers thought that only experimental research could support the concept of causality. For example, nurses are interested in discovering what causes anxiety in many settings. If we can uncover the causes, we could develop interventions that would prevent or decrease the anxiety. Causality makes it necessary to order events chronologically; that is, if we find in a randomly assigned experiment that event 1 (stress) occurs before event 2 (anxiety) and that those in the stressed group were anxious whereas those in the unstressed group were not, we can say that the hypothesis of stress causing anxiety is supported by these empirical observations. If these results were found in a nonexperimental study where some subjects underwent the stress of surgery and were anxious and others did not have surgery and were not anxious, we would say that there is an association or relationship between stress (surgery) and anxiety. But on the basis of the results of a nonexperimental study, we could not say that the stress of surgery caused the anxiety.

QSEN EVIDENCE-BASED PRACTICE TIPS

Studies that use nonexperimental designs often precede and provide the foundation for building a program of research that leads to experimental designs that test the effectiveness of nursing interventions.

Many variables (e.g., anxiety) that nurse researchers wish to study cannot be manipulated, nor would it be wise or ethical to manipulate them. Yet there is a need to have studies that can assert a predictive or causal sequence. In light of this need, many nurse researchers are using several analytical techniques that can explain the relationships among variables to establish predictive or causal links. These analytical techniques are called *causal modeling, model testing,* and *associated causal analysis techniques* (Kline, 2011; Plichta & Kelvin, 2013).

When reading studies, you also will find the terms *path analysis,* LISREL, *analysis of covariance structures, structural equation modeling (SEM),* and *hierarchical linear modeling (HLM)* to describe the statistical techniques (see Chapter 16) used in these studies. These terms do not designate the design of a study, but are statistical tests that are used in many nonexperimental designs to predict how precisely a dependent variable can be predicted based on an independent variable. For example, SEM was used to understand risk and promotive factors for youth violence and bullying in a sample of US seventh grade students who completed a survey containing items about future expectations, attitudes towards violence, past 30-day bullying experiences, and violent behavior. SEM was used to establish a model of how the variables related to one another. The findings supported the hypothesis that more positive future expectations would be related to lower levels of both physical and relational bullying and that relational bullying would be mediated by attitudes towards violence (Stoddard et al., 2015). This sophisticated design aids understanding of bullying behavior and the positive aspects of early adolescents' lives that may help them avoid such behavior and provide useful direction for professionals like school nurses and other school-based mental health professionals when developing interventions focused on decreasing bullying. Sometimes researchers want to make a forecast or prediction about how patients will respond to an intervention or a disease process or how successful individuals will be in a particular setting or field of specialty. In this case, a model may be tested to assess which physical activity scores were not significant.

Many nursing studies test models. The statistics used in model-testing studies are advanced, but you should be able to read the article, understand the purpose of the study, and determine if the model generated was logical and developed with a solid basis from the literature and past research. This section cites several studies that conducted sound tests of theoretical models.

HELPFUL HINT

Nonexperimental research studies have progressed to the point where prediction models are often used to explore or test relationships between independent and dependent variables.

ADDITIONAL TYPES OF QUANTITATIVE METHODS

Other types of quantitative studies complement the science of research. The additional research methods provide a means of viewing and interpreting phenomena that give further breadth and knowledge to nursing science and practice. The additional types include methodological research, secondary analysis, and mixed methods.

Methodological Research

Methodological research is the development and evaluation of data collection instruments, scales, or techniques. As you will find in Chapters 14 and 15, methodology greatly influences research and the evidence produced.

The most significant and critically important aspect of methodological research addressed in measurement development is called **psychometrics**. Psychometrics focuses on the theory and development of measurement instruments (such as questionnaires) or measurement techniques (such as observational techniques) through the research process. Nurse researchers have used the principles of psychometrics to develop and test measurement instruments that focus on nursing phenomena. Many of the phenomena of interest to practice and research are intangible, such as interpersonal conflict, resilience, quality of life, coping, and symptom experience. The intangible nature of various phenomena—yet the recognition of the need to measure them—places methodological research in an important position. Methodological research differs from other designs of research in two ways. First, it does not include all of the research process steps as discussed in Chapter 1. Second, to implement its techniques, the researcher must have a sound knowledge of psychometrics or must consult with a researcher knowledgeable in psychometric techniques. The methodological researcher is not interested in the relationship of the independent variable and dependent variable or in the effect of an independent variable on a dependent variable. The methodological researcher is interested in identifying an intangible construct (concept) and making it tangible with a paper-and-pencil instrument or observation protocol.

A methodological study basically includes the following steps:

- Defining the concept or behavior to be measured
- Formulating the instrument's items
- Developing instructions for users and respondents
- Testing the instrument's reliability and validity

These steps require a sound, specific, and exhaustive literature review to identify the theories underlying the concept. The literature review provides the basis of item formulation. Once the items have been developed, the researcher assesses the tool's reliability and validity (see Chapter 15). As an example of methodological research, Rini (2016) identified that the concept of a women's experience of childbirth had not been adequately measured. In order to measure this concept, Rini's (2016) review of the literature and an earlier concept analysis provided the basis for the development of the instrument, the Women's Experience in Childbirth Survey (WECS). The instrument was developed in order to "provide a comprehensive measure of a women's perception of the childbirth experience and its effects on maternal and neonatal outcomes" (Rini, 2016, p. 269). Having developed a conceptual definition, Rini followed through by testing the instrument for reliability and validity (see Chapter 15). Common considerations that researchers incorporate into methodological research are outlined in Table 10.3. Many more examples of methodological research can be found in the research literature. The specific procedures of methodological research are beyond the scope of this book, but you are urged to closely review the instruments used in studies.

Secondary Analysis

Secondary analysis is also not a design but rather a research method in which the researcher takes previously collected and analyzed data from *one* study and reanalyzes the data or a subset of the data for a *secondary* purpose. The original study may be either an experimental or a nonexperimental design. As large data sets become more available, secondary analysis has become more prominent and a useful methodology for answering questions related to population health issues. Data for secondary analysis may be derived from a large clinical trial and data available through large health care organizations and databases. For example, Knight and colleagues (2016) conducted a secondary analysis of data from a larger observational prospective study (DeVon et al., 2014). The aim of the secondary analysis was to identify common trajectories of symptom severity in the 6 months following an ED visit for potential acute coronary syndrome (ACS). In the parent study, a convenience sample of participants was recruited from the ED of four academic medical centers and one community hospital. Data from a total of 1005 male (62.6%) and female (37.4%) participants with a mean age of 60.2 years (SD = 14.17 years) were analyzed for common trajectories of symptom severity using the validated 13-item ACS Symptom Checklist. Findings from this secondary analysis identified seven types of trajectories across eight symptoms, labeled "tapering off," "mild/persistent," "moderate/worsening," "moderate/improving," "late onset," and "severe/improving." Trajectories differed by age, gender, and diagnosis. The data from this study allowed further in-depth exploration of distinct symptoms trajectories in the 6 months after an ED visit for potential ACS. This has the potential to improve clinical assessment of ongoing symptoms and patient education.

TABLE 10.3 Common Considerations in the Development of Measurement Tools

Consideration	Example
A well-constructed scale, test, or interview schedule should consist of an objective, standardized measure of a behavior that has been clearly defined.	Rini (2016) provided a comprehensive literature review and definitions of the concepts that she operationalized for the WECS.
Observations should be made on a small but carefully chosen sampling of the behavior of interest, thus permitting the reader to feel confident that the samples are representative.	Rini (2016) piloted the instrument with 11 mothers to determine the clarity and sufficiently of the items as well as a preferred scaling method (Likert or Semantic Differential Scale).
An instrument should be standardized. It should be a set of uniform items and response possibilities, uniformly administered and scored.	Based on the initial pilot test of the instrument. The 49-item scale was developed using a 5-point Likert scale. Thirteen of the items are reversed scored and the answers summed. A higher score indicates a more positive birth experience. Potential scores range from 49 to 245.
The items should be unambiguous; clear-cut, concise, exact statements with only one idea per item.	A pilot study was conducted to evaluate the WECS items and the administration procedures. The pilot data indicated that several items needed to be dropped.
The item types should be limited in the type of variations. Subjects who are expected to shift from one type of item to another may fail to provide a true response as a result of the distraction of making such a change.	Mixing true-or-false items with questions that require a yes-or-no response and items that provide a response format of five possible answers is conducive to a high level of measurement error. The WECS contained only a 5-point Likert scale.
Items should not provide irrelevant clues. Unless carefully constructed, an item may furnish an indication of the expected response or answer. Furthermore, the correct answer or expected response to one item should not be given by another item.	An item that provides a clue to the expected answer may contain value words that convey cultural expectations, such as the following: "A good wife enjoys caring for her home and family."
Instruments should not be made difficult by requiring unnecessarily complex or exact operations. Furthermore, the difficulty of an instrument should be appropriate to the level of the subjects being assessed. Limiting each item to one concept or idea helps accomplish this objective.	A test constructed to evaluate learning in an introductory course in research methods may contain an item that is inappropriate for the designated group, such as the following: "A nonlinear transformation of data to linear data is a useful procedure before testing a hypothesis of curvilinearity."
An instrument's diagnostic, predictive, or measurement value depends on the degree to which it serves as an indicator of a relatively broad and significant behavior area, known as the universe of content for the behavior. A behavior must be clearly defined before it can be measured. The extent to which test items appear to accomplish this objective is an indication of the instrument's content and/or construct validity.	The WECS development included establishment of acceptable content validity. The WECS items were submitted to a panel of experts of a nurse midwife, two maternal infant nursing instructors and a nurse with instrument development experience. The Content Validity Index = 0.75–1.0, which means that the items are deemed to reflect the universe of content related to collaborative trust. Construct validity was established using factor analysis.
An instrument should adequately cover the defined behavior. A primary consideration is whether the number and nature of items are adequate. If there are too few items, the accuracy or reliability of the measure must be questioned.	Rini (2016) presented a complete overview of the validity and reliability testing for the scale and provided a detailed discussion of the findings and needed future testing.
The measure must prove its worth empirically through tests of reliability and validity.	A researcher should demonstrate that a scale is accurate and measures what it purports to measure (see Chapter 15). Rini (2016) provided the data on the reliability and validity testing of the WECS scale.

WECS, Women's experience in childbirth survey.

Identification of at-risk patients can target specific subpopulations for individualized education, post-ED discharge support and evidence-based symptom management plans, and gender differences in risky sexual behavior among urban adolescents exposed to violence.

Mixed Methods

Over the years, **mixed methods** have been defined in various ways. Historically mixed methods included the use of multimethod research or thought, which means including in one study use of a variety of data sources, such as use of different investigators, use of multiple theories in one study, or use of multiple methods (Denzin, 1978). Over the years these terms and methods have been refined and clarified (Johnson et al., 2007). The definition and core characteristics that integrate the diverse meaning of mixed methods research are as follows:

In mixed methods, the researcher:

- "Based on the research question collects and analyzes rigorously both qualitative and quantitative data
- Mixes the two forms of data concurrently by combining the data
- Gives priority to one or both forms of data in terms of emphasis
- Uses the procedures of both in one study or in multiple phases of a program of study
- Frames the procedures within philosophical worldviews and theoretical lenses
- Combines the procedures into specific research designs that direct the plan for conducting the study" (Creswell & Plano Clark, 2011, pp. 5–6).

The order of data collection in a mixed methods study varies depending on the question that a researcher wishes to answer. In a mixed methods study the quantitative data may be collected simultaneously with the qualitative data, or one may follow the other. Studying a question using both methods can contribute to a better understanding of an area of research. An example of a mixed methods study was completed by Christian and colleagues (2016). The aim of the study was to assess the feasibility of overcoming barriers to physical activity in a group of teenagers over a period of 1 year using a voucher system of rewards. The qualitative portion of the study included three focus groups on three different occasions at baseline, 6 months, and post-intervention 1 year. The purpose of the groups was to understand the effects of physical activity, fitness, and motivation, as well as barriers to the use of the vouchers during the study with students and teachers. The quantitative portion included the use of an aerobic fitness test, a self-reported activity scale, and a physical activity measure using an accelerometer. The measurement instruments and interviews were administered on three occasions over a year. The design of this study allowed the research team to assess how well the voucher program supported physical activity, aerobic fitness, and increased motivation using multiple methods in a group of adolescents. The study's findings supported that the use of vouchers provided access to more physical activity, increased socialization, and improved fitness activity in the adolescents during the year.

There is a diversity of opinion on how to evaluate mixed methods studies. Evaluation can include analyzing the quantitative and qualitative designs of the study separately, or as proposed by Creswell and Plano Clark (2011), there should be a separate set of criteria for mixed methods studies dependent on the designs and methods used.

HELPFUL HINT

As you read the literature, you will find labels such as *outcomes research, needs assessments, evaluation research,* and *quality assurance.* These studies are not designs per se. These studies use either experimental or nonexperimental designs. Studies with these labels are designed to test the effectiveness of health care techniques, programs, or interventions. When reading such a research study, the reader should assess which design was used and if the principles of the design, sampling strategy, and analysis are consistent with the study's purpose.

APPRAISAL FOR EVIDENCE-BASED PRACTICE NONEXPERIMENTAL DESIGNS

Criteria for appraising nonexperimental designs are presented in the Critical Appraisal Criteria box. When appraising nonexperimental research designs, you should keep in mind that such designs offer the researcher a lower level of control and an increased risk of bias. The level of evidence provided by nonexperimental designs is not as strong as evidence generated by experimental designs; however, there are other important clinical research questions that need to be answered beyond the testing of interventions and experimental or quasi-experimental designs.

The first step in critiquing nonexperimental designs is to determine which type of design was used in the study. Often a statement describing the design of the study appears in the abstract and in the methods section of the report. If such a statement is not present, you should closely examine the paper for evidence of which type of design was employed. You should be able to discern that either a survey or a relationship design was used. For example, you would expect an investigation of self-concept development in children from birth to 5 years of age to be a relationship study using a cohort/prospective/longitudinal design. If a cohort/prospective/longitudinal study was used, you should assess for possible threats to internal validity or bias, such as mortality, testing, and instrumentation. Potential threats to internal or external validity should be recognized by the researchers at the end of the study and, in particular, the limitations section.

Next, evaluate the literature review of the study to determine if a nonexperimental design was the most appropriate approach to the research question or hypothesis. For example, many studies on pain (e.g., intensity, severity, perception) are suggestive of a relationship between pain and any of the independent variables (diagnosis, coping style, and ethnicity) under consideration where the independent variable cannot be manipulated. As such, these studies suggest a nonexperimental correlational, longitudinal/prospective/cohort, a retrospective/ex post facto/case control, or a cross-sectional design. Investigators will use one of these designs to examine the relationship between the variables in naturally occurring groups. Sometimes you may think that it would have been more appropriate if the investigators had used an experimental or a quasi-experimental design. However, you must recognize that pragmatic or ethical considerations also may have guided the researchers in their choice of design (see Chapters 8 through 18).

CRITICAL APPRAISAL CRITERIA

Nonexperimental Designs

1. Based on the theoretical framework, is the rationale for the type of design appropriate?
2. How is the design congruent with the purpose of the study?
3. Is the design appropriate for the research question or hypothesis?
4. Is the design suited to the data collection methods?
5. Does the researcher present the findings in a manner congruent with the design used?
6. Does the research go beyond the relational parameters of the findings and erroneously infer cause-and-effect relationships between the variables?
7. Where appropriate, how does the researcher discuss the threats to internal validity (bias) and external validity (generalizability)?
8. How does the author identify the limitations of the study?
9. Does the researcher make appropriate recommendations about the applicability based on the strength and quality of evidence provided by the nonexperimental design and the findings?

Finally, the factor or factors that actually influence changes in the dependent variable can be ambiguous in nonexperimental designs. As with all complex phenomena, multiple factors can contribute to variability in the subjects' responses. When an experimental design is not used for controlling some of these extraneous variables that can influence results, the researcher must strive to provide as much control as possible within the context of a nonexperimental design, to decrease bias. For example, when it has not been possible to randomly assign subjects to treatment groups as an approach to controlling an independent variable, the researchers will use strict inclusion and exclusion criteria and calculate an adequate sample size using power analysis that will support a valid testing of the research question or hypothesis (see Chapter 12). Threats to internal and external validity or potential sources of bias represent a major influence when interpreting the findings of a nonexperimental study because they impose limitations to the generalizability of the results. It is also important to remember that prediction of patient clinical outcomes is of critical value for clinical researchers. Nonexperimental designs can be used to make predictions if the study is designed with an adequate sample size (see Chapter 12), collects data consistently, and uses reliable and valid instruments (see Chapter 15).

If you are appraising methodological research, you need to apply the principles of reliability and validity (see Chapter 15). A secondary analysis needs to be reviewed from several perspectives. First, you need to understand if the researcher followed sound scientific logic in the secondary analysis completed. Second, you need to review the original study that the data were extracted from to assess the reliability and validity of the original study. Even though the format and methods vary, it is important to remember that all research has a central goal: to answer questions scientifically and provide the strongest, most consistent evidence possible, while controlling for potential bias.

KEY POINTS

- Nonexperimental designs are used in studies that construct a picture or make an account of events as they naturally occur. Nonexperimental designs can be classified as either survey studies or relationship/difference studies.

- Survey studies and relationship/difference studies are both descriptive and exploratory in nature.
- Survey research collects detailed descriptions of existing phenomena and uses the data either to justify current conditions and practices or to make more intelligent plans for improving them.
- Correlational studies examine relationships.
- Developmental studies are further broken down into categories of cross-sectional studies, cohort/longitudinal/prospective studies, and case control/retrospective/ex post facto studies.
- Methodological research, secondary analysis, and mixed methods are examples of other means of adding to the body of nursing research. Both the researcher and the reader must consider the advantages and disadvantages of each design.
- Nonexperimental research designs do not enable the investigator to establish cause-and-effect relationships between the variables. Consumers must be wary of nonexperimental studies that make causal claims about the findings unless a causal modeling technique is used.
- Nonexperimental designs also offer the researcher the least amount of control. Threats to validity impose limitations on the generalizability of the results and as such should be fully assessed by the critical reader.
- The critiquing process is directed toward evaluating the appropriateness of the selected nonexperimental design in relation to factors, such as the research problem, theoretical framework, hypothesis, methodology, and data analysis and interpretation.
- Though nonexperimental designs do not provide the highest level of evidence (Level I), they do provide a wealth of data that become useful pieces for formulating both Level I and Level II studies that are aimed at developing and testing nursing interventions.

CRITICAL THINKING CHALLENGES

- IPE The mid-term assignment for your interprofessional research course is to critically appraise an assigned study on the relationship of perception of pain severity and quality of life in advanced cancer patients. You and your nursing student colleagues think it is a cross-sectional design, but your medical student colleagues think it is a quasi-experimental design because it has several specific hypotheses. How would each group of students support their argument, and how would they collaborate to resolve their differences?
- You are completing your senior practicum on a surgical unit, and for preconference your student group has just completed a search for studies related to the effectiveness of handwashing in decreasing the incidence of nosocomial infections, but the studies all use an ex post facto/case control design. You want to approach the nurse manager on the unit to present the evidence you have collected and critically appraised, but you are concerned about the strength of the evidence because the studies all use a nonexperimental design. How would you justify that this is the "best available evidence"?
- You are a member of a journal club at your hospital. Your group is interested in the effectiveness of smoking cessation interventions provided by nurses. An electronic search indicates that 12 individual research studies and one meta-analysis meet your inclusion criteria. Would your group begin with critically appraising the 12 individual studies or the one meta-analysis? Provide rationale for your choice, including

consideration of the strength and quality of evidence provided by individual studies versus a meta-analysis.

- A patient in a primary care practice who had a history of a "heart murmur" called his nurse practitioner for a prescription for an antibiotic before having a periodontal (gum) procedure. When she responded that according to the new American Heart Association (AHA) clinical practice guideline, antibiotic prophylaxis is no longer considered appropriate for his heart murmur, the patient got upset, stating, "But I always take antibiotics! I want you to tell me why I should believe this guideline. How do I know my heart will not be damaged by listening to you?" What is the purpose of a clinical practice guideline, and how would you as a nurse practitioner respond to this patient?

REFERENCES

Bender, M., Williams, M., Su, W., et al. (2016). Clinical nurse leader integrated care delivery to improve care quality: Factors influencing perceived success. *Journal of Nursing Scholarship*, *48*(4), 414–422.

Campbell, D. T., & Stanley, J. C. (1963). *Experimental and quasi-experimental designs for research.* Chicago, IL: Rand-McNally.

Christian, D., Todd, C., Hill, R., et al. (2016). Active children through incentive vouchers-evaluation (ACTIVE): A mixed methods feasibility study. *BMC Public Health*, *16*, 890.

Creswell, J. W., & Plano Clark, V. L. (2011). *Designing and conducting mixed methods research.* Thousand Oaks, CA: Sage Publications.

DeVon, H. A., Burke, L. A., Nelson, H., et al. (2014). Disparities in patients presenting to the emergency department with potential acute coronary syndrome: It matters if you are black or white. *Heart & Lung*, *43*, 270–277.

Denzin, N. K. (1978). *The research act: A theoretical introduction to sociological methods.* New York: McGraw Hill.

Fessele, K. L., Hayat, M. J., Mayer, D. K., & Atkins, R. L. (2016). Factors associated with unplanned hospitalizations among patients with nonmetastatic colorectal cancers intended for treatment in ambulatory settings. *Nursing Research*, *65*(1), 24–33.

Hawthorne, D. M., Youngblut, J. M., & Brooten, D. (2016). Parent spirituality, grief, and mental health at 1 and 3 months after their infant's/child's death in an intensive care unit. *Journal of Pediatric Nursing*, *31*, 73–80.

Johnson, R.B., Onwuegbuzie, A. J., & Turner, L.A. (2007). Toward a definition of mixed methods research. *Journal of Mixed Methods Research*, *1*(2), 122–133.

Kline, R. (2011). *Principles and practices of structural equation modeling* (3rd ed.). New York, NY: Guilford Press.

Knight, E. P., Shea, K., Rosenfeld, A. G., et al. (2016). Symptom trajectories after an emergency department visit for potential acute coronary syndrome. *Nursing Research*, *65*(4), 268–289.

Koc, Z., & Cinarli, T. (2015). Cervical cancer, human papillomavirus, and vaccination. *Nursing Research*, *64*(6), 452–465.

Kousha, T., & Castner, J. (2016). The air quality health index and emergency department visits for otitis media. *Journal of Nursing Scholarship*, *48*(2), 163–171.

Lee, B., Fan, J., Hung, C., et al. (2016). Illness representations of injury: a comparison of patients and their caregivers. *Journal of Nursing Scholarship*, *48*(3), 254–264.

Lee, C. E., Von Ah, D., Szuck, B., & Lau, Y. J. (2016). Determinants of physical activity maintenance in breast cancer survivors after a community-based intervention. *Oncology Nursing Forum*, *43*(1), 93–102.

Nyamathi, A., Salem, B. E., Zhang, S., et al. (2015). Nursing case management, peer coaching, and hepatitis A and B vaccine completion among homeless men recently released on parole; randomized clinical trial. *Nursing Research*, *64*(3), 177–189.

Nyamathi, A. M., Zhang, S. X, Wall, S., et al. (2016). Drug use and multiple sex partners among homeless ex-offenders: secondary findings from an experimental study. *Nursing Research*, *65*(3), 179–190.

Plichta, S., & Kelvin, E. (2013). *Munro's statistical methods for health care research* (6th ed.). Philadelphia: Lippincott, Williams & Wilkins.

Rini, E. V. (2016). The development and psychometric analysis of the women's experience in childbirth survey. *Journal of Nursing Measurement*, *124*(2), 268–280.

Stoddard, S. A., Varela, J. J., & Zimmerman, M. A. (2015). Future expectations, attitude, toward violence, and bullying perpetration during early adolescence. *Nursing Research*, *64*(6), 422–433.

Turner-Sack, A. M., Menna, R., Setchell, S. R., et al. (2016). Psychological functioning, post-traumatic growth, and coping in parents and siblings of adolescent cancer survivors. *Oncology Nursing Forum*, *43*(1), 48–56.

Go to Evolve at **http://evolve.elsevier.com/LoBiondo/** for review questions, critiquing exercises, and additional research articles for practice in reviewing and critiquing.

11

Systematic Reviews and Clinical Practice Guidelines

Geri LoBiondo-Wood

Go to Evolve at **http://evolve.elsevier.com/LoBiondo/** for review questions, critiquing exercises, and additional research articles for practice in reviewing and critiquing.

LEARNING OUTCOMES

After reading this chapter, you should be able to do the following:

- Describe the types of research reviews.
- Describe the components of a systematic review.
- Differentiate between a systematic review, meta-analysis, and integrative review.
- Describe the purpose of clinical guidelines.
- Differentiate between an expert- and an evidence-based clinical guideline.
- Critically appraise systematic reviews and clinical practice guidelines.

KEY TERMS

AGREE II
clinical practice guidelines
effect size
evidence-based practice guidelines
expert-based practice guidelines
forest plot
integrative review
meta-analysis
systematic review

The breadth and depth of clinical research has grown. As the number of studies focused on a similar area conducted by multiple research teams has increased, it has become important to have a means of organizing and assessing the quality, quantity, and consistency among the findings of a group of like studies. The previous chapters have introduced the types of qualitative and quantitative designs and how to critique these studies for quality and applicability to practice. The purpose of this chapter is to acquaint you with systematic reviews and clinical guidelines that assess multiple studies focused on the same clinical question, and how these reviews and guidelines can support evidence-based practice. Terminology used to define systematic reviews and clinical guidelines has changed as this area of research and literature assessment has grown. The definitions used in this textbook are consistent with the definitions from the Cochrane Collaboration and the Preferred Reporting for Systematic Reviews and Meta-Analyses (PRISMA) Group (Higgins & Green, 2011; Moher et al., 2009; Stroup et al., 2000). Systematic reviews and clinical guidelines are critical and meaningful for the development of quality improvement practices.

SYSTEMATIC REVIEW TYPES

A **systematic review** is a summation and assessment of research studies found in the literature based on a clearly focused question that uses systematic and explicit criteria and methods to identify, select, critically appraise, and analyze relevant data from the selected studies to summarize the findings in a focused area (Liberati et al., 2009; Moher et al., 2009; Moher, Shamseer, et al., 2015). Statistical methods may or may not be used to analyze the studies reviewed. Multiple terms and methods are used to systematically review the literature, depending on the review's purpose. See Box 11.1 for the components of a systematic review. Some terms are used interchangeably. The terms *systematic review* and *meta-analysis* are often used interchangeably or together. The only review type that can be labeled a **meta-analysis** is one that reviewed studies using statistical methods. When evaluating a systematic review, it is important to assess how well each of the studies in the review minimized bias or maintained the elements of control (see Chapters 8 and 9).

You will also find reviews of an area of research or theory synthesis termed **integrative reviews**. *Integrative reviews* critically appraise the literature in an area but without a statistical analysis and are the broadest category of review (Whittemore, 2005; Whittemore & Knafl, 2005). Recently new types of reviews have been developed. These include rapid reviews, scoping reviews, and realist reviews (Moher, Stewart, et al., 2015). Systematic, integrative, and additional types of reviews are not designs per se, but methods for searching and integrating the literature related to a specific clinical issue. These methods take the

BOX 11.1 Systematic Review Components With or Without Meta-Analysis

Introduction

Review of rationale and a clear clinical question (PICO)

Methods

Information sources, databases used, and search strategy identified: how studies were selected and data extracted as well as the variables extracted and defined

Description of methods used to assess risk of bias, summary measures identified (e.g., risk, ratio); identification of how data are combined, if studies are graded, what quality appraisal system was used (see Chapters 1, 17, and 18)

Results

Number of studies screened and characteristics, risk of bias within studies; if a meta-analysis there will be a synthesis of results including confidence intervals, risk of bias for each study, and all outcomes considered

Discussion

Summary of findings, including the strength, quality, quantity, and consistency of the evidence for each outcome

Any limitations of the studies; conclusions and recommendations of findings for practice

Funding

Sources of funding for the systematic review

CRITICAL THINKING DECISION PATH

Completing a Systematic Review

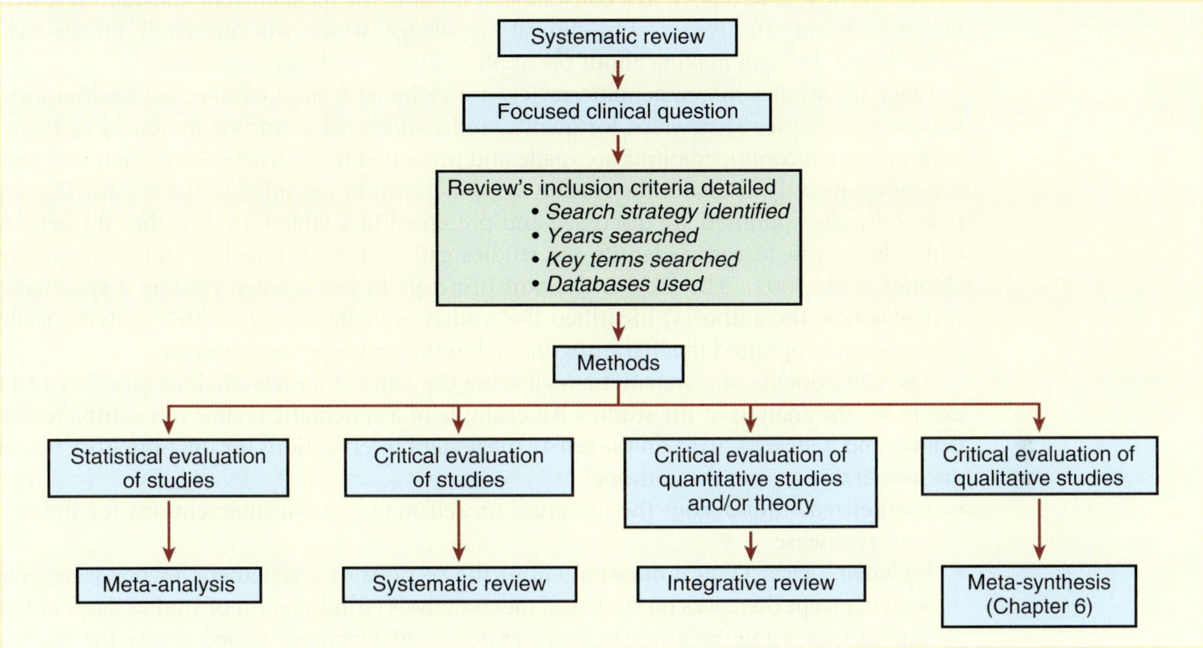

results of many studies in a specific area; assess the studies critically for reliability and validity (quality, quantity, and consistency) (see Chapters 1, 7, 17, and 18); and synthesize findings to inform practice. No matter what type of review you are reading, it is important that the authors have clearly detailed the methods that were used and that those methods can be replicated (Moher, Stewart, et al., 2015). Meta-analysis provides Level I evidence as the studies in the review are statistically analyzed and integrates the results of many studies. Systematic reviews and meta-analyses also grade the level of design or evidence of the studies reviewed. The Critical Thinking Decision Path outlines the path for completing a systematic review.

SYSTEMATIC REVIEW

A systematic review is a summary of a search of quantitative studies that use similar designs based on a focused clinical question (PICO). The goal is to assess the strength and quality of the evidence found in the literature on a clinical subject. The review uses rigorous inclusion and exclusion criteria, an explicit reproducible methodology to identify all studies that meet the eligibility criteria, and an assessment of the validity of the findings from the included studies (Moher et al., 2009). The goal is to bring together all of the studies related to a focused clinical question in order to assess the strength and quality of the evidence provided by the chosen studies in relation to:

- Sampling issues
- Internal validity (bias) threats
- External validity

- Data analysis
- Applicability of findings to practice

The purpose is to report, in a consolidated fashion, the most current and valid research on intervention effectiveness and clinical knowledge, which will ultimately inform evidence-based decision making about the applicability of findings to practice.

Once the studies in a systematic review are gathered from a comprehensive literature search (see Chapter 3), assessed for quality, and synthesized according to quality or focus, then practice recommendations are made and presented in an article. More than one person independently evaluates the studies to be included or excluded in the review. The articles critically appraised are discussed and presented in a table format within the article, which helps you to easily identify the studies gathered for the review and their quality (Moher et al., 2009). The most important principle to assess when reading a systematic review is how the author(s) identified the studies evaluated and how they systematically reviewed and appraised the literature that led to the reviewers' conclusions.

The components of a systematic review are the same as a meta-analysis (see Box 11.1) except for the analysis of the studies. An example of a systematic review was completed by Conley and Redeker (2016) on the self-management interventions for inflammatory bowel disease. In this review, the authors:

- Synthesized studies from the literature on self-management interventions for inflammatory disease
- Included a clear clinical question; all of the sections of a systematic review were presented, except there was no statistical meta-analysis (combination of studies data) of the studies as a whole because the interventions and outcomes varied across the studies reviewed
- Summarized studies according to the health-related outcomes and assessed for quality

Each study in this review was considered *individually, not analyzed collectively,* for its sample size, effect size, and its contribution to knowledge in the area based on a set of criteria. Although systematic reviews are highly useful, they also have to be reviewed for potential bias and carefully critiqued for scientific rigor.

META-ANALYSIS

A **meta-analysis** is a systematic summary using *statistical techniques* to assess and combine studies of the same design to obtain a precise estimate of *effect* (impact of an intervention on the dependent variable/outcomes or association between variables). The terms meta-analysis and systematic review are often used interchangeably. The main difference is *only* a meta-analysis includes a statistical assessment of the studies reviewed. A meta-analysis treats all the studies reviewed as one large data set in order to obtain a precise estimate of the effect (impact) of the results (outcomes) of the studies in the review.

Meta-analysis uses a rigorous process of summary and determines the impact of a number of studies rather than the impact derived from a single study alone (see Chapter 10). After the clinical question is identified and the search of the review of published and unpublished literature is completed, a meta-analysis is conducted in two phases:

Phase I: The data are extracted (i.e., outcome data, sample sizes, quality of the studies, and measures of variability from the identified studies).

Phase II: The decision is made as to whether it is appropriate to calculate what is known as a pooled average result (effect) of the studies reviewed.

Effect sizes are calculated using the difference in the average scores between the intervention and control groups from each study (Cochrane Handbook of Systematic Reviews for Interventions, 2016). Each study is considered a unit of analysis. A meta-analysis takes the effect size (see Chapter 12) from each of the studies reviewed to obtain an estimate of the population (or the whole) to create a single effect size of all the studies. Thus the **effect size** is an estimate of how large of a difference there is between intervention and control groups in the *summarized* studies. **Example:** ➤ The meta-analysis in Appendix E studied the question "What is the impact of nurse-led clinics (NLCs) on the mortality and morbidity of patients with cardiovascular disease (CVD)?" In this review, the authors synthesized the literature from studies on the effectiveness of NLCs in terms of mortality and morbidity outcomes (Al-Mallah et al., 2015). The studies that assessed this question were reviewed and each weighted for its impact or effect on improving mortality and morbidity. This estimate helps health care providers decide which intervention, if any, was more useful for improving well-being. Detailed components of a systematic review with or without meta-analysis (Moher et al., 2009) are listed in Box 11.1.

In addition to calculating effect sizes, meta-analyses use multiple statistical methods to present and depict the data from studies reviewed (see Chapters 19 and 20). One of these methods is a **forest plot**, sometimes called a blobbogram. A forest plot graphically depicts the results of analyzing a number of studies. Fig. 11.1 is an example of a forest plot from Al-Mallah and colleagues' meta-analysis (Al-Mallah et al., 2015; Appendix E, Fig. 2, Box A). This review identified that the available evidence suggests a favorable effect of NLCs on all-cause mortality, rate of major adverse cardiac events, and adherence to medications in patients with CVD.

QSEN EVIDENCE-BASED PRACTICE TIP

Evidence-based practice methods such as meta-analysis increase your ability to manage the ever-increasing volume of information produced to develop the best evidence-based practices.

All cause mortality

	Nurse Clinic		Control			Odds Ratio
Study or Subgroup	Events	Total	Events	Total	Weight	M-H, Random, 95% CI
Campbell1998	22	673	25	670	10.7%	0.87 [0.49, 1.56]
Cupples	13	317	29	300	8.0%	0.40 [0.20, 0.78]
DeBusk	12	293	10	292	5.0%	1.20 [0.51, 2.83]
Delaney	100	673	128	670	44.3%	0.74 [0.55, 0.98]
Goodman	2	94	4	94	1.2%	0.49 [0.09, 2.74]
Haskell	3	145	3	155	1.4%	1.07 [0.21, 5.39]
Jolly	15	277	23	320	8.1%	0.74 [0.38, 1.45]
Khanal	47	617	45	616	20.2%	1.05 [0.68, 1.60]
Lapointe	2	57	4	56	1.2%	0.47 [0.08, 2.69]
Total (95% CI)		**3146**		**3173**	**100.0%**	**0.78 [0.65, 0.95]**
Total events	216		271			

Heterogeneity: $Tau^2 = 0.00$; $Chi^2 = 7.65$, df = 8 (P = 0.47); $I^2 = 0\%$
Test for overall effect: Z = 2.52 (P = 0.01)

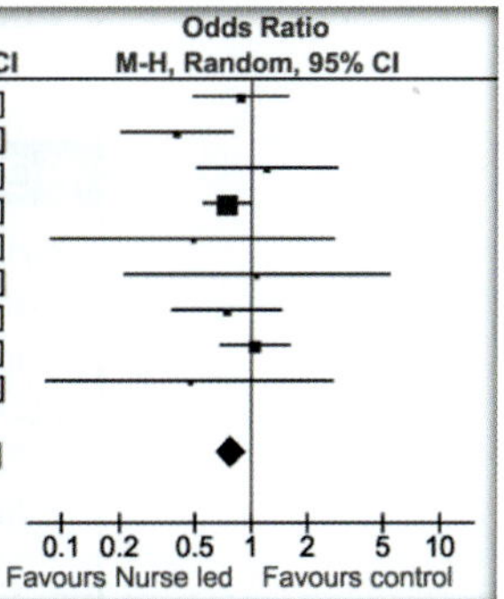

FIG 11.1 An example of a forest plot. (Adapted from Al-Mallah, M. H., Farah, I., Al-Madani, W., et al. [2015]. The impact of nurse-led clinics on the mortality and morbidity of patients with cardiovascular diseases: A systematic review and meta-analysis. *Journal of Cardiovascular Nursing, 31*[1], 89–95.)

Fig. 11.1 displays nine studies that compared all-cause mortality in nurse-led groups versus the control groups (usual care). Each study analyzed is listed. To the right of the listed study is a horizontal line that identifies the effect size estimate for each study. The box on the vertical line represents the effect size of each study, and the diamond is the effect or significance of the combined studies. The boxes to the left of the zero line mean that NLC care was favored or produced a significant effect. The box to the right of the line indicates studies in which usual care was not favored or significant. The diamond is a more precise estimate of the interventions as it combines the data from all the studies. The exemplar provided is basic, as meta-analysis is a sophisticated methodology. For a fuller understanding, several references are provided (Borenstein et al., 2009; da Costa & Juni, 2014; Higgins & Green, 2011); see also Chapters 19 and 20.

A well-done meta-analysis assesses for bias in studies and provides clinicians a means of evaluating the merit of a body of clinical research. The Cochrane Library published by the Cochrane Collaboration provides a repository of sound meta-analyses. **Example:** ➤ Martineau and colleagues (2016) completed a meta-analysis to assess the use of vitamin D to prevent asthma exacerbation and improve asthma control in children and adults. The report presents an introduction, details of the methods used to search the literature (databases, search terms, and years), data extraction, and analysis. The report also includes an evidence table of the studies reviewed, a description of how the data were summarized, results of the meta-analysis, a forest plot of the reviewed studies (see Chapter 19), conclusions, and implications for practice and research.

COCHRANE COLLABORATION

The largest repository of meta-analyses is the Cochrane Collaboration/Review. The Cochrane Collaboration prepares and maintains a body of systematic reviews that focus on health care interventions (Box 11.2). The reviews are found in the Cochrane Database of Systematic Reviews. The Cochrane Collaboration collaborates with a wide range of health care individuals with different skills and backgrounds for developing reviews. These partnerships assist with developing reviews that minimize bias while keeping current with assessment of health care interventions, promoting access to the database, and ensuring the quality of the reviews (Cochrane Handbook for Systematic Reviews, 2016). The steps of a Cochrane Report mirror those of a meta-analysis except for the inclusion of a plain

BOX 11.2 Cochrane Review Sections

- Review information: Authors and contact person
- Abstract
- Plain language summary
- The review
  - Background of the question
  - Objectives of the search
  - Methods for selecting studies for review
  - Type of studies reviewed
- Types of participants, types of intervention, types of outcomes in the studies
  - Search methods for finding studies
- Data collection
- Analysis of the located studies, including effect sizes
- Results including description of studies, risk of bias, intervention effects
- Discussion
- Implications for research and practice
- References and tables to display the data
- Supplementary information (e.g., appendices, data analysis)

BOX 11.3 Cochrane Library Databases

- Cochrane Database of Systematic Reviews: Full-text Cochrane reviews
- DARE: Critical assessments and abstracts of other systematic reviews that conform to quality criteria
- CENTRAL: Information of studies published in conference proceedings and other sources not available in other databases
- CMR: Bibliographic information on articles and books on reviewing research and methodological studies

CENTRAL, Cochrane Central Register of Controlled Trials; *CMR,* Cochrane Methodology Register; *DARE,* Database of Abstracts of Review of Effects.

language summary. This useful feature is a straightforward summary of the meta-analysis. The Cochrane Library also publishes several other useful databases (Box 11.3).

INTEGRATIVE REVIEW

You will also find critical reviews of an area of research without a statistical analysis or a theory synthesis, termed **integrative reviews.** An integrative review is the broadest category of review (Whittemore, 2005; Whittemore & Knafl, 2005). It can include theoretical literature, research literature, or both. An integrative review may include methodology studies, a theory review, or the results of differing research studies with wide-ranging clinical implications (Whittemore, 2005). An integrative review can include quantitative or qualitative research, or both. Statistics are not used to summarize and generate conclusions about the studies. Several examples of an integrative review are found in Box 11.4. Recommendations for future research are suggested in each review.

REPORTING GUIDELINES: SYSTEMATIC REVIEWS AND META-ANALYSIS

Systematic reviews and meta-analysis publications are found widely in the research literature. As these resources present an accumulation of potentially clinically relevant knowledge, there was also a need to develop a standard for what information should be included in these reviews. There are several guidelines available for reporting systematic reviews.

BOX 11.4 Integrative Review Examples

- Brady and colleagues (2014) published an integrative review on the management and effects of steroid-induced hyperglycemia in hospitalized patients with cancer with or without preexisting diabetes. This review included a purpose, description of the methods used (databases searched, years included), key terms used, and parameters of the search. These components allow others to evaluate and replicate the search. Eighteen studies that assessed steroid-induced hyperglycemia in hospitalized patients with cancer were reviewed in the text and via a table format.
- Kestler and LoBiondo-Wood (2012) published an integrative review of symptom experience in children and adolescents with cancer. The review was a follow-up of a 2003 review published by Docherty (2003) and was completed to assess the progress that has been made since the 2003 research publication on the symptoms of pediatric oncology patients. The review included a description of the search strategy used including databases, years searched, terms used, and the results of the search. Literature on each symptom was described, and a table of the 52 studies reviewed was included.

These are the PRISMA (Moher et al., 2009) and MOOSE (Meta-analysis of Observational Studies in Epidemiology) (Stroup et al., 2000). A review of these guidelines will help you critically read meta-analyses and interpret if there is any bias in the review.

TOOLS FOR EVALUATING INDIVIDUAL STUDIES

As the importance of practicing from a base of evidence has grown, so has the need to have tools or instruments available that can assist practitioners in evaluating studies of various types. When evaluating studies for clinical evidence, it is first important to assess if the study is valid. At the end of each chapter of this text are critiquing questions that will aid you in assessing if studies are valid and if the results are applicable to your practice. In addition to these questions, there are standardized appraisal tools that can assist with appraising the evidence. The Center for Evidence Based Medicine (CEBM), whose focus is on teaching critical appraisal, developed tools known as Critical Appraisal Tools that provide an evidence-based approach for assessing the quality, quantity, and consistency of specific study designs (CEBM, 2016). These instruments are part of an international network that provides consumers with specific questions to help assess study quality. Each checklist has a number of general questions as well as design-specific questions. The tools center on assessing a study's methodology, validity, and reliability. The questions focus on the following:

1. Does this study address a clearly focused question?
2. Did the study use valid methods to address the question?
3. Are the valid results of the study important?
4. Are these valid, important results applicable to my patient or population?

There are four critical appraisal worksheets with targeted questions relevant to a specific design. The checklist with instructions can be found at http://www.cebm.net/critical appraisal. The design-specific **CEBM** tools with critical evaluative information for each design are available online and include:

- Systematic reviews
- Randomized controlled studies
- Diagnostic studies
- Prognosis

CLINICAL PRACTICE GUIDELINES

Clinical practice guidelines are systematically developed statements or recommendations that link research and practice and serve as a guide for practitioners. Guidelines have been developed to assist in bridging practice and research. Guidelines are developed by professional organizations, government agencies, institutions, or convened expert panels. Guidelines provide clinicians with an algorithm for clinical management or decision making for specific diseases (e.g., colon cancer) or treatments (e.g., pain management). Not all guidelines are well developed, and, like research, they must be assessed before implementation (see Chapter 9). Guidelines should present scope and purpose of the practice, detail who the development group included, demonstrate scientific rigor, be clear in their presentation, demonstrate clinical applicability, and demonstrate editorial independence. An example is the National Comprehensive Cancer Network, which is an interdisciplinary consortium of 21 cancer centers around the world. Interdisciplinary groups develop practice guidelines for practitioners and education guidelines for patients. These guidelines are accessible at www.nccn.org.

Practice guidelines can be either expert-based or evidence-based. **Evidence-based practice guidelines** are those developed using a scientific process. This process includes first assembling a multidisciplinary group of experts in a specific field. This group is charged with completing a rigorous search of the literature and completing an evidence table that summarizes the quality and strength of the evidence from which the practice guideline is derived (see Chapters 19 and 20). For various reasons, not all areas of clinical practice have a sufficient research base; therefore, **expert-based practice guidelines** are developed. Expert-based guidelines depend on having a group of nationally known experts in the field who meet and solely use opinions of experts along with whatever research evidence is developed to date. If limited research is available for such a guideline, a rationale should be presented for the practice recommendations.

Many national organizations develop clinical practice guidelines. It is important to know which one to apply to your patient population. **Example:** ➤ There are numerous evidence-based practice guidelines developed for the management of pain. These guidelines are available from organizations such as the Oncology Nurses Society, American Academy of Pediatrics, National Comprehensive Cancer Network, National Cancer Institute, American College of Physicians, and American Academy of Pain Medicine. You need to be able to evaluate each of the guidelines and decide which is the most appropriate for your patient population.

The Agency for Healthcare Research and Quality supports the National Guideline Clearinghouse (NGC). The NGC's mission is to provide health care professionals from all disciplines with objective, detailed information on clinical practice guidelines that are disseminated, implemented, and issued. The NGC encourages groups to develop guidelines for implementation via their site; it is a very useful site for finding well-developed clinical guidelines on a wide range of health- and illness-related topics. Specific guidelines can be found on the AHRQ Effective Health Care Program website.

IPE HIGHLIGHT

When evaluating a Clinical Practice Guideline (CPG), it is important for an interprofessional team to use an evidence-based critical appraisal tool like AGREE II to determine the strength and quality of the CPG for applicability to practice.

EVALUATING CLINICAL PRACTICE GUIDELINES

As evidence-based practice guidelines proliferate, it becomes increasingly important that you critique these guidelines with regard to the methods used for guideline formulation and consider how they might be used in practice. Critical areas that should be assessed when critiquing evidence-based practice guidelines include the following:

- Date of publication or release and authors
- Endorsement of the guideline
- Clear purpose of what the guideline covers and patient groups for which it was designed
- Types of evidence (research, theoretical) used in guideline formulation
- Types of research included in formulating the guideline (e.g., "We considered only randomized and other prospective controlled trials in determining efficacy of therapeutic interventions.")

- Description of the methods used in grading the evidence
- Search terms and retrieval methods used to acquire evidence used in the guideline
- Well-referenced statements regarding practice
- Comprehensive reference list
- Review of the guideline by experts
- Whether the guideline has been used or tested in practice and, if so, with what types of patients and in which types of settings

Evidence-based practice guidelines that are formulated using rigorous methods provide a useful starting point for understanding the evidence base of practice. However, more research may be available since the publication of the guideline, and refinements may be needed. Although information in well-developed, national, evidence-based practice guidelines are a helpful reference, it is usually necessary to localize the guideline using institution-specific evidence-based policies, procedures, or standards before application within a specific setting.

There are several tools for appraising the quality of clinical practice guidelines. The **Appraisal of Guidelines Research and Evaluation II (AGREE II)** instrument is one of the most widely used to evaluate the applicability of a guideline to practice (Brouwers et al., 2010, AGREE Collaboration). The AGREE II was developed to assist in evaluating guideline quality, provide a methodological strategy for guideline development, and inform practitioners about what information should be reported in guidelines and how it should be reported. The AGREE II is available online. The instrument focuses on six domains, with a total of 23 questions rated on a seven-point scale and two final assessment items that require the appraiser to make overall judgments of the guideline based on how the 23 items were rated. Along with the instrument itself, the AGREE Enterprise website offers guidance on tool usage and development. The AGREE II has been tested for reliability and validity. The guideline assesses the following components of a practice guideline:

1. Scope and purpose of the guideline
2. Stakeholder involvement
3. Rigor of the guideline development
4. Clarity and presentation of the guideline
5. Applicability of the guideline to practice
6. Demonstrated editorial independence of the developers

CRITICAL APPRAISAL CRITERIA

Systematic Reviews

1. Does the PICO question match the studies included in the review?
2. Are the review methods clearly stated and comprehensive?
3. Are the dates of the review's inclusion clear and relevant to the area reviewed?
4. Are the inclusion and exclusion criteria for studies in the review clear and comprehensive?
5. What criteria were used to assess each of the studies in the review for quality and scientific merit?
6. If studies were analyzed individually, were the data clear?
7. Were the methods of study combination clear and appropriate?
8. If the studies were reviewed collectively, how large was the effect?
9. Are the clinical conclusions drawn from the studies relevant and supported by the review?

Clinical practice guidelines, although they are systematically developed and make explicit recommendations for practice, may be formatted differently. Practice guidelines should reflect the components listed. Guidelines can be located on an organization's website, at the AHRQ, on the NGC website (www.AHRQ.gov), or on MEDLINE (see Chapters 3 and 20). Well-developed guidelines are constructed using the principles of a systematic review.

APPRAISAL FOR EVIDENCE-BASED PRACTICE SYSTEMATIC REVIEWS AND CLINICAL GUIDELINES

For each of the review methods described—systematic, meta-analysis, integrative, and clinical guidelines—think about each method as one that progressively sifts and sorts research studies and the data until the highest quality of evidence is used to arrive at the conclusions. First the researcher combines the results of all the studies based on a focused, specific question. The studies that do not meet the inclusion criteria are then excluded and the data assessed for quality. This process is repeated sequentially, excluding studies until only the studies of highest quality available are included in the analysis. An alteration in the overall results as an outcome of this sorting and separating process suggests how sensitive the conclusions are to the quality of studies included (Whittemore, 2005). No matter which type of review is completed, it is important to understand that the research studies reviewed still must be examined through your evidence-based practice lens. This means that evidence that you have derived through your critical appraisal and synthesis or derived through other researchers' reviews must be integrated with an individual clinician's expertise and patients' wishes.

You should note that a researcher who uses any of the systematic review methods of combining evidence does not conduct the original studies or analyze the data from each study, but rather takes the data from all the published studies and synthesizes the information by following a set of systematic steps. Systematic methods for combining evidence are used to synthesize both nonexperimental and experimental research studies.

Finally, evidence-based practice requires that you determine—based on the strength and quality of the evidence provided by the systematic review coupled with your clinical expertise and patient values—whether or not you would consider a change in practice. For example, the meta-analysis by Al-Mallah and colleagues (2015) in Appendix E details the

CRITICAL APPRAISAL CRITERIA

Critiquing Clinical Guidelines

1. Is the date of publication or release current?
2. Are the authors of the guideline clear and appropriate to the guideline?
3. Is the clinical problem and purpose clear in terms of what the guideline covers and patient groups for which it was designed?
4. What types of evidence were used in formulating the guideline, and are they appropriate to the topic?
5. Is there a description of the methods used to grade the evidence?
6. Were the search terms and retrieval methods used to acquire research and theoretical evidence used in the guideline clear and relevant?
7. Is the guideline well-referenced and comprehensive?
8. Are the recommendations in the guideline sourced according to the level of evidence for its basis?
9. Has the guideline been reviewed by experts in the appropriate field of discipline?
10. Who funded the guideline development?

important findings from the literature, some of which could be used in nursing practice and some that need further research.

Systematic reviews that use multiple randomized controlled trials (RCTs) to combine study results offer stronger evidence (Level I) in estimating the magnitude of an effect for an intervention (see Chapter 2, Table 2.3). The strength of evidence provided by systematic reviews is a key component for developing a practice based on evidence. The qualitative counterpart to systematic reviews is *meta-synthesis*, which uses qualitative principles to assess qualitative research and is described in Chapter 6.

KEY POINTS

- A systematic review is a summary of a search of quantitative studies that use similar designs based on a PICO question.
- A meta-analysis is a systematic summary of studies using statistical techniques to assess and combine studies of the same design to obtain a precise estimate of the impact of an intervention.
- The terms *systematic review* and *meta-analysis* are used interchangeably, but only a meta-analysis includes a statistical assessment of the studies reviewed.
- An integrative review is the broadest category of reviews and can include a theoretical literature review, or a review of both quantitative and qualitative research literature.
- The Cochrane Collaboration prepares and maintains a body of up-to-date systematic reviews focused on health care interventions.
- There are standardized tools available for evaluating individual studies. An example of such tools are available from the Centre for Evidence Based Medicine.
- Clinical practice guidelines are systematically developed statements or recommendations that link research and practice. There are two types of clinical practice guidelines: evidence-based practice guidelines and expert-based practice guidelines.
- Evidence-based guidelines are practice guidelines developed by experts who assess the research literature for the quality and strength of the evidence for an area of practice.
- Expert-based guidelines are developed typically by a nationally known group of experts in an area using opinions of experts along with whatever research evidence is available to date.
- The Appraisal of Guidelines Research and Evaluation II is a tool for appraising the quality of clinical practice guidelines.

CRITICAL THINKING CHALLENGES

- An assignment for your research class is to critically appraise the systematic review in Appendix E by Malwallah and colleagues using the Systematic Review Critical Appraisal Tool from the Center for Evidence-based Medicine (CEBM) using the following link, www.cebm.net, to determine whether the effect size reveals a significant difference between the intervention and control group in the summarized studies. How does the effect size pertain to applicability of findings to practice.
- IPE Your interprofessional primary care team is asked to write an evidence-based policy that will introduce depression screening as a required part of the admission protocol in your practice. Debate the pros and cons of considering the evidence to inform your protocol provided by a meta-analysis of 10 RCT studies with a combined sample size of $n = 859$, in comparison to 10 individual RCTs, only 2 of which have a sample size of $n = 100$.

- Explain why it is important to have an interprofessional team conducting a systematic review.

REFERENCES

Al-Mallah, M. H., Farah, I., Al-Madani, W., et al. (2015). The impact of nurse-led clinics on the mortality and morbidity of patients with cardiovascular diseases: A systematic review and meta-analysis. *Journal of Cardiovascular Nursing*, *31*(1), 89–95.

Borenstein, M., Hedges, L. V., Higgins, J. P. T., & Rothstein, H. R. (2009). *Introduction to meta-analysis.* United Kingdom: Wiley.

Brady, V. J., Grimes, D., Armstrong, T., & LoBiondo-Wood, G. (2014). Management of steroid-induced hyperglycemia in hospitalized patients with cancer: A review. *Oncology Nursing Forum*, *41*, E355–E365.

Brouwers, M., Kho, M. E., Browman, G. P., et al. for the AGREE Next Steps Consortium. (2010). AGREE II: Advancing guideline development, reporting and evaluation in healthcare. *Canadian Medical Association Journal*, *182*, E839–E842. doi:10.1503/090449.

Center for Evidence-Based Medicine Critical Appraisal Tools. (2016). www.cebm.net/critical-appraisal.

Cochrane Handbook for Systematic Reviews. (2016). http://www.cochrane-handbook.org.

Conley, S., & Redeker, N. (2016). A systematic review of management interventions for inflammatory bowel disease. *Journal of Nursing Scholarship*, *48*(2), 118–127.

da Costa, B. R., & Juni, P. (2014). Systematic reviews and meta-analyses of randomized trials: Principles and pitfalls. *European Heart Journal*, *35*, 3336–3345.

Docherty, S. L. (2003). Symptom experiences of children and adolescents with cancer. *Annual Review Nursing Research*, *21*(2), 123–149.

Higgins, J. P. T., & Green, S. (2011). *Cochrane handbook for systematic reviews of interventions version* 5.1.0. http://www.cochrane-handbook.org.

Kestler, S. A., & LoBiondo-Wood, G. (2012). Review of symptom experiences in children and adolescents with cancer. *Cancer Nursing*, *35*(2), E31–E49. doi:10.1097/NCC.0b013e3182207a2a.

Liberati, A., Altman, D. G., Tetzlaff, J., et al. (2009). The PRISMA statement for reporting systematic reviews and meta-analyses of studies that evaluate health care interventions: Explanation and elaboration. *Annuals of Internal Medicine*, *151*(4), w65–w94.

Martineau, A. R., Cates, C. J., Urashima, M., et al. (2016). Vitamin D for the management of asthma. *Cochrane Database of Systematic Reviews*, *9*, CD011511. doi:10.1002/14651858.CD011511.pub2.

Moher, D., Liberati, A., Tetzlaff, J., & Altman, D. G. (2009). Preferred reporting items for systematic reviews and meta-analyses: The PRISMA statement. *PLOS Medicine*, *62*(10), 1006–1012. doi:10.1016/j.jclinepi.2009.06.005.

Moher, D., Shamseer, L., Clarke, M., et al. (2015). Preferred reporting items for systematic review and meta-analysis protocols (PRISMA—P) 2015 Statement. *Systematic Reviews*, *4*(1), 1.

Moher, D., Stewart, L., & Shekelle, P. (2015). All in the family: Systematic reviews, rapid reviews, scoping reviews, realist reviews and more. *Systematic Reviews*, *4*, 183.

Stroup, D. F., Berlin, J. A., Morton, S. C., et al. (2000). Meta-analysis of observational studies in epidemiology: A proposal for reporting. Meta-analysis of observational studies in epidemiology (MOOSE) group. *The Journal of the American Medical Association*, *283*, 2008–2012.

Whittemore, R. (2005). Combining evidence in nursing research: Methods and implications. *Nursing Research*, *54*(1), 56–62.

Whittemore, R., & Knafl, K. (2005). The integrative review: Updated methodology. *Journal of Advanced Nursing*, *52*(5), 546–553.

Go to Evolve at **http://evolve.elsevier.com/LoBiondo/** for review questions, critiquing exercises, and additional research articles for practice in reviewing and critiquing.

12

Sampling

Judith Haber

Go to Evolve at **http://evolve.elsevier.com/LoBiondo/** for review questions, critiquing exercises, and additional research articles for practice in reviewing and critiquing.

LEARNING OUTCOMES

After reading this chapter, you should be able to do the following:

- Identify the purpose of sampling.
- Define *population, sample,* and *sampling.*
- Compare a population and a sample.
- Discuss the importance of inclusion and exclusion criteria.
- Define *nonprobability* and *probability sampling.*
- Identify the types of nonprobability and probability sampling strategies.
- Compare the advantages and disadvantages of nonprobability and probability sampling strategies.
- Discuss the contribution of nonprobability and probability sampling strategies to strength of evidence provided by study findings.
- Discuss the factors that influence sample size.
- Discuss potential threats to internal and external validity as sources of sampling bias.
- Use the critical appraisal criteria to evaluate the "Sample" section of a research report.

KEY TERMS

accessible population
convenience sampling
data saturation
delimitations
element
eligibility criteria
exclusion criteria
inclusion
multistage (cluster) sampling
network (snowball) sampling
nonprobability sampling
pilot study
population
probability sampling
purposive sampling
quota sampling
random selection
representative sample
sample
sampling
sampling frame
sampling unit
simple random sampling
snowballing
stratified random sampling
target population

The sampling section of a study is usually found in the "Methods" section of a research article. You will find it important to understand the sampling process and the elements that contribute to a researcher using the most appropriate sampling strategy for the type of research being conducted. Equally important is knowing how to critically appraise the sampling section of a study to identify how the strengths and weaknesses of the sampling process contributed to the overall strength and quality of evidence provided by the findings of a study.

When you are critically appraising the sampling section of a study, the threats to internal and external validity as sources of bias need to be considered (see Chapter 8). Your evaluation of the sampling section is very important in your overall critical appraisal of a study's findings and applicability to practice.

Sampling is the process of selecting representative units of a population in a study. Many problems in research cannot be solved without employing rigorous sampling procedures. **Example:** ➤ When testing the effectiveness of a medication for patients with type 2 diabetes, the drug is administered to a sample of the population for whom the drug is potentially appropriate. The researcher must come to conclusions without giving the drug to every patient with diabetes or laboratory animal. Because human lives are at stake, the researcher cannot afford to arrive casually at conclusions that are based on the first dozen patients available for study.

The impact of arriving at conclusions that are not accurate or making generalizations from a small nonrepresentative sample is much more severe in research than in everyday life. Essentially, researchers sample representative segments of the population because it is rarely feasible or necessary to sample the entire population of interest to obtain relevant information.

This chapter will familiarize you with the basic concepts of sampling as they primarily pertain to the principles of quantitative research design, nonprobability and probability sampling, sample size, and the related critical appraisal process. Sampling issues that relate to qualitative research designs are discussed in Chapters 5, 6, and 7.

SAMPLING CONCEPTS

Population

A **population** is a well-defined set with specified properties. A population can be composed of people, animals, objects, or events. Examples of populations might be all of the female patients older than 65 years admitted to a specific hospital for congestive heart failure (CHF) during the year 2017, all of the children with asthma in the state of New York, or all of the men and women with a diagnosis of clinical depression in the United States. These examples illustrate that a population may be broadly defined and potentially involve millions of people or narrowly specified to include only several hundred people.

The population criteria establish the **target population**—that is, the entire set of cases about which the researcher would like to make generalizations. A target population might include all undergraduate nursing students enrolled in accelerated baccalaureate programs in the United States. Because of time, money, and personnel, however, it is often not feasible to pursue a study using a target population.

An **accessible population**, one that meets the target population criteria and that is available, is used instead. **Example:** ➤ An accessible population might include all full-time accelerated baccalaureate students attending school in Oregon. Pragmatic factors must also be considered when identifying a potential population of interest.

It is important to know that a population is not restricted to humans. It may consist of hospital records; blood, urine, or other specimens taken from patients at a clinic; historical documents; or laboratory animals. **Example:** ➤ A population might consist of all the $HgbA_{1C}$ blood test specimens collected from patients in the City Hospital diabetes clinic or all of the patient charts on file who had been screened during pregnancy for HIV infection. A population can be defined in a variety of ways. The basic unit of the population must be clearly defined because the generalizability of the findings will be a function of the population criteria.

Inclusion and Exclusion Criteria

When reading a research report, you should consider whether the researcher has identified the population characteristics that form the basis for the inclusion (eligibility) or exclusion (delimitations) criteria used to select the sample—whether people, objects, or events. The terms **inclusion** or **eligibility criteria** and **exclusion criteria** or **delimitations** define characteristics that limit the population to a homogenous group of subjects. The population characteristics that provide the basis for inclusion (eligibility) criteria should be evident in the sample—that is, the characteristics of the population and the sample should be congruent in order to assess the representativeness of the sample. Examples of inclusion or eligibility criteria and exclusion criteria or delimitations include the following:

- gender
- age
- marital status
- socioeconomic status
- religion
- ethnicity
- level of education
- age of children
- health status
- diagnosis

Think about the concept of inclusion or eligibility criteria applied to a study where the subjects are patients. **Example:** ➤ Participants in a study investigating the effectiveness of a nurse practitioner (NP) delivered symptom management intervention for patients initiating chemotherapy for nonmetastatic cancer compared to standard oncology care. The aim was to reduce patient reported symptom burden by facilitating patient-NP collaboration and early management of symptoms (Traeger et al., 2015). Participants had to meet the following inclusion (eligibility) criteria:

1. Age: At least 18 years
2. Newly diagnosed with Stage I to Stage III breast cancer (BC), lung cancer (LC), or colorectal cancer (CRC)
3. Scheduled to initiate chemotherapy for nonmetastatic disease
4. Able to respond to questionnaires in English

Inclusion and exclusion criteria are established to control for extraneous variability or bias that would limit the strength of evidence contributed by the sampling plan in relation to the study's design. Each inclusion or exclusion criterion should have a rationale, presumably related to a potential contaminating effect on the dependent variable. **Example:** ➤ Subjects were excluded from this study if they had:

- A concurrent cognitive or psychiatric condition or substance abuse problem that would prevent adherence to the protocol
- Evidence of metastatic cancer
- Had already received chemotherapy for their malignancy

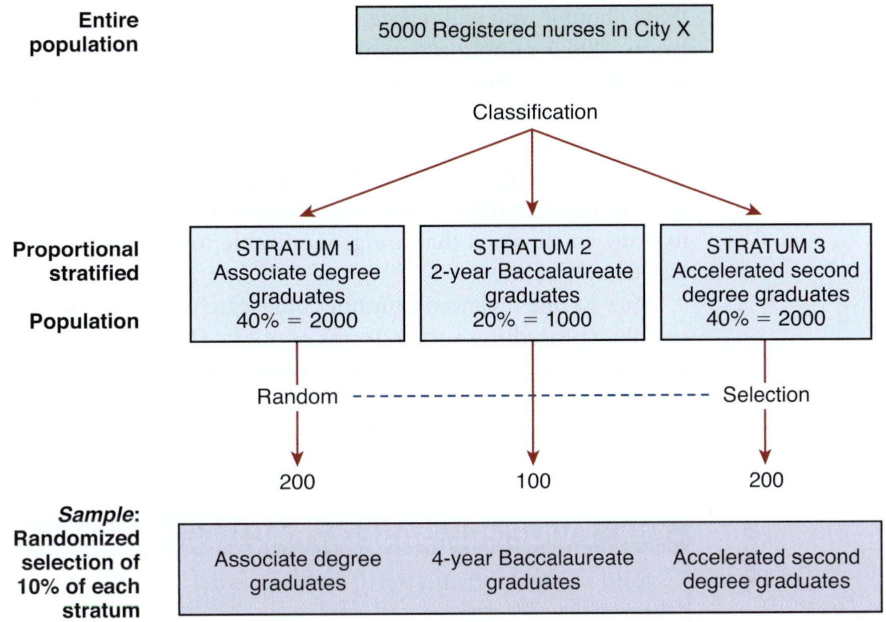

FIG 12.1 Subject selection using a proportional stratified random sampling strategy.

The careful establishment of sample inclusion or exclusion criteria will increase a study's precision and strength of evidence, thereby contributing to the accuracy and generalizability of the findings (see Chapter 8). Fig. 12.1 provides an example of a flow chart that illustrates how potential study participants were screened using the above inclusion (eligibility) and exclusion criteria for enrollment in the NP delivered symptom management intervention study by Traeger and colleagues (2015).

HELPFUL HINT

Researchers may not clearly identify the population under study, or the population is not clarified until the "Discussion" section when the effort is made to discuss the group (population) to which the study findings can be generalized.

Samples and Sampling

Sampling is the selection of a portion or subset of the designated population that represents the entire population. A **sample** is a set of elements that make up the population; an **element** is the most basic unit about which information is collected. The most common element in nursing research is individuals, but other elements (e.g., places, objects) can form the basis of a sample or population. **Example:** ➤ A researcher was planning a study that investigated barriers that may underlie the decline in girls' physical activity (PA), beginning at the onset of adolescence. Eight midwestern US schools were randomly assigned to either receive a multicomponent PA intervention called "Girls on the Move" or serve as a control. The schools were identified as the sampling units rather than the treatment alone (Vermeesch et al., 2015). The purpose of sampling is to increase a study's efficiency. If you think about it, you will realize that it is not feasible to examine every element in the population. When sampling is done properly, the researcher can draw inferences and make generalizations about the population without examining each element in the population. Sampling procedures identify specific selection criteria to ensure that the characteristics of the phenomena of interest will be, or are likely to be, present in all of the units being studied. The researcher's efforts to ensure that the sample is representative of the target population strengthens the evidence generated by the sample, which allows the researcher to draw conclusions that are generalizable to the population and applicable to practice (see Chapter 8).

After having reviewed a number of research studies, you will recognize that samples and sampling procedures vary in terms of merit. The foremost criterion in appraising a sample is its representativeness. A **representative sample** is one whose key characteristics closely match those of the population. If 70% of the population in a study of child-rearing practices consisted of women and 40% were full-time employees, a representative sample should reflect these characteristics in the same proportions.

QSEN EVIDENCE-BASED PRACTICE TIP

Consider whether the choice of participants was biased, thereby influencing the strength of evidence provided by the outcomes of the study.

TYPES OF SAMPLES

Sampling strategies are generally grouped into two categories: nonprobability sampling and probability sampling. In **nonprobability sampling**, elements are chosen by nonrandom methods. The drawback of this strategy is that there is no way of estimating each element's probability of being included in a particular sample. Essentially, there is no way of ensuring that every element has a chance for inclusion in a nonprobability sample.

Probability sampling uses some form of random selection when the sample is chosen. This type of sample enables the researcher to estimate the probability that each element of the population will be included in the sample. Probability sampling is the more rigorous type of sampling strategy and is more likely to result in a representative sample. A summary of sampling strategies appears in Table 12.1 and is discussed in the following sections.

QSEN EVIDENCE-BASED PRACTICE TIP

Determining whether the sample is representative of the population being studied will influence your interpretation of the evidence provided by the findings and decision making about their relevance to the patient population and practice setting.

HELPFUL HINT

A research article may not be explicit about the sampling strategy used. If the sampling strategy is not specified, assume that a convenience sample was used for a quantitative study and a purposive sample was used for a qualitative study.

TABLE 12.1 Summary of Sampling Strategies

Sampling Strategy	Ease of Drawing Sample	Risk of Bias	Representativeness of Sample
Nonprobability			
Convenience	Easy	Greater than any other sampling strategy	Because samples tend to be self-selecting, representativeness is questionable
Quota	Relatively easy	Contains unknown source of bias that affects external validity	Builds in some representativeness by using knowledge about population of interest
Purposive	Relatively easy	Bias increases with greater heterogeneity of population; conscious bias is also a danger	Very limited ability to generalize because sample is handpicked
Probability			
Simple random	Time consuming	Low	Maximized; probability of nonrepresentativeness decreases with increased sample size
Stratified random	Time consuming	Low	Enhanced
Cluster	Less or more time consuming depending on the strata	Subject to more sampling errors than simple or stratified	Less representative than simple or stratified

Nonprobability Sampling

Because of lack of random selection, the findings of studies using nonprobability sampling are less generalizable than those using a probability sampling strategy, and they tend to produce less representative samples. When a nonprobability sample is carefully chosen to reflect the target population through the careful use of inclusion and exclusion criteria and adequate sample size, you can have more confidence in the sample's representativeness and the external validity of the findings (see Chapter 8). The three major types of nonprobability sampling are convenience, quota, and purposive sampling strategies.

Convenience Sampling

Convenience sampling is the use of the most readily accessible persons or objects as subjects. The subjects may include volunteers, the first 100 patients admitted to hospital X with a particular diagnosis, all of the people enrolled in program Y during the month of September, or all of the students enrolled in course Z at a particular university during 2014. The subjects are convenient and accessible to the researcher and are thus called a *convenience sample.* **Example:** ➤ A study evaluating an NP-led intensive behavioral treatment program for obesity implemented in an adult primary care practice used a convenience sample of obese adults (18 years and older) who were primary care patients of a patient-centered medical home (PCMH) practice who met the eligibility criteria and volunteered to participate in the study (Thabault et al., 2016).

The advantage of a convenience sample is that generally it is easier to obtain subjects. The researcher will still have to be concerned with obtaining a sufficient number of subjects who meet the inclusion criteria. The major disadvantage of a convenience sample is that the risk of bias is greater than in any other type of sample (see Table 12.1). The fact that convenience samples use voluntary participation increases the probability of researchers recruiting those people who feel strongly about the issue being studied, which may favor certain outcomes. In this case, ask yourself the following as you think about the strength and quality of evidence contributed by the sampling component of a study:

- What motivated some people to participate and others not to participate (self-selection)?
- What kind of data would have been obtained if nonparticipants had also responded?
- How representative are the people who did participate in relation to the population?
- What kind of confidence can you have in the evidence provided by the findings?

Researchers may recruit subjects in clinic settings, stop people on a street corner to ask their opinion on some issue, place advertisements in the newspaper, or place signs in local churches, community centers, or supermarkets, indicating that volunteers are needed for a particular study. To assess the degree to which a convenience sample approximates a random sample, the researcher checks for the representativeness of the convenience sample by comparing the sample to population percentages and, in that way, assesses the extent to which bias is or is not evident (Sousa et al., 2004).

Because acquiring research subjects is a problem that confronts many researchers, innovative recruitment strategies may be used. A unique method of accessing and recruiting subjects is the use of online computer networks (e.g., disease-specific chat rooms, blogs, and bulletin boards). **Example:** ➤ In the study by Traeger et al. (2015) that implemented a nursing intervention to enhance outpatient chemotherapy symptom management, trained staff screened chemotherapy schedules and electronic health record data to identify all potential participants. When you appraise a study you should recognize that the convenience sampling strategy, although most common, is the weakest sampling strategy with regard to strength of evidence and generalizability (external validity) unless it is followed by random assignment to groups, as you will find in studies that are randomized clinical trials (RCT) (see Chapter 9). When a convenience sample is used, caution should be exercised in interpreting the data and assessing the researcher's comments about the external validity and applicability of the findings (see Chapter 8).

Quota Sampling

Quota sampling refers to a form of nonprobability sampling in which subjects who meet the inclusion criteria are recruited and consecutively enrolled until the target sample size is reached. The study by Traeger and colleagues provides an example of quota sampling when trained study coordinators approached eligible chemotherapy patients during their first chemotherapy visit to introduce the study, obtained informed consent, and enrolled interested and eligible consecutive patients until the target enrollment was reached.

Sometimes knowledge about the population of interest is used to build some representativeness into the sample (see Table 12.1). A quota sample can identify the strata of the population and proportionally represents the strata in the sample. **Example:** ➤ The data in Table 12.2 reveal that 40% of the 5000 nurses in city X are associate degree graduates, 20% are 4-year baccalaureate degree graduates, and 40% are accelerated second-degree baccalaureate graduates. Each stratum of the population should be proportionately represented in the sample. In this case, the researcher used a proportional quota sampling strategy and decided to sample 10% of a population of 5000 (i.e., 500 nurses). Based on the proportion of each stratum in the population, 200 associate degree graduates, 100 4-year baccalaureate graduates, and 200 accelerated baccalaureate graduates were the quotas

TABLE 12.2 **Numbers and Percentages of Students in Strata of a Quota Sample of 5000 Graduates of Nursing Programs in City X**

	Associate Degree Graduates	4-year Baccalaureate Degree Graduates	Accelerated Baccalaureate Degree Graduates
Population	2000 (40%)	1000 (20%)	2000 (40%)
Strata	200	100	200

established for the three strata. The researcher recruited subjects who met the study's eligibility criteria until the quota for each stratum was filled. In other words, once the researcher obtained the necessary 200 associate degree graduates, 100 4-year baccalaureate degree graduates, and 200 accelerated baccalaureate degree graduates, the sample was complete.

The characteristics chosen to form the strata are selected according to a researcher's knowledge of the population and the literature review. The criterion for selection should be a variable that reflects important differences in the dependent variables under investigation. Age, gender, religion, ethnicity, medical diagnosis, socioeconomic status, level of completed education, and occupational rank are among the variables that are likely to be important stratifying variables in nursing research studies.

The researcher systematically ensures that proportional segments of the population are included in the sample. The quota sample is not randomly selected (i.e., once the proportional strata have been identified, the researcher recruits and enrolls subjects until the quota for each stratum has been filled) but does increase the sample's representativeness. This sampling strategy addresses the problem of overrepresentation or underrepresentation of certain segments of a population in a sample.

As you critically appraise a study, your aim is to determine whether the sample strata appropriately reflect the population under consideration and whether the stratifying variables are homogeneous enough to ensure a meaningful comparison of differences among strata. Establishment of strict inclusion and exclusion criteria and using power analysis to determine appropriate sample size increase the rigor of a quota sampling strategy by creating homogeneous subject categories that facilitate making meaningful comparisons across strata.

Purposive Sampling

Purposive sampling is a common strategy. The researcher selects subjects who are considered to be typical of the population. Purposive sampling can be found in both quantitative and qualitative studies. When a researcher is considering the sampling strategy for a randomized clinical trial focusing on a specific diagnosis or patient population, the sampling strategy is often purposive in nature. In such studies the researcher first purposively selects subjects who are then randomized to groups.

Purposive sampling is commonly used in qualitative research studies. **Example:** ➤ The objective of the qualitative study by van Dijk et al. (2015) was to examine how patients assign a number to their currently experienced postoperative pain. They selected a purposive sample of patients who had surgery the day before and were experiencing postoperative pain with a score of at least 4 on the Numeric Rating Scale (NRS). Subjects were selected until the new information obtained did not provide further insight into the themes or no new themes emerged (data saturation; see Chapters 5, 6, and 14). A purposive sample is used also when a highly unusual group is being studied, such as a population with a rare genetic disease (e.g., Huntington chorea). In this case, the researcher would describe the sample characteristics precisely to ensure that the reader will have an accurate picture of the subjects in the sample.

Today, computer networks (e.g., online services) can be a valuable resource in helping researchers access and recruit subjects for purposive samples. Online support group bulletin boards that facilitate recruitment of subjects for purposive samples exist for people with cancer, rheumatoid arthritis, multiple sclerosis, human immunodeficiency virus/acquired immunodeficiency syndrome (HIV/AIDS), postpartum depression, Lyme disease, and many others.

The researcher who uses a purposive sample assumes that errors of judgment in overrepresenting or underrepresenting elements of the population in the sample will tend to balance out. As indicated in Table 12.1, there may be conscious bias in the selection of subjects; the ability to generalize from the evidence provided by the findings is very limited. Box 12.1 lists examples of when a purposive sample may be appropriate.

Network Sampling

Network sampling, sometimes referred to as **snowballing**, is used for locating samples that are difficult or impossible to locate in other ways. This strategy takes advantage of social networks and the fact that friends tend to have characteristics in common. When a few subjects with the necessary eligibility criteria are found, the researcher asks for their assistance in getting in touch with others with similar criteria. **Example:** ➤ Online computer networks, as described in the section on purposive sampling and in this last example, can be used to assist researchers in acquiring otherwise difficult to locate subjects, thereby taking advantage of the networking or snowball effect. In a study that aimed to gain consensus from experts on the priorities for clinical nursing and midwifery research in southern and eastern African countries, the researchers used contacts with networks of regional nursing colleagues and leaders, snowball sampling, to compile a list of potential research experts who met the inclusion criteria and agreed to participate by responding to the Delphi research priority survey. To expand their network of experts, they asked survey respondents for referrals to others who met the criteria and might be willing to participate. Surveys were sent to the new potential participants who were identified (Sun et al., 2015).

BOX 12.1 Criteria for Use of a Purposive Sampling Strategy

- Effective pretesting of newly developed instruments with a purposive sample of divergent types of people
- Validation of a scale or test with a known-group technique
- Collection of exploratory data in relation to an unusual or highly specific population, particularly when the total target population remains an unknown to the researcher
- Collection of descriptive data (e.g., as in qualitative studies) that seek to describe the lived experience of a particular phenomenon (e.g., postpartum depression, caring, hope, surviving childhood sexual abuse)
- Focus of the study population relates to a specific diagnosis (e.g., type 1 diabetes, ovarian cancer) or condition (e.g., legal blindness, terminal illness) or demographic characteristic (e.g., same-sex twin pairs)

> **HELPFUL HINT**
>
> When convenience or purposive sampling is used as the first step in recruiting a sample for a randomized clinical trial, as illustrated in Fig. 12.1, it is followed by random assignment of subjects to an intervention or control group, which increases the generalizability of the findings.

Probability Sampling

The primary characteristic of **probability sampling** is the random selection of elements from the population. **Random selection** occurs when each element of the population has an equal and independent chance of being included in the sample. When probability sampling is used, you have greater confidence that the sample is representative of the population being studied rather than biased. Three commonly used probability sampling strategies are simple random, stratified random, and cluster.

Random selection of sample subjects should not be confused with randomization or random assignment of subjects. The latter, discussed earlier in this chapter and in Chapter 8, refers to the assignment of subjects to either an experimental or a control group on a random basis. Random assignment is most closely associated with RCT.

Simple Random Sampling

Simple random sampling is a carefully controlled process. The researcher defines the population (a set), lists all of the units of the population (a **sampling frame**), and selects a sample of units (a subset) from which the sample will be chosen. **Example:** ➤ If American hospitals specializing in the treatment of cancer were the sampling unit, a list of all such hospitals would be the sampling frame. If certified school nurses constituted the accessible population, a list of those nurses would be the sampling frame.

Once a list of the population elements has been developed, the best method of selecting a random sample is to use a computer program that generates the order in which the random selection of subjects is to be carried out.

The advantages of simple random sampling are as follows:

- Sample selection is not subject to the conscious biases of the researcher.
- Representativeness of the sample in relation to the population characteristics is maximized.
- Differences in the characteristics of the sample and the population are purely a function of chance.
- Probability of choosing a nonrepresentative sample decreases as the size of the sample increases.

Example: ➤ Simple random sampling was used in a study testing the feasibility of collecting hair for cortisol measurement from a probability sample of 516 racially and socioeconomically diverse urban adolescents aged 11 to 17 years participating in a larger prospective study on adolescent health and well-being (Ford et al., 2016). The sampling frame was based on a combination of eligible households and public school data from the study area. The addresses were sorted by zip code, and random replicates of 500 participants were drawn. The randomly selected households were contacted to solicit participation in the study.

The major disadvantage of simple random sampling is that it can be a time-consuming and inefficient method of obtaining a random sample. **Example:** ➤ Consider the task of listing all of the baccalaureate nursing students in the United States. With random sampling, it may also be impossible to obtain an accurate or complete listing of every element in the population. **Example:** ➤ Imagine trying to obtain a list of all suicides in New York City for the year 2016. It often is the case that although suicide may have been the cause of death, another cause (e.g., cardiac failure) appears on the death certificate. It would be difficult to estimate how many elements of the target population would be eliminated from consideration. The issue of bias would definitely enter the picture despite the researcher's best efforts. In the final analysis, you, as the evaluator of a research article, must be cautious about generalizing from findings, even when random sampling is the stated strategy or if the target population has been difficult or impossible to list completely.

QSEN EVIDENCE-BASED PRACTICE TIP

When thinking about applying study findings to your clinical practice, consider whether the participants making up the sample are similar to your own patients.

Stratified Random Sampling

Stratified random sampling requires that the population be divided into strata or subgroups as illustrated in Fig. 12.1. The subgroups or subsets that the population is divided into are homogeneous. An appropriate number of elements from each subset are randomly selected on the basis of their proportion in the population. The goal of this strategy is to achieve a greater degree of representativeness. Stratified random sampling is similar to the proportional stratified quota sampling strategy discussed earlier in the chapter. The major difference is that stratified random sampling uses a random selection procedure for obtaining sample subjects.

The population is stratified according to any number of attributes, such as age, gender, ethnicity, religion, socioeconomic status, or level of education completed. The variables selected to form the strata should be adaptable to homogeneous subsets with regard to the attributes being studied. **Example:** ➤ A study by Wong et al. (2016) examined whether high-comorbidity patients had larger increases in primary care provider (PCP) visits attributable to primary care medical home (PCMH) implementation in a large integrated health system in comparison to other patients enrolled in primary care. The data were obtained from the Veterans Health Association (VHA) Corporate Data Warehouse (CDW), which contains comprehensive administrative data tracking patient utilization, demographics, and clinical measures including ICD-9 diagnostic codes. For each quarter of the study, they identified a 1% random sample of all VHA primary care patients in the database that quarter. The final sample consisted of 8.4 million patient quarter observations. All analyses were stratified by age group (under 65 and age 65+), comorbidity burden score, and outpatient visits. As illustrated in Table 12.1, several advantages to a stratified random sampling strategy include (1) representativeness of the sample is enhanced; (2) researcher has a valid basis for making comparisons among subsets; and (3) researcher is able to oversample a disproportionately small stratum to adjust for their underrepresentation, statistically weigh the data accordingly, and continue to make legitimate comparisons.

The obstacles encountered by a researcher using this strategy include (1) difficulty of obtaining a population list containing complete critical variable information, (2) time-consuming effort of obtaining multiple enumerated lists, (3) challenge of enrolling proportional strata, and (4) time and money involved in carrying out a large-scale study using a stratified sampling strategy.

Multistage Sampling (Cluster Sampling)

Multistage (cluster) sampling involves a successive random sampling of units (clusters) that progress from large to small and meet sample eligibility criteria. The first-stage **sampling unit** consists of large units or clusters. The second-stage sampling unit consists of smaller units or clusters. Third-stage sampling units are even smaller. **Example:** ➤ If a sample of critical care nurses is desired, the first sampling unit would be a random sample of hospitals, obtained from an American Hospital Association list, that meet the eligibility criteria (e.g., size, type). The second-stage sampling unit would consist of a list of critical care nurses practicing at each hospital selected in the first stage (i.e., the list obtained from the vice president for nursing at each hospital). The criteria for inclusion in the list of critical care nurses would be as follows:

1. Certified as a Certified Critical Care Registered Nurse (CCRN) with at least 3 years' experience as a critical care nurse
2. At least 75% of the CCRN's time spent in providing direct patient care in a critical care unit
3. Full-time employment at the hospital

The second-stage sampling unit would obtain a random selection of 10 CCRNs from each hospital who met the previously mentioned eligibility criteria.

When multistage sampling is used in relation to large national surveys, states are used as the first-stage sampling unit; followed by successively smaller units such as counties, cities, districts, and blocks as the second-stage sampling unit; and finally households as the third-stage sampling unit.

Sampling units or clusters can be selected by simple random or stratified random sampling methods. **Example:** ➤ Sun et al. (2015) conducted a survey using the Delphi method to gain consensus about regional clinical nursing and midwifery research priorities from experts in participating eastern and southern African countries. Clinical nursing and midwifery experts from 13 countries participated in the first round of the survey by completing the electronic survey, and experts from 14 countries participated in the second round. This approach to multistage sampling was chosen because the electronic format facilitates obtaining consensus from a large panel of experts in a wide geographic region by providing anonymity, eliminating the potential for leaders to dominate the process, and providing a chance in Round 2 to change their mind after considering the group opinion. The main advantage of cluster sampling, as illustrated in Table 12.1, is that it can be more economical in terms of time and money than other types of probability sampling. There are two major disadvantages: (1) more sampling errors tend to occur than with simple random or stratified random sampling, and (2) appropriate handling of the statistical data from cluster samples is very complex. When you are critically appraising a study, you will need to consider whether the use of cluster sampling is justified in light of the research design, as well as other pragmatic matters, such as economy.

QSEN EVIDENCE-BASED PRACTICE TIP

The sampling strategy, whether probability or nonprobability, must be appropriate to the design and evaluated in relation to the level of evidence provided by the design.

CRITICAL THINKING DECISION PATH

Assessing the Relationship Between the Type of Sampling Strategy and the Appropriate Generalizability

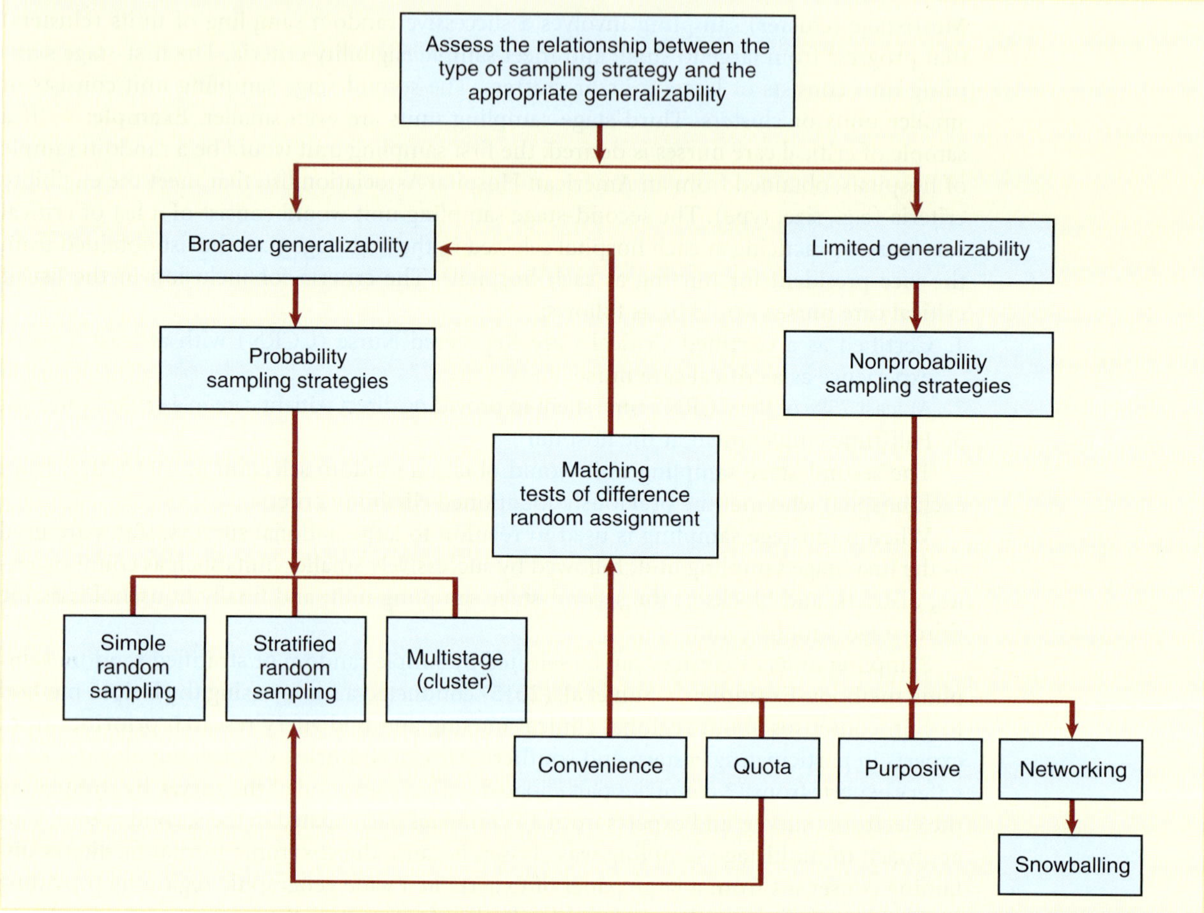

The Critical Thinking Decision Path illustrates the relationship between the type of sampling strategy and the appropriate generalizability.

SAMPLE SIZE

There is no single rule that can be applied to the determination of a sample's size. When arriving at an estimate of sample size, many factors, such as the following, must be considered:

- Type of design
- Type of sampling procedure
- Type of formula used for estimating optimum sample size
- Degree of precision required
- Heterogeneity of the attributes under investigation

- Relative frequency that the phenomenon of interest occurs in the population (i.e., a common versus a rare health problem)
- Projected cost of using a particular sampling strategy

HELPFUL HINT

Look for a brief discussion of a study's sampling strategy in the "Methods" section of a research article. Sometimes there is a separate subsection with the heading "Sample," "Subjects," or "Study Participants." A statistical description of the characteristics of the actual sample often does not appear until the "Results" section of a research article. You may also find a table in the Results section that summarizes the sample characteristics using descriptive statistics (see Chapter 14).

The sample size should be determined before a study is conducted. A general rule is always to use the largest sample possible. The larger the sample, the more representative of the population it is likely to be; smaller samples produce less accurate results.

One exception to this principle occurs when using qualitative designs. In this case, sample size is not predetermined. Sample sizes in qualitative research tend to be small because of the large volume of verbal data that must be analyzed and because this type of design tends to emphasize intensive and prolonged contact with subjects (Speziale & Carpenter, 2011). Subjects are added to the sample until **data saturation** is reached (i.e., new data no longer emerge during the data-collection process). Fittingness of the data is a more important concern than representativeness of subjects (see Chapters 5, 6, and 7).

Another exception is in the case of a **pilot study**, which is defined as a small sample study conducted as a prelude to a larger scale study that is often called the "parent study." The pilot study is typically a smaller scale of the parent study, with similar methods and procedures that yield preliminary data to determine the feasibility of conducting a larger scale study and establish that sufficient scientific evidence exists to justify subsequent, more extensive research.

The principle of "larger is better" holds true for both probability and nonprobability samples. Results based on small samples (under 10) tend to be unstable—the values fluctuate from one sample to the next, and it is difficult to apply statistics meaningfully. Small samples tend to increase the probability of obtaining a markedly nonrepresentative sample. As the sample size increases, the mean more closely approximates the population values, thus introducing fewer sampling errors.

IPE HIGHLIGHT

Remember to have your interprofessional Journal Club evaluate the appropriateness of the generalizations made about the studies you critically appraise in light of the sampling procedure and any sources of bias that affect applicability of the findings to your patient population.

It is possible to estimate the sample size needed with the use of a statistical procedure known as power analysis (Cohen, 1988). Power analysis is an advanced statistical technique that is commonly used by researchers and is a requirement for external funding. When it is not used, you will have less confidence provided by the findings because the study may be based on a sample that is too small. A researcher may commit a type II error of accepting a null hypothesis when it should have been rejected if the sample is too small (see Chapter 16). No matter how high a research design is located on the evidence hierarchy (e.g., Level II—experimental design consisting of a randomized clinical trial), the findings of a study and their generalizability are weakened when power analysis is not calculated to ensure an adequate sample size to determine the effect of the intervention.

It is beyond the scope of this chapter to describe this complex procedure in great detail, but a simple example will illustrate its use. Nyamathi and colleagues (2015) wanted to assess the impact of three interventions: peer coaching with nurse case management (PC-NCM), peer coaching (PC), and usual care (UC) on completion of hepatitis A and B vaccination series. How would a research team such as Nyamathi and colleagues know the appropriate number of subjects that should be used in the study? When using power analysis, the researcher must estimate how large an impact (effect) will be observed between the three intervention groups (i.e., to test differences among PC-NCM, PC, and UC groups in terms of vaccination completion rates). If a moderate difference is expected, a conventional effect size of .20 is assumed. With a significance level of .05, a total of 114 participants would be needed for each intervention group to detect a statistically significant difference between the groups with a power of .80. The total sample in this study ($n = 600$) exceeded the minimum number of 114 per intervention group.

HELPFUL HINT

Remember to evaluate the appropriateness of the generalizations made about the study findings in light of the target population, the accessible population, the type of sampling strategy, and the sample size.

When calculating sample size using power analysis, the total sample size needs to consider that attrition, or dropouts, will occur and build in approximately 15% extra subjects to make sure that the ability to detect differences between groups or the effect of an intervention remains intact. When expected differences are large, it does not take a very large sample to ensure that differences will be revealed through statistical analysis.

When critically appraising a study, you should evaluate the sample size in terms of the following: (1) how representative the sample is relative to the target population, and (2) to whom the researcher wishes to generalize the study's results. The goal is to have a sample as representative as possible with as little sampling error as possible. Unless representativeness is ensured, all the data in the world become inconsequential. When an appropriate sample size, including power analysis for calculation of sample size, and sampling strategy have been used, you can feel more confident that the sample is representative of the accessible population rather than biased (Fig. 12.2) and the potential for generalizability of findings is greater (see Chapter 8).

QSEN EVIDENCE-BASED PRACTICE TIP

Research designs and types of samples are often linked. When a nonprobability purposive sampling strategy is used to recruit participants to a study using an experimental design, you would expect random assignment of subjects to an intervention or control group to follow.

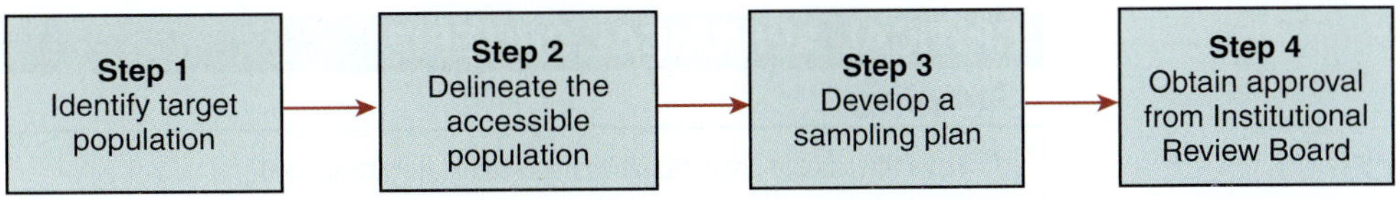

FIG 12.2 Summary of general sampling procedure.

APPRAISAL FOR EVIDENCE-BASED PRACTICE SAMPLING

The criteria for critical appraisal of a study's sample are presented in the Critical Appraisal Criteria box. As you evaluate the sample section of a study, you must raise two questions:

1. If this study were to be replicated, would there be enough information presented about the nature of the population, the sample, the sampling strategy, and sample size of another investigator to carry out the study?
2. What are the sampling threats to internal and external validity that are sources of bias?

The answers to these questions highlight the important link of the sample to the findings and the strength of the evidence used to make clinical decisions about the applicability of the findings to clinical practice (see Chapter 8).

In Chapter 8, we talked about how selection effect as a threat to internal validity could occur in studies where a convenience, quota, or purposive sampling strategy was used. In these studies, individuals themselves decide whether or not to participate. Subject mortality or attrition is another threat to internal validity related to sampling (see Chapter 8). Mortality is the loss of subjects from the study, usually from the first data-collection point to the second. If the subjects who remain in the study are different from those who drop out, the results can be affected. When more of the subjects in one group drop out than the other group, the results can also be influenced. It is common for journals to require authors reporting on research results to include a flow chart that diagrams the screening, recruitment, enrollment, random assignment, and attrition process and results. Threats to external validity related to sampling are concerned with the generalizability of the results to other populations. Generalizability depends on who actually participates in a study. Not everyone who is approached meets the inclusion criteria, agrees to enroll, or completes the study. Bias in sample representativeness and generalizability of findings are important sampling issues that have generated national concern because the presence of these factors decreases confidence in the evidence provided by the findings and limits applicability. Historically, many of the landmark adult health studies (e.g., the Framingham heart study, the Baltimore longitudinal study on aging) excluded women as subjects. Despite the all-male samples, the findings of these studies were generalized from males to all adults, in spite of the lack of female representation in the samples. Similarly, the use of largely European-American subjects in clinical trials limits the identification of variant responses to interventions or drugs in ethnic or racially distinct groups (Ward, 2003). Findings based on European-American data cannot be generalized to African Americans, Asians, Hispanics, or any other cultural group.

CRITICAL APPRAISAL CRITERIA

Sampling

1. Have the sample characteristics been completely described?
2. Can the parameters of the study population be inferred from the description of the sample?
3. To what extent is the sample representative of the population as defined?
4. Are the eligibility/inclusion criteria for the sample clearly identified?
5. Have sample exclusion criteria/delimitations for the sample been established?
6. Would it be possible to replicate the study population?
7. How was the sample selected? Is the method of sample selection appropriate?
8. What kind of bias, if any, is introduced by this sampling method?
9. Is the sample size appropriate? How is it substantiated?
10. Are there indications that rights of subjects have been ensured?
11. Does the researcher identify limitations in generalizability of the findings from the sample to the population? Are they appropriate?
12. Is the sampling strategy appropriate for the design of the study and level of evidence provided by the design?
13. Does the researcher indicate how replication of the study with other samples would provide increased support for the findings?

When appraising the sample of a study, you must remember that despite the use of a carefully controlled sampling procedure that minimizes error, there is no guarantee that the sample will be representative. Factors such as sample heterogeneity and subject dropout may jeopardize the representativeness of the sample despite the most stringent random sampling procedure.

When a purposive sample is used in experimental and quasi-experimental studies, you should determine whether or how the subjects were randomly assigned to groups. If criteria for random assignment have not been followed, you have a valid basis for being cautious about the strength of evidence provided by the proposed conclusions of the study.

Although random selection may be the ideal in establishing the representativeness of a study population, more often realistic barriers (e.g., institutional policy, inaccessibility of subjects, lack of time or money, and current state of knowledge in the field) necessitate the use of nonprobability sampling strategies. Many important research questions that are of interest to nursing do not lend themselves to probability sampling. A well-designed, carefully controlled study using a nonprobability sampling strategy can yield accurate and meaningful evidence that makes a significant contribution to nursing's scientific body of knowledge.

The greatest difficulty in nonprobability sampling stems from the fact that not every element in the population has an equal chance of being represented. Therefore it is likely that some segment of the population will be systematically underrepresented. If the population is homogeneous on critical characteristics, such as age, gender, socioeconomic status, and diagnosis, systematic bias will not be very important. Few of the attributes that researchers are interested in, however, are sufficiently homogeneous to make sampling bias an irrelevant consideration.

Basically you will decide whether the sample size for a quantitative study is appropriate and its size is justifiable. You want to make sure that the researcher indicated how the sample size was determined. The method of arriving at the sample size and the rationale should be briefly mentioned. In the study designed to examine the role of resilience in the relationships of hallucination and delusion-like experiences to psychological distress in a nonclinical population, the sample was selected through a stratified cluster sampling procedure (Barahmand & Ahmad, 2016). The sampling frame consisted of 11,000 students. The power analysis indicated that based on a 5% margin of error and a 95% confidence level and expecting the sample proportion to be 50%, a sample size of at least 372 individuals (3.38% of the population) was needed to detect a significant difference. To allow for data loss through mortality, data loss, or incomplete answers, a sample of 440 individuals (4% of the population) were enrolled in the study. When appraising qualitative research designs, you also apply criteria related to sampling strategies that are relevant for a particular type of qualitative study. In general, sampling strategies for qualitative studies are purposive because the study of specific phenomena in their natural setting is emphasized; any subject belonging to a specified group is considered to represent that group. Keep in mind that qualitative studies will not discuss predetermining sample size or method of arriving at sample size. Rather, sample size will tend to be small and a function of data saturation. Finally, evidence that the rights of human subjects have been protected should appear in the "Sample" section of the research report and probably consists of no more than one sentence. Remember to evaluate whether permission was obtained from an institutional review board that reviewed the study relative to the maintenance of ethical research standards (see Chapter 13).

KEY POINTS

- Sampling is a process that selects representative units of a population for study. Researchers sample representative segments of the population because it is rarely feasible or necessary to sample entire populations of interest to obtain accurate and meaningful information.
- Researchers establish eligibility criteria; these are descriptors of the population and provide the basis for selection of a sample. Eligibility criteria, which are also referred to as delimitations, include the following: age, gender, socioeconomic status, level of education, religion, and ethnicity.
- The researcher must identify the target population (i.e., the entire set of cases about which the researcher would like to make generalizations). Because of the pragmatic constraints, however, the researcher usually uses an accessible population (i.e., one that meets the population criteria and is available).
- A sample is a set of elements that makes up the population.
- A sampling unit is the element or set of elements used for selecting the sample. The foremost criterion in appraising a sample is the representativeness or congruence of characteristics with the population.
- Sampling strategies consist of nonprobability and probability sampling.
- In nonprobability sampling, the elements are chosen by nonrandom methods. Types of nonprobability sampling include convenience, quota, and purposive sampling.
- Probability sampling is characterized by the random selection of elements from the population. In random selection, each element in the population has an equal and independent chance of being included in the sample. Types of probability sampling include simple random, stratified random, and multistage sampling.
- Sample size is a function of the type of sampling procedure being used, the degree of precision required, the type of sample estimation formula being used, the heterogeneity

of the study attributes, the relative frequency of occurrence of the phenomena under consideration, and cost.

- Criteria for drawing a sample vary according to the sampling strategy. Systematic organization of the sampling procedure minimizes bias. The target population is identified, the accessible portion of the target population is delineated, permission to conduct the research study is obtained, and a sampling plan is formulated.
- When critically appraising a research report, the sampling plan needs to be evaluated for its appropriateness in relation to the particular research design and level of evidence generated by the design.
- Completeness of the sampling plan is examined in light of potential replicability of the study. The critiquer appraises whether the sampling strategy is the strongest plan for the particular study under consideration.
- An appropriate systematic sampling plan will maximize the efficiency of a research study. It will increase the strength, accuracy, and meaningfulness of the evidence provided by the findings and enhance the generalizability of the findings from the sample to the population.

CRITICAL THINKING CHALLENGES

- How do inclusion and exclusion criteria contribute to increasing the strength of evidence provided by the sampling strategy of a research study?
- Why is it important for a researcher to use power analysis to calculate sample size? How does adequate sample size affect subject mortality, representativeness of the sample, the researcher's ability to detect a treatment effect, and your ability to generalize from the study findings to your patient population?
- How does a flow chart such as the one in Fig. 12.1 of the Thomas article in Appendix A contribute to the strength and quality of evidence provided by the findings of research study and their potential for applicability to practice?
- IPE Your interprofessional team member argues that a random sample is always better, even if it is small and represents ONLY one site. Another team member counters that a very large convenience sample with random assignment to groups representing multiple sites can be very significant. Which colleague would you defend and why? How would each scenario affect the strength and quality of evidence provided by the findings?
- Your research classmate argues that a random sample is always better, even if it is small and represents only one site. Another student counters that a very large convenience sample representing multiple sites can be very significant. Which classmate would you defend and why? How would each scenario affect the strength and quality of evidence provided by the findings?

REFERENCES

Barahmand, U., & Ahmad, R. H. S. (2016). Psychotic-like experiences and psychological distress: the role of resilience. *Journal of the American Psychiatric Nurses Association*, *22*(4), 312–319.

Cohen, J. (1988). *Statistical power analysis for the behavioral sciences* (2nd ed.). New York, NY: Academic Press.

Ford, J. L., Boch, S. J., & McCarthy, D. O. (2016). Feasibility of hair collection for cortisol measurement in population research on adolescent health. *Nursing Research*, *65*(3), k249–k255.

Nyamathi, A., Salem, B. E., Zhang, S., et al. (2015). Nursing case management, peer coaching, and hepatitis A and B vaccine completion among homeless men recently released on parole; Randomized clinical trial. *Nursing Research*, *64*(3), 177–189.

Sousa, V. D., Zauszniewski, J. A., & Musil, C. M. (2004). How to determine whether a convenience sample represents the population. *Applied Nursing Research*, *17*(2), 130–133.

Speziale, S., & Carpenter, D. R. (2011). *Qualitative research in nursing* (4th ed.). Philadelphia, PA: Lippincott.

Sun, C., Dohrn, J., Klopper, H., et al. (2015). Clinical nursing and midwifery research priorities in eastern and southern African countries: Results from a Delphi Survey. *Nursing Research*, *64*(6), 466–475.

Thabault, P. J., Burke, P. J., & Ades, P. A. (2016). Intensive behavioral treatment weight loss program in an adult primary care practice. *Journal of the American Association of Nurse Practitioners*, *28*, 249–257.

Traeger, L., McDonnell, T. M., McCarty, C. E., et al. (2015). Nursing intervention to enhance outpatient chemotherapy symptom management: patient reported outcomes of a randomized controlled trial. *Cancer*, *121*, 3905–3913.

Van Dijk, J. F. M., Vervoort, S. C. J. M., van Wijck, A. J. M., et al. (2016). Postoperative patients perspectives on rating pain: A qualitative study. *International Journal of Nursing Studies*, *53*, 260–269.

Vermeesch, A. L., Ling, J., Voskull, V. R., et al. (2015). Biological and sociocultural differences in perceived barriers to physical activity among firth-to-seventh grade urban girls. *Nursing Research*, *64*(5), 342–350.

Ward, L. S. (2003). Race as a variable in cross-cultural research. *Nursing Outlook*, *51*(3), 120–125.

Wong, E. S., Rosland, A. M., Fihn, S. D., & Nelson, K. M. (2016). Patient-centered medical home implementation in the veterans' health administration and primary care use: differences by patient co-morbidity burden. *Journal of General Internal Medicine*, *31*(12), 1467–1474.

Go to Evolve at **http://evolve.elsevier.com/LoBiondo/** for review questions, critiquing exercises, and additional research articles for practice in reviewing and critiquing.

13

Legal and Ethical Issues

Judith Haber and Geri LoBiondo-Wood

Go to Evolve at **http://evolve.elsevier.com/LoBiondo/** for review questions, critiquing exercises, and additional research articles for practice in reviewing and critiquing.

LEARNING OUTCOMES

After reading this chapter, you should be able to do the following:

- Describe the historical background that led to the development of ethical guidelines for the use of human subjects in research.
- Identify the essential elements of an informed consent form.
- Evaluate the adequacy of an informed consent form.
- Describe the institutional review board's role in the research review process.
- Identify populations of subjects who require special legal and ethical research considerations.
- Describe the nurse's role as patient advocate in research situations.
- Critique the ethical aspects of a research study.

KEY TERMS

anonymity
assent
beneficence
confidentiality
consent
ethics
informed consent
institutional review boards
justice
respect for persons
risk/benefit ratio

The focus of this chapter is the legal and ethical considerations that must be addressed before, during, and after the conduct of research. Informed consent, institutional review boards (IRBs), and research involving vulnerable populations—elderly people, pregnant women, children, and prisoners—are discussed. The nurse's role as patient advocate, whether functioning as researcher, caregiver, or research consumer, is addressed.

ETHICAL AND LEGAL CONSIDERATIONS IN RESEARCH: A HISTORICAL PERSPECTIVE

Ethical and legal considerations with regard to research first received attention after World War II, when the US Secretary of State and Secretary of War learned that the trials for war criminals would focus on justifying the atrocities committed by Nazi physicians as "medical research." The American Medical Association appointed a group to develop a code of ethics for research that would serve as a standard for judging the medical atrocities committed on concentration camp prisoners.

The resultant Nuremberg Code and its definitions of the terms *voluntary, legal capacity, sufficient understanding,* and *enlightened decision* have been the subject of numerous court cases and presidential commissions involved in setting ethical standards in research (Amdur & Bankert, 2011). The code requires informed consent in all cases but makes no provisions for any special treatment of children, the elderly, or the mentally incompetent. In the United States, federal guidelines for the ethical conduct of research were developed in the 1970s. Despite the safeguards provided by the federal guidelines, some of the most atrocious, and hence memorable, examples of unethical research took place in the United States as recently as the 1990s. These examples are highlighted in Table 13.1. They are sad reminders of our

TABLE 13.1 Highlights of Unethical Research Studies Conducted in the United States

Research Study	Year(s)	Focus of Study	Ethical Principle Violated
Hyman vs. Jewish Chronic Disease Hospital case	1965	Doctors injected cancer-ridden aged and senile patients with their own cancer cells to study the rejection response.	Informed consent was not obtained. There was no indication that the study was reviewed and approved by an ethics committee. The two physicians claimed they did not wish to evoke emotional reactions or refusals to participate by informing the subjects of the nature of the study (Hershey & Miller, 1976).
Ivory Coast, Africa, AIDS/AZT case	1994	In a study supported by the US government and conducted in the Ivory Coast, Dominican Republic, and Thailand, some pregnant women infected with HIV were given placebo pills rather than AZT, a drug known to prevent mothers from passing on the virus. Babies were in danger of contracting HIV unnecessarily.	Subjects who consented to participate and randomized to the control group were denied access to a medication regimen with a known benefit. This violates a subjects' right to fair treatment and protection (French, 1997; Wheeler, 1997).
Midgeville, Georgia, case	1969	Investigational drugs were used on mentally disabled children without first obtaining the opinion of a psychiatrist.	There was no review of the study protocol or institutional approval of the program before implementation (Levine, 1986).
Tuskegee, Alabama, Syphilis Study	1932–1973	For 40 years the US Public Health Service conducted a study using two groups of poor black male sharecroppers. One group included those who had untreated syphilis; the other group was judged to be free of the disease. Treatment was withheld from the group having syphilis even after penicillin became available and accepted as effective treatment. Steps were taken to prevent the subjects from obtaining it. Researchers wanted to study the untreated disease.	Many subjects who consented to participate were not informed about the purpose and procedures of the research. Others were unaware that they were subjects. The degree of risk outweighed the potential benefit. Withholding of known effective treatment violates the subjects' right to fair treatment and protection from harm (Levine, 1986).

Continued

TABLE 13.1 Highlights of Unethical Research Studies Conducted in the United States—cont'd

Research Study	Year(s)	Focus of Study	Ethical Principle Violated
San Antonio Contraceptive Study	1969	This study examined side effects of oral contraceptives in 76 impoverished Mexican-American women who were randomly assigned to an experimental group receiving birth control pills or a control group receiving placebos. Subjects were not informed about the placebo and pregnancy risk; 11 subjects became pregnant, 10 of whom were in the placebo control group.	Informed consent principles were violated; full disclosure of potential risk, harm, results, or side effects was not evident in the informed consent document. The potential risk outweighed the benefits of the study. The subjects' right to fair treatment and protection from harm was violated (Levine, 1986).
Willowbrook Hospital Study	1972	Mentally incompetent children ($n = 350$) were not admitted to Willowbrook Hospital, a residential treatment facility, unless parents consented to their children being subjects in a study examining the natural history of infectious hepatitis and the effect of gamma globulin. Children were deliberately infected with the hepatitis virus under various conditions. Some received gamma globulin; others did not.	The principle of voluntary consent was violated. Parents were coerced to consent to their children's participation as research subjects. Subjects or their guardians have a right to self-determination—that is, they should be free of constraint, coercion, or undue influence of any kind.
UCLA Schizophrenia Medication Study	1983	The study examined the effects of withdrawing psychotropic medications of 50 patients being treated for schizophrenia; 23 subjects suffered severe relapses after their medication was stopped. The study's goal was to determine if some schizophrenics might do better without medications that had deleterious side effects.	Although subjects signed an informed consent, they were not informed how severe their relapses might be, or that they could suffer worsening symptoms with each recurrence. Informed consent principles violated; full disclosure of potential risk, harm, results, or side effects was not evident in informed consent form. Potential risks outweighed the study's benefits. The subjects' right to fair treatment and protection from harm was violated (Hilts, 1995).

own tarnished research heritage and illustrate the human consequences of not adhering to ethical research standards.

In 1973 the first set of proposed regulations on the protection of human subjects were published. The most important provision was a regulation mandating that an institutional review board must review and approve all studies. In 1974, the National Commission for the Protection of Human Subjects of Biomedical and Behavioral Research was created. A major charge brought forth by the commission was to identify the basic principles that should underlie the conduct of biomedical and behavioral research involving human subjects and to develop guidelines to ensure that research is conducted in accordance with those principles (Amdur & Bankert, 2011). Three ethical principles were identified as relevant to the conduct of research involving human subjects: the principles of **respect for persons**, **beneficence**, and **justice** (Box 13.1). Included in the report called the Belmont Report, these principles provided the basis for regulations affecting research (National

BOX 13.1 Basic Ethical Principles Relevant to the Conduct of Research

Respect for Persons

People have the right to self-determination and to treatment as autonomous agents. Thus they have the freedom to participate or not participate in research. Persons with diminished autonomy are entitled to protection.

Beneficence

Beneficence is an obligation to do no harm and maximize possible benefits. Persons are treated in an ethical manner, decisions are respected, they are protected from harm, and efforts are made to secure their well-being.

Justice

Human subjects should be treated fairly. An injustice occurs when a benefit to which a person is entitled is denied without good reason or when a burden is imposed unduly.

Commission for the Protection of Human Subjects of Biomedical and Behavioral Research, 1978).

The US Department of Health and Human Services (USDHHS) also developed a set of regulations which have been revised several times (USDHHS, 2009). They include:

- General requirements for informed consent
- Documentation of informed consent
- IRB review of research proposals
- Exempt and expedited review procedures for certain kinds of research
- Criteria for IRB approval of research

Protection of Human Rights

Human rights are the claims and demands that have been justified in the eyes of an individual or by a group of individuals. The term refers to the rights outlined in the American Nurses Association (ANA, 2001) guidelines:

1. Right to self-determination
2. Right to privacy and dignity
3. Right to anonymity and confidentiality
4. Right to fair treatment
5. Right to protection from discomfort and harm

These rights apply to all involved in research, including research team members who may be involved in data collection, practicing nurses involved in the research setting, and subjects participating in the study. As you read a research article, you must realize that any issues highlighted in Table 13.2 should have been addressed and resolved before a research study is approved for implementation.

Procedures for Protecting Basic Human Rights

Informed Consent

Elements of informed consent illustrated by the ethical principles of respect and by its related right to self-determination are outlined in Box 13.2 and Table 13.2. It is critical to note that informed consent is not just giving a potential subject a consent form, but is a *process* that the researcher completes with each subject. Informed consent is documented by a consent form that is given to prospective subjects and contains standard elements.

TABLE 13.2 **Protection of Human Rights**

Definition	Violation of Basic Human Right	Example
Right to Self-Determination		
Based on the principle of respect for persons, people should be treated as autonomous with the freedom to choose without external controls. An autonomous agent is one who is informed about a proposed study and allowed to choose to participate or not; subjects have the right to withdraw from a study without penalty. Subjects with diminished autonomy are entitled to protection. They are more vulnerable because of age, legal or mental incompetence, terminal illness, or confinement to an institution. Justification for use of vulnerable subjects must be provided.	A subject's right to self-determination is violated through use of coercion, covert data collection, and deception. • Coercion occurs when an overt threat of harm or excessive reward is presented to ensure compliance. • Covert data collection occurs when people become subjects and are exposed to research treatments without their knowledge. • Deception occurs when subjects are actually misinformed about the research's purpose. • Potential for violation of the right to self-determination is greater for subjects with diminished autonomy; they have decreased ability to give informed consent and are vulnerable.	Subjects may feel that their care will be adversely affected if they refuse to participate in research. The Jewish Chronic Disease Hospital Study (see Table 13.1) is an example in which patients and their doctors did not know that cancer cells were being injected. In the Milgrim (1963) study, subjects were deceived when asked to administer electric shocks to another person; the person was really an actor who pretended to feel the shocks. Subjects administering the shocks were very stressed by participating in this study, although they were not administering shocks at all. The Willowbrook Study (see Table 13.1) is an example of how coercion was used to obtain parental consent of vulnerable mentally retarded children who would not be admitted to the institution unless the children participated in a study in which they were deliberately injected with the hepatitis virus.
Right to Privacy and Dignity		
Based on the principle of respect, privacy is the freedom of a person to determine the time, extent, and circumstances under which private information is shared or withheld from others.	The Privacy Act (1974) was instituted to protect subjects from such violations. These occur most frequently during data collection when invasive questions are asked that might result in loss of job or dignity, or might create embarrassment and mental distress. It also may occur when subjects are unaware that information is being shared with others.	Subjects may be asked personal questions such as the following: "Were you sexually abused as a child?" "Do you use drugs?" "What are your sexual preferences?" When questions are asked using hidden microphones or hidden tape recorders, the subjects' privacy is invaded because they have no knowledge that the data are being shared with others. Subjects also have a right to control access of others to their records.
Right to Anonymity and Confidentiality		
Based on the principle of respect, **anonymity** exists when a subject's identity cannot be linked, even by the researcher, with their individual responses.	Anonymity is violated when the subjects' responses can be linked with their identity.	Subjects are given a code number instead of using names for identification purposes. Subjects' names are never used when reporting findings.
Confidentiality means that individual identities of subjects will not be linked to the information they provide and will not be publicly divulged.	Confidentiality is breached when a researcher, either by accident or by direct action, allows an unauthorized person to gain access to study data that contains subjects' identity information or responses that create a potentially harmful situation for subjects.	Breaches of confidentiality with regard to sexual preference, income, drug use, prejudice, or personality variables can be harmful to subjects. Data are analyzed as group data so individuals cannot be identified by their responses.

TABLE 13.2 Protection of Human Rights—cont'd

Definition	Violation of Basic Human Right	Example
Right to Fair Treatment		
Based on the principle of justice, people should be treated fairly and receive what they are due or owed. Fair treatment is equitable subject selection and treatment during a study, including selection of subjects for reasons directly related to the problem studied vs. convenience, compromised position, or vulnerability. Also included is fair treatment of subjects during a study, including fair distribution of risks and benefits regardless of age, race, or socioeconomic status.	Injustices with regard to subject selection have occurred as a result of social, cultural, racial, and gender biases in society. Historically, research subjects often have been obtained from groups of people who were regarded as having less "social value," such as the poor, prisoners, slaves, the mentally incompetent, and the dying. Often subjects were treated carelessly, without consideration of physical or psychological harm.	The Tuskegee Syphilis Study (1973), the Jewish Chronic Disease Study (1965), the San Antonio Contraceptive Study (1969), and the Willowbrook Study (1972) (see Table 13.1) all provide examples related to unfair subject selection. Investigators should not be late for data collection appointments, should terminate data collection on time, should not change agreed-on procedures or activities without consent, and should provide agreed-on benefits such as a copy of the study findings or a participation fee.
Right to Protection from Discomfort and Harm		
Based on the principle of beneficence, people must take an active role in promoting good and preventing harm in the world around them, as well as in research studies. Discomfort and harm can be physical, psychological, social, or economic in nature. There are five categories of studies based on levels of harm and discomfort: 1. No anticipated effects 2. Temporary discomfort 3. Unusual level of temporary discomfort 4. Risk of permanent damage 5. Certainty of permanent damage	Subjects' right to be protected is violated when researchers know in advance that harm, death, or disabling injury will occur and thus the benefits do not outweigh the risk.	Temporary physical discomfort involving minimal risk includes fatigue or headache, and emotional discomfort including travel expenses incurred to and from the data collection site. Studies examining sensitive issues, such as rape, incest, or spouse abuse, might cause unusual levels of temporary discomfort by opening up current and/or past traumatic experiences. In these situations, researchers assess distress levels and provide debriefing sessions during which the subject may express feelings and ask questions. The researcher makes referrals for professional intervention. Studies having the potential to cause permanent damage are more likely to be medical rather than nursing in nature. A recent clinical trial of a new drug, a recombinant activated protein C (rAPC) (Zovan) for treatment of sepsis, was halted when interim findings from the Phase III clinical trials revealed a reduced mortality rate for the treatment group vs. the placebo group. Evaluation of the data led to termination of the trial to make available a known beneficial treatment to all patients. In some research, such as the Tuskegee Syphilis Study or the Nazi medical experiments, subjects experienced permanent damage or death.

BOX 13.2 Elements of Informed Consent

1. Title of protocol
2. Invitation to participate
3. Basis for subject selection
4. Overall purpose of study
5. Explanation of procedures
6. Description of risks and discomforts
7. Potential benefits
8. Alternatives to participation
9. Financial obligations
10. Assurance of confidentiality
11. In case of injury compensation
12. HIPAA disclosure
13. Subject withdrawal
14. Offer to answer questions
15. Concluding consent statement
16. Identification of investigators

Informed consent is a legal principle that means that potential subjects understand the implications of participating in research and they knowingly agree to participate (Amdur & Bankert, 2011). Informed consent (USDHHS, 2009; Food and Drug Administration [FDA], 2012a) is defined as follows:

> *The knowing consent of an individual or his/her legally authorized representative, under circumstances that provide the prospective subject or representative sufficient opportunity to consider whether or not to participate without undue inducement or any element of force, fraud, deceit, duress, or other forms of constraint or coercion.*

No investigator may involve a person as a research subject before obtaining the legally effective informed consent of a subject or legally authorized representative. The study must be explained to all potential subjects, including the study's purpose; procedures; risks, discomforts, and benefits; and expected duration of participation (i.e., when the study's procedures will be implemented, how many times, and in what setting). Potential subjects must also be informed about any appropriate alternative procedures or treatments, if any, that might be advantageous to the subject. For example, in the Tuskegee Syphilis Study, the researchers should have disclosed that penicillin was an effective treatment for syphilis. Any compensation for subjects' participation must be delineated when there is more than minimal risk through disclosure about medical treatments and/or compensation that is available if injury occurs.

IPE HIGHLIGHT

It is important for your team to remember that the right to personal privacy may be more difficult to protect when researchers are carrying out qualitative studies because of the small sample size and the subjects' verbatim quotes are often used in the findings/results section of the research article to highlight the findings.

Prospective subjects must have time to decide whether to participate in a study. The researcher must not coerce the subject into participating, nor may researchers collect data on subjects who have explicitly refused to participate in a study. An ethical violation of this principle is illustrated by the halting of eight experiments by the US Food and Drug Administration (FDA) at the University of Pennsylvania's Institute for Human Gene Therapy 4 months after the death of an 18-year-old man, Jesse Gelsinger, who received experimental treatment as part of the institute's research. The institute could not document that all patients had been informed of the risks and benefits of the procedures. Furthermore, some patients who received the therapy should have been considered ineligible because their illnesses were more severe than allowed by the clinical protocols. Mr. Gelsinger had a non-life-threatening genetic disorder that permits toxic amounts of ammonia to build up in the liver. Nevertheless, he volunteered for an experimental treatment in which normal genes were implanted directly into his liver, and he subsequently died of multiple organ failure. The institute failed to report to the FDA that two patients in the same trial as Mr. Gelsinger had suffered severe side effects, including inflammation of the liver as a result of the treatment. This should have triggered a halt to the trial (Brainard & Miller, 2000). Of course, subjects may discontinue participation or withdraw from a study at any time without penalty or loss of benefits.

HELPFUL HINT

Research reports rarely provide readers with detailed information regarding the degree to which the researcher adhered to ethical principles, such as informed consent, because of space limitations in journals that make it impossible to describe all aspects of a study. Failure to mention procedures to safeguard subjects' rights does not necessarily mean that such precautions were not taken.

The language of the consent form must be understandable. The reading level should be no higher than eighth grade for adults, in lay language, and the avoidance of technical terms should be observed (USDHHS, 2009). Subjects should not be asked to waive their rights or release the investigator from liability for negligence. The elements for an informed consent form are listed in Box 13.2.

Investigators obtain **consent** through personal discussion with potential subjects. This process allows the person to obtain immediate answers to questions. However, consent forms, which are written in narrative or outline form, highlight elements that both inform and remind subjects of the nature of the study and their participation (Amdur & Bankert, 2011).

Assurance of anonymity and confidentiality (defined in Table 13.2) is conveyed in writing and describes how confidentiality of the subjects' records will be maintained. The right to privacy is also protected through protection of individually identifiable health information (IIHI). The USDHHS developed the following guidelines to help researchers, health care organizations, health care providers, and academic institutions determine when they can use and disclose IIHI:

- IIHI has to be "de-identified" under the HIPAA Privacy Rule.
- Data are part of a limited data set, and a data use agreement with the researcher is in place.
- A potential subject provides authorization for the researcher to use and disclose protected health information (PHI).
- A waiver or alteration of the authorization requirement is obtained from the IRB.
- The consent form must be signed and dated by the subject. The presence of witnesses is not always necessary but does constitute evidence that the subject actually signed the form. If the subject is a minor or is physically or mentally incapable of signing the consent, the legal guardian or representative must sign. The investigator also signs the form to indicate commitment to the agreement.

A copy of the signed informed consent is given to the subject. The researcher maintains the original for their records. Some research, such as a retrospective chart audit, may not require informed consent—only institutional approval. In some cases, when minimal risk is involved, the investigator may have to provide the subject only with an information sheet and verbal explanation. In other cases, such as a volunteer convenience sample, completion and return of research instruments provide evidence of consent. The IRB will help advise on exceptions to these guidelines, and there are cases in which the IRB might grant waivers or amend its guidelines in other ways. The IRB makes the final determination regarding the most appropriate documentation format. You should note whether and what kind of evidence of informed consent has been provided in a research article.

HELPFUL HINT

Researchers may not obtain written, informed consent when the major means of data collection is through self-administered questionnaires. The researcher usually assumes implied consent in such cases—that is, the return of the completed questionnaire reflects the respondent's voluntary consent to participate.

Institutional Review Boards

IRBs are boards that review studies to assess that ethical standards are met in relation to the protection of the rights of human subjects. The National Research Act (1974) requires that agencies such as universities, hospitals, and other health care organizations (e.g., managed care companies) where the conduct of biomedical or behavioral research involving human subjects is conducted must submit an application with assurances that they have an IRB, sometimes called a human subjects' committee, that reviews the research projects and protects the rights of the human subjects (Food and Drug Administration [FDA], 2012b). At agencies where no federal grants or contracts are awarded, there is usually a review mechanism similar to an IRB process, such as a research advisory committee. The National Research Act requires that the IRBs have at least five members of various research backgrounds to promote complete and adequate study reviews. The members must be qualified by virtue of their expertise and experience and reflect professional, gender, racial, and cultural diversity. Membership must include one member whose concerns are primarily nonscientific (lawyer, clergy, ethicist) and at least one member from outside the agency. IRB members have mandatory training in scientific integrity and prevention of scientific misconduct, as do the principal investigator of a study and their research team members. In an effort to protect research subjects, the HIPAA Privacy Rule has made IRB requirements much more stringent for researchers (Code of Federal Regulations, Part 46, 2009).

The IRB is responsible for protecting subjects from undue risk and loss of personal rights and dignity. The **risk/benefit ratio**, the extent to which a study's benefits are maximized and the risks are minimized such that the subjects are protected from harm, is always a major consideration. For a research proposal to be eligible for consideration by an IRB, it must already have been approved by a departmental review group, such as a nursing research committee that attests to the proposal's scientific merit and congruence with institutional policies, procedures, and mission. The IRB reviews the study's protocol to ensure that it meets the requirements of ethical research that appear in Box 13.3.

IRBs provide guidelines that include steps to be taken to receive IRB approval. For example, guidelines for writing a standard consent form or criteria for qualifying for an expedited rather than a full IRB review may be made available. The IRB has the authority to approve research, require modifications, or disapprove a research study. A researcher must receive IRB approval before beginning to conduct research. IRBs have the authority to

BOX 13.3 Code of Federal Regulations for IRB Approval of Research Studies

To approve research, the IRB must determine that the following has been satisfied:

1. Risks to subjects are minimized.
2. Risks to subjects are reasonable in relation to anticipated benefits.
3. Selection of the subjects is equitable.
4. Informed consent must be and will be sought from each prospective subject or the subject's legally authorized representative.
5. Informed consent form must be properly documented.
6. Where appropriate, the research plan makes adequate provision for monitoring the data collected to ensure subject safety.
7. There are adequate provisions to protect subjects' privacy and the confidentiality of data.
8. Where some or all of the subjects are likely to be vulnerable to coercion or undue influence, additional safeguards are included.

audit, suspend, or terminate approval of research that is not conducted in accordance with IRB requirements or that has been associated with unexpected serious harm to subjects.

IRBs also have mechanisms for reviewing research in an expedited manner when the risk to research subjects is minimal (Code of Federal Regulations, 2009). Keep in mind that although a researcher may determine that a project involves minimal risk, the IRB makes the final determination, and the research may not be undertaken until approved. A full list of research categories eligible for expedited review is available from any IRB office. Examples include the following:

- Prospective collection of specimens by noninvasive procedure (e.g., buccal swab, deciduous teeth, hair/nail clippings)
- Research conducted in established educational settings in which subjects are de-identified
- Research involving materials collected for clinical purposes
- Research on taste, food quality, and consumer acceptance
- Collection of excreta and external secretions, including sweat
- Recording of data on subjects 18 years or older, using noninvasive procedures routinely employed in clinical practice
- Voice recordings
- Study of existing data, documents, records, pathological specimens, or diagnostic data

An expedited review does not automatically exempt the researcher from obtaining informed consent, and most importantly, the department or agency mechanisms retains the final judgment as to whether or not a study may be exempt.

When critiquing research, it is important to be conversant with current regulations to determine whether ethical standards have been met. The Critical Thinking Decision Path illustrates the ethical decision-making process an IRB might use in evaluating the risk/benefit ratio of a research study.

Protecting Basic Human Rights of Vulnerable Groups

Researchers are advised to consult their agency's IRB for the most recent federal and state rules and guidelines when considering research involving vulnerable groups who may have diminished autonomy, such as the elderly, children, pregnant women, the unborn, those

CRITICAL THINKING DECISION PATH

Evaluating the Risk/Benefit Ratio of a Research Study

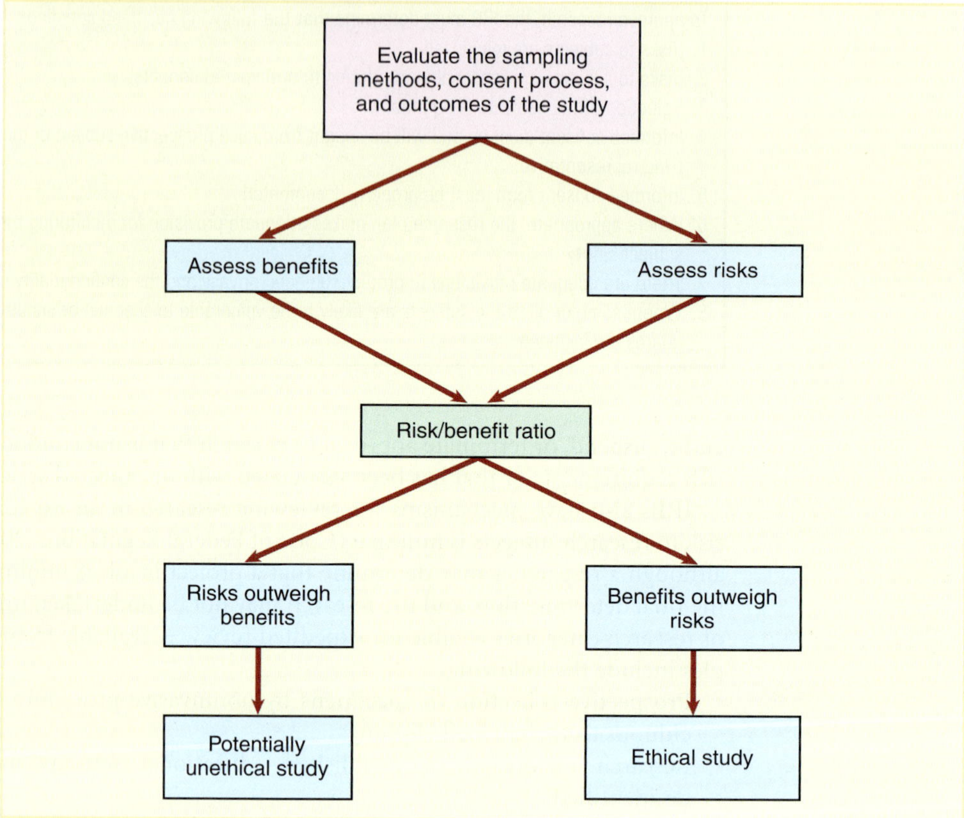

who are emotionally or physically disabled, prisoners, the deceased, students, and persons with AIDS. In addition, researchers should consult the IRB before planning research that potentially involves an oversubscribed research population, such as organ transplantation patients or AIDS patients, or "captive" and convenient populations, such as prisoners. It should be emphasized that use of special populations does not preclude undertaking research; extra precautions must be taken to protect their rights.

Research With Children. The age of majority differs from state to state, but there are some general rules for including children as subjects (Title 45, CFR46 Subpart D, USDHHS, 2009). Usually a child can **assent** between the ages of 7 and 18 years. Research in children requires parental permission and child assent. **Assent** contains the following fundamental elements:

1. A basic understanding of what the child will be expected to do and what will be done to the child
2. A comprehension of the basic purpose of the research
3. An ability to express a preference regarding participation

In contrast to assent, **consent** requires a relatively advanced level of cognitive ability. Informed consent reflects competency standards requiring abstract appreciation and reasoning regarding the information provided. The federal guidelines have specific criteria and standards that must be met for children to participate in research. If the research involves more than minimal risk and does not offer direct benefit to the individual child, both parents must give permission. When individuals reach maturity, usually at age 18 years, they may render their own consent. They may do so at a younger age if they have been legally declared emancipated minors. Questions regarding this are addressed by the IRB and/or research administration office and not left to the discretion of the researcher to answer.

Research With Pregnant Women, Fetuses, and Neonates. Research with pregnant women, fetuses, and neonates requires additional protection but may be conducted if specific criteria are met (HHS Code of Federal Regulations, Title 45, CFR46 Subpart B, 2009). Decisions are made relative to the direct or indirect benefit or lack of benefit to the pregnant woman and the fetus. For example, pregnant women may be involved in research if the research suggests the prospect of direct benefit to the pregnant women and fetus by providing data for assessing risks to pregnant women and fetuses. If the research suggests the prospect of direct benefit to the fetus solely, then both the mother and father must provide consent.

Research With Prisoners. The federal guidelines also provide guidance to IRBs regarding research with prisoners. These guidelines address the issues of allowable research, understandable language, adequate assurances that participation does not affect parole decisions, and risks and benefits (HHS Code of Federal Regulations, Title 45 Part 46, Subpart C, 2009).

Research With the Elderly. Elderly individuals have been historically and are potentially vulnerable to abuse and as such require special consideration. There is no issue if the potential subject can supply legally effective informed consent. Competence is not a clear issue. The complexity of the study may affect one's ability to consent to participate. The capacity to obtain informed consent should be assessed in each individual for each research protocol being considered. For example, an elderly person may be able to consent to participate in a simple observational study but not in a clinical drug trial. The issue of the necessity of requiring the elderly to provide consent often arises, and each situation must be evaluated for its potential to preserve the rights of this population.

No vulnerable population may be singled out for study because it is convenient. For example, neither people with mental illness nor prisoners may be studied because they are an available and convenient group. Prisoners may be studied if the studies pertain to them—that is, studies concerning the effects and processes of incarceration. Similarly, people with mental illness may participate in studies that focus on expanding knowledge about psychiatric disorders and treatments. Students also are often a convenient group. They must not be singled out as research subjects because of convenience; the research questions must have some bearing on their status as students. In all cases, the burden is on the investigator to show the IRB that it is appropriate to involve vulnerable subjects in research.

HELPFUL HINT

Keep in mind that researchers rarely mention explicitly that the study participants were vulnerable subjects or that special precautions were taken to appropriately safeguard the human rights of this vulnerable group. Research consumers need to be attentive to the special needs of groups who may be unable to act as their own advocates or are unable to adequately assess the risk/benefit ratio of a research study.

APPRAISAL FOR EVIDENCE-BASED PRACTICE LEGAL AND ETHICAL ASPECTS OF A RESEARCH STUDY

Research reports do not contain detailed information regarding the ways in which the investigator adhered to the legal and ethical principles presented in this chapter. Lack of written evidence regarding the protection of human rights does not imply that appropriate steps were not taken.

The Critical Appraisal Criteria box provides guidelines for evaluating the legal and ethical aspects of a study. When reading a study, due to space constraints, you will not see all areas explicitly addressed in the article. Box 13.4 provides examples of statements in research articles that illustrate the brevity with which the legal and ethical component of a study is reported.

Information about the legal and ethical considerations of a study is usually presented in the methods section of an article. The subsection on the sample or data-collection methods is the most likely place for this information. The author most often indicates in a sentence that informed consent was obtained and that approval from an IRB was granted. To protect subject and institutional privacy, the locale of the study frequently is described in general terms in the sample subsection of the report. For example, the article might state that data were collected at a 1000-bed tertiary care center in the southwest, without mentioning its name. Protection of subject privacy may be explicitly addressed by statements indicating that anonymity or confidentiality of data was maintained or that grouped data were used in the data analysis.

CRITICAL APPRAISAL CRITERIA

Legal and Ethical Issues

1. Was the study approved by an IRB or other agency committees?
2. Is there evidence that informed consent was obtained from all subjects or their representatives? How was it obtained?
3. Were the subjects protected from physical or emotional harm?
4. Were the subjects or their representatives informed about the purpose and nature of the study?
5. Were the subjects or their representatives informed about any potential risks that might result from participation in the study?
6. Is the research study designed to maximize the benefit(s) to human subjects and minimize the risks?
7. Were subjects coerced or unduly influenced to participate in this study? Did they have the right to refuse to participate or withdraw without penalty? Were vulnerable subjects used?
8. Were appropriate steps taken to safeguard the privacy of subjects? How have data been kept anonymous and/or confidential?

BOX 13.4 Examples of Legal and Ethical Content in Published Research Reports Found in the Appendices

- "The study was approved by the Institutional Review Board (IRB) from the university, the 4 recruitment facilities and the State Department of Health prior to recruitment of study participants" (Hawthorne et al., 2016, p. 76).
- "Following institutional ethics approvals from the University of Windsor in Ontario, Canada and the University of Western Ontario, Canada data were collected from the pediatric oncology patients" (Turner-Sack et al., 2016, p. 50).

When considering the special needs of vulnerable subjects, you should be sensitive to whether the special needs of groups, unable to act on their own behalf, have been addressed. For instance, has the right of self-determination been addressed by the informed consent protocol identified in the research report?

When qualitative studies are reported, verbatim quotes from informants often are incorporated into the findings section of the article. In such cases, you will evaluate how effectively the author protected the informant's identity, either by using a fictitious name or by withholding information such as age, gender, occupation, or other potentially identifying data (see Chapters 5, 6, and 7 for ethical issues related to qualitative research).

It should be apparent from the preceding sections that although the need for guidelines for the use of human subjects in research is evident and the principles themselves are clear, there are many instances when you must use your best judgment both as a patient advocate and as a research consumer when evaluating the ethical nature of a research project. When conflicts arise, you must feel free to raise suitable questions with appropriate resources and personnel. In an institution these may include contacting the researcher first and then, if there is no resolution, the director of nursing research and the chairperson of the IRB. In cases where ethical considerations in a research article are in question, clarification from a colleague, agency, or IRB is indicated. You should pursue your concerns until satisfied that the patient's rights and your rights as a professional nurse are protected.

KEY POINTS

- Ethical and legal considerations in research first received attention after World War II during the Nuremberg Trials, from which developed the Nuremberg Code. This became the standard for research guidelines protecting the human rights of research subjects.
- The Belmont Report discusses three basic ethical principles (respect for persons, beneficence, and justice) that underlie the conduct of research involving human subjects.
- Protection of human rights includes (1) right to self-determination, (2) right to privacy and dignity, (3) right to anonymity and confidentiality, (4) right to fair treatment, and (5) right to protection from discomfort and harm.
- Procedures for protecting human rights include gaining informed consent, which illustrates the ethical principle of respect, and obtaining IRB approval, which illustrates the ethical principles of respect, beneficence, and justice.
- Special consideration should be given to studies involving vulnerable populations, such as children, the elderly, prisoners, and those who are mentally or physically disabled.
- Nurses must be knowledgeable about the legal and ethical components of research so they can evaluate whether a researcher has ensured protection of patient rights.

CRITICAL THINKING CHALLENGES

- A state government official interested in determining the number of infants infected with the human immunodeficiency virus (HIV) has approached your hospital to participate in a state-wide funded study. The protocol will include the testing of all newborns for HIV, but the mothers will not be told that the test is being done, nor will they be told the results. Using the basic ethical principles found in Box 13.2, defend or refute the practice. How will the findings of the proposed study be affected if the protocol is carried out?

- As a research consumer, what kind of information related to the legal and ethical aspects of a research study would you expect to see written about in a published research study? How does that differ from the data the researcher would have to prepare for an IRB submission?
- A randomized clinical trial (RCT) testing the effectiveness of a new Lyme disease vaccine is being conducted as a multisite RCT. There are two vaccine intervention groups, each of which is receiving a different vaccine, and one control group that is receiving a placebo. Using the information in Table 13.2, identify the conditions under which the RCT is halted due to potential legal and ethical issues to subjects.
- IPE Your interprofessional QI team is asked to do a presentation about risk/benefit ratio and how it influences clinical decision making and resource allocation in your clinical organization.

REFERENCES

Amdur, R., & Bankert, E. A. (2011). *Institutional Review Board: Member Handbook.* (3rd ed.). Boston, MA: Jones & Bartlett.

American Nurses Association. (2001). *Code for nurses with interpretive statements.* Kansas City, MO: Author.

Brainard, J., & Miller, D. W. (2000). U.S. regulators suspend medical studies at two universities. *Chronicle of Higher Education*, A30.

Code of Federal Regulations (2009), Part 46, Vol. 1. http://www.accessdata.fda.gov/scripts/cdrh/cfdocs/cfcfr/cfresearch.cfm

French, H. W. (1997, October 9). AIDS research in Africa: Juggling risks and hopes. *New York Times*, A1–A12.

Hawthorne, D., Youngblut, J. M., & Brooten, D. (2016). Parent spirituality, grief, and mental health at 1 and 3 months after their infant's/child's death in an intensive care unit. *Journal of Pediatric Nursing, 31*, 73–80.

Hershey, N., & Miller, R. D. (1976). *Human experimentation and the law.* Germantown, MD: Aspen.

Hilts, P. J. (1995, March 9). Agency faults a UCLA study for suffering of mental patients. *New York Times*, A1–A11.

Levine, R. J. (1986). *Ethics and regulation of clinical research* (2nd ed.). Baltimore, MD-Munich, Germany: Urban & Schwartzenberg.

National Commission for the Protection of Human Subjects of Biomedical and Behavioral Research. (1978). *Belmont report: ethical principles and guidelines for research involving human subjects, DHEW pub no 05.* Washington, DC: US Government Printing Office, 78–0012.

Turner-Sack, A. M., Menna, R., Setchell, S. R., et al. (2016). Psychological functioning, post-treatment growth, and coping in parents and siblings of adolescent cancer survivors, *43*(1), 48–56.

US Department of Health and Human Services (USDHHS). (2009). 45 CFR 46. *Code of Federal Regulations: protection of human subjects.* Washington, DC: Author.

US Food and Drug Administration (FDA). (2012a). *A guide to informed consent, Code of Federal Regulations, Title 21, Part 50.* www.fda.gov/oc/ohrt/irbs/informedconsent.html.

US Food and Drug Administration (FDA). (2012b). *Institutional Review Boards, Code of Federal Regulations, Title 21, Part 56.* www.fda.gov/oc/ohrt/irbs/appendixc.html.

Wheeler, D. L. (1997). Three medical organizations embroiled in controversy over use of placebos in AIDS studies abroad. *Chronicle of Higher Education*, A15–A16.

Go to Evolve at **http://evolve.elsevier.com/LoBiondo/** for review questions, critiquing exercises, and additional research articles for practice in reviewing and critiquing.

14

Data Collection Methods

Susan Sullivan-Bolyai and Carol Bova

Go to Evolve at **http://evolve.elsevier.com/LoBiondo/** for review questions, critiquing exercises, and additional research articles for practice in reviewing and critiquing.

LEARNING OUTCOMES

After reading this chapter, you should be able to do the following:

- Define the types of data collection methods used in research.
- List the advantages and disadvantages of each data collection method.
- Compare how specific data collection methods contribute to the strength of evidence in a study.
- Identify potential sources of bias related to data collection.
- Discuss the importance of intervention fidelity in data collection.
- Critically evaluate the data collection methods used in published research studies.

KEY TERMS

anecdotes
closed-ended questions
concealment
consistency
content analysis
debriefing
demographic data
existing data
field notes
intervention
interview guide
interviews
Likert scales
measurement
measurement error
objective
observation
open-ended questions
operational definition
participant observation
physiological data
questionnaires
random error
reactivity
respondent burden
scale
scientific observation
self-report
systematic
systematic error

Nurses are always collecting information (or data) from patients. We collect data on blood pressure, age, weight, and laboratory values as part of our daily work. Data collected for practice purposes and for research have several key differences. Data collection procedures in research must be **objective**, free from the researchers' personal biases, attitudes, and beliefs, and **systematic**. **Systematic** means that everyone who is involved in the data collection process collects the data from each subject in a uniform, consistent, or standard way. This is called **fidelity.** When reading a study, the data collection methods should be identifiable, transparent, and repeatable. Thus, when reading the research literature to inform your evidence-based practice, there are several issues to consider regarding data collection methods.

It is important that researchers carefully define the *concepts* or *variables* they measure. The process of translating a concept into a measurable variable requires the development of an **operational definition.** An operational definition is how the researcher measures each variable. **Example:** ➤ Turner-Sack and colleagues (2016) (see Appendix D) conceptually defined *coping* for adolescents (cancer survivors) and their siblings as active, emotion-focused avoidant and acceptance coping; for parents, the definition was similar but slightly different, with active, social support, and emotion-focused avoidant and acceptance coping. They operationally defined *coping* as measured by the COPE, a measurement scale that assesses coping in adolescents and adults.

The purpose of this chapter is to familiarize you with the ways that researchers collect data from subjects. The chapter provides you with the tools for evaluating data collection procedures commonly used in research, their strengths and weaknesses, how consistent data collection operations (fidelity) can increase study rigor and decrease bias that affects study internal and external validity (see Chapter 8), and how useful each technique is for providing evidence for nursing practice. This information will help you critique the research literature and decide whether the findings provide evidence that is applicable to your practice setting.

MEASURING VARIABLES OF INTEREST

Largely the success of a study depends on the *fidelity* (consistency and quality) of the data collection methods or measurement used. Determining what **measurement** to use in a study may be the most difficult and time-consuming step in study design. Thus, the process of evaluating and selecting the instruments to measure variables of interest is of critical importance to the potential success of the study.

As you read research articles and the data collection techniques used, look for **consistency** with the study's aim, hypotheses, setting, and population. Data collection may be viewed as a two-step process. First, the researcher chooses the study's data collection method(s). An algorithm that influences a researcher's choice of data collection methods is diagrammed in the Critical Thinking Decision Path. The second step is deciding if the measurement scales are reliable and valid. Reliability and validity of instruments are discussed in Chapter 15 (for quantitative research) and in Chapter 6 (for qualitative research).

DATA COLLECTION METHODS

When reading a study, be aware that investigators decide early in the process whether they need to collect their own data or whether data already exist in the form of records or databases. This decision is based on a thorough literature review and the availability of existing data. If the researcher determines that no data exist, new data can be collected through **observation**, **self-report** (interviewing or questionnaires), or by collecting **physiological data** using standardized instruments or testing procedures (e.g., laboratory tests, x-rays). **Existing data** can be collected by extracting data from medical records or local, state, and national databases. Each of these methods has a specific purpose, as well as pros and cons inherent in its use. It is important to remember that all data collection methods rely on the ability of the researcher to standardize these procedures to increase data accuracy and reduce measurement error.

CRITICAL THINKING DECISION PATH

Consumer of Research Literature Review

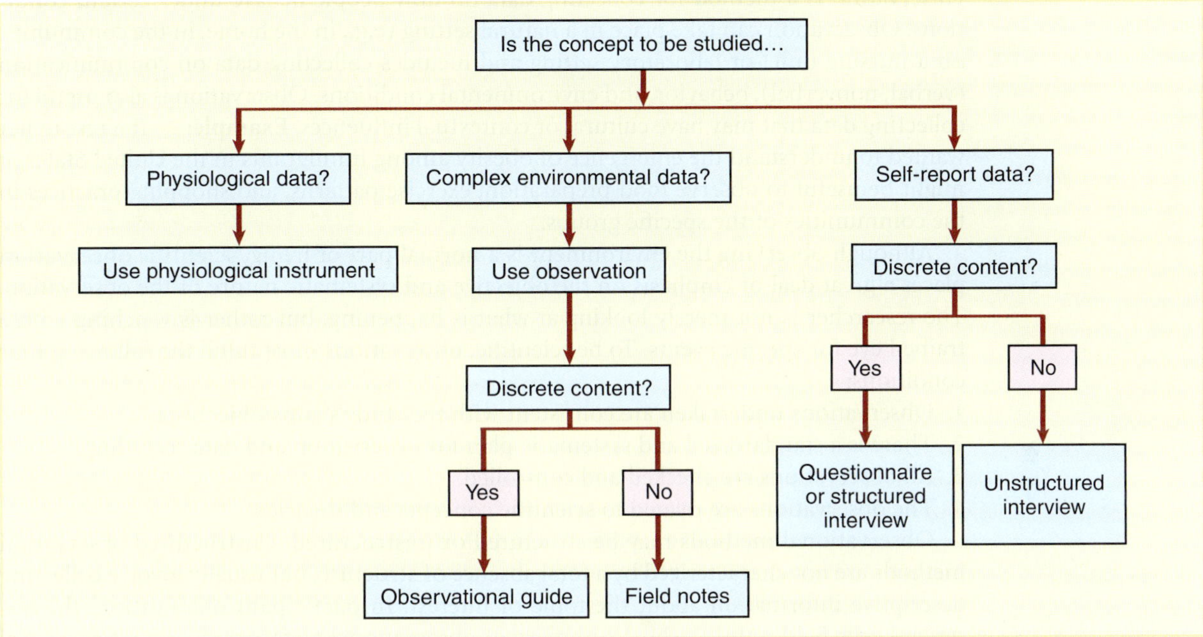

Measurement error is the difference between what really exists and what is measured in a study. Every study has some amount of measurement error. Measurement error can be random or systematic (see Chapter 15). **Random error** occurs when scores vary in a random way. Random error occurs when data collectors do not use standard procedures to collect data consistently among all subjects in a study. **Systematic error** occurs when scores are incorrect but in the same direction. An example of systematic error occurs when all subjects were weighed using a weight scale that is under by 3 pounds for all subjects in the study. Researchers attempt to design data collection methods that will be consistently applied across all subjects and time points to reduce measurement error.

HELPFUL HINT

Remember that the researcher may not always present complete information about the way the data were collected, especially when established instruments were used. To learn about the instrument that was used in greater detail, you may need to consult the original article describing the instrument.

To help decipher the quality of the data collection section in a research article, we will discuss the three main methods used for collecting data: observation, self-report, and physiological measurement.

QSEN EVIDENCE-BASED PRACTICE TIP

It is difficult to place confidence in a study's findings if the data collection methods are not consistent.

Observational Methods

Observation is a method for collecting data on how people behave under certain conditions. Observation can take place in a natural setting (e.g., in the home, in the community, on a nursing unit) or laboratory setting and includes collecting data on communication (verbal, nonverbal), behavior, and environmental conditions. Observation is also useful for collecting data that may have cultural or contextual influences. **Example:** ➤ If a researcher wanted to understand the emergence of obesity among immigrants in the United States, it might be useful to observe food preparation, exercise patterns, and shopping practices in the communities of the specific groups.

Although observing the environment is a normal part of living, **scientific observation** places a great deal of emphasis on the objective and systematic nature of the observation. The researcher is not merely looking at what is happening, but rather is watching with a trained eye for specific events. To be scientific, observations must fulfill the following four conditions:

1. Observations undertaken are consistent with the study's aims/objectives.
2. There is a standardized and systematic plan for observation and data recording.
3. All observations are checked and controlled.
4. The observations are related to scientific concepts and theories.

Observational methods may be structured or unstructured. Unstructured observation methods are not characterized by a total absence of structure, but usually involve collecting descriptive information about the topic of interest. In **participant observation**, the observer keeps **field notes** (a short summary of observations) to record the activities, as well as the observer's interpretations of these activities. *Field notes* usually are not restricted to any particular type of action or behavior; rather, they represent a narrative set of written notes intended to paint a picture of a social situation in a more general sense. Another type of unstructured observation is the use of anecdotes. **Anecdotes** are summaries of a particular observation that usually focus on the behaviors of interest and frequently add to the richness of research reports by illustrating a particular point (see Chapters 5 and 6 for more on qualitative data collection strategies). Structured observations involve specifying in advance what behaviors or events are to be observed. Typically standardized forms are used for record keeping and include categorization systems, checklists, or rating scales. Structured observation relies heavily on the formal training and standardization of the observers (see Chapter 15 for an explanation of interrater reliability).

Observational methods can also be distinguished by the role of the observer. The observer's role is determined by the amount of interaction between the observer and those being observed. These methods are illustrated in Fig. 14.1. **Concealment** refers to whether the subjects know they are being observed. Concealment has ethical implications for the study. Whether concealment is permitted in a study will be decided by an institutional review board. The decision will be based on the potential risk to the subjects, the scientific rationale for the concealment, as well as the plan to debrief the participants about the concealment once the study is completed. **Intervention** deals with whether the observer provokes actions from those who are being observed. Box 14.1 describes the basic types of observational roles implemented by the observer(s). These are distinguishable by the amount of concealment or intervention implemented by the observer.

Observing subjects without their knowledge may violate assumptions of informed consent, and therefore researchers face ethical problems with this approach. However,

		Concealment	
		Yes	No
Intervention	Yes	Researcher hidden An intervention	Researcher open An intervention
	No	Researcher hidden No intervention	Researcher open No intervention

FIG 14.1 Types of observational roles in research.

sometimes there is no other way to collect such data, and the data collected are unlikely to have negative consequences for the subject. In these cases, the disadvantages of the study are outweighed by the advantages. Further, the problem is often handled by informing subjects after the observation, allowing them the opportunity to refuse to have their data included in the study and discussing any questions they might have. This process is called **debriefing**.

When the observer is neither concealed nor intervening, the ethical question is not a problem. Here the observer makes no attempt to change the subjects' behavior and informs them that they are to be observed. Because the observer is present, this type of observation allows a greater depth of material to be studied than if the observer is separated from the subject by an artificial barrier, such as a one-way mirror. **Participant observation** is a commonly used observational technique in which the researcher functions as a part of a social group to study the group in question. The problem with this type of observation is **reactivity** (also referred to as the Hawthorne effect), or the distortion created when the subjects change behavior because they know they are being observed.

BOX 14.1 Basic Types of Observational Roles

1. *Concealment without intervention.* The researcher watches subjects without their knowledge and does not provoke the subject into action. Often such concealed observations use hidden television cameras, audio recording devices, or one-way mirrors. This method is often used in observational studies of children and their parents. You may be familiar with rooms with one-way mirrors in which a researcher can observe the behavior of the occupants of the room without being observed by them. Such studies allow for the observation of children's natural behavior and are often used in developmental research.
2. *Concealment with intervention.* Concealed observation with intervention involves staging a situation and observing the behaviors that are evoked in the subjects as a result of the intervention. Because the subjects are unaware of their participation in a research study, this type of observation has fallen into disfavor and rarely is used in nursing research.
3. *No concealment without intervention.* The researcher obtains informed consent from the subject to be observed and then simply observes his or her behavior.
4. *No concealment with intervention.* No concealment with intervention is used when the researcher is observing the effects of an intervention introduced for scientific purposes. Because the subjects know they are participating in a research study, there are few problems with ethical concerns; however, *reactivity* is a problem in this type of study.

QSEN EVIDENCE-BASED PRACTICE TIP

When reading a research report that uses observation as a data collection method, note evidence of consistency across data collectors through use of interrater reliability (see Chapter 15) data. When this is present, it increases your confidence that the data were collected systematically.

Scientific observation has several advantages, the main one being that observation may be the only way for the researcher to study the variable of interest. **Example:** ➤ What people say they do often may not be what they really do. Therefore, if the study is designed to obtain substantive findings about human behavior, observation may be the only way to ensure the validity of the findings. In addition, no other data collection method can match the depth and variety of information that can be collected when using these techniques. Such techniques also are quite flexible in that they may be used in both experimental and nonexperimental designs. As with all data collection methods, observation also has its disadvantages. Data obtained by observational techniques are vulnerable to observer bias. Emotions, prejudices, and values can influence the way behaviors and events are observed and recorded. In general, the more the observer needs to make inferences and judgments about what is being observed, the more likely it is that distortions will occur. Thus in judging the adequacy of observation methods, it is important to consider how observation forms were constructed and how observers were trained and evaluated.

Ethical issues can also occur if subjects are not fully aware that they are being observed. For the most part, it is best to inform subjects of the study's purpose and the fact that they are being observed. However, in certain circumstances, informing the subjects will change behaviors (Hawthorne effect; see Chapter 8). **Example:** ➤ If a nurse researcher wanted to study hand-washing frequency in a nursing unit, telling the nurses that they were being observed for their rate of hand washing would likely increase the hand-washing rate and thereby make the study results less valid. Therefore, researchers must carefully balance full disclosure of all research procedures with the ability to obtain valid data through observational methods.

IPE HIGHLIGHT

It is important for members of your team to remember to look for evidence of fidelity, that data collectors and those carrying out the intervention were trained on how to collect data and/or implement an intervention consistently. It is also important to determine that there was periodic supervision to make sure that the consistency was maintained.

Self-Report Methods

Self-report methods require subjects to respond directly to either **interviews** or **questionnaires** about their experiences, behaviors, feelings, or attitudes. Self-report methods are commonly used in nursing research and are most useful for collecting data on variables that cannot be directly observed or measured by physiological instruments. Some variables commonly measured by self-report in nursing research studies include quality of life, satisfaction with nursing care, social support, pain, resilience, and functional status.

The following are some considerations when evaluating self-report methods:

- *Social desirability.* There is no way to know for sure if a subject is telling the truth. People are known to respond to questions in a way that makes a favorable impression.

Example: ➤ If a nurse researcher asks patients to describe the positive and negative aspects of nursing care received, the patient may want to please the researcher and respond with all positive responses, thus introducing bias into the data collection process. There is no way to tell whether the respondent is telling the truth or responding in a socially desirable way, so the accuracy of self-report measures is always open for scrutiny.

- *Respondent burden* is another concern for researchers who use self-report (Ulrich et al., 2012). **Respondent burden** occurs when the length of the questionnaire or interview is too long or the questions are too difficult to answer in a reasonable amount of time considering respondents' age, health condition, or mental status. It also occurs when there are multiple data collection points, as in longitudinal studies when the same questionnaires have to be completed multiple times. Respondent burden can result in incomplete or erroneous answers or missing data, jeopardizing the validity of the study findings.

Interviews and Questionnaires

Interviews are a method of data collection where a data collector asks subjects to respond to a set of open-ended or closed-ended questions as described in Box 14.2. Interviews are used in both quantitative and qualitative research, but are best used when the researcher may need to clarify the task for the respondent or is interested in obtaining more personal information from the respondent.

Open-ended questions allow more varied information to be collected and require a qualitative or content analysis method to analyze responses (see Chapter 6). **Content analysis** is a method of analyzing narrative or word responses to questions and either counting similar responses or grouping the responses into themes or categories (also used in qualitative research). Interviews may take place face to face, over the telephone, or online via a web-based format.

Questionnaires are paper-and-pencil instruments designed to gather data from individuals about knowledge, attitudes, beliefs, and feelings. Questionnaires, like interviews, may be open-ended or closed-ended, as presented in Box 14.2. Questionnaires are most useful when there is a finite set of questions. Individual items in a questionnaire must be clearly written so that the intent of the question and the nature of the response options are clear. Questionnaires may be composed of individual items that measure different variables

BOX 14.2 Uses for Open-Ended and Closed-Ended Questions

- **Open-ended questions** are used when the researcher wants the subjects to respond in their own words or when the researcher does not know all of the possible alternative responses. Interviews that use open-ended questions often use a list of questions and probes called an **interview guide**. Responses to the interview guide are often audio-recorded to capture the subject's responses. An example of an open-ended question is used for the interview in Appendix D.
- **Closed-ended questions** are structured, fixed-response items with a fixed number of responses. Closed-ended questions are best used when the question has a finite number of responses and the respondent is to choose the one closest to the correct response. Fixed-response items have the advantage of simplifying the respondent's task but result in omission of important information about the subject. Interviews that use closed-ended questions typically record a subject's responses directly on the questionnaire. An example of a closed-ended item is found in Box 14.3.

or concepts (e.g., age, race, ethnicity, and years of education) or scales. Survey researchers rely almost entirely on questionnaires for data collection.

Questionnaires can be referred to as instruments, measures, scales, or tools. When multiple items are used to measure a single concept, such as quality of life or anxiety, and the scores on those items are combined mathematically to obtain an overall score, the questionnaire or measurement instrument is called a **scale**. The important issue is that each of the items must measure the same concept or variable. An intelligence test is an example of a scale that combines individual item responses to determine an overall quantification of intelligence.

Scales can have subscales or total scale scores. For instance, in the study by Turner-Sack and colleagues (2016) (see Appendix D), the COPE scale has four separate subscales to measure coping for adolescents (cancer survivors) and their siblings, and four for parents with subjects responding to a four-point scale ranging from 1 to 4, with 1 indicating "I usually do not do this" and 4 indicating "I usually do this a lot." The investigators also added a religious coping subscale for adolescents and siblings and parents. Higher scores reflect more use of that particular type of coping strategy. The response options for scales are typically lists of statements on which respondents indicate, for example, whether they "strongly agree," "agree," "disagree," or "strongly disagree." This type of response option is called a **Likert-type scale**.

QSEN EVIDENCE-BASED PRACTICE TIP

Scales used in research should have evidence of adequate reliability and validity so that you feel confident that the findings reflect what the researcher intended to measure (see Chapter 15).

Box 14.3 shows three items from a survey of nursing job satisfaction. The first item is closed-ended and uses a Likert scale response format. The second item is also closed-ended, and it forces respondents to choose from a finite number of possible answers. The third item is open-ended, and respondents use their own words to answer the question, allowing an unlimited number of possible answers. Often researchers use a combination of Likert-type, closed-ended, and open-ended questions when collecting data in nursing research.

Turner-Sack and colleagues (2016; see Appendix D) used all self-report instruments to examine differences among adolescents, siblings, and parents and their psychological functioning, post-traumatic growth, and coping strategies. They also collected **demographic data**. Demographic data includes information that describes important characteristics about the subjects in a study (e.g., age, gender, race, ethnicity, education, marital status). It is important to collect demographic data in order to describe and compare different study samples so you can evaluate how similar the sample is to your patient population.

When reviewing articles with numerous questionnaires, remember (especially if the study deals with vulnerable populations) to assess if the author(s) addressed potential respondent burden such as:

- Reading level (eighth grade)
- Questionnaire font size (14-point font)
- Need to read and assist some subjects
- Time it took to complete the questionnaire (30 minutes)
- Multiple data collection points

BOX 14.3 Examples of Open-Ended and Closed-Ended Questions

Open-Ended Questions

Please list the three most important reasons why you chose to stay in your current job:

1. ____________
2. ____________
3. ____________

Closed-Ended Questions (Likert Scale)

How satisfied are you with your current position?

1	2	3	4	5
Very satisfied	Moderately satisfied	Undecided	Moderately dissatisfied	Very dissatisfied

Closed-Ended Questions

On average, how many patients do you care for in 1 day?

1. 1 to 3
2. 4 to 6
3. 7 to 9
4. 10 to 12
5. 13 to 15
6. 16 to 18
7. 19 to 20
8. More than 20

This information is very important for judging the respondent burden associated with study participation. It is important to examine the benefits and caveats associated with using interviews and questionnaires as self-report methods. Interviews offer some advantages over questionnaires. The response rate is almost always higher with interviews, and there are fewer missing data, which helps reduce bias.

HELPFUL HINT

Remember, sometimes researchers make trade-offs when determining the measures to be used. **Example:** A researcher may want to learn about an individual's attitudes regarding job satisfaction; however, practicalities may preclude using an interview, so a questionnaire may be used instead.

Another advantage of the interview is that vulnerable populations such as children, the blind, and those with low literacy may not be able to fill out a questionnaire. With an interview, the data collector knows who is giving the answers. When questionnaires are mailed, for example, anyone in the household could be the person who supplies the answers. Interviews also allow for some safeguards, such as clarifying misunderstood questions, and observing and recording the level of the respondent's understanding of the questions. In addition, the researcher has flexibility over the order of the questions.

With questionnaires, the respondent can answer questions in any order. Sometimes changing the order of the questions can change the response. Finally, interviews allow for richer and more complex data to be collected. This is particularly so when open-ended responses are sought. Even when closed-ended response items are used, interviewers can probe to understand why a respondent answered in a particular way.

Questionnaires also have certain advantages. They are much less expensive to administer than interviews that require hiring and thoroughly training interviewers. Thus if a researcher has a fixed amount of time and money, a larger and more diverse sample can be obtained with questionnaires. Questionnaires may allow for more confidentiality and anonymity with sensitive issues that participants may be reluctant to discuss in an interview. Finally, the fact that no interviewer is present assures the researcher and the reader that there will be no interviewer bias. *Interviewer bias* occurs when the interviewer unwittingly leads the respondent to answer in a certain way. This problem can be especially pronounced in studies that use open-ended questions. The tone used to ask the question and/or nonverbal interviewer responses such as a subtle nod of the head could lead a respondent to change an answer to correspond with what the researcher wants to hear.

Finally, the use of Internet-based self-report data collection (both interviewing and questionnaire delivery) has gained momentum. The use of an online format is economical and can capture subjects from different geographic areas without the expense of travel or mailings. Open-ended questions are already typed and do not require transcription, and closed-ended questions can often be imported directly into statistical analysis software, and therefore reduce data entry mistakes. The main concerns with Internet-based data collection procedures involve the difficulty of ensuring informed consent (e.g., Is checking a box indicating agreement to participate the same thing as signing an informed consent form?) and the protection of subject anonymity, which is difficult to guarantee with any Internet-based venue. In addition, the requirement that subjects have computer access limits the use of this method in certain age groups and populations. However, the advantages of increased efficiency and accuracy make Internet-based data collection a growing trend among nurse researchers.

Physiological Measurement

Physiological data collection involves the use of specialized equipment to determine the physical and biological status of subjects. Such measures can be *physical*, such as weight or temperature; *chemical*, such as blood glucose level; *microbiological*, as with cultures; or *anatomical*, as in radiological examinations. What separates these data collection procedures from others used in research is that they require special equipment to make the observation.

Physiological or biological measurement is particularly suited to the study of many types of nursing problems. **Example:** ➤ Examining different methods for taking a patient's temperature or blood pressure or monitoring blood glucose levels may yield important information for determining the effectiveness of certain nursing monitoring procedures or interventions. However, it is important that the method be applied consistently to all subjects in the study. **Example:** ➤ Nurses are quite familiar with taking blood pressure measurements. However, for research studies that involve blood pressure measurement, the process must be standardized (Bern et al., 2007; Pickering et al., 2005). The subject must be positioned (sitting or lying down) the same way for a specified period of time, the same blood pressure instrument must be used, and often multiple blood pressure measurements are taken under the same conditions to obtain an average value.

The advantages of using physiological data collection methods include the objectivity, precision, and sensitivity associated with these measures. Unless there is a technical malfunction, two readings of the same instrument taken at the same time by two different nurses are likely to yield the same result. Because such instruments are intended to measure the variable being studied, they offer the advantage of being precise and sensitive enough to pick up subtle variations in the variable of interest. It is also unlikely that a subject in a study can deliberately distort physiological information.

Physiological measurements are not without inherent disadvantages and include the following:

- Some instruments may be quite expensive to obtain and use.
- Physiological instruments often require specialized training to be used accurately.

- The variable of interest may be altered as a result of using the instrument. **Example:** ➤ An individual's blood pressure may increase just because a health care professional enters the room (called *white coat syndrome*).
- Although thought as being nonintrusive, the presence of some types of devices might change the measurement. **Example:** ➤ The presence of a heart rate monitoring device might make some patients anxious and increase their heart rate.
- All types of measuring devices are affected in some way by the environment. A simple thermometer can be affected by the subject drinking something hot or smoking a cigarette immediately before the temperature is taken. Thus it is important to consider whether the researcher controlled such environmental variables in the study.

Existing Data

All of the data collection methods discussed thus far concern the ways that researchers gather new data to study phenomena of interest. Sometimes existing data can be examined in a new way to study a problem. The use of records (e.g., medical records, care plans, hospital records, death certificates) and databases (e.g., US Census, National Cancer Database, Minimum Data Set for Nursing Home Resident Assessment and Care Screening) are frequently used to answer research questions about clinical problems. Typically, this type of research design is referred to as *secondary analysis.*

The use of available data has advantages. First, data are already collected, thus eliminating subject burden and recruitment problems. Second, most databases contain large populations; therefore sample size is rarely a problem and random sampling is possible. Larger samples allow the researcher to use more sophisticated analytic procedures, and random sampling enhances generalizability of findings. Some records and databases collect standardized data in a uniform way and allow the researcher to examine trends over time. Finally, the use of available records has the potential to save significant time and money.

On the other hand, institutions may be reluctant to allow researchers to have access to their records. If the records are kept so that an individual cannot be identified (known as de-identified data), this is usually not a problem. However, the Health Insurance Portability and Accountability Act (HIPAA), a federal law, protects the rights of individuals who may be identified in records (Bova et al., 2012; see Chapter 13). Recent escalation in the computerization of health records has led to discussion about the desirability of access to such records for research. Currently, it is not clear how much computerized health data will be readily available for research purposes.

Another problem that affects the quality of available data is that the researcher has access only to those records that have survived. If the records available are not representative of all of the possible records, the researcher may have to make an intelligent guess as to their accuracy. **Example:** ➤ A researcher might be interested in studying socioeconomic factors associated with the suicide rate. Frequently, these data are underreported because of the stigma attached to suicide, so the records would be biased.

QSEN EVIDENCE-BASED PRACTICE TIP

Critical appraisal of any data collection method includes evaluating the appropriateness, objectivity, and consistency of the method employed.

CONSTRUCTION OF NEW INSTRUMENTS

Sometimes researchers cannot locate an instrument with acceptable reliability and validity to measure the variable of interest (see Chapter 15). In this situation, a new instrument or scale must be developed.

Instrument development is complex and time consuming. It consists of the following steps:

- Define the concept to be measured.
- Clarify the target population.
- Develop the items.
- Assess the items for content validity.
- Develop instructions for respondents and users.
- Pretest and pilot test the items.
- Estimate reliability and validity.

Defining the concept to be measured requires that the researcher develop expertise in the concept, which includes an extensive review of the literature and of all existing measurements that deal with related concepts. The researcher will use all of this information to synthesize the available knowledge so that the construct can be defined.

Once defined, the individual items measuring the concept can be developed. The researcher will develop many more items than are needed to address each aspect of the concept. The items are evaluated by a panel of experts in the field to determine if the items measure what they are intended to measure (content validity) (see Chapter 15). Items will be eliminated if they are not specific to the concept. In this phase, the researcher needs to ensure consistency among the items, as well as consistency in testing and scoring procedures.

Finally, the researcher pilot tests the new instrument to determine the quality of the instrument as a whole (reliability and validity), as well as the ability of each item to discriminate among individual respondents (variance in item response). Pilot testing can also yield important evidence about the reading level (too low or too high), length of the instrument (too short or too long), directions (clear or not clear), response rate (the percent of potential subjects who return a completed scale), and the appropriateness of culture or context. The researcher also may administer a related instrument to see if the new instrument is sufficiently different from the older one (construct validity). Instrument development and testing is an important part of nursing science because our ability to evaluate evidence related to practice depends on measuring nursing phenomena in a clear, consistent, and reliable way.

APPRAISAL FOR EVIDENCE-BASED PRACTICE DATA COLLECTION METHODS

Assessing the adequacy of data collection methods is an important part of evaluating the results of studies that provide evidence for clinical practice. The data collection procedures provide a snapshot of the rigor with which the study was conducted. From an evidence-based practice perspective, you can judge if the data collection procedures would fit within your clinical environment and with your patient population. The manner in which the data were collected affects the study's internal and external validity. A well-developed methods section of a study decreases bias in the findings. A key element for evidence-based practice is if the procedures were consistently completed. Also consider the following:

- If observation was used, was an observation guide developed, and were the observers trained and supervised until there was a high level of interrater reliability? How was the training confirmed periodically throughout the study to maintain fidelity and decrease bias?
- Was a data collection procedure manual developed and used during the study?
- If the study tested an intervention, were there interventionist and data collector training?
- If a physiological instrument was used, was the instrument properly calibrated throughout the study and the data collected in the same manner from each subject?
- If there were missing data, how were the data accounted for?

Some of these details may be difficult to discern in a research article, due to space limitations imposed by the journal. Typically, the interview guide, questionnaires, or scales are not available for review. However, research articles should indicate the following:

- Type(s) of data collection method used (self-report, observation, physiological, or existing data)
- Evidence of training and supervision for the data collectors and interventionists
- Consistency with which data collection procedures were applied across subjects
- Any threats to internal validity or bias related to issues of instrumentation or testing
- Any sources of bias related to external validity issues, such as the Hawthorne effect
- Scale reliability and validity discussed
- Interrater reliability across data collectors and time points (if observation was used)

When you review the data collection methods section of a study, it is important to think about the data strength and quality of the evidence. You should have confidence in the following:

- An appropriate data collection method was used
- Data collectors were appropriately trained and supervised
- Data were collected consistently by all data collectors
- Respondent burden, reactivity, and social desirability was avoided

You can critically appraise a study in terms of data collection bias being minimized, thereby strengthening potential applicability of the evidence provided by the findings. Because a research article does not always provide all of the details, it is not uncommon to contact the researcher to obtain added information that may assist you in using results in practice. Some helpful questions to ask are listed in the Critical Appraisal Criteria box.

CRITICAL APPRAISAL CRITERIA

Data Collection Methods

1. Are all of the data collection instruments clearly identified and described?
2. Are operational definitions provided and clear?
3. Is the rationale for their selection given?
4. Is the method used appropriate to the problem being studied?
5. Were the methods used appropriate to the clinical situation?
6. Was a standardized manual used to guide data collection?
7. Were all data collectors adequately trained and supervised?
8. Are the data collection procedures the same for all subjects?

Observational Methods

1. Who did the observing?
2. Were the observers trained to minimize bias?
3. Was there an observation guide?

Continued

4. Were the observers required to make inferences about what they saw?
5. Is there any reason to believe that the presence of the observers affected the subject's behavior?
6. Were the observations performed using the principles of informed consent?
7. Was interrater agreement between observers established?

Self-Report: Interviews

1. Is the interview schedule described adequately enough to know whether it covers the topic?
2. Is there clear indication that the subjects understood the task and the questions?
3. Who were the interviewers, and how were they trained?
4. Is there evidence of interviewer bias?

Self-Report: Questionnaires

1. Is the questionnaire described well enough to know whether it covers the topic?
2. Is there evidence that subjects were able to answer the questions?
3. Are the majority of the items appropriately closed-ended or open-ended?

Physiological Measurement

1. Is the instrument used appropriate to the research question or hypothesis?
2. Is a rationale given for why a particular instrument was selected?
3. Is there a provision for evaluating the accuracy of the instrument?

Existing Data: Records and Databases

1. Are the existing data used appropriately, considering the research question and hypothesis being studied?
2. Are the data examined in such a way as to provide new information?
3. Is there any indication of selection bias in the available records?

KEY POINTS

- Data collection methods are described as being both objective and systematic. The data collection methods of a study provide the operational definitions of the relevant variables.
- Types of data collection methods include observational, self-report, physiological, and existing data. Each method has advantages and disadvantages.
- Physiological measurement involves the use of technical instruments to collect data about patients' physical, chemical, microbiological, or anatomical status. They are suited to studying patient clinical outcomes and how to improve the effectiveness of nursing care. Physiological measurements are objective, precise, and sensitive. Expertise, training, and consistent application of these tests or procedures are needed to reduce the measurement error associated with this data collection method.
- Observational methods are used in nursing research when the variables of interest deal with events or behaviors. Scientific observation requires preplanning, systematic recording, controlling the observations, and providing a relationship to scientific theory. This method is best suited to research problems that are difficult to view as a part of a whole. The advantages of observational methods are that they provide flexibility to measure many types of situations and they allow for depth and breadth of information to be collected. Disadvantages include that data may be distorted as a result of the observer's presence and observations may be biased by the person who is doing the observing.
- Interviews are commonly used data collection methods in nursing research. Either open-ended or closed-ended questions may be used when asking the subject questions.

The form of the question should be clear to the respondent, free of suggestion, and grammatically correct.

- Questionnaires, or paper-and-pencil tests, are useful when there are a finite number of questions to be asked. Questions need to be clear and specific. Questionnaires are less costly in terms of time and money to administer to large groups of subjects, particularly if the subjects are geographically widespread. Questionnaires also can be completely anonymous and prevent interviewer bias.
- Existing data in the form of records or large databases are an important source for research data. The use of available data may save the researcher considerable time and money when conducting a study. This method reduces problems with subject recruitment, access, and ethical concerns. However, records and available data are subject to problems of authenticity and accuracy.

CRITICAL THINKING CHALLENGES

- When a researcher opts to use observation as the data collection method, what steps must be taken to minimize bias?
- In a randomized clinical trial investigating the differential effect of an educational video intervention in comparison to a telephone counseling intervention, data were collected at four different hospitals by four different data collectors. What steps should the researcher take to ensure intervention fidelity?
- What are the strengths and weaknesses of collecting data using existing sources such as records, charts, and databases?
- IPE Your interprofessional Journal Club just finished reading the research article by Nyamathi and colleagues in Appendix A. As part of your critical appraisal of this study, your team needed to identify the strengths and weaknesses of the data collection section. Discuss the sources of bias in the data collection procedures and evidence of fidelity.
- How does a training manual decrease the possibility of introducing bias into the data collection process, thereby increasing intervention fidelity?

REFERENCES

Bern, L., Brandt, M., Mbelu, N., et al. (2007). Differences in blood pressure values obtained with automated and manual methods in medical inpatients. *MEDSURG Nursing*, *16*, 356–361.

Bova, C., Drexler, D., & Sullivan-Bolyai, S. (2012). Reframing the influence of HIPAA on research. *Chest*, *141*, 782–786.

Pickering, T., Hall, J., Appel, L., et al. (2005). Recommendations for blood pressure measurement in humans and experimental animals: part 1: blood pressure measurement in humans: a statement for professionals from the Subcommittee of Professional and Public Education of the American Heart Association Council on High Blood Pressure Research. *Hypertension*, *45*, 142–161.

Turner-Sack, A., Menna, R., Setchell, S., et al. (2016). Psychological functioning, post-traumatic growth, and coping in parents and siblings of adolescent cancer survivors. *Oncology Nursing Forum*, *43*, 48–56. doi:10.1188/16.ONF.48-56.

Ulrich, C. M., Knafl, K. A., Ratcliffe, S. J., et al. (2012). Developing a model of the benefits and burdens of research participation in cancer clinical trials. *American Journal of Bioethics Primary Research*, *3*(2), 10–23.

Go to Evolve at **http://evolve.elsevier.com/LoBiondo/** for review questions, critiquing exercises, and additional research articles for practice in reviewing and critiquing.

15

Reliability and Validity

Geri LoBiondo-Wood and Judith Haber

Go to Evolve at **http://evolve.elsevier.com/LoBiondo/** for review questions, critiquing exercises, and additional research articles for practice in reviewing and critiquing.

LEARNING OUTCOMES

After reading this chapter, you should be able to do the following:

- Discuss how measurement error can affect the outcomes of a study.
- Discuss the purposes of reliability and validity.
- Define *reliability.*
- Discuss the concepts of stability, equivalence, and homogeneity as they relate to reliability.
- Compare and contrast the estimates of reliability.
- Define *validity.*
- Compare and contrast content, criterion-related, and construct validity.
- Identify the criteria for critiquing the reliability and validity of measurement tools.
- Use the critical appraisal criteria to evaluate the reliability and validity of measurement tools.
- Discuss how reliability and validity contribute to the strength and quality of evidence provided by the findings of a research study.

KEY TERMS

chance (random) errors
concurrent validity
construct
construct validity
content validity
content validity index
contrasted-groups (known-groups) approach
convergent validity
criterion-related validity
Cronbach's alpha
divergent/discriminant validity
equivalence
error variance
face validity
factor analysis
homogeneity
hypothesis-testing approach
internal consistency
interrater reliability
item to total correlations
kappa
Kuder-Richardson (KR-20) coefficient
Likert scale
observed test score
parallel or alternate form reliability
predictive validity
reliability
reliability coefficient
split-half reliability
stability
systematic (constant) error
test-retest reliability
validity

The measurement of phenomena is a major concern of nursing researchers. Unless measurement instruments validly (accurately) and reliably (consistently) reflect the concepts of the theory being tested, conclusions drawn from a study will be invalid or biased. Issues of reliability and validity are of central concern to researchers, as well as to appraisers of research. From either perspective, the instruments that are used in a study must be evaluated. Researchers often face the challenge of developing new instruments and, as part of that process, establishing the reliability and validity of those instruments.

When reading studies, you must assess the reliability and validity of the instruments to determine the soundness of these selections in relation to the concepts (concepts are often called **constructs** in instrument development studies) or variables under study. The appropriateness of instruments and the extent to which reliability and validity are demonstrated have a profound influence on the strength of the findings and the extent to which bias is present. Invalid measures produce invalid estimates of the relationships between variables, thus introducing bias, which affects the study's internal and external validity. As such, the assessment of reliability and validity is an extremely important critical appraisal skill for assessing the strength and quality of evidence provided by the design and findings of a study and its applicability to practice.

This chapter examines the types of reliability and validity and demonstrates the applicability of these concepts to the evaluation of instruments in research and evidence-based practice.

RELIABILITY, VALIDITY, AND MEASUREMENT ERROR

Reliability is the ability of an instrument to measure the attributes of a variable or construct *consistently.* **Validity** is the extent to which an instrument measures the attributes of a concept *accurately*. To understand reliability and validity, you need to understand potential errors related to instruments. Researchers may be concerned about whether the scores that were obtained for a sample of subjects were consistent, true measures of the behaviors and thus an accurate reflection of the differences among individuals. The extent of variability in test scores that is attributable to error rather than a true measure of the behaviors is the **error variance.** Error in measurement can occur in multiple ways.

An **observed test score** that is derived from a set of items actually consists of the true score plus error (Fig. 15.1). The error may be either chance or random error, or it may be

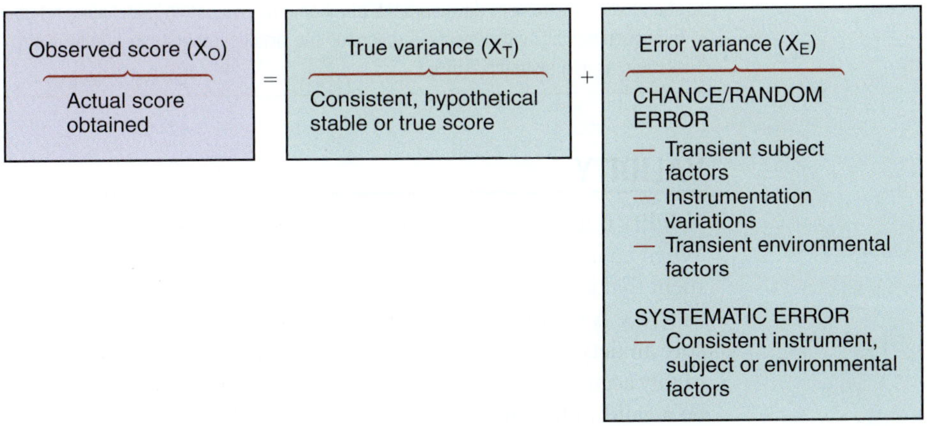

FIG 15.1 Components of observed scores.

systematic or constant error. Validity is concerned with systematic error, whereas reliability is concerned with random error. **Chance** or **random errors** are errors that are difficult to control (e.g., a respondent's anxiety level at the time of testing). Random errors are unsystematic in nature; they are a result of a transient state in the subject, the context of the study, or the administration of an instrument. **Example:** ➤ Perceptions or behaviors that occur at a specific point in time (e.g., anxiety) are known as state or transient characteristics and are often beyond the awareness and control of the examiner. Another example of random error is in a study that measures blood pressure. Random error resulting in different blood pressure readings could occur by misplacement of the cuff, not waiting for a specific time period before taking the blood pressure, or placing the arm randomly in relationship to the heart while measuring blood pressure.

Systematic or **constant error** is measurement error that is attributable to relatively stable characteristics of the study sample that may bias their behavior and/or cause incorrect instrument calibration. Such error has a systematic biasing influence on the subjects' responses and thereby influences the validity of the instruments. For instance, level of education, socioeconomic status, social desirability, response set, or other characteristics may influence the validity of the instrument by altering measurement of the "true" responses in a systematic way. **Example:** ➤ A subject is completing a survey examining attitudes about caring for elderly patients. If the subject wants to please the investigator, items may constantly be answered in a socially desirable way rather than reflecting how the individual actually feels, thus making the estimate of validity inaccurate. Systematic error occurs also when an instrument is improperly calibrated. Consider a scale that consistently gives a person's weight at 2 pounds less than the actual body weight. The scale could be quite reliable (i.e., capable of reproducing the precise measurement), but the result is consistently invalid.

The concept of error is important when appraising instruments in a study. The information regarding the instruments' reliability and validity is found in the instrument or measures section of a study, which can be separately titled or appear as a subsection of the methods section of a research report, unless the study is a psychometric or instrument development study (see Chapter 10).

HELPFUL HINT

Research articles vary considerably in the amount of detail included about reliability and validity. When the focus of a study is instrument development, psychometric evaluation—including reliability and validity data—is carefully documented and appears throughout the article rather than briefly in the "Instruments" or "Measures" section, as in a research article.

VALIDITY

Validity is the extent to which an instrument measures the attributes of a concept accurately. When an instrument is valid, it reflects the concept it is supposed to measure. A valid instrument that is supposed to measure anxiety does so; it does not measure another concept, such as stress. A measure can be reliable but not valid. Let's say that a researcher wanted to measure anxiety in patients by measuring their body temperatures. The researcher could obtain highly accurate, consistent, and precise temperature recordings, but such a measure may not be a valid indicator of anxiety. Thus the high reliability of an instrument is not necessarily congruent with evidence of validity. A valid instrument, however, is reliable. An instrument cannot validly measure a variable if it is erratic, inconsistent, or inaccurate. There are three types of validity that vary according to the kind of information provided and the purpose of the instrument (i.e., *content, criterion-related,* and *construct validity*). As you appraise research articles, you will want to evaluate whether sufficient evidence of validity is present and whether the type of validity is appropriate to the study's design and the instruments used in the study.

As you read the instruments or measures sections of studies, you will notice that validity data are reported much less frequently than reliability data. DeVon and colleagues (2007) note that adequate validity is frequently claimed, but rarely is the method specified. This lack of reporting, largely due to publication space constraints, shows the importance of critiquing the quality of the instruments and the conclusions (see Chapters 14 and 17).

QSEN EVIDENCE-BASED PRACTICE TIP

Selecting instruments that have strong evidence of validity increases your confidence in the study findings—that the researchers actually measured what they intended to measure.

Content Validity

Content validity represents the universe of content or the domain of a given variable/construct. The universe of content provides the basis for developing the items that will adequately represent the content. When an investigator is developing an instrument and issues of content validity arise, the concern is whether the measurement instrument and the items it contains are representative of the content domain that the researcher intends to measure. The researcher begins by defining the concept and identifying the attributes or dimensions of the concept. The items that reflect the concept and its domain are developed.

The formulated items are submitted to content experts who judge the items. **Example:** ➤ Researchers typically request that the experts indicate their agreement with the scope of the items and the extent to which the items reflect the concept under consideration. Box 15.1 provides an example of content validity.

BOX 15.1 Published Examples of Content Validity and Content Validity Index

Content Validity

An expert panel of key stakeholders assisted with validation of the items on the adherence subscale on the modified version of the Fidelity Checklist. To determine adherence items, the expert panel of key stakeholders identified items that were deemed mandatory for clinicians to cover during the intervention. The mandatory items were used to develop the adherence subscale. Through in-person discussion, key stakeholders arrived at a 100% agreement on the relevance of each item of the adherence subscale, ensuring the content validity of both the intervention and the adherence subscale (Clark et al., 2016).

Content Validity Index

For the Chinese Illness Perception Questionnaire Revised Trauma (the Chinese IPQ-Revised-Trauma), the Item-level Content Validity Index (I-CVI) was calculated by a panel of five trauma content experts. An average of 88% for all subscale items was scored by the experts, indicating that the validity of the score was reguaranteed. A few words were fixed after expert checking. The ratings were on a four-point scale with a response format of 1 = *not relevant* to 4 = *highly relevant.* The I-CVI for each item was computed based on the percentage of experts giving a rating of 3 or 4, indicating item relevance (Lee et al., 2016).

Another method used to establish content validity is the **content validity index** (CVI). The CVI moves beyond the level of agreement of a panel of expert judges and calculates an index of interrater agreement or relevance. This calculation gives a researcher more confidence or evidence that the instrument truly reflects the concept or construct. When reading the instrument section of a research article, note that the authors will comment if a CVI was used to assess content validity. When reading a psychometric study that reports the development of an instrument, you will find great detail and a much longer section indicating how exactly the researchers calculated the CVI and the acceptable item cutoffs. In the scientific literature there has been discussion of accepting a CVI of 0.78 to 1.0, depending on the number of experts (DeVon et al., 2007; Lynn, 1986). An example from a study that used CVI is presented in Box 15.1. A subtype of content validity is **face validity**, which is a rudimentary type of validity that basically verifies that the instrument gives the appearance of measuring the concept. It is an intuitive type of validity in which colleagues or subjects are asked to read the instrument and evaluate the content in terms of whether it appears to reflect the concept the researcher intends to measure.

QSEN EVIDENCE-BASED PRACTICE TIP

If face and/or content validity, the most basic types of validity, was (or were) the only type(s) of validity reported in a research article, you would not appraise the measurement instrument(s) as having strong psychometric properties, which would negatively influence your confidence about the study findings.

Criterion-Related Validity

Criterion-related validity indicates to what degree the subject's performance on the instrument and the subject's actual behavior are related. The criterion is usually the second measure, which assesses the same concept under study. Two forms of **criterion-related validity** are **concurrent and predictive.**

Concurrent validity refers to the degree of correlation of one test with the scores of another more established instrument of the same concept when both are administered at the same time. A high correlation coefficient indicates agreement between the two measures and evidence of concurrent validity.

Predictive validity refers to the degree of correlation between the measure of the concept and some future measure of the same concept. Because of the passage of time, the correlation coefficients are likely to be lower for predictive validity studies. Examples of concurrent and predictive validity as they appear in research articles are illustrated in Box 15.2.

Construct Validity

Construct validity is based on the extent to which a test measures a theoretical construct, attribute, or trait. It attempts to validate the theory underlying the measurement by testing of the hypothesized relationships. Testing confirms or fails to confirm the relationships that are predicted between and/or among concepts and, as such, provides more or less support for the construct validity of the instruments measuring those concepts. The establishment of construct validity is complex, often involving several studies and approaches. The hypothesis-testing, factor analytical, convergent and divergent, and contrasted-groups approaches are discussed in the following sections. Box 15.3 provides examples of different types of construct validity as it is reported in published research articles.

BOX 15.2 Published Examples of Reported Criterion-Related Validity

Concurrent Validity

The Patient-Reported Outcomes Measurement Information System Fatigue-Short Form (PROMIS-SF) consists of seven items that measure both the experience of fatigue and the interference of fatigue on daily activities over the past week (NIH, 2007). Concurrent validity of the PROMIS-SF was established through correlations between the PROMIS-SF and the Multidimensional Fatigue Symptom Inventory-Short Form (MFSI-SF), as well as the Brief Fatigue Inventory (BFI). Correlations between the PROMIS-SF and the MFSI-SF ranged from $r = 0.70$ to 0.85, and correlations between the PROMIS-F-SF and the BFI ranged from $r = 0.60$ to 0.71. Correlations between measures of like constructs are expected to be strong. As all three were measures of fatigue, strong correlations were expected and provided evidence of concurrent validity (Ameringer et al., 2016).

Predictive Validity

In a study modifying the Champion Health Belief Model Scale (Champion, 1993) to fit with prostate cancer screening (PCS), translate it into Arabic, and test the psychometric properties of the Champion Health Belief Model Scale for Prostate Cancer Screening (CHBMS-PCS), the predictive validity of the Arabic version was established by using regression analysis (Chapter 16) to predict the combined predictive effect of all seven subscales of the CHBMS-PCS on the performance of the PCS. All of the subscales were found to be significantly correlated and predictive for the performance of the PCS at the $p < .05$ level or less (Abudas et al., 2016).

BOX 15.3 Published Examples of Reported Construct Validity

Contrasted Groups (Known Groups)

In the study to examine the psychometric properties of the Patient-Reported Outcomes Measurement Information System Fatigue Short-Form across diverse populations, known group validity was established by correlating the four study samples' levels of fatigue (e.g., fibromyalgia, sickle cell disease, cardio metabolic risk, pregnancy) with healthy controls. The study samples had significantly higher levels of fatigue than the healthy controls (Ameringer et al., 2016).

Convergent Validity

"**Convergent construct validity** of the Spiritual Coping Strategies Scale (SCS) subscales is supported by correlations of 0.40 with the well-established Spiritual Well Being instrument (Baldacchino & Bulhagiar, 2003). In this study, parents' subscales internal consistencies at T1 and T2 were $r = 0.87$ to 0.90 for religious activities and $r = 0.80$ to 0.82 for spiritual activities" (Hawthorne et al., 2016; Appendix B).

Divergent (Discriminant) Validity

Pearson correlations between the Patient-Reported Outcomes Measurement Information System Fatigue Short-Form (PROMIS-F-SF), and the Perceived Stress Scale (PSS) and depressive symptoms (CES-D) were calculated to assess the discriminant validity. Since correlations between measures of constructs that are related but not alike are expected to be weak to moderate, correlations between the PROMIS-F-SF and CES-D ranged from $r = 0.45$ to 0.64 and the PROMIS-F-SF and the PSS ranged from $r = 0.37$ to 0.62 supported the discriminant validity of the PROMIS-F-SF (Ameringer et al., 2016).

Factor Analysis

In a study assessing nurses' perceived leadership abilities during episodes of clinical deterioration, Hart and colleagues (2016) did psychometric testing of the Clinical Deterioration Leadership Ability Scale (CDLAS). Construct validity was supported by a Principal Components Analysis with varimax rotation. The factor analysis determined a 1-factor structure with factor loadings that ranged from 0.655 to 0.792; exceeding the factor loading cutoff of 0.40, this factor was named leadership abilities.

Hypothesis Testing

In a study assessing nurses' perceived leadership abilities during episodes of clinical deterioration, it was hypothesized that nurses with 11 or more years of practice experience would score significantly higher on the Clinical Deterioration Leadership Ability Scale (CDLAS) than nurses with 10 years or less of practice experience. A statistically significant difference in CDLAS mean *t-test* scores ($p = 0.047$) supported this hypothesis, thereby providing evidence of construct validity (Hart et al., 2016).

Hypothesis-Testing Approach

When the **hypothesis-testing approach** is used, the investigator uses the theory or concept underlying the measurement instruments to validate the instrument. The investigator does this by developing hypotheses regarding the behavior of individuals with varying scores on the measurement instrument, collecting data to test the hypotheses, and making inferences on the basis of the findings concerning whether the rationale underlying the instrument's construction is adequate to explain the findings and thereby provide support for evidence of construct validity (see Box 15.2).

Convergent and Divergent Approaches

Strategies for assessing construct validity include convergent and divergent approaches. **Convergent validity**, sometimes called **concurrent validity**, refers to a search for other measures of the construct. Sometimes two or more instruments that theoretically measure the same construct are identified, and both are administered to the same subjects. A correlational analysis (i.e., test of relationship; see Chapter 16) is performed. If the measures are positively correlated, convergent validity is said to be supported.

Divergent validity, sometimes called **discriminant validity**, uses measurement approaches that differentiate one construct from others that may be similar. Sometimes researchers search for instruments that measure the opposite of the construct. If the divergent measure is negatively related to other measures, validity for the measure is strengthened.

HELPFUL HINT

When validity data about the measurements used in a study are not included in a research article, you have no way of determining whether the intended concept is actually being captured by the measurement. Before you use the results in such a case, it is important to go back to the original primary source to check the instrument's validity.

Contrasted-Groups Approach

When the **contrasted-groups approach** (sometimes called the **known-groups approach**) is used to test construct validity, the researcher identifies two groups of individuals who are suspected to score extremely high or low in the characteristic being measured by the instrument. The instrument is administered to both the high-scoring and the low-scoring group, and the differences in scores are examined. If the instrument is sensitive to individual differences in the trait being measured, the mean performance of these two groups should differ significantly and evidence of construct validity would be supported. A *t* test or analysis of variance could be used to statistically test the difference between the two groups (see Box 15.2 and Chapter 16).

QSEN EVIDENCE-BASED PRACTICE TIP

When the instruments used in a study are presented, note whether the sample(s) used to develop the measurement instrument(s) is (are) similar to your patient population.

Factor Analytical Approach

A final approach to assessing construct validity is **factor analysis**. This is a procedure that gives the researcher information about the extent to which a set of items measures the same underlying concept (variable) of a construct. Factor analysis assesses the degree to which the individual items on a scale truly cluster around one or more concepts. Items designed to measure the same concept should load on the same factor; those designed to measure different concepts should load on different factors (Anastasi & Urbina, 1997; Furr & Bacharach, 2008; Nunnally & Bernstein, 1993). This analysis, as illustrated in the example in Box 15.2, will also indicate whether the items in the instrument reflect a single construct or several constructs.

The Critical Thinking Decision Path will help you assess the appropriateness of the type of validity and reliability selected for use in a particular study.

CRITICAL THINKING DECISION PATH

Determining the Appropriate Type of Validity and Reliability Selected for a Study

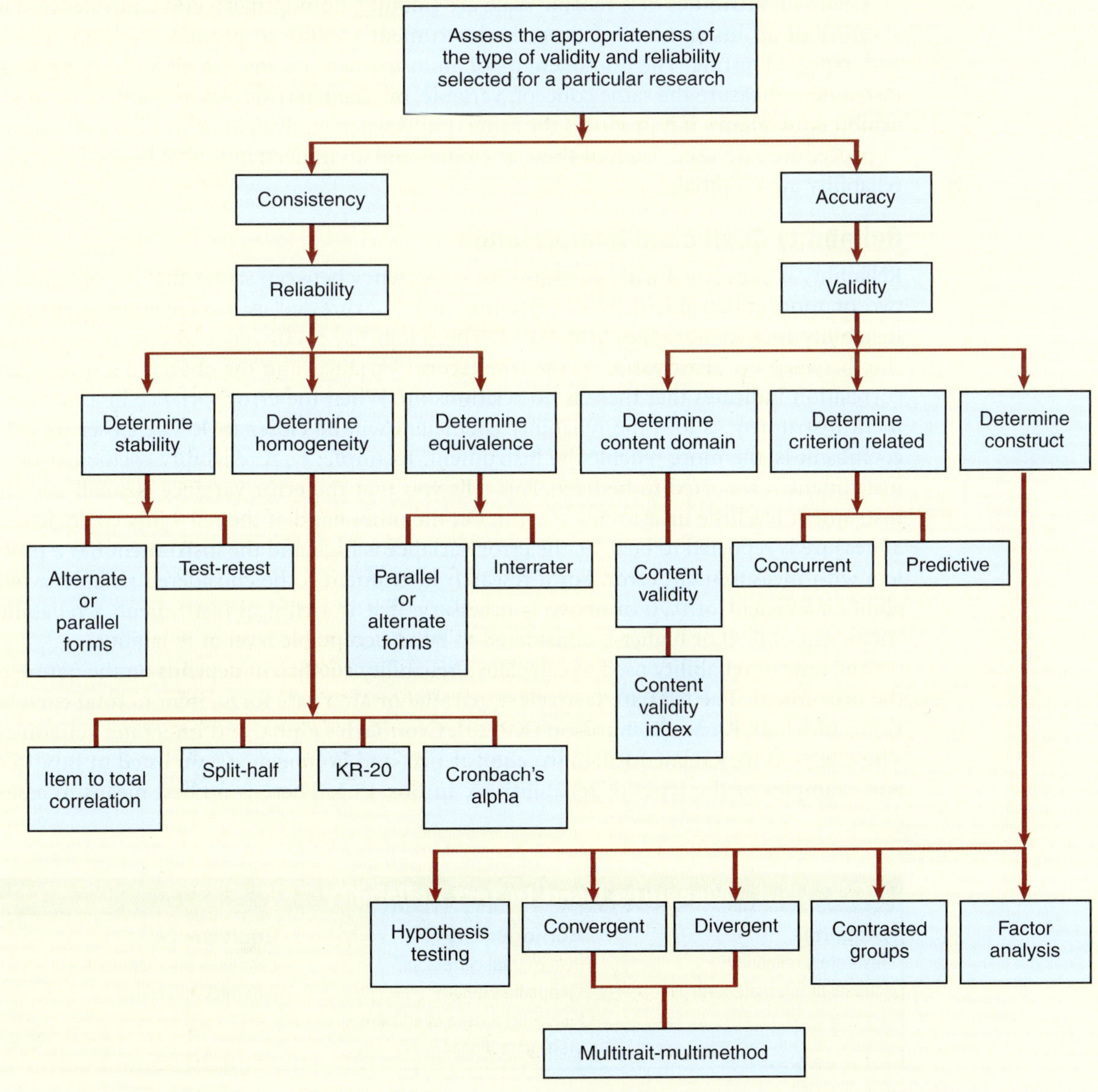

RELIABILITY

Reliable people are those whose behavior can be relied on to be consistent and predictable. Likewise, the **reliability** of an instrument is defined as the extent to which the instrument produces the same results if the behavior is repeatedly measured with the same scale. Reliability is concerned with consistency, accuracy, precision, stability, equivalence, and homogeneity. Concurrent with the questions of validity or after they are answered, you ask about the reliability of the instrument. Reliability refers to the proportion of consistency to inconsistency in measurement. In other words, if we use the same or comparable instruments on more than one occasion to measure a set of behaviors that ordinarily remains relatively constant, we would expect similar results if the instruments are reliable.

The main attributes of a reliable scale are stability, homogeneity, and equivalence. The **stability** of an instrument refers to the instrument's ability to produce the same results with repeated testing. The **homogeneity** of an instrument means that all of the items in an instrument measure the same concept, variable, or characteristic. An instrument is said to exhibit **equivalence** if it produces the same results when equivalent or parallel instruments or procedures are used. Each of these attributes and an understanding of how to interpret reliability are essential.

Reliability Coefficient Interpretation

Reliability is concerned with the degree of consistency between scores that are obtained at two or more independent times of testing and is expressed as a correlation coefficient. Reliability coefficient ranges from 0 to 1. The **reliability coefficient** expresses the relationship between the error variance, the true (score) variance, and the observed score. A zero correlation indicates that there is no relationship. When the error variance in a measurement instrument is low, the reliability coefficient will be closer to 1. The closer to 1 the coefficient is, the more reliable the instrument. **Example:** ➤ A reliability coefficient of an instrument is reported to be 0.89. This tells you that the error variance is small and the instrument has little measurement error. On the other hand, if the reliability coefficient of a measure is reported to be 0.49, the error variance is high and the instrument has a problem with measurement error. For a research instrument to be considered reliable, a reliability coefficient of 0.70 or above is necessary. If it is a clinical instrument, a reliability coefficient of 0.90 or higher is considered to be an acceptable level of reliability.

The tests of reliability used to calculate a reliability coefficient depends on the nature of the instrument. The tests are **test-retest**, **parallel or alternate form**, **item to total correlation**, **split-half**, **Kuder-Richardson (KR-20)**, **Cronbach's alpha**, and **interrater reliability**. These tests as they relate to stability, equivalence, and homogeneity are listed in Box 15.4, and examples of the types of reliability are in Box 15.5. There is no best means to assess

BOX 15.4 Measures Used to Test Reliability

Stability	Homogeneity	Equivalence
Test-retest reliability	Item to total correlation	Parallel or alternate form
Parallel or alternate form	Split-half reliability	Interrater reliability
	Kuder-Richardson coefficient	
	Cronbach's alpha	

BOX 15.5 Published Examples of Reported Reliability

Internal Consistency

In a study by Bhandari and Kim (2016) investigating self-care behaviors of Nepalese adults with type 2 diabetes, self-care behaviors were measured by the DMSE scale (Bijl et al., 1999). Cronbach's alpha was 0.81 in a study of European adults with type 2 DM (Bijl et al., 1999); it was 0.86 in the current study.

Test-Retest Reliability

In a study by Ganz and colleagues (2016) that examined whether nurses fully implement their scope of practice, the Implementation of Scope of Practice Scale, developed by the researchers for the study, established strong test-retest reliability ($r = 0.92$) by administering the scale at baseline and again 3 weeks later.

Kuder-Richardson (KR-20)

A study by Jessee and Tanner (2016) aimed to develop a Clinical Coaching Interactions Inventory, a tool to evaluate one-to-one teaching, verbal questioning, and feedback behaviors of clinical faculty and/or preceptors interacting with students in clinical settings. The teaching-questioning dimension demonstrated Kuder-Richardson Formula 20 (KR-20) of 0.70 overall, 0.63 for the faculty version, and 0.71 for the staff nurse preceptor version. The inventory is composed of binary items (e.g., Yes/No), and therefore a lower KR-20 reliability estimate is not unexpected and a KR-20 reliability estimate can still be considered acceptable.

Interrater Reliability and Kappa

In the Johansson and colleagues (2016) study evaluating the oral health status of older adults in Sweden receiving elder care, the ROAG-J was used to assess oral health by evaluating the condition of the voice, lips, oral mucosa, tongue, gums, teeth, saliva, swallowing, and any prostheses. Moderate to good interrater reliability was reported for the trained examiners (mean kappa estimate 0.59); interrater reproducibility (kappa estimate 1.00) and high sensitivity and specificity within elderly care in previous studies have been reported (Anderson et al., 2002; Ribeiro et al., 2014).

Item to Total

Abuadas and colleagues (2016) examined the item-to-total correlations as part of the assessment of reliability for the Arabic version of the Champion's Health Belief Model Scales for Prostate Cancer Screening (CHBMS-PCS). The aim was to identify poorly functioning items on the CHBMS-PCS. A cutoff score of 0.30 was established; all of the corrected item-to-total correlations were greater than 0.30 and ranged from 0.60 to 0.79. This indicated that the scale items have distinguishing consistency with each other. This was reinforced by the Cronbach's alpha coefficient for the total scale of 0.87.

reliability. The reliability method that the researcher uses should be consistent with the study's aim and the instrument's format.

Stability

An instrument is stable or exhibits **stability** when the same results are obtained on repeated administration of the instrument. Measurement over time is important when an instrument is used in a longitudinal study and therefore used on several occasions. Stability is also a consideration when a researcher is conducting an intervention study that is designed to effect a change in a specific variable. In this case, the instrument is administered and then again later, after the experimental intervention has been completed. The tests that are used to estimate stability are test-retest and parallel or alternate form.

Test-Retest Reliability

Test-retest reliability is the administration of the same instrument to the same subjects under similar conditions on two or more occasions. Scores from repeated testing are compared. This comparison is expressed by a correlation coefficient, usually a Pearson *r* (see Chapter 16). The interval between repeated administrations varies and depends on the variable being measured. **Example:** ➤ If the variable that the test measures is related to the developmental stages in children, the interval between tests should be short. The amount of time over which the variable was measured should also be identified in the study.

> **HELPFUL HINT**
>
> When a longitudinal design with multiple data collection points is being conducted, look for evidence of test-retest or parallel form reliability.

Parallel or Alternate Form

Parallel or **alternate form reliability** is applicable and can be tested only if two *comparable forms* of the *same* instrument exist. Not many instruments have a parallel form, so it is unusual to find examples in the literature. It is similar to test-retest reliability in that the same individuals are tested within a specific interval, but it differs because a *different* form of the *same* test is given to the subjects on the second testing. **Parallel forms** or tests contain the same types of items that are based on the same concept, but the wording of the items is different. The development of parallel forms is desired if the instrument is intended to measure a variable for which a researcher believes that "test-wiseness" will be a problem (see Chapter 8). **Example:** ➤ Consider a study to establish the reliability and validity of the Social Attribution Task-Multiple Choice (SAT-MC), a measurement instrument of geometric figures designed to assess implicit social attribution formation while reducing verbal and cognitive demands required of other common measures (Johannesen et al., 2013). The authors conducted a comparable analysis of the SAT-MC and the new SAT-MC II, a comparable form created for repeated testing to decrease threats to internal validity related to practice effect. External validation measures between the two forms were nearly identical, with evidence supporting convergent and divergent validity. Practically speaking, it is difficult to develop alternate forms of an instrument when one considers the many issues of reliability and validity. If alternate forms of a test exist, they should be highly correlated if the measures are to be considered reliable.

Internal Consistency/Homogeneity

Another attribute of an instrument related to reliability is the **internal consistency** or **homogeneity**. In this case, the items within the scale reflect or measure the same concept. This means that the items within the scale correlate or are complementary to each other. This also means that a scale is unidimensional. A unidimensional scale is one that measures one concept, such as self-efficacy. Box 15.5 provides several examples of how internal consistency is reported. Internal consistency can be assessed using one of four methods: item to total correlations, split-half reliability, Kuder-Richardson (KR-20) coefficient, or Cronbach's alpha.

> **QSEN EVIDENCE-BASED PRACTICE TIP**
>
> When the characteristics of a study sample differ significantly from the sample in the original study, check to see if the researcher has reestablished the reliability of the instrument with the current sample.

Item to Total Correlations

Item to total correlations measure the relationship between each of the items and the total scale. When item to total correlations are calculated, a correlation for each item on the scale is generated (Table 15.1). Items that do not achieve a high correlation may be deleted from the instrument. Usually in a research study, all of the item to total correlations are not reported unless the study is a report of a methodological study. The lowest and highest correlations are typically reported.

Cronbach's Alpha

The fourth and most commonly used test of internal consistency is **Cronbach's alpha**, which is used when a measurement instrument uses a Likert scale. Many scales used to measure psychosocial variables and attitudes have a Likert scale response format. A **Likert scale** format asks the subject to respond to a question on a scale of varying degrees of intensity between two extremes. The two extremes are anchored by responses ranging from "strongly agree" to "strongly disagree" or "most like me" to "least like me." The points between the two extremes may range from 1 to 4, 1 to 5, or 1 to 7. Subjects are asked to identify the response closest to how they feel. Cronbach's alpha simultaneously compares each item in the scale with the others. A total score is then used in the data analysis as illustrated in Table 15.1. Alphas above 0.70 are sufficient evidence for supporting the internal consistency of the instrument. Fig. 15.2 provides examples of items from an instrument that use a Likert scale format.

TABLE 15.1 Examples of Cronbach's Alpha From the Alhusen Study (Appendix B)

Dimensions	Original	Sample 1	Sample 2	Sample 3
Negative reactivity	0.90	0.89	0.90	0.92
Task persistence	0.90	0.89	0.91	0.92
Approach/withdrawal	0.88	0.84	0.86	0.92
Activity	0.85	0.80	0.86	0.92

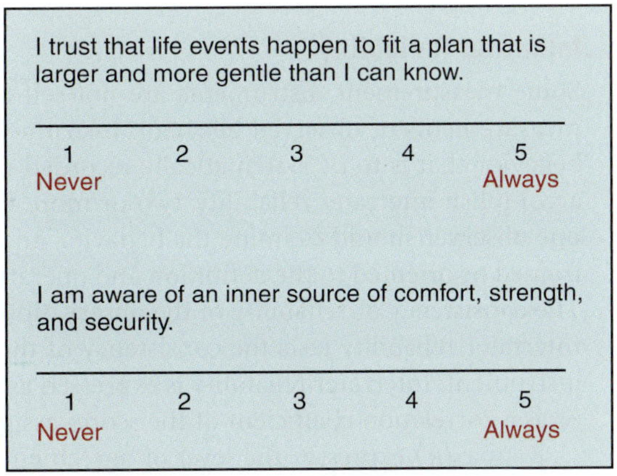

FIG 15.2 Examples of a Likert scale. (Redrawn from Roberts, K. T., & Aspy, C. B. (1993). Development of the serenity scale. *Journal of Nursing Measurement, 1*(2), 145–164.)

Split-Half Reliability

Split-half reliability involves dividing a scale into two halves and making a comparison. The halves may be odd-numbered and even-numbered items or may be a simple division of the first from the second half, or items may be randomly selected into halves that will be analyzed opposite one another. The split-half method provides a measure of consistency. The two halves of the test or the contents in both halves are assumed to be comparable, and a reliability coefficient is calculated. If the scores for the two halves are approximately equal, the test may be considered reliable. See Box 15.5 for an example.

Kuder-Richardson (KR-20) Coefficient

The **Kuder-Richardson (KR-20) coefficient** is the estimate of homogeneity used for instruments that have a dichotomous response format. A dichotomous response format is one in which the question asks for a "yes/no" or "true/false" response. The technique yields a correlation that is based on the consistency of responses to all the items of a single form of a test that is administered one time. The minimum acceptable KR-20 score is $r = 0.70$ (see Box 15.5).

> **IPE HIGHLIGHT**
>
> Your team is critically appraising a research study reporting on an innovative intervention for reducing risk for hospital acquired pressure ulcers. Data are collected using observation and multiple observers. You want to find evidence that the observers have been trained until there is a high level of interrater reliability so that you are confident that they were observing the subjects' skin according to standardized criteria and completing their Checklist ratings in a consistent way across observers.

Equivalence

Equivalence either is the consistency or agreement among observers using the same measurement instrument or is the consistency or agreement between alternate forms of an instrument. An instrument is thought to demonstrate equivalence when two or more observers have a high percentage of agreement of an observed behavior or when alternate forms of a test yield a high correlation. There are two methods to test equivalence: interrater reliability and alternate or parallel form.

Interrater Reliability

Some measurement instruments are not self-administered questionnaires but are direct measurements of observed behavior. Instruments that depend on direct observation of a behavior that is to be systematically recorded must be tested for **interrater reliability**. To accomplish interrater reliability, two or more individuals should make an observation, or one observer should examine the behavior on several occasions. The observers should be trained or oriented to the definition and operationalization of the behavior to be observed. The consistency or reliability of the observations among observers is extremely important. Interrater reliability tests the consistency of the observer rather than the reliability of the instrument. Interrater reliability is expressed as a percentage of agreement between scorers or as a correlation coefficient of the scores assigned to the observed behaviors.

Kappa (κ) expresses the level of agreement observed beyond the level that would be expected by chance alone. κ ranges from $+1$ (total agreement) to 0 (no agreement). A κ of

0.80 or better indicates good interrater reliability. κ between 0.80 and 0.68 is considered acceptable/substantial agreement; less than 0.68 allows tentative conclusions to be drawn at times when lower levels are accepted (McDowell & Newell, 1996) (see Box 15.5).

QSEN EVIDENCE-BASED PRACTICE TIP

Interrater reliability is an important approach to minimizing bias.

Parallel or Alternate Form

Parallel or alternate form was described in the discussion of stability in this chapter. Use of parallel forms is a measure of stability and equivalence. The procedures for assessing equivalence using parallel forms are the same.

CLASSIC TEST THEORY VERSUS ITEM RESPONSE THEORY

The methods of reliability and validity described in this chapter are considered classical test theory (CTT) methods. There are newer methods that you will find described in research articles under the category of item response theory (IRT). The two methods share basic characteristics, but some feel that IRT methods are superior for discriminating test items. Several terms and concepts linked with IRT are Rasch models and one (or two) parameter logistic models. The methodology of these methods is beyond the scope of this text, but several references are cited for future use (DeVellis, 2012; Furr & Bacharach, 2008).

HOW VALIDITY AND RELIABILITY ARE REPORTED

When reading a research article, a lengthy discussion of how the different types of reliability and validity were obtained will typically not be found. What is found in the methods section is the instrument's title, a definition of the concept/construct that it measures, and a sentence or two about discussion is appropriate. Examples of what you will see include the following:

- "Tedeschi and Calhoun (1996) reported an internal consistency coefficient of 0.9 for the full scale the PTG (Post-traumatic Growth Inventory) for the full scale and a test-retest reliability of 0.71 after two months. Yaskowich (2003) reported an internal consistency for the full scale of the modified PTGI in a sample of 35 adolescent cancer survivors. The internal consistency of the modified PTGI was 0.94 for survivors and siblings and 0.96 for parents in the current study" (Turner-Sack et al., 2016, p. 51; Appendix D).
- The Connor-Davidson Resilience Scale (CD-RISC) reports the "Cronbach's alpha for the full scale is reported to be .89 and item-total correlations range from .30 to .70. The CD-RISC possess good validity and reliability in the Iranian population (Khoshouei, 2009) and Cronbach's alpha for the scale in the current study was .93" (Barahmand & Ahmad, 2016).
- "Content, construct, and criterion-related validity has been documented for the Bakas Caregiving Outcomes Scale (BCOS) that measures Life changes (e.g., Changes in social functioning, subjective well-being, and physical health). Evidence of internal consistency reliability has been documented in primary care and with stroke care givers. The Cronbach alpha for the BCOS in this study was 0.87" (Bakas et al., 2015).

APPRAISAL FOR EVIDENCE-BASED PRACTICE RELIABILITY AND VALIDITY

Reliability and validity are crucial aspects in the critical appraisal of a measurement instrument. Criteria for critiquing reliability and validity are presented in the Critical Appraisal Criteria box. When reviewing a research article, you need to appraise each instrument's reliability and validity. In a research article, the reliability and validity for each measure should be presented or a reference should be provided where it was described in more detail. If this information is not been presented at all, you must seriously question the merit and use of the instrument and the evidence provided by the study's results.

The amount of information provided for each instrument will vary depending on the study type and the instrument. In a psychometric study (an instrument development study) you will find great detail regarding how the researchers established the reliability and validity of the instrument. When reading a research article in which the instruments are used to test a research question or hypothesis, you may find only brief reference to the type of reliability and validity of the instrument. If the instrument is a well-known, reliable, and valid instrument, it is not uncommon that only a passing comment may be made, which is appropriate. **Example:** ➤ In the study by Vermeesch and colleagues (2015) examining biological and sociocultural differences in perceived barriers to physical activity among fifth to seventh grade urban girls, the researchers noted acceptable face, content and construct validity, and reliability estimated by Cronbach's alpha of 0.78 have been reported (Robbins et al., 2008, 2009). As in the previously provided example, authors often will cite a reference that you can locate if you are interested in detailed data about the instrument's reliability or validity. If a study does not use reliable and valid questionnaires, you need to consider the sources of bias that may exist as threats to internal or external validity. It is very difficult to place confidence in the evidence generated by a study's findings if the measures used did not have established validity and reliability. The following discussion highlights key areas related to reliability and validity that should be evident as you read a research article.

The investigator determines which type of reliability procedures need to be used in the study, depending on the nature of the measurement instrument and how it will be used.

CRITICAL APPRAISAL CRITERIA

Reliability and Validity

1. Was an appropriate method used to test the reliability of the instrument?
2. Is the reliability of the instrument adequate?
3. Was an appropriate method(s) used to test the validity of the instrument?
4. Is the validity of the measurement instrument adequate?
5. If the sample from the developmental stage of the instrument was different from the current sample, were the reliability and validity recalculated to determine if the instrument is appropriate for use in a different population?
6. What kinds of threats to internal and/or external validity are presented by weaknesses in reliability and/or validity?
7. Are strengths and weaknesses of the reliability and validity of the instruments appropriately addressed in the "Discussion," "Limitations," or "Recommendations" sections of the report?
8. How do the reliability and/or validity affect the strength and quality of the evidence provided by the study findings?

Example: ➤ If the instrument is to be administered twice, you would expect to read that test-retest reliability was used to establish the stability of the instrument. If an alternate form has been developed for use in a repeated-measures design, evidence of alternate form reliability should be presented to determine the equivalence of the parallel forms. If the degree of internal consistency among the items is relevant, an appropriate test of internal consistency should be presented. In some instances, more than one type of reliability will be presented, but as you assess the instruments section of a research report, you should determine whether all are appropriate. **Example:** ➤ The Kuder-Richardson formula implies that there is a single right or wrong answer, making it inappropriate to use with scales that provide a format of three or more possible responses. In the latter case, another formula is applied, such as Cronbach's coefficient alpha. Another important consideration is the acceptable level of reliability, which varies according to the type of test. Reliability coefficients of 0.70 or higher are desirable. The validity of an instrument is limited by its reliability; that is, less confidence can be placed in scores from tests with low reliability coefficients.

Satisfactory evidence of validity will probably be the most difficult item for you to ascertain. It is this aspect of measurement that is most likely to fall short of meeting the required criteria. Page count limitations often account for this brevity. Detailed validity data usually are only reported in studies focused on instrument development; therefore validity data are mentioned only briefly or, sometimes, not at all. The most common type of reported validity is content validity. When reviewing a study, you want to find evidence of content validity. Once again, you will find the detailed reporting of content validity and the CVI in psychometric studies; Box 15.2 provides a good example of how content validity is reported in a psychometric study. Such procedures provide you with assurance that the instrument is psychometrically sound and that the content of the items is consistent with the conceptual framework and construct definitions. In studies where several instruments are used, the reporting of content validity is either absent or very brief.

Construct validity and criterion-related validity are more precise statistical tests of whether the instrument measures what it is supposed to measure. Ideally an instrument should provide evidence of content validity, as well as criterion-related or construct validity, before one invests a high level of confidence in the instrument. You will see evidence that the reliability and validity of a measurement instrument are reestablished periodically, as you can see in the examples that appear in Boxes 15.2 to 15.5. You would expect to see the strengths and weaknesses of instrument reliability and validity presented in the "Discussion," "Limitations," and/or "Recommendations" sections of an article. In this context, the reliability and validity might be discussed in terms of bias—that is, threats to internal and/or external validity that affect the study findings. **Example:** ➤ In the study by Hart and colleagues (2016), evaluating the psychometric properties of the Clinical Deterioration Leadership Ability Scale (CDLAS), the authors note that despite satisfactory reliability and validity findings, limitations include the homogeneous sample of mostly white, female registered nurses practicing in one integrated five hospital health system in the southeast United States. This sample limits the generalizability of the results to other populations. The authors suggest that further research is needed with diverse groups of nurses in multiple geographic locations. In addition, further research should focus on conducting test-retest reliability to further establish the psychometric properties of the CDLAS.

The findings of any study in which the reliability and validity are sparse does limit generalizability of the findings, but also adds to our knowledge regarding future research directions. Finally, recommendations for improving future studies in relation to instrument reliability and validity may be proposed.

As you can see, the area of reliability and validity is complex. You should not feel intimidated by the complexity of this topic; use the guidelines presented in this chapter to systematically assess the reliability and validity aspects of a research study. Collegial dialogue is also an approach for evaluating the merits and shortcomings of an existing, as well as a newly developed, instrument that is reported in the nursing literature. Such an exchange promotes the understanding of methodologies and techniques of reliability and validity, stimulates the acquisition of a basic knowledge of psychometrics, and encourages the exploration of alternative methods of observation and use of reliable and valid instruments in clinical practice.

KEY POINTS

- Reliability and validity are crucial aspects of conducting and critiquing research.
- Validity is the extent to which an instrument measures the attributes of a concept accurately. Three types of validity are content validity, criterion-related validity, and construct validity.
- The choice of a method for establishing reliability or validity is important and is made by the researcher on the basis of the characteristics of the measurement instrument and its intended use.
- Reliability is the ability of an instrument to measure the attributes of a concept or construct consistently. The major tests of reliability are test-retest, parallel or alternate form, split-half, item to total correlation, Kuder-Richardson, Cronbach's alpha, and interrater reliability.
- The selection of a method for establishing reliability or validity depends on the characteristics of the instrument, the testing method that is used for collecting data from the sample, and the kinds of data that are obtained.
- Critical appraisal of instrument reliability and validity in a research report focuses on internal and external validity as sources of bias that contribute to the strength and quality of evidence provided by the findings.

CRITICAL THINKING CHALLENGES

- Discuss the types of validity that must be established before you invest a high level of confidence in the measurement instruments used in a research study.
- What are the major tests of reliability? Why is it important to establish the appropriate type of reliability for a measurement instrument?
- A journal club just finished reading the research report by Thomas and colleagues in Appendix A. As part of their critical appraisal of this study, they needed to identify the strengths and weaknesses of the reliability and validity section of this research report. If you were a member of this journal club, how would you assess the reliability and validity of the instruments used in this study?
- How does the strength and quality of evidence related to reliability and validity influence the applicability of findings to clinical practice?

- IPE When your QI Team finds that a researcher does not report reliability or validity data, which threats to internal and/or external validity should your team consider? In your judgment, how would these threats affect your evaluation of the strength and quality of evidence provided by the study and your team's confidence in applying the findings to practice?

REFERENCES

Abuadas, M. H., Petro-Nustas, W., Albikawi, Z. F., & Nabolski, M. (2016). Transcultural adaptation and validation of Champion's health belief model scales for prostate cancer screening. *Journal of Nursing Measurement, 24*(2), 296–313.

Ameringer, S., Elswick, R. K. Jr., Menzies, V., et al. (2016). Psychometric evaluation of the patient-reported outcomes measurement information system fatigue-short form across diverse populations. *Nursing Research, 65*(4), *279k–289k.*

Anastasi, A., & Urbina, S. (1997). *Psychological testing* (7th ed.). New York, NY: Macmillan.

Bakas, T., Austin, J. K., Habermann, B., et al. (2015). Telephone assessment and skill-building kit for stroke caregivers; A randomized controlled clinical trial. *Stroke, 46*, 3478–3487.

Baldacchino, D. R., & Bulhagiar, A. (2003). Psychometric evaluation of the spiritual coping strategies in English, Maltese: Back translation and bilingual versions. *Journal of Advanced Nursing, 42*, 558–570.

Barahmand, U., & Ahmad, R. H. S. (2016). Psychotic-like experiences and psychological distress: The role of resilience. *Journal of the American Psychiatric Nurses Association, 22*(4), 312–319.

Bhandari, P., & Kim, M. (2016). Self-care behaviors of Nepalese adults with type 2 diabetes: A mixed methods analysis. *Nursing Research, 65*(3), 202–214.

Bijl, J. V., Peolgeest-Eeltink, A. V., & Shortbridge-Baggett, L. (1999). The psychometric properties of the diabetes management self-efficacy scale for patients with type 2 diabetes mellitus. *Journal of Advanced Nursing, 30*, 352–359.

Champion, V. L. (1993). Instrument refinement for breast cancer screening behaviors. *Nursing Research, 42*(3), 139–143.

Clark, A., Breitenstein, S., Martsolf, D. S., & Winstanley, E. L. (2016). Assessing fidelity of a community-based opioid overdose prevention program: Modification of the fidelity checklist. *Journal of Nursing Scholarship, 48*(4), 378–377.

DeVon, F. A., Block, M. E., Moyle-Wright, P., et al. (2007). A psychometric toolbox for testing validity and reliability. *Journal of Nursing Scholarship, 39*(2), 155–164.

DeVellis, R. F. (2012). *Scale development: Theory and applications.* Los Angeles, CA: Sage Publications.

Furr, M. R., & Bacharach, V. R. (2008). *Psychometrics: An introduction.* Los Angeles, CA: Sage Publications.

Ganz, F.D., Toren, O., & Fadion, F. (2016). Factors associated with full implementation of scope of practice. *Journal of Nursing Scholarship, 48*(3), 285–293.

Hart, P. L., Spiva, L. A., & Mareno, N. (2016). Clinical deterioration leadership ability scale: A psychometric study. *Journal of Nursing Measurement, 24*(2), 314–322.

Hawthorne, D. M., Youngblut, J. M., & Brooten, D. (2016). Parent spirituality, grief, and mental health at 1 and 3 months after their infant's/child's death in an intensive care unit. *Journal of Pediatric Nursing, 31*, 73–80.

Johansson, I., Jansson, H., & Lindmark, U. (2016). Oral health status of older adults in Sweden receiving elder care: Findings from nursing assessments. *Nursing Research, 65*(3), 215–223.

Johannesen, J. K., Lurie, J. B., Fiszdon, J. M., & Bell, M. D. (2013). The social attribution task-multiple choice (SAT-MC): A psychometric and equivalence study of an alternate form. *ISRN Psychiatry, 2013*, 1–9.

Khoshouei, M. S. (2009). Psychometric evaluation of the Connor-Davidson resilience scale (CD-RISC) using Iranian students. *International Journal of Testing*, *9*(1), 60–66.

Lee, C. E., Von Ah, D., Szuck, B., & Lau, Y. J. (2016). Determinants of physical activity maintenance in breast cancer survivors after a community-based intervention. *Oncology Nursing Forum*, *43*(1), 93–102.

Lynn, M. R. (1986). Determination and quantification of content validity. *Nursing Research*, *35*, 382–385.

McDowell, I., & Newell, C. (1996). *Measuring health: A guide to rating scales and questionnaires*. New York, NY: Oxford Press.

Nunnally, J. C., & Bernstein, I. H. (1993). *Psychometric theory* (3rd ed.). New York, NY: McGraw-Hill.

Robbins, L. B., Sikorski, A., Hamel, L.M., et al. (2009). Gender comparisons of perceived benefits of and barriers to physical activity in middle school youth. *Research in Nursing and Health*, *32*, 163–176.

Robbins, L. B., Sikorski, A., & Morely, B. (2008). Psychometric assessment of the adolescent physical activity perceived benefits and barriers scale. *Journal of Nursing Measurement*, *16*, 98–112.

Tedeschi, R. G., & Calhoun, L. G. (1996). The post-traumatic growth inventory: Measuring the positive legacy of trauma. *Journal of Traumatic Stress*, *9*, 455k–471k.

Turner-Sack, A. M., Menna, R., Setchell, S.R., et al. (2016). Psychological functioning, post-traumatic growth, and coping in parents and siblings of adolescent cancer survivors. *Oncology Nursing Forum*, *43*(1), 48–56.

Vermeesch, A. L., Ling, J., Voskull, V. R., et al. (2015). Biological and sociocultural differences in perceived barriers to physical activity among fifth-to-seventh-grade urban girls. *Nursing Research*, *64*(5), 342–350.

Yaskowich, E. (2003). Posttraumatic growth in children and adolescents with cancer. *Digital Dissertation*, *63*, 3948.

Go to Evolve at **http://evolve.elsevier.com/LoBiondo/** for review questions, critiquing exercises, and additional research articles for practice in reviewing and critiquing.

16

Data Analysis: Descriptive and Inferential Statistics

Susan Sullivan-Bolyai and Carol Bova

Go to Evolve at **http://evolve.elsevier.com/LoBiondo/** for review questions, critiquing exercises, and additional research articles for practice in reviewing and critiquing.

LEARNING OUTCOMES

After reading this chapter, you should be able to do the following:

- Differentiate between descriptive and inferential statistics.
- State the purposes of descriptive statistics.
- Identify the levels of measurement in a study.
- Describe a frequency distribution.
- List measures of central tendency and their use.
- List measures of variability and their use.
- State the purpose of inferential statistics.
- Explain the concept of probability as it applies to the analysis of sample data.
- Distinguish between a type I and type II error and its effect on a study's outcome.
- Distinguish between parametric and nonparametric tests.
- List some commonly used statistical tests and their purposes.
- Critically appraise the statistics used in published research studies.
- Evaluate the strength and quality of the evidence provided by the findings of a research study and determine applicability to practice.

KEY TERMS

analysis of covariance
analysis of variance
categorical variable
chi-square (χ^2)
continuous variable
correlation
degrees of freedom
descriptive statistics
dichotomous variable
factor analysis
Fisher exact probability test
frequency distribution
inferential statistics
interval measurement
levels of measurement
level of significance (alpha level)
mean
measures of central tendency
measures of variability
median
measurement
modality
mode
multiple analysis of variance
multiple regression
multivariate statistics
nominal measurement
nonparametric statistics
normal curve
null hypothesis
ordinal measurement
parameter
parametric statistics
Pearson correlation coefficient (Pearson *r*; Pearson product moment correlation coefficient)
percentile
probability
range
ratio measurement
sampling error

Continued

KEY TERMS—cont'd

scientific hypothesis
standard deviation
statistic
t statistic
type I error
type II error

It is important to understand the principles underlying statistical methods used in quantitative research. This understanding allows you to critically analyze the results of research that may be useful in practice. Researchers link the statistical analyses they choose with the type of research question, design, and level of data collected.

As you read a research article, you will find a discussion of the statistical procedures used in both the methods and results sections. In the methods section, you will find the planned statistical analyses. In the results section, you will find the data generated from testing the hypotheses or research questions. The data are analyzed using both descriptive and inferential statistics.

Procedures that allow researchers to describe and summarize data are known as **descriptive statistics**. Descriptive statistics include measures of central tendency, such as mean, median, and mode; measures of variability, such as range and standard deviation (SD); and some correlation techniques, such as scatter plots. For example, Nyamathi and colleagues (2015; Appendix A) used descriptive statistics to inform the reader about the 345 subjects who were eligible for the HAV/HBV vaccine in their study (51% African American, 31% Latino, 59% not married, with a mean education of 11.6 years).

Statistical procedures that allow researchers to estimate how reliably they can make *predictions* and *generalize* findings based on the data are known as **inferential statistics**. Inferential statistics are used to analyze the data collected, test hypotheses, and answer the research questions in a research study. With inferential statistics, the researcher is trying to draw conclusions that extend beyond the study's data.

This chapter describes how researchers use descriptive and inferential statistics in studies. This will help you determine the appropriateness of the statistics used and to interpret the strength and quality of the reported findings, as well as the clinical significance and applicability of the results for your evidence-based practice.

LEVELS OF MEASUREMENT

Measurement is the process of assigning numbers to variables or events according to rules. Every variable in a study that is assigned a specific number must be similar to every other variable assigned that number. The measurement level is determined by the nature of the object or event being measured. Understanding the **levels of measurement** is an important first step when you evaluate the statistical analyses used in a study. There are four levels of measurement: nominal, ordinal, interval, and ratio (Table 16.1). The level of measurement of each variable determines the statistic that can be used to answer a research question or test a hypothesis. The higher the level of measurement, the greater the flexibility the researcher has in choosing statistical procedures. The following Critical Thinking Decision Path illustrates the relationship between levels of measurement and the appropriate use of descriptive statistics.

TABLE 16.1 **Level of Measurement Summary Table**

Measurement	Description	Measures of Central Tendency	Measures of Variability
Nominal	Classification	Mode	Modal percentage, range, frequency distribution
Ordinal	Relative rankings	Mode, median	Range, percentile, frequency distribution
Interval	Rank ordering with equal intervals	Mode, median, mean	Range, percentile, standard deviation
Ratio	Rank ordering with equal intervals and absolute zero	Mode, median, mean	All

CRITICAL THINKING DECISION PATH

Descriptive Statistics

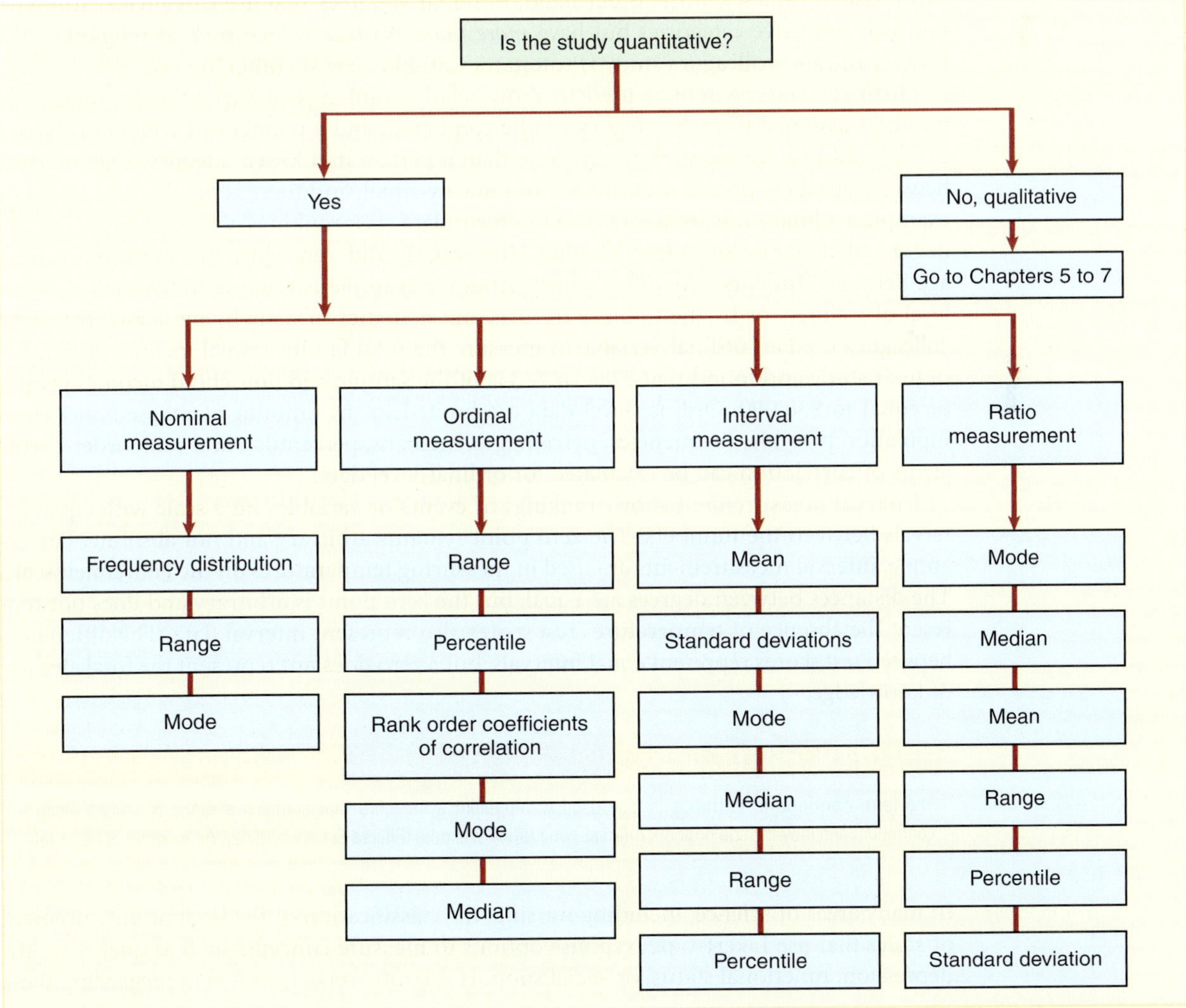

Nominal measurement is used to classify variables or events into categories. The categories are mutually exclusive; the variable or event either has or does not have the characteristic. The numbers assigned to each category are only labels; such numbers do not indicate more or less of a characteristic. Nominal-level measurement is used to categorize a sample on such information as gender, marital status, or religious affiliation. For example, Hawthorne and colleagues (2016; Appendix B) measured race using a nominal level of measurement. Nominal-level measurement is the lowest level and allows for the least amount of statistical manipulation. When using nominal-level variables, the frequency and percent are typically calculated. For example, Hawthorne and colleagues (2016) found that among their sample of mothers, 44% were black, non-Hispanic; 37% Hispanic; and 19% white, non-Hispanic.

A variable at the nominal level can also be categorized as either a **dichotomous** or a **categorical variable**. A **dichotomous** (nominal) **variable** is one that has *only two true values*, such as true/false or yes/no. For example, in the Turner-Sack and colleagues (2016; Appendix D) study the variable gender (male/female) is dichotomous because it has only two possible values. On the other hand, nominal variables that are **categorical** still have mutually exclusive categories but have *more than two true values,* such as religion in the Hawthorne and colleagues study (Protestant, Catholic, Jewish, other, none).

Ordinal measurement is used to show relative rankings of variables or events. The numbers assigned to each category can be compared, and a member of a higher category can be said to have more of an attribute than a person in a lower category. The intervals between numbers on the scale are not necessarily equal, and there is no absolute zero. For example, ordinal measurement is used to formulate class rankings, where one student can be ranked higher or lower than another. However, the difference in actual grade point average between students may differ widely. Another example is ranking individuals by their level of wellness or by their ability to carry out activities of daily living. Hawthorne and colleagues used an ordinal variable to measure the total family annual income of families in their study and found that 37% (n = 34) of the sample had household incomes greater or equal to $50,000. Ordinal-level data are limited in the amount of mathematical manipulation possible. Frequencies, percentages, medians, percentiles, and rank order coefficients of correlation can be calculated for ordinal-level data.

Interval measurement shows rankings of events or variables on a scale with equal intervals between the numbers. The zero point remains arbitrary and not absolute. For example, interval measurements are used in measuring temperatures on the Fahrenheit scale. The distances between degrees are equal, but the zero point is arbitrary and does not represent the absence of temperature. Test scores also represent interval data. The differences between test scores represent equal intervals, but a zero does not represent the total absence of knowledge.

HELPFUL HINT

The term **continuous variable** is also used to represent a measure that contains a range of values along a continuum and may include ordinal-, interval-, and ratio-level data (Plichta & Kelvin, 2012). An example is heart rate.

In many areas of science, including nursing, the classification of the level of measurement of scales that use Likert-type response options to measure concepts such as quality of life, depression, functional status, or social support is controversial, with some regarding these measurements as ordinal and others as interval. You need to be aware of this controversy and look at each study individually in terms of how the data are analyzed. Interval-level data allow more manipulation of data, including the addition and subtraction of numbers and the calculation of means. This additional manipulation is why many argue for classifying behavioral scale data as interval level. For example, Turner-Sack and colleagues (2016) used the Brief Symptom Inventory (BSI) to evaluate psychological distress of adolescent cancer survivors and siblings. The BSI has 53 items and uses a five-point Likert scale from 0 (not at all) to 4 (extremely), with higher scores indicating greater psychological distress. They reported the mean BSI score as 47.31 for cancer survivors and 48.94 for siblings.

Ratio measurement shows rankings of events or variables on scales with equal intervals and absolute zeros. The number represents the actual amount of the property the object possesses. Ratio measurement is the highest level of measurement, but it is most often used in the physical sciences. Examples of ratio-level data that are commonly used in nursing research are height, weight, pulse, and blood pressure. All mathematical procedures can be performed on data from ratio scales. Therefore, the use of any statistical procedure is possible as long as it is appropriate to the design of the study.

HELPFUL HINT

Descriptive statistics assist in summarizing data. The descriptive statistics calculated must be appropriate to the purpose of the study and the level of measurement.

DESCRIPTIVE STATISTICS

Frequency Distribution

One way of organizing descriptive data is by using a frequency distribution. In a **frequency distribution** the number of times each event occurs is counted. The data can also be grouped and the frequency of each group reported. Table 16.2 shows the results of an examination given to a class of 51 students. The results of the examination are reported in several ways. The columns on the left give the raw data tally and the frequency for each grade, and the columns on the right give the grouped data tally and grouped frequencies.

When data are grouped, it is necessary to define the size of the group or the interval width so that no score will fall into two groups and each group will be mutually exclusive. The grouping of the data in Table 16.2 prevents overlap; each score falls into only one group. The grouping should allow for a precise presentation of the data without a serious loss of information.

Information about frequency distributions may be presented in the form of a table, such as Table 16.2, or in graphic form. Fig. 16.1 illustrates the most common graphic forms: the histogram and the frequency polygon. The two graphic methods are similar in that both plot scores, or percentages of occurrence, against frequency. The greater the number of points plotted, the smoother the resulting graph. The shape of the resulting graph allows for observations that further describe the data.

Measures of Central Tendency

Measures of central tendency are used to describe the pattern of responses among a sample. Measures of central tendency include the mean, median, and mode. They yield a single number that describes the middle of the group and summarize the members of a

TABLE 16.2 Frequency Distribution

INDIVIDUAL			GROUP		
Score	**Tally**	**Frequency**	**Score**	**Tally**	**Frequency**
90	I	1	>89	I	1
88	I	1	—	—	—
86	I	1	80–89	IIIII IIIII IIIII	15
84	IIIII I	6	—	—	—
82	II	2	70–79	IIIII IIIII IIIII IIIII III	23
80	IIIII	5	—	—	—
78	IIIII	5	—	—	—
76	I	1	60–69	IIIII IIIII	10
74	IIIII II	7	—	—	—
72	IIIII IIII	9	<59	II	2
70	I	1	—	—	—
68	III	3	—	—	—
66	II	2	—	—	—
64	IIII	4	—	—	—
62	I	1	—	—	—
60	—	0	—	—	—
58	I	1	—	—	—
56		0	—	—	—
54	I	1	—	—	—
52		0	—	—	—
50		0	—	—	—
Total		51	—	—	51

Mean, 73.1; standard deviation, 12.1; median, 74; mode, 72; range, 36 (54–90).

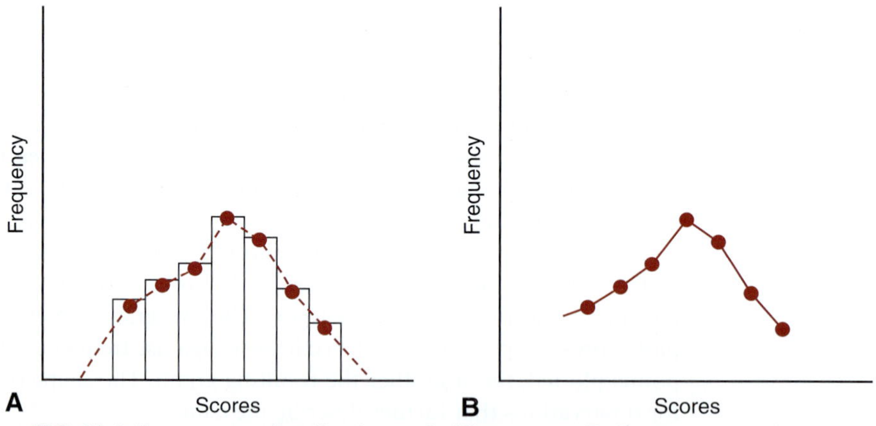

FIG 16.1 Frequency distributions. **A,** Histogram. **B,** Frequency polygon.

sample. Each measure of central tendency has a specific use and is most appropriate to specific kinds of measurement and types of distributions.

The **mean** is the arithmetical average of all the scores (add all of the values in a distribution and divide by the total number of values) and is used with interval or ratio data. The mean is the most widely used measure of central tendency. Most statistical tests of significance use the mean. The mean is affected by every score and can change greatly with extreme scores, especially in studies that have a limited sample size. The mean is generally considered the single best point for summarizing data when using interval- or ratio-level data. You can find the mean in research reports by looking for the symbol $\bar{x}$.

The **median** is the score where 50% of the scores are above it and 50% of the scores are below it. The median is not sensitive to extremes in high and low scores. It is best used when the data are skewed (see the Normal Distribution section in this chapter) and the researcher is interested in the "typical" score. For example, if age is a variable and there is a wide range with extreme scores that may affect the mean, it would be appropriate to also report the median. The median is easy to find either by inspection or by calculation and can be used with ordinal-, interval-, and ratio-level data.

The **mode** is the most frequent value in a distribution. The mode is determined by inspection of the frequency distribution (not by mathematical calculation). For example, in Table 16.2 the mode would be a score of 72 because nine students received this score and it represents the score that was attained by the greatest number of students. It is important to note that a sample distribution can have more than one mode. The number of modes contained in a distribution is called the **modality** of the distribution. It is also possible to have no mode when all scores in a distribution are different. The mode is most often used with nominal data but can be used with all levels of measurement. The mode cannot be used for calculations, and it is unstable; that is, the mode can fluctuate widely from sample to sample from the same population.

HELPFUL HINT

Of the three measures of central tendency, the mean is the affected by every score and the most useful. The mean can only be calculated with interval and ratio data.

When you examine a study, the measures of central tendency provide you with important information about the distribution of scores in a sample. If the distribution is symmetrical and unimodal, the mean, median, and mode will coincide. If the distribution is skewed (asymmetrical), the mean will be pulled in the direction of the long tail of the distribution and will differ from the median. With a skewed distribution, all three statistics should be reported.

HELPFUL HINT

Measures of central tendency are descriptive statistics that describe the characteristics of a sample.

Normal Distribution

The concept of the **normal distribution** is based on the observation that data from repeated measures of interval- or ratio-level data group themselves about a midpoint in a distribution in a manner that closely approximates the normal curve illustrated in Fig. 16.2.

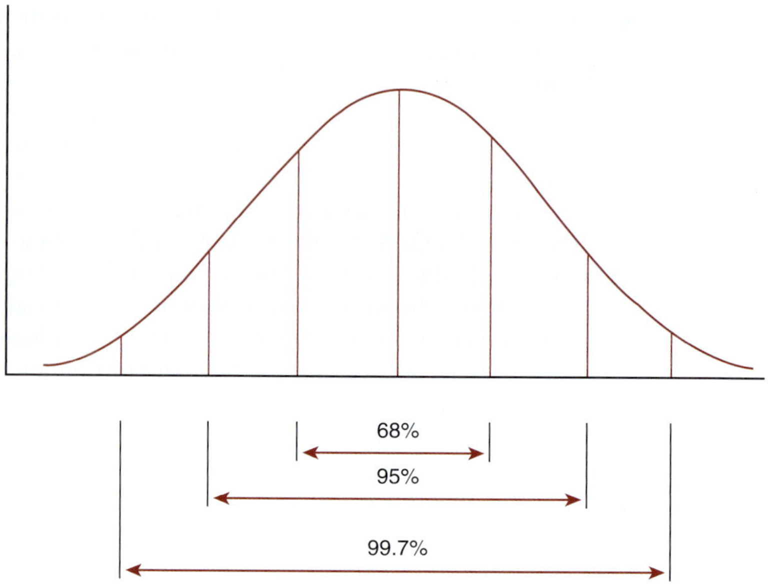

FIG 16.2 The normal distribution and associated standard deviations.

The **normal curve** is one that is symmetrical about the mean and is unimodal. The mean, median, and mode are equal. An additional characteristic of the normal curve is that a fixed percentage of the scores fall within a given distance of the mean. As shown in Fig. 16.2, about 68% of the scores or means will fall within 1 SD of the mean, 95% within 2 SD of the mean, and 99.7% within 3 SD of the mean. The presence or absence of a normal distribution is a fundamental issue when examining the appropriate use of inferential statistical procedures.

QSEN EVIDENCE-BASED PRACTICE TIP

Inspection of descriptive statistics for the sample will indicate whether the sample data are skewed.

Interpreting Measures of Variability

Variability or dispersion is concerned with the spread of data. **Measures of variability** answer questions such as: "Is the sample homogeneous (similar) or heterogeneous (different)?" If a researcher measures oral temperatures in two samples, one sample drawn from a healthy population and one sample from a hospitalized population, it is possible that the two samples will have the same mean. However, it is likely that there will be a wider range of temperatures in the hospitalized sample than in the healthy sample. Measures of variability are used to describe these differences in the dispersion of data. As with measures of central tendency, the various measures of variability are appropriate to specific kinds of measurement and types of distributions.

HELPFUL HINT

The descriptive statistics related to variability will enable you to evaluate the homogeneity or heterogeneity of a sample.

The **range** is the simplest but most unstable measure of variability. Range is the difference between the highest and lowest scores. A change in either of these two scores would change the range. The range should always be reported with other measures of variability. The range in Table 16.2 is 36, but this could easily change with an increase or decrease in the high score of 90 or the low score of 54. Turner-Sack and colleagues (2016; Appendix D) reported the range of BSI scores among their sample of adolescent cancer survivors (range = 25 to 79).

A **percentile** represents the percentage of cases a given score exceeds. The median is the 50% percentile, and in Table 16.2 it is a score of 74. A score in the 90th percentile is exceeded by only 10% of the scores. The zero percentile and the 100th percentile are usually dropped.

The **standard deviation** (SD) is the most frequently used measure of variability, and it is based on the concept of the normal curve (see Fig. 16.2). It is a measure of average deviation of the scores from the mean and as such should always be reported with the mean. The SD considers all scores and can be used to interpret individual scores. The SD is used in the calculation of many inferential statistics.

HELPFUL HINT

Many measures of variability exist. The SD is the most useful because it helps you visualize how the scores disperse around the mean.

INFERENTIAL STATISTICS

Inferential statistics allow researchers to test hypotheses about a population using data obtained from probability samples. Statistical inference is generally used for two purposes: to estimate the probability that the statistics in the sample accurately reflect the population parameter and to test hypotheses about a population.

A **parameter** is a characteristic of a *population,* whereas a **statistic** is a characteristic of a *sample.* We use statistics to estimate population parameters. Suppose we randomly sample 100 people with chronic lung disease and use an interval-level scale to study their knowledge of the disease. If the mean score for these subjects is 65, the mean represents the sample statistic. If we were able to study every subject with chronic lung disease, we could calculate an average knowledge score, and that score would be the parameter for the population. As you know, a researcher rarely is able to study an entire population, so inferential statistics provide evidence that allows the researcher to make statements about the larger population from studying the sample.

CRITICAL THINKING DECISION PATH

Inferential Statistics—Difference Questions

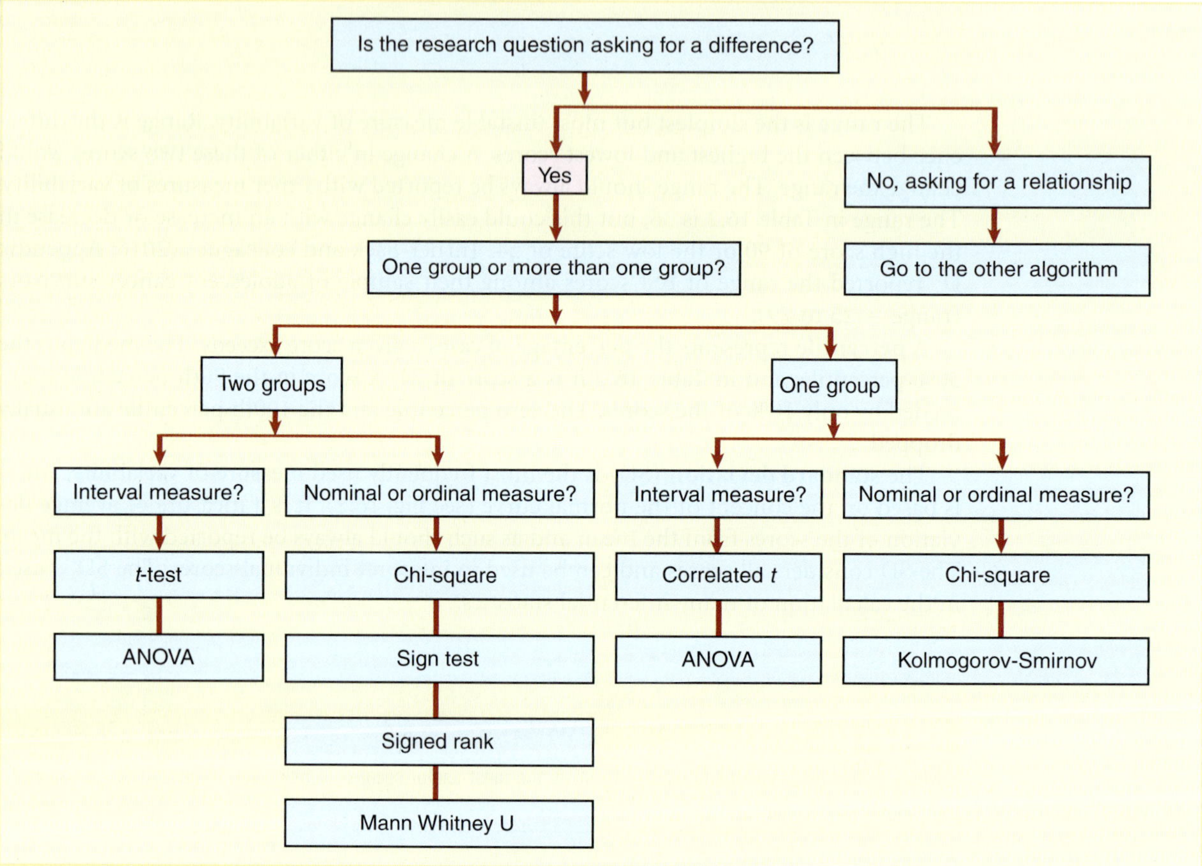

The example given alludes to two important qualifications of how a study must be conducted so that inferential statistics may be used. First, it was stated that the sample was selected using probability methods (see Chapter 12). Because you are already familiar with the advantages of probability sampling, it should be clear that if we wish to make statements about a population from a sample, that sample must be representative. All procedures for inferential statistics are based on the assumption that the sample was drawn with a known probability. Second, the scale used has to be at either an interval or a ratio level of measurement. This is because the mathematical operations involved in calculating inferential statistics require this higher level of measurement. It should be noted that in studies that use nonprobability methods of sampling, inferential statistics are also used. To compensate for the use of nonprobability sampling methods, researchers use techniques such as sample size estimation using power analysis. The following two Critical Thinking Decision Paths examine inferential statistics and provide matrices that researchers use for statistical decision making.

CRITICAL THINKING DECISION PATH

Inferential Statistics—Relationship Questions

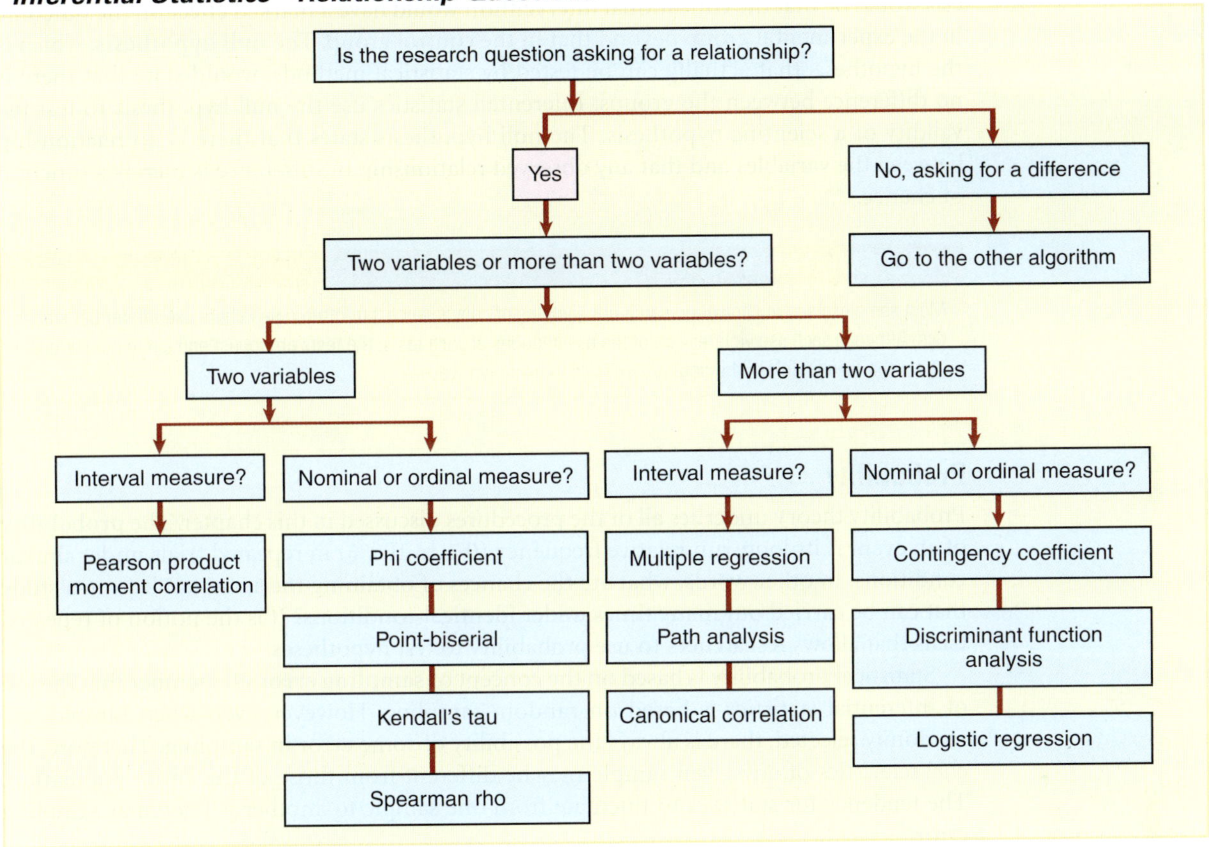

Hypothesis Testing

Inferential statistics are used for hypothesis testing. Statistical hypothesis testing allows researchers to make objective decisions about the data from their study. The use of statistical hypothesis testing answers questions such as the following: "How much of this effect is the result of chance?" "How strongly are these two variables associated with each other?" "What is the effect of the intervention?"

IPE HIGHLIGHT

Members of your interprofessional team may have diverse data analysis preparation. Capitalizing on everybody's background, try to figure out whether the statistical tests chosen for the studies your team is critically appraising are appropriate for the design, type of data collection, and level of measurement.

The procedures used when making inferences are based on principles of negative inference. In other words, if a researcher studied the effect of a new educational program for patients with chronic lung disease, the researcher would actually have two hypotheses: the scientific hypothesis and the null hypothesis. The research or **scientific hypothesis** is that which the researcher believes will be the outcome of the study. In our example, the scientific hypothesis would be that the educational intervention would have a marked effect on the outcome in the experimental group beyond that in the control group. The **null hypothesis**, which is the hypothesis that actually can be tested by statistical methods, would state that there is no difference between the groups. Inferential statistics use the null hypothesis to test the validity of a scientific hypothesis. The null hypothesis states that there is no relationship between the variables and that any observed relationship or difference is merely a function of chance.

HELPFUL HINT

Most samples used in clinical research are samples of convenience, but often researchers use inferential statistics. Although such use violates one of the assumptions of such tests, the tests are robust enough to not seriously affect the results unless the data are skewed in unknown ways.

Probability

Probability theory underlies all of the procedures discussed in this chapter. The **probability** of an event is its long-run relative frequency (0% to 100%) in repeated trials under similar conditions. In other words, what are the chances of obtaining the same result from a study that can be carried out many times under identical conditions? It is the notion of repeated trials that allows researchers to use probability to test hypotheses.

Statistical probability is based on the concept of **sampling error**. Remember that the use of inferential statistics is based on random sampling. However, even when samples are randomly selected, there is always the possibility of some error in sampling. Therefore, the characteristics of any given sample may be different from those of the entire population. The tendency for statistics to fluctuate from one sample to another is known as sampling error.

QSEN EVIDENCE-BASED PRACTICE TIP

The strength and quality of evidence are enhanced by repeated trials that have consistent findings, thereby increasing generalizability of the findings and applicability to clinical practice.

Type I and Type II Errors

Statistical inference is always based on incomplete information about a population, and it is possible for errors to occur. There are two types of errors in statistical inference—type I and type II errors. A **type I error** occurs when a researcher rejects a null hypothesis when it is actually true (i.e., accepts the premise that there is a difference when actually there is no difference between groups). A **type II error** occurs when a researcher accepts a null hypothesis that is actually false (i.e., accepts the premise that there is no difference between the groups when a difference actually exists). The relationship of the two types of errors is shown in Fig. 16.3.

When critiquing a study to see if there is a possibility of a type I error having occurred (rejecting the null hypothesis when it is actually true), one should consider the reliability

Conclusion of test of significance	REALITY	
	Null hypothesis is true	Null hypothesis is not true
Not statistically significant	Correct conclusion	Type II error
Statistically significant	Type I error	Correct conclusion

FIG 16.3 Outcome of statistical decision making.

and validity of the instruments used. For example, if the instruments did not accurately measure the intervention variables, one could conclude that the intervention made a difference when in reality it did not. It is critical to consider the reliability and validity of all the measurement instruments reported (see Chapter 15). For example, Turner-Sack and colleagues (2016) reported the reliability of the BSI in their sample and found it was reliable, as evidenced by a Cronbach's alpha, of 0.97 for survivors and siblings and 0.98 for parents (refer to Chapter 15 to review scale reliability). This gives the reader greater confidence in the study's results.

In a practice discipline, type I errors usually are considered more serious because if a researcher declares that differences exist where none are present, the potential exists for patient care to be affected adversely. Type II errors (accepting the null hypothesis when it is false) often occur when the sample is too small, thereby limiting the opportunity to measure *the treatment effect*, the true difference between two groups. A larger sample size improves the ability to *detect the treatment effect*—that is, the difference between two groups. If no significant difference is found between two groups with a large sample, it provides stronger evidence (than with a small sample) not to reject the null hypothesis.

Level of Significance

The researcher does not know when an error in statistical decision making has occurred. It is possible to know only that the null hypothesis is indeed true or false if data from the total population are available. However, the researcher can control the risk of making type I errors by setting the level of significance before the study begins (a priori).

The **level of significance (alpha level)** is the probability of making a type I error, the probability of rejecting a true null hypothesis. The minimum level of significance acceptable for most research is .05. If the researcher sets alpha, or the level of significance, at .05, the researcher is willing to accept the fact that if the study were done 100 times, the decision to reject the null hypothesis would be wrong 5 times out of those 100 trials. As is sometimes the case, if the researcher wants to have a smaller risk of rejecting a true null hypothesis, the level of significance may be set at .01. In this case the researcher is willing to be wrong only once in 100 trials.

The decision as to how strictly the alpha level should be set depends on how important it is to avoid errors. For example, if the results of a study are to be used to determine whether a great deal of money should be spent in an area of patient care, the researcher may decide that the accuracy of the results is so important that an alpha level of .01 is needed. In most studies, however, alpha is set at .05.

Perhaps you are thinking that researchers should always use the lowest alpha level possible to keep the risk of both types of errors at a minimum. Unfortunately, decreasing the risk of making a type I error increases the risk of making a type II error. Therefore the researcher always has to accept more of a risk of one type of error when setting the alpha level.

HELPFUL HINT

Decreasing the alpha level acceptable for a study increases the chance that a type II error will occur. When a researcher is doing many statistical tests, the probability of some of the tests being significant increases as the number of tests increases. Therefore, when a number of tests are being conducted, the researcher may decrease the alpha level to .01.

Clinical and Statistical Significance

It is important for you to realize that there is a difference between statistical significance and clinical significance. When a researcher tests a hypothesis and finds that it is statistically significant, it means that the finding is unlikely to have happened by chance. For example, if a study was designed to test an intervention to help a large sample of patients lose weight, and the researchers found that a change in weight of 1.02 pounds was statistically significant, one might find this questionable because few would say that a change in weight of just over 1 pound would represent a clinically significant difference. Therefore as a consumer of research it is important for you to evaluate the clinical significance as well as the statistical significance of findings.

Some people believe that if findings are not statistically significant, they have no practical value. However, knowing that something does not work is important information to share with the scientific community. Nonsupported hypotheses provide as much information about the intervention as supported hypotheses. Nonsignificant results (sometimes called negative findings) force the researcher to return to the literature and consider alternative explanations for why the intervention did not work as planned.

QSEN EVIDENCE-BASED PRACTICE TIP

You will study the results to determine whether the new treatment is effective, the size of the effect, and whether the effect is clinically important.

Parametric and Nonparametric Statistics

Tests of significance may be parametric or nonparametric. **Parametric statistics** have the following attributes:

1. Involve the estimation of at least one population parameter
2. Require measurement on at least an interval scale
3. Involve certain assumptions about the variables being studied

One important assumption is that the variable is normally distributed in the overall population.

In contrast to parametric tests, **nonparametric statistics** are not based on the estimation of population parameters, so they involve less restrictive assumptions about the underlying distribution. Nonparametric tests usually are applied when the variables have been measured on a nominal or ordinal scale, or when the distribution of scores is severely skewed.

HELPFUL HINT

Just because a researcher has used nonparametric statistics does not mean that the study is not useful. The use of nonparametric statistics is appropriate when measurements are not made at the interval level or the variable under study is not normally distributed.

There has been some debate about the relative merits of the two types of statistical tests. The moderate position taken by most researchers and statisticians is that nonparametric statistics are best used when data are not at the interval level of measurement, when the sample is small, and data do not approximate a normal distribution. However, most researchers prefer to use parametric statistics whenever possible (as long as data meet the assumptions) because they are more powerful and more flexible than nonparametric statistics.

Tables 16.3 and 16.4 list the commonly used inferential statistics. The test used depends on the level of the measurement of the variables in question and the type of hypothesis being studied. These statistics test two types of hypotheses: that there is a difference between groups (see Table 16.3) or that there is a relationship between two or more variables (see Table 16.4).

QSEN EVIDENCE-BASED PRACTICE TIP

Try to discern whether the test chosen for analyzing the data was chosen because it gave a significant *p* value. A statistical test should be chosen on the basis of its appropriateness for the type of data collected, not because it gives the answer that the researcher hoped to obtain.

TABLE 16.3 Tests of Differences Between Means

Level of Measurement	One Group	TWO GROUPS: Related	TWO GROUPS: Independent	More Than Two Groups
Nonparametric				
Nominal	Chi-square	Chi-square Fisher exact probability	Chi-square	Chi-square
Ordinal	Kolmogorov-Smirnov	Sign test Wilcoxon matched pairs Signed rank	Chi-square Median test Mann-Whitney *U* test	Chi-square
Parametric				
Interval or ratio	Correlated *t* ANOVA (repeated measures)	Correlated *t*	Independent *t* ANOVA	ANOVA ANCOVA MANOVA

ANOVA, Analysis of variance; *ANCOVA,* analysis of covariance; *MANOVA,* multiple analysis of variance.

TABLE 16.4 Tests of Association

Level of Measurement	Two Variables	More Than Two Variables
Nonparametric		
Nominal	Phi coefficient Point-biserial	Contingency coefficient
Ordinal	Kendall's tau Spearman rho	Discriminant function analysis
Parametric		
Interval or ratio	Pearson *r*	Multiple regression Path analysis Canonical correlation

Tests of Difference

The type of test used for any particular study depends primarily on whether the researcher is examining differences in one, two, or three or more groups and whether the data to be analyzed are nominal, ordinal, or interval (see Table 16.3). Suppose a researcher has conducted an experimental study (see Chapter 9). What the researcher hopes to determine is that the two randomly assigned groups are different after the introduction of the experimental treatment. If the measurements taken are at the interval level, the researcher would use the *t* test to analyze the data. If the *t* statistic was found to be high enough as to be unlikely to have occurred by chance, the researcher would reject the null hypothesis and conclude that the two groups were indeed more different than would have been expected on the basis of chance alone. In other words, the researcher would conclude that the experimental treatment had the desired effect.

QSEN EVIDENCE-BASED PRACTICE TIP

Tests of difference are most commonly used in experimental and quasi-experimental designs that provide Level II and Level III evidence.

The ***t* statistic** tests whether two group means are different. Thus this statistic is used when the researcher has two groups, and the question is whether the mean scores on some measure are more different than would be expected by chance. To use this test, the dependent variable (DV) must have been measured at the interval or ratio level, and the two groups must be independent. By independent we mean that nothing in one group helps determine who is in the other group. If the groups are related, as when samples are matched, and the researcher also wants to determine differences between the two groups, a paired or correlated *t* test would be used. The **degrees of freedom** (represents the freedom of a score's value to vary given what is known about the other scores and the sum of scores; often $df = N - 1$) are reported with the *t* statistic and the probability value (p). Degrees of freedom is usually abbreviated as *df*.

The *t* statistic illustrates one of the major purposes of research in nursing—to demonstrate that there are differences between groups. Groups may be naturally occurring collections, such as gender, or they may be experimentally created, such as the treatment and control groups. Sometimes a researcher has more than two groups, or measurements are taken more than once, and then **analysis of variance** (ANOVA) is used. ANOVA is similar to the *t* test. Like the *t* statistic, ANOVA tests whether group means differ, but rather than testing each pair of means separately, ANOVA considers the variation between groups and within groups.

HELPFUL HINT

A research report may not always contain the test that was done. You can find this information by looking at the tables. For example, a table with *t* statistics will contain a column for "*t*" values, and an ANOVA table will contain "*F*" values.

Analysis of covariance (ANCOVA) is used to measure differences among group means, but it also uses a statistical technique to equate the groups under study on an important variable. Another expansion of the notion of ANOVA is **multiple analysis of variance** (MANOVA), which also is used to determine differences in group means, but it is used when there is more than one DV.

Nonparametric Statistics

When data are at the nominal level and the researcher wants to determine whether groups are different, the researcher uses the **chi-square (χ^2)**. Chi-square is a nonparametric statistic used to determine whether the frequency in each category is different from what would be expected by chance. As with the *t* test and ANOVA, if the calculated chi-square is high enough, the researcher would conclude that the frequencies found would not be expected on the basis of chance alone, and the null hypothesis would be rejected. Although this test is quite robust and can be used in many different situations, it cannot be used to compare frequencies when samples are small and expected frequencies are less than six in each cell. In these instances the **Fisher exact probability test** is used.

When the data are ranks, or are at the ordinal level, researchers have several other nonparametric tests at their disposal. These include the *Kolmogorov-Smirnov test*, the *sign test*, the *Wilcoxon matched pairs test*, the *signed rank test for related groups*, the *median test*, and the *Mann-Whitney U test for independent groups*. Explanation of these tests is beyond the scope of this chapter; those readers who desire further information should consult a general statistics book.

HELPFUL HINT

Chi-square is the test of difference commonly used for nominal level demographic variables such as gender, marital status, religion, ethnicity, and others.

Tests of Relationships

Researchers often are interested in exploring the *relationship* between two or more variables. Such studies use statistics that determine the **correlation**, or the degree of association, between two or more variables. Tests of the relationships between variables are sometimes considered to be descriptive statistics when they are used to describe the magnitude and direction of a relationship of two variables in a sample and the researcher does not wish to make statements about the larger population. Such statistics also can be inferential when they are used to test hypotheses about the correlations that exist in the target population.

QSEN EVIDENCE-BASED PRACTICE TIP

You will often note that in the results or findings section of a research study, parametric (e.g., *t* tests, ANOVA) and nonparametric (e.g., chi-square, Fisher exact probability test) measures will be used to test differences among variables depending on their level of measurement. For example, chi-square may be used to test differences among nominal level demographic variables, *t* tests will be used to test the hypotheses or research questions about differences between two groups, and ANOVA will be used to test differences among groups when there are multiple comparisons.

Null hypothesis tests of the relationships between variables assume that there is no relationship between the variables. Thus when a researcher rejects this type of null hypothesis, the conclusion is that the variables are in fact related. Suppose a researcher is interested in the relationship between the age of patients and the length of time it takes them to recover from surgery. As with other statistics discussed, the researcher would design a study to collect the appropriate data and then analyze the data using measures of association. In this example, age and length of time until recovery would be considered interval-level measurements. The researcher would use a test called the **Pearson correlation coefficient**, **Pearson *r***, or **Pearson product moment correlation coefficient**. Once the Pearson *r* is calculated, the researcher consults the distribution for this test to determine whether the value obtained is likely to have occurred by chance. Again, the research reports both the value of the correlation and its probability of occurring by chance.

Correlation coefficients can range in value from −1.0 to +1.0 and also can be zero. A zero coefficient means that there is no relationship between the variables. *A perfect positive correlation* is indicated by a +1.0 coefficient, and a *perfect negative correlation* by a −1.0 coefficient. We can illustrate the meaning of these coefficients by using the example from the previous paragraph. If there were no relationship between the age of the patient and the time required for the patient to recover from surgery, the researcher would find a correlation of zero. However, if the correlation was +1.0, it would mean that the older the patient, the longer the recovery time. A negative coefficient would imply that the younger the patient, the longer the recovery time.

Of course, relationships are rarely perfect. The magnitude of the relationship is indicated by how close the correlation comes to the absolute value of 1. Thus a correlation of −.76 is just as strong as a correlation of +.76, but the direction of the relationship is opposite. In addition, a correlation of .76 is stronger than a correlation of .32. When a researcher tests hypotheses about the relationships between two variables, the test considers whether the magnitude of the correlation is large enough not to have occurred by chance. This is the meaning of the probability value or the *p* value reported with correlation coefficients. As with other statistical tests of significance, the larger the sample, the greater the likelihood of finding a significant correlation. Therefore researchers also report the *df* associated with the test performed.

Nominal and ordinal data also can be tested for relationships by nonparametric statistics. When two variables being tested have only two levels (e.g., male/female; yes/no), the *phi coefficient* can be used to test relationships. When the researcher is interested in the relationship between a nominal variable and an interval variable, the *point-biserial correlation* is used. *Spearman rho* is used to determine the degree of association between two sets of ranks, as is *Kendall's tau*. All of these correlation coefficients may range in value from −1.0 to +1.0.

> **QSEN EVIDENCE-BASED PRACTICE TIP**
>
> Tests of relationship are usually associated with nonexperimental designs that provide Level IV evidence. Establishing a strong statistically significant relationship between variables often lends support for replicating the study to increase the consistency of the findings and provide a foundation for developing an intervention study.

Advanced Statistics

Nurse researchers are often interested in health problems that are very complex and require that we analyze many different variables at once using advanced statistical procedures called **multivariate statistics**. Computer software has made the use of multivariate statistics quite accessible to researchers. When researchers are interested in understanding more about a problem than just the relationship between two variables, they often use a technique called **multiple regression**, which measures the relationship between one interval-level DV and several independent variables (IVs). Multiple regression is the expansion of correlation to include more than two variables, and it is used when the researcher wants to determine what variables contribute to the explanation of the DV and to what degree. For example, a researcher may be interested in determining what factors help women decide to breastfeed their infants. A number of variables, such as the mother's age, previous experience with breastfeeding, number of other children, and knowledge of the advantages of breastfeeding, might be measured and analyzed to see whether they separately and together predict the duration of breastfeeding. Such a study would require the use of multiple regression.

Another advanced technique often used in nursing research is **factor analysis**. There are two types of factor analysis, exploratory and confirmatory factor analysis. Exploratory factor analysis is used to reduce a set of data so that it may be easily described and used. It is also used in the early phases of instrument development and theory development. Factor analysis is used to determine whether a scale actually measured the concepts that it is intended to measure. Confirmatory factor analysis resembles structural equation modeling and is used in instrument development to examine construct validity and reliability and to compare factor structures across groups (Plichta & Kelvin, 2012).

Many studies use statistical modeling procedures to answer research questions. Causal modeling is used most often when researchers want to test hypotheses and theoretically derived relationships. *Path analysis, structured equation modeling (SEM), and linear structural relations analysis (LISREL)* are different types of modeling procedures used in nursing research.

Many other statistical techniques are available for nurse researchers. It is beyond the scope of this chapter to review all statistical analyses available. You should consider having several statistical texts available to you as you sort through the evidence reported in studies that are important to your clinical practice (e.g., Field, 2013; Plichta & Kelvin, 2012).

APPRAISAL FOR EVIDENCE-BASED PRACTICE DESCRIPTIVE AND INFERENTIAL STATISTICS

Nurses are challenged to understand the results of studies that use sophisticated statistical procedures. Understanding the principles that guide statistical analysis is the first step in this process. Statistics are used to describe the samples of studies and to test for hypothesized differences or associations in the sample. Knowing the characteristics of the sample of a study allows you to determine whether the results are potentially useful for your patients. For example, if a study sample was primarily white with a mean age of 42 years (SD 2.5), the findings may not be applicable if your patients are mostly elderly and African American. Cultural, demographic, or clinical factors of an elderly population of a different ethnic group may contribute to different results. Thus understanding the descriptive statistics of a study will assist you in determining the applicability of findings to your practice setting.

Statistics are also used to test hypotheses. Inferential statistics used to analyze data and the associated significance level (p values) indicate the likelihood that the association or difference found in a study is due to chance or to a true difference among groups. The closer the p value is to zero, the less likely the association or difference of a study is due to chance. Thus inferential statistics provide an objective way to determine if the results of the study are likely to be a true representation of reality. However, it is still important for you to judge the clinical significance of the findings. Was there a big enough effect (difference between the experimental and control groups) to warrant changing current practice?

The systematic review and meta-analysis by Al-Mallah and colleagues (2016; Appendix E) provides an excellent example of how a meta-analysis (the summarization of many studies)

CRITICAL APPRAISAL CRITERIA

Descriptive and Inferential Statistics

1. Were appropriate descriptive statistics used?
2. What level of measurement was used to measure each of the major variables?
3. Is the sample size large enough to prevent one extreme score from affecting the summary statistics used?
4. What descriptive statistics are reported?
5. Were these descriptive statistics appropriate to the level of measurement for each variable?
6. Are there appropriate summary statistics for each major variable (e.g., demographic variables) and any other relevant data?
7. Does the hypothesis indicate that the researcher is interested in testing for differences between groups or in testing for relationships? What is the level of significance?
8. Does the level of measurement permit the use of parametric statistics?
9. Is the size of the sample large enough to permit the use of parametric statistics?
10. Has the researcher provided enough information to decide whether the appropriate statistics were used?
11. Are the statistics used appropriate to the hypothesis, the research question, the method, the sample, and the level of measurement?
12. Are the results for each of the research questions or hypotheses presented clearly and appropriately?
13. If tables and graphs are used, do they agree with the text and extend it, or do they merely repeat it?
14. Are the results understandable?
15. Is a distinction made between clinical significance and statistical significance? How is it made?

can help us understand the mortality and morbidity of patients who are cared for at nurse-led clinics.

QSEN EVIDENCE-BASED PRACTICE TIP

A basic understanding of statistics will improve your ability to think about the effect of the IV on the DV and related patient outcomes for your patient population and practice setting.

There are a few steps to follow when critiquing the statistics used in studies (see the Critical Appraisal Criteria box). Before a decision can be made as to whether the statistics that were used make sense, it is important to return to the beginning of the research study and review the purpose of the study. Just as the hypotheses or research questions should flow from the purpose of a study, so should the hypotheses or research questions suggest the type of analysis that will follow. The hypotheses or the research questions should indicate the major variables that are expected to be tested and presented in the "Results" section. Both the summary descriptive statistics and the results of the inferential testing of each of the variables should be in the "Results" section with appropriate information.

After reviewing the hypotheses or research questions, you should proceed to the "Methods" section. Next, try to determine the level of measurement for each variable. From this information it is possible to determine the measures of central tendency and variability that should be used to summarize the data. For example, you would not expect to see a mean used as a summary statistic for the nominal variable of gender. In all likelihood, gender would be reported as a frequency distribution. However, you would expect to find a mean and SD for a variable that used a questionnaire. The means and SD should be provided for measurements performed at the interval level. The sample size is another aspect of the "Methods" section that is important to review when evaluating the researcher's use of descriptive statistics. The sample is usually described using descriptive summary statistics. Remember, the larger the sample, the less chance that one outlying score will affect the summary statistics. It is also important to note whether the researchers indicated that they did a power analysis to estimate the sample size needed to conduct the study.

If tables or graphs are used, they should agree with the information presented in the text. Evaluate whether the tables and graphs are clearly labeled. If the researcher presents grouped frequency data, the groups should be logical and mutually exclusive. The size of the interval in grouped data should not obscure the pattern of the data, nor should it create an artificial pattern. Each table and graph should be referred to in the text, but each should add to the text—not merely repeat it.

The following are some simple steps for reading a table:

1. Look at the title of the table and see if it matches the purpose of the table.
2. Review the column headings and assess whether the headings follow logically from the title.
3. Look at the abbreviations used. Are they clear and easy to understand? Are any nonstandard abbreviations explained?
4. Evaluate whether the statistics contained in the table are appropriate to the level of measurement for each variable.

After evaluating the descriptive statistics, inferential statistics can then be evaluated. The best place to begin appraising the inferential statistical analysis of a research study is with the hypothesis or research question. If the hypothesis or research question indicates that a relationship will be found, you should expect to find tests of correlation. If the study is experimental or quasi-experimental, the hypothesis or research question would indicate that the author is looking for significant differences between the groups studied, and you would expect to find statistical tests of differences between means that test the effect of the intervention. Then as you read the "Methods" section of the paper, again consider what level of measurement the author has used to measure the important variables. If the level of measurement is interval or ratio, the statistics most likely will be parametric statistics. On the other hand, if the variables are measured at the nominal or ordinal level, the statistics used should be nonparametric. Also consider the size of the sample, and remember that samples have to be large enough to permit the assumption of normality. If the sample is quite small (e.g., 5 to 10 subjects), the researcher may have violated the assumptions necessary for inferential statistics to be used. Thus the important question is whether the researcher has provided enough justification to use the statistics presented.

Finally, consider the results as they are presented. There should be enough data presented for each hypothesis or research question studied to determine whether the researcher actually examined each hypothesis or research question. The tables should accurately reflect the procedure performed and be in harmony with the text. For example, the text should not indicate that a test reached statistical significance while the tables indicate that the probability value of the test was above .05. If the researcher has used analyses that are not discussed in this text, you may want to refer to a statistics text to decide whether the analysis was appropriate to the hypothesis or research question and the level of measurement.

There are two other aspects of the data analysis section that you should appraise. The results of the study in the text of the article should be clear. In addition, the author should attempt to make a distinction between the clinical and statistical significance of the evidence related to the findings. Some results may be statistically significant, but their clinical importance may be doubtful in terms of applicability for a patient population or clinical setting. If this is so, the author should note it. Alternatively, you may find yourself reading a research study that is elegantly presented, but you come away with a "So what?" feeling. From an evidence-based practice perspective, a significant hypothesis or research question should contribute to improving patient care and clinical outcomes. The important question to ask is "What is the strength and quality of the evidence provided by the findings of this study and their applicability to practice?"

Note that the critical analysis of a research paper's statistical analysis is not done in a vacuum. It is possible to judge the adequacy of the analysis only in relationship to the other important aspects of the paper: the problem, the hypotheses, the research question, the design, the data collection methods, and the sample. Without consideration of these aspects of the research process, the statistics themselves have very little meaning.

KEY POINTS

- Descriptive statistics are a means of describing and organizing data gathered in research.
- The four levels of measurement are nominal, ordinal, interval, and ratio. Each has appropriate descriptive techniques associated with it.
- Measures of central tendency describe the average member of a sample. The mode is the most frequent score, the median is the middle score, and the mean is the arithmetical average of the scores. The mean is the most stable and useful of the measures of central

tendency and, combined with the standard deviation, forms the basis for many of the inferential statistics.

- The frequency distribution presents data in tabular or graphic form and allows for the calculation or observations of characteristics of the distribution of the data, including skew symmetry, and modality.
- In nonsymmetrical distributions, the degree and direction of the off-center peak are described in terms of positive or negative skew.
- The range reflects differences between high and low scores.
- The SD is the most stable and useful measure of variability. It is derived from the concept of the normal curve. In the normal curve, sample scores and the means of large numbers of samples group themselves around the midpoint in the distribution, with a fixed percentage of the scores falling within given distances of the mean. This tendency of means to approximate the normal curve is called the sampling distribution of the means.
- Inferential statistics are a tool to test hypotheses about populations from sample data.
- Because the sampling distribution of the means follows a normal curve, researchers are able to estimate the probability that a certain sample will have the same properties as the total population of interest. Sampling distributions provide the basis for all inferential statistics.
- Inferential statistics allow researchers to estimate population parameters and to test hypotheses. The use of these statistics allows researchers to make objective decisions about the outcome of the study. Such decisions are based on the rejection or acceptance of the null hypothesis, which states that there is no relationship between the variables.
- If the null hypothesis is accepted, this result indicates that the findings are likely to have occurred by chance. If the null hypothesis is rejected, the researcher accepts the scientific hypothesis that a relationship exists between the variables that is unlikely to have been found by chance.
- Statistical hypothesis testing is subject to two types of errors: type I and type II.
- A type I error occurs when the researcher rejects a null hypothesis that is actually true.
- A type II error occurs when the researcher accepts a null hypothesis that is actually false.
- The researcher controls the risk of making a type I error by setting the alpha level, or level of significance; however, reducing the risk of a type I error by reducing the level of significance increases the risk of making a type II error.
- The results of statistical tests are reported to be significant or nonsignificant. Statistically significant results are those whose probability of occurring is less than .05 or .01, depending on the level of significance set by the researcher.
- Commonly used parametric and nonparametric statistical tests include those that test for differences between means, such as the *t* test and ANOVA, and those that test for differences in proportions, such as the chi-square test.
- Tests that examine data for the presence of relationships include the Pearson *r*, the sign test, the Wilcoxon matched pairs, signed rank test, and multiple regression.
- The most important aspect of critiquing statistical analyses is the relationship of the statistics employed to the problem, design, and method used in the study. Clues to the appropriate statistical test to be used by the researcher should stem from the researcher's hypotheses. The reader also should determine if all of the hypotheses have been presented in the paper.
- A basic understanding of statistics will improve your ability to think about the level of evidence provided by the study design and findings and their relevance to patient outcomes for your patient population and practice setting.

CRITICAL THINKING CHALLENGES

- When reading a research study, what is the significance of applying findings if a nurse researcher made a type I error in statistical inference?
- What is the relationship between the level of measurement a researcher uses and the choice of statistics used? As you read a research study, identify the statistics, level of measurement, and the associated level of evidence provided by the design.
- When reviewing a study you find the sample size provided does not seem adequate. Before you make this final decision, think about how the design type (e.g., pilot study, intervention study), data collection methods, the number of variables, and the sensitivity of the data collection instruments can affect your decision.
- IPE When your team finishes critically appraising a research study, those team members responsible for the critique report that the findings are not statistically significant. Consider how those findings are or are not applicable to your practice.

REFERENCES

Al-Mallah, M. H., Faraf, I., Al-Madani, W., et al. (2016). The impact of nurse-led clinics on mortality and morbidity of patients with cardiovascular diseases: a systematic review and meta-analysis. *Journal of Cardiovascular Nursing*, *31*, 89–95. doi:10.1097/JCN.0000000000000224.

Field, A. (2013). *Discovering statistics using SPSS* (4th ed.). Thousand Oaks, CA: Sage.

Hawthorne, D. M., Youngblut, J. M., & Brooten, D. (2016). Parent spirituality, grief, and mental health at 1-year and 3 months after their infant's/child's death in an intensive care unit. *Journal of Pediatric Nursing*, *31*, 73–80. doi:org/10.1016/j.pedn.2015.07.008.

Nyamathi, A., Salem, B. E., Zhang, S., et al. (2015). Nursing care management, peer coaching, and hepatitis A and B vaccine completion among homeless men recently released on parole. *Nursing Research*, *64*, 177–189. doi:10.1097/NNR.0000000000000083.

Plichta, S. B., & Kelvin, E. (2012). *Munro's statistical methods for health care research* (6th ed.). Philadelphia, PA: Lippincott Williams & Wilkins.

Turner-Sack, A. M., Menna, R., Setchell, S. R., et al. (2016). Psychological functioning, post traumatic growth, and coping in parents and siblings of adolescent cancer survivors. *Oncology Nursing Forum*, *43*, 48–57. doi:10.1188/16.ONF.48-56.

Go to Evolve at **http://evolve.elsevier.com/LoBiondo/** for review questions, critiquing exercises, and additional research articles for practice in reviewing and critiquing.

17

Understanding Research Findings

Geri LoBiondo-Wood

Go to Evolve at http://evolve.elsevier.com/LoBiondo/ for review questions, critiquing exercises, and additional research articles for practice in reviewing and critiquing.

LEARNING OUTCOMES

After reading this chapter, you should be able to do the following:

- Discuss the difference between the "Results" and the "Discussion" sections of a research study.
- Determine if findings are objectively discussed.
- Describe how tables and figures are used in a research report.
- List the criteria of a meaningful table.
- Identify the purpose and components of the "Discussion" section.
- Discuss the importance of including generalizability and limitations of a study in the report.
- Determine the purpose of including recommendations in the study report.
- Discuss how the strength, quality, and consistency of evidence provided by the findings are related to a study's results, limitations, generalizability, and applicability to practice.

KEY TERMS

confidence interval
findings
generalizability
limitations
recommendations

The ultimate goal of nursing research is to develop knowledge that advances evidence-based nursing practice and quality patient care. From a clinical application perspective, analysis, interpretation, discussion, and generalizability of the results become highly important pieces of the research study. After the analysis of the data, the researcher puts the final pieces of the jigsaw puzzle together to view the total picture with a critical eye. This process is analogous to evaluation, the last step in the nursing process. You may view these last sections as an easier step for the investigator, but it is here that a most critical and creative process comes to the forefront. In the final sections of the report, after the statistical procedures have been applied, the researcher relates the findings to the research question, hypotheses, theoretical framework, literature, methods, and analyses; reviews the findings for any potential bias; and makes decisions about the application of the findings to future research and practice.

The final sections of published studies are generally titled "Results" and "Discussion." Other topics, such as conclusions, limitations of findings, recommendations, and implications for future research and nursing practice, may be addressed separately or included in these sections. The presentation format is a function of the author's and the journal's stylistic considerations. The function of these final sections is to integrate all aspects of the research process, as well as to discuss, interpret, and identify the limitations, the threats related to bias, and the generalizability relevant to the investigation, thereby furthering evidence-based practice. The process that both an investigator and you use to assess the results of a study is depicted in the Critical Thinking Decision Path.

The goal of this chapter is to introduce the purpose and content of the final sections of a research study where data are presented, interpreted, discussed, and generalized.

FINDINGS

The **findings** of a study are the results, conclusions, interpretations, recommendations, and implications for future research and nursing practice, which are addressed by separating the presentation into two major areas. These two areas are the results and the discussion of the results. The "Results" section focuses on the results or statistical findings of a study, and the "Discussion" section focuses on the remaining topics. For both sections, the rule applies—as it does to all other sections of a report—that the content must be presented clearly, concisely, and logically.

QSEN EVIDENCE-BASED PRACTICE TIP

Evidence-based practice is an active process that requires you to consider how, and if, research findings are applicable to your patient population and practice setting.

Results

The "Results" section of a study is the data-bound section of the report and is where the quantitative data or numbers generated by the descriptive and inferential statistical tests are presented. Other headings that may be used for the results section are "Statistical Analyses," "Data Analysis," or "Analysis." The results of the data analysis set the stage for the interpretation or discussion and the limitations sections that follow the results. The "Results" section should reflect analysis of each research question and/or hypothesis tested. The information from each hypothesis or research question should be sequentially presented. The tests used to analyze the data should be identified. If the exact test that was used is not explicitly stated, the values obtained should be noted. The researcher does this by providing the numerical values of the statistics and stating the specific test value and probability level achieved (see Chapter 16). **Examples** ➤ of these statistical results can be found in Table 17.1. The numbers are important, but there is much more to the research process than the numbers. They are one piece of the whole. Chapter 16 conceptually presents the meanings of the numbers found in studies. Whether you only superficially understand statistics or have an in-depth knowledge of statistics, it should be obvious that the results are clearly stated, and the presence or lack of statistically significant results should be noted.

TABLE 17.1 Examples of Reported Statistical Results

Statistical Test	Examples of Reported Results
Mean	$m = 118.28$
Standard deviation	SD = 62.5
Pearson correlation	$r = .49, P < .01$
Analysis of variance	$F = 3.59, df = 2, 48, P < .05$
t test	$t = 2.65, P < .01$
Chi-square	$\chi^2 = 2.52, df = 1, P < .05$

CRITICAL THINKING DECISION PATH

Assessing Study Results

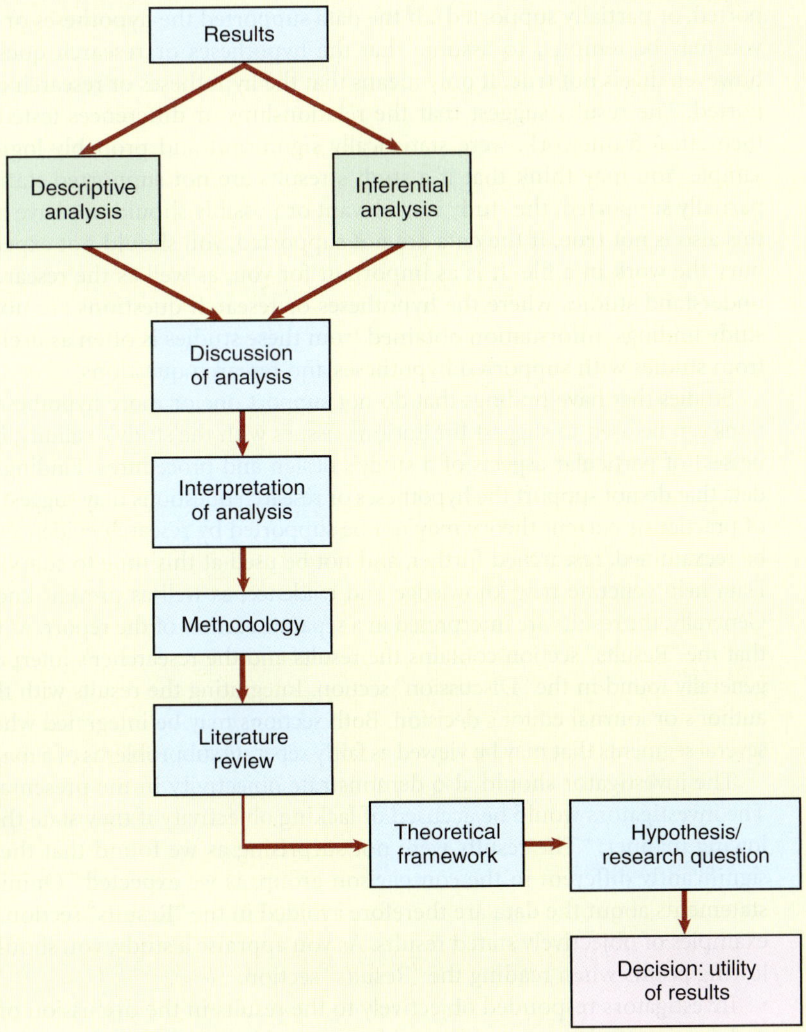

HELPFUL HINT

In the results section of a research report, the descriptive statistics results are generally presented first; then the inferential results of each hypothesis or research question that was tested are presented.

At times the researchers will begin the "Results" or "Data Analysis" section by identifying the name of the statistical software program they used to analyze the data. This is not a statistical test but a computer program specifically designed to analyze a variety of statistical tests. **Example:** ➤ Li and colleagues (2016) state that "SPSS version 22.0 software and *Mplus7* were used for the statistical analysis" (see Chapter 16). Information on the statistical tests used is presented after this information.

The researcher will present the data for all of the hypotheses tested or research questions asked (e.g., whether the hypotheses or research questions were accepted, rejected, supported, or partially supported). If the data supported the hypotheses or research questions, you may be tempted to assume that the hypotheses or research questions were *proven;* however, this is not true. It only means that the hypotheses or research questions were supported. The results suggest that the relationships or differences tested, derived from the theoretical framework, were statistically significant and probably logical for that study's sample. You may think that if a study's results are not supported statistically or are only partially supported, the study is irrelevant or possibly should not have been published, but this also is not true. If the data are not supported, you should not expect the researcher to bury the work in a file. It is as important for you, as well as the researcher, to review and understand studies where the hypotheses or research questions are not supported by the study findings. Information obtained from these studies is often as useful as data obtained from studies with supported hypotheses and research questions.

Studies that have findings that do not support one or more hypotheses or research questions can be used to suggest **limitations** (issues with the study's validity, bias, or study weaknesses) of particular aspects of a study's design and procedures. Findings from studies with data that do not support the hypotheses or research questions may suggest that current modes of practice or current theory may not be supported by research evidence and therefore must be reexamined, researched further, and not be used at this time to support practice changes. Data help generate new knowledge and evidence, as well as prevent knowledge stagnation. Generally, the results are interpreted in a separate section of the report. At times, you may find that the "Results" section contains the results and the researcher's interpretations, which are generally found in the "Discussion" section. Integrating the results with the discussion is the author's or journal editor's decision. Both sections may be integrated when a study contains several segments that may be viewed as fairly separate subproblems of a major overall problem.

The investigator should also demonstrate objectivity in the presentation of the results. The investigators would be accused of lacking objectivity if they state the results in the following manner: "The results were not surprising as we found that the mean scores were significantly different in the comparison group, as we expected." Opinions or reactionary statements about the data are therefore avoided in the "Results" section. Box 17.1 provides examples of objectively stated results. As you appraise a study, you should consider the following points when reading the "Results" section:

- Investigators responded objectively to the results in the discussion of the findings.
- Investigators interpreted the evidence provided by the results, with a careful reflection on all aspects of the study that preceded the results. Data presented are summarized.

BOX 17.1 Examples of Results Section

- "Parents' psychological distress was positively associated with age ($r = 0.53$, $P < 0.01$) and avoidant coping (e.g., denial, disengagement) ($r = 0.53$, $P < 0.01$)" (Turner-Sack et al., 2016).
- "Bereaved fathers' greater use of spiritual activities was significantly related to lower symptoms of grief (despair, detachment and disorganization at T1 and T2 [Table 2])" (Hawthorne et al., 2012).

Much data are generated, but only the critical summary numbers for each test are presented. Examples of summarized demographic data are the means and standard deviations of age, education, and income. Including all data is too cumbersome. The results should be viewed as a summary.

- Reduction of data is provided in the text and through the use of tables and figures. Tables and figures facilitate the presentation of large amounts of data.
- Results for the descriptive and inferential statistics for each hypothesis or research question are presented. No data are omitted, even if they are not significant. Untoward events during the course of the study should be reported.

In their study, Hawthorne and colleagues (2016) developed tables to present the results visually. Table 17.2 provides a portion of the descriptive results about the subjects' demographics. Table 17.3 provides the correlations among the study's variables. Tables allow researchers to provide a more visually thorough explanation and discussion of the results. If tables and figures are used, they must be concise. Although the article's text is the major mode of communicating the results, the tables and figures serve a supplementary but independent role. The role of tables and figures is to report results with some detail that the investigator does not explore in the text. This does not mean that tables and figures should not be mentioned in the text. The amount of detail that an author uses in the text to describe the specific tabled data varies according to the needs of the author. A good table is one that meets the following criteria:

- Supplements and economizes the text
- Has precise titles and headings
- Does not repeat the text

TABLE 17.2 Description of the Sample

Characteristic	Mothers (n = 114)	Fathers (n = 51)
Age [*m* (SD)]	31.1 (7.73)	36.8 (9.32)
Race [*n* (%)]		
White non-Hispanic	22 (19)	14 (28)
Black non-Hispanic	50 (44)	16 (31)
Hispanic	42 (37)	21 (41)
Education [*n* (%)]		
Less than high school	12 (11)	7 (14)
High school graduate	31 (27)	13 (25)
Some college	36 (32)	12 (24)
College degree	35 (30)	19 (37)

From Hawthorne, D. M., Youngblut, J. M., & Brooten, D. (2016). Parent spirituality, grief, and mental health at 1 and 3 months after their infant's/child's death in an intensive care unit. *Journal of Pediatric Nursing, 31*, 73–80.

TABLE 17.3 Correlations of Parents' Use of Spiritual and Religious Activities With Grief, Mental Health, and Personal Growth at 1 (T1) and 3 (T2) Months Post-Death

		SPIRITUAL ACTIVITIES		RELIGIOUS ACTIVITIES	
Parent Outcome	Time Point	Mothers (n = 108)	Fathers (n = 50)	Mothers (n = 108)	Fathers (n = 50)
Grief					
Despair	T1	−.54**	−.47**	−.18	−.32**
	T2	−.51**	−.29*	−.11	−.15
Detachment	T1	−.56**	−.61**	−.19	−.26*
	T2	−.53**	−.35**	−.02	−.10
Disorganization	T1	−.41**	−.43**	−.02	−.25*
	T2	−.55**	−.23*	−.02	−.10
Depression	T1	−.54**	−.46**	−.19	−.27*
	T2	−.55**	−.39**	−.14	−.01
PTSD	T1	−.30**	−.29	−.10	−.12
	T2	−.35**	−.07	−.08	−.03
Personal growth	T1	−.51**	.51**	.42**	.10
	T2	−.64**	.49**	.37**	.31**

*$P < .05$.
**$P < .01$.
From Hawthorne, D. M., Youngblut, J. M., & Brooten, D. (2016). Parent spirituality, grief, and mental health at 1 and 3 months after their infant's/child's death in an intensive care unit. *Journal of Pediatric Nursing, 31,* 73–80.

Tables are found in each of the studies in the appendices. Each of these tables helps to economize and supplement the text clearly, with precise data that help you to visualize the variables quickly and to assess the results.

QSEN EVIDENCE-BASED PRACTICE TIP

As you reflect on the results of a study, think about how the results fit with previous research on the topic and the strength and quality of available evidence on which to base clinical practice decisions.

Discussion

In this section, the investigator interprets and discusses the study's results. The researcher makes the data come alive and gives meaning to and provides interpretations for the numbers in quantitative studies or the concepts in qualitative studies. This discussion section contains a discussion of the findings, the study's **limitations**, and **recommendations** for practice and future research. At times these topics are separated as stand-alone sections of the research report, or they may be integrated under the title of "Discussion." You may ask where the investigator extracted the meaning that is applied in this section. If the researcher does the job properly, you will find a return to the beginning of the study. The researcher returns to the earlier points in the study where the purpose, objective, and research question and/or a hypothesis was identified, and independent and dependent variables were linked on the basis of a theoretical framework and literature review (see Chapters 3 and 4). It is in this section that the researcher discusses

- Both the supported and nonsupported data
- Limitations or weaknesses (threats to internal or external validity) of a study in light of the design, sample, instruments, data collection procedures, and fidelity
- How the theoretical framework was supported or not supported
- How the data may suggest additional or previously unrealized findings
- Strength and quality of the evidence provided by the study and its findings interpreted in relation to its applicability to practice and future research

Even if the data are supported, this is not the final word. Statistical significance is not the endpoint of a researcher's thinking; statistically significant but low *P* values may not be indicative of research breakthroughs. It is important to think beyond statistical significance to clinical significance. This means that statistical significance in a study does not always indicate that the results of a study are clinically significant. A key step in the process of evaluation is the ability to critically analyze beyond the test of significance by assessing a research study's applicability to practice. Chapters 19 through 21 review the methods used to analyze the usefulness and applicability of research findings. Within nursing and health care literature, discussion of clinical significance, evidence-based practice, and quality improvement are focal points (Titler, 2012). As indicated throughout this text, many important pieces in the research puzzle must fit together for a study to be evaluated as a well-done study. The evidence generated by the findings of a study is appraised in order to validate current practice or support the need for a change in practice. Results of unsupported hypotheses or research questions do not require the investigator to go on a fault-finding tour of each piece of the study—this can become an overdone process. All research studies have weaknesses as well as strengths. The final discussion is an attempt to identify the strengths as well as the weaknesses or bias of the study.

HELPFUL HINT

A well-written "Results" section is systematic, logical, concise, and drawn from all of the analyzed data. The writing in the "Results" section should allow the data to reflect the testing of the research questions and hypotheses. The length of this section depends on the scope and breadth of the analysis.

Researchers and appraisers should accept statistical significance with prudence. Statistically significant findings are not the sole means of establishing a study's merit. Remember that accepting statistical significance means accepting that the sample mean is the same as the population mean. Statistical significance is a measure of assessment that, if true, does not automatically support the merit to a study and, if untrue, does not necessarily negate the value of a study (see Chapter 12). Another method to assess the merit of a study and determine whether the findings from one study can be generalized is to calculate a **confidence interval**. A confidence interval quantifies the uncertainty of a statistic or the probable value range within which a population parameter is expected to lie (see Chapter 19). The process used to calculate a confidence interval is beyond the scope of this text, but references are provided for further explanation (Altman, 2005; Altman et al., 2005; Kline, 2004). Other aspects, such as the sample, instruments, data collection methods, and fidelity, must also be considered.

Whether the results are or are not statistically supported, in this section, the researcher returns to the conceptual/theoretical framework and analyzes each step of the research process to accomplish a discussion of the following issues:

- Suggest what the possible or actual problems are in the study.
- Whether findings are supported or not supported, the researcher is obliged to review the study's processes.
- Was the theoretical thinking correct? (See Chapters 3 and 4.)
- Was the correct design chosen? (See Chapters 9 and 10.)
- In terms of sampling methods (see Chapter 12), was the sample size adequate? Were the inclusion and exclusion criteria delineated well?
- Did any bias arise during the course of the study; that is, threats to internal and external validity? (See Chapter 8.)
- Was data collection consistent, and did it exhibit fidelity? (See Chapter 14.)
- Were the instruments sensitive to what was being tested? Were they reliable and valid? (See Chapters 14 and 15.)
- Were the analysis choices appropriate? (See Chapter 16.)

The purpose of this section is not to show humility or one's technical competence but rather to enable you to judge the validity of the interpretations drawn from the data and the general worth of the study. It is in this section of the report that the researcher ties together all the loose ends of the study and returns to the beginning to assess if the findings support, extend, or counter the theoretical framework of the study. It is from this point that you can begin to think about clinical relevance, the need for replication, or the germination of an idea for further research. The researcher also includes generalizability and recommendations for future research, as well as a summary or a conclusion.

Generalizations (**generalizability**) are inferences that the data are representative of similar phenomena in a population beyond the study's sample. Rarely, if ever, can one study be a recommendation for action. Beware of research studies that may overgeneralize. Generalizations that draw conclusions and make inferences for a specific group within a particular situation and at a particular time are appropriate. An **example** ➤ of such a limitation is drawn from the study conducted by Hawthorne and colleagues (2016; Appendix B). The researchers appropriately noted the following:

> *There are several additional limitations of the study. At 1 and 3 months post-death, parents were in early stages of grieving. Thus, these findings may not be applicable to parents who are later in the grieving process.*

This type of statement is important for consumers of research. It helps to guide our thinking in terms of a study's clinical relevance and also suggests areas for research. One study does not provide all of the answers, nor should it. In fact, the risk versus the benefit of the potential change in practice must be considered in terms of the strength and quality of the evidence (see Chapter 19). The greater the risk involved in making a change in practice, the stronger the evidence needs to be to justify the merit of implementing a practice change. The final steps of evaluation are critical links to the refinement of practice and the generation of future research. Evaluation of research, like evaluation of the nursing process, is not the last link in the chain but a connection between the strength of the evidence that may serve to improve patient care and inform clinical decision making and support an evidence-based practice.

BOX 17.2 Examples of Research Recommendations and Practice Implications

Research Recommendations

- "The findings support the need to continue examining the effects of childhood and adolescent cancer on the entire family. Additional studies would benefit from having all members of each family participate to obtain a true family systems perspective on the impact of childhood and adolescent cancer" (Turner-Sack et al., 2016).
- "Further research is needed to determine if any changes, whether negative or positive, occurred in parents' use of religious and spiritual activities to cope and the effect on their grief response, mental health and personal growth in the later stages of bereavement" (Hawthorne et al., 2016).

Practice Implications

- "The results from this longitudinal study with a racially and ethnically diverse sample provide evidence for healthcare professionals about the importance of spiritual coping activities for bereaved mothers and fathers" (Hawthorne et al., 2016).
- "Healthcare providers have contact not only with their patients, but also with their patients' family members. These findings demonstrate the need to be aware of the potential impact of cancer on all family members" (Turner-Sack et al., 2016).

IPE HIGHLIGHT

Your team should remember the saying that a good study is one that raises more questions than it answers. So your team should not view a researcher's review of a study's limitations and recommendations for future research as evidence of the researcher's lack of research skills. Rather, it reflects the next steps in building a strong body of evidence.

The final element that the investigator integrates into the "Discussion" is the recommendations. The **recommendations** are the investigator's suggestions for the study's application to practice, theory, and further research. This requires the investigator to reflect on the following questions:

- What contribution does this study make to clinical practice?
- What are the strengths, quality, and consistency of the evidence provided by the findings?
- Does the evidence provided in the findings validate current practice or support the need for change in practice?

Box 17.2 provides **examples** of recommendations for future research and implications for nursing practice. This evaluation places the study into the realm of what is known and what needs to be known before being used. Nursing knowledge and evidence-based practice have grown tremendously over the last century through the efforts of many nurse researchers and scholars.

APPRAISAL FOR EVIDENCE-BASED PRACTICE RESEARCH FINDINGS

The "Results" and the "Discussion" sections are the researcher's opportunity to examine the logic of the hypothesis (or hypotheses) or research question(s) posed, the theoretical framework, the methods, and the analysis (see the critical appraisal criteria box). This final section requires as much logic, conciseness, and specificity as employed in the preceding steps of the research process. You should be able to identify statements of the type of analysis that was used and whether the data statistically supported the hypothesis or research question. These statements should be straightforward and should not reflect bias (see Tables 17.2 and 17.3). Auxiliary data or serendipitous findings also may be presented. If such auxiliary findings are presented, they should be as dispassionately presented as the hypothesis and research question data.

The statistical test(s) used should also be noted. The numerical value of the obtained data should also be presented (see Tables 17.1 to 17.3). The presentation of the tests, the numerical values found, and the statements of support or nonsupport should be clear, concise, and systematically reported. For illustrative purposes that facilitate readability, the researchers should present extensive findings in tables. If the findings were not supported, you should—as the researcher did—attempt to identify, without finding fault, possible methodological problems (e.g., sample too small to detect a treatment effect).

From a consumer perspective, the "Discussion" section at the end of a research article is very important for determining the potential application to practice. The "Discussion" section should interpret the study's data for future research and implications for practice, including its strength, quality, gaps, limitations, and conclusions of the study. Statements reflecting the underlying theory are necessary, whether or not the hypotheses were supported. Included in this discussion are the limitations for practice. This discussion should reflect each step of the research process and potential threats to internal validity or bias and external validity or generalizability.

This last presentation can help you begin to rethink clinical practice, provoke discussion in clinical settings (see Chapters 19 and 20), and find similar studies that may support or refute the phenomena being studied to more fully understand the problem.

CRITICAL APPRAISAL CRITERIA

Research Findings

1. Are the results of each of the hypotheses presented?
2. Is the information regarding the results concisely and sequentially presented?
3. Are the tests that were used to analyze the data presented?
4. Are the results presented objectively?
5. If tables or figures are used, do they meet the following standards?
   a. They supplement and economize the text.
   b. They have precise titles and headings.
   c. They are not repetitious of the text.
6. Are the results interpreted in light of the hypotheses, research questions, and theoretical framework, and all of the other steps that preceded the results?
7. If the hypotheses or research questions are supported, does the investigator provide a discussion of how the theoretical framework was supported?
8. How does the investigator attempt to identify the study's weaknesses (i.e., threats to internal and external validity) and strengths, as well as suggest possible solutions for the research area?
9. Does the researcher discuss the study's clinical relevance?
10. Are any generalizations made, and if so, are they within the scope of the findings or beyond the findings?
11. Are any recommendations for future research stated or implied?
12. What is the study's strength of evidence?

One study alone does not lead to a practice change. Evidence-based practice and quality improvement require you to critically read and understand each study—that is, the quality of the study, the strength of the evidence generated by the findings and its consistency with other studies in the area, and the number of studies that were conducted in the area. This assessment along with the active use of clinical judgment and patient preference leads to evidence-based practice.

KEY POINTS

- The analysis of the findings is the final step of a study. It is in this section that the results will be presented in a straightforward manner.
- All results should be reported whether or not they support the hypothesis. Tables and figures may be used to illustrate and condense data for presentation.
- Once the results are reported, the researcher interprets the results. In this presentation, usually titled "Discussion," readers should be able to identify the key topics being discussed. The key topics, which include an interpretation of the results, are the limitations, generalizations, implications, and recommendations for future research.
- The researcher draws together the theoretical framework and makes interpretations based on the findings and theory in the section on the interpretation of the results. Both statistically supported and unsupported results should be interpreted. If the results are not supported, the researcher should discuss the results, reflecting on the theory as well as possible problems with the methods, procedures, design, and analysis.
- The researcher should present the limitations or weaknesses of the study. This presentation is important because it affects the study's generalizability. The generalizations or inferences about similar findings in other samples also are presented in light of the findings.
- Be alert for sweeping claims or overgeneralizations. An overextension of the data can alert the consumer to possible researcher bias.
- The recommendations provide the consumer with suggestions regarding the study's application to practice, theory, and future research. These recommendations provide a final perspective on the utility of the investigation.
- The strength, quality, and consistency of the evidence provided by the findings are related to the study's limitations, generalizability, and applicability to practice.

CRITICAL THINKING CHALLENGES

- Do you agree or disagree with the statement that "a good study is one that raises more questions than it answers"? Support your perspective with examples.
- As the number of resources such as the Cochrane Library, meta-analysis, systematic reviews, and evidence-based reports in journals grow, why is it necessary to be able to critically read and appraise the studies within the reports yourself? Justify your answer.
- IPE Engage your interprofessional team in a debate to defend or refute the following statement. "All results should be reported and interpreted whether or not they support the research question or hypothesis." If all findings are not reported, how would this affect the applicability of findings to your patient population and practice setting?
- How does a clear understanding of a study's discussion of the findings and implications for practice help you rethink your practice?

REFERENCES

Altman, D. G. (2005). Why we need confidence intervals. *World Journal of Surgery*, *29*, 554–556.

Altman, D. G., Machin, D., Bryant, T., & Gardener, S. (2005). *Statistics with confidence: confidence intervals and statistical guidelines* (2nd ed.). London, UK: BMJ Books.

Hawthorne, D. M., Youngblut, J. M., & Brooten, D. (2016). Parent spirituality, grief, and mental health at 1 and 3 months after their infant's/child's death in an intensive care unit. *Journal of Pediatric Nursing*, *31*, 73–80.

Kline, R. B. (2004). *Beyond significance testing: reforming data analysis methods in behavioral research* (1st ed.). Washington, DC: American Psychological Association.

Li, J., Zhuang, H., Luo, Y., & Zhang, R. (2016). Perceived transcultural self-efficacy of nurses in general hospitals in Guangzhiou, China. *Nursing Research*, *65*(5), 371–379.

Titler, M. G. (2012). Nursing science and evidence-based practice. *Western Journal of Nursing Research*, *33*(3), 291–295.

Turner-Sack, A. M., Menna, R., Setchell, S. R., et al. (2016). Psychological functioning, post traumatic growth, and coping in parent and siblings of adolescent cancer survivors. *Oncology Nursing Forum*, *43*(1), 48–56.

Go to Evolve at **http://evolve.elsevier.com/LoBiondo/** for review questions, critiquing exercises, and additional research articles for practice in reviewing and critiquing.

18

Appraising Quantitative Research

Deborah J. Jones

Go to Evolve at **http://evolve.elsevier.com/LoBiondo/** for review questions, critiquing exercises, and additional research articles for practice in reviewing and critiquing.

LEARNING OUTCOMES

After reading this chapter, you should be able to do the following:

- Identify the purpose of the critical appraisal process.
- Describe the criteria for each step of the critical appraisal process.
- Describe the strengths and weaknesses of a research report.
- Assess the strength, quality, and consistency of evidence provided by a quantitative research report.
- Discuss applicability of the findings of a research report for evidence-based nursing practice.
- Conduct a critique of a research report.

The critical appraisal and interpretation of the findings of a research article is an acquired skill that is important for nurses to master as they learn to determine the usefulness of the published literature. As we strive to make recommendations to change or support nursing practice, it is important for you to be able to assess the strengths and weaknesses of a research report.

Critical appraisal is an evaluation of the strength and quality, as well as the weaknesses, of the study, not a "criticism" of the work, per se. It provides a structure for reviewing and evaluating the sections of a research study. This chapter presents critiques of two quantitative studies, a randomized controlled trial (RCT) and a descriptive study, according to the critical appraisal criteria shown in Table 18.1. These studies provide Level II and Level IV evidence.

As reinforced throughout each chapter of this book, it is not only important to conduct and read research, but to actively use research findings to inform evidence-based practice. As nurse researchers increase the depth (quality) and breadth (quantity) of studies, the data to support evidence-informed decision making regarding applicability of clinical interventions that contribute to quality outcomes are more readily available. This chapter presents critiques of two studies, each of which tests research questions reflecting different quantitative designs. Criteria used to help you in judging the relative merit of a research study are found in previous chapters. An abbreviated set of critical appraisal questions

TABLE 18.1 Summary of Major Content Sections of a Research Report and Related Critical Appraisal Guidelines

Section	Critical Appraisal Questions to Guide Evaluation
Background and Significance (see Chapters 2 and 3)	Does the background and significance section make it clear why the proposed study was conducted?
Research Question and Hypothesis (see Chapter 2)	1. What research question(s) or hypothesis (or hypotheses) are stated, and are they appropriate to express a relationship (or difference) between an independent and a dependent variable? 2. Has the research question(s) or hypothesis (or hypotheses) been placed in the context of an appropriate theoretical framework? 3. Has the research question(s) or hypothesis (or hypotheses) been substantiated by adequate experiential and scientific background material? 4. Has the purpose, aim(s), or goal(s) of the study been substantiated? 5. Is each research question or hypothesis specific to one relationship so that each can be either supported or not supported? 6. Given the level of evidence suggested by the research question, hypothesis, and design, what is the potential applicability to practice?
Review of the Literature (see Chapters 3 and 4)	1. Does the search strategy include an appropriate and adequate number of databases and other resources to identify key published and unpublished research and theoretical resources? 2. Is there an appropriate theoretical/conceptual framework that guides development of the research study? 3. Are both primary source theoretical and research literature used? 4. What gaps or inconsistencies in knowledge or research does the literature uncover so that it builds on earlier studies? 5. Does the review include a summary/critique of the studies that includes the strengths and weakness or limitations of the study? 6. Is the literature review presented in an organized format that flows logically? 7. Is there a synthesis summary that presents the overall strengths and weaknesses and arrives at a logical conclusion that generates hypotheses or research questions?
Methods	
Internal and External Validity (see Chapter 8)	1. What are the controls for the threats to internal validity? Are they appropriate? 2. What are the controls for the threats to external validity? Are they appropriate? 3. What are the sources of bias, and are they dealt with appropriately? 4. How do the threats to internal and external validity affect the strength and quality of evidence? 5. Was the fidelity of the intervention maintained, and if so, how?
Research Design (see Chapters 9 and 10)	1. What type of design is used in the study? 2. Is the rationale for the design appropriate? 3. Does the design used seem to flow from the proposed research question(s) or hypothesis (or hypotheses), theoretical framework, and literature review? 4. What types of controls are provided by the design that increase or decrease bias?
Sampling (see Chapter 12)	1. What type of sampling strategy is used? Is it appropriate for the design? 2. How was the sample selected? Was the strategy used appropriate for the design? 3. Does the sample reflect the population as identified in the research question or hypothesis? 4. Is the sample size appropriate? How is it substantiated? Was a power analysis necessary? 5. To what population may the findings be generalized?
Legal-Ethical Issues (see Chapter 13)	1. How have the rights of subjects been protected? 2. What indications are given that institutional review board approval has been obtained? 3. What evidence is given that informed consent of the subjects has been obtained?

TABLE 18.1 Summary of Major Content Sections of a Research Report and Related Critical Appraisal Guidelines—cont'd

Section	Critical Appraisal Questions to Guide Evaluation
Data Collection Methods and Procedures (see Chapter 14)	1. Physiological measurement: a. Is a rationale given for why a particular instrument or method was selected? If so, what is it? b. What provision is made for maintaining accuracy of the instrument and its use, if any? 2. Observation: a. Who did the observing? b. How were the observers trained and supervised to minimize bias? c. Was there an observation guide? d. Was interrater reliability calculated? e. Is there any reason to believe that the presence of observers affected the behavior of the subjects? 3. Interviews: a. Who were the interviewers? How were they trained and supervised to minimize bias? b. Is there any evidence of interview bias, and if so, what is it? How does it affect the strength and quality of evidence? 4. Instruments: a. What is the type and/or format of the instruments (e.g., Likert scale)? b. Are the operational definitions provided by the instruments consistent with the conceptual definition(s)? c. Is the format appropriate for use with this population? d. What type of bias is possible with self-report instruments? 5. Available data and records: a. Are the records or data sets used appropriate for the research question(s) or hypothesis (or hypotheses)? b. What sources of bias are possible with use of records or existing data sets? 6. Overall, how was intervention fidelity maintained?
Reliability and Validity (see Chapter 15)	1. Was an appropriate method used to test the reliability of the instrument(s)? 2. Was the reliability and validity of the instrument(s) adequate? 3. Was the appropriate method(s) used to test the validity of the instrument(s)? 4. Have the strengths and weaknesses related to reliability and validity of the instruments been presented? 5. What kinds of threats to internal and external validity are presented as weaknesses in reliability and/or validity? 6. How do the reliability and/or validity affect the strength and quality of evidence provided by the study findings?
Data Analysis (see Chapter 16)	1. Were the descriptive or inferential statistics appropriate to the level of measurement for each variable? 2. Are the inferential statistics appropriate for the type of design, research question(s), or hypothesis (or hypotheses)? 3. If tables or figures are used, do they meet the following standards? a. They supplement and economize the text. b. They have precise titles and headings. c. They do not repeat the text. 4. Did testing of the research question(s) or hypothesis (or hypotheses) clearly support or not support each research question or hypothesis?

Continued

TABLE 18.1 Summary of Major Content Sections of a Research Report and Related Critical Appraisal Guidelines—cont'd

Section	Critical Appraisal Questions to Guide Evaluation
Conclusions, Implications, and Recommendations (see Chapter 17)	1. Are the results of each research question or hypothesis presented objectively? 2. Is the information regarding the results concisely and sequentially presented? 3. If the data are supportive of the hypothesis or research question, does the investigator provide a discussion of how the theoretical framework was supported? 4. How does the investigator attempt to identify the study's weaknesses and limitations (e.g., threats to internal and external validity) and strengths and suggest possible research solutions in future studies? 5. Does the researcher discuss the study's relevance to clinical practice? 6. Are any generalizations made, and if so, are they made within the scope of the findings? 7. Are any recommendations for future research stated or implied?
Applicability to Nursing Practice (see Chapter 17)	1. What are the risks/benefits involved for patients if the findings are applied in practice? 2. What are the costs/benefits of applying the findings of the study? 3. Do the strengths of the study outweigh the weaknesses? 4. What are the strength, quality, and consistency of evidence provided by the study findings? 5. Are the study findings applicable in terms of feasibility? 6. Are the study findings generalizable? 7. Would it be possible to replicate this study in another clinical setting?

presented in Table 18.1 summarize detailed criteria found at the end of each chapter and are used as a critical appraisal guide for the two sample research critiques in this chapter. These critiques are included to illustrate the critical appraisal process and the potential applicability of research findings to clinical practice, thereby enhancing the evidence base for nursing practice.

For clarification, you are encouraged to return to earlier chapters for the detailed presentation of each step of the research process, key terms, and the critical appraisal criteria associated with each step of the research process. The criteria and examples in this chapter apply to quantitative studies using experimental and nonexperimental designs.

STYLISTIC CONSIDERATIONS

When you are reading research, it is important to consider the type of journal in which the article is published. Some journals publish articles regarding the conduct, methodology, or results of research studies (e.g., *Nursing Research*). Other journals (e.g., *Journal of Obstetric, Gynecologic, and Neonatal Research*) publish clinical, educational, and research articles. The author decides where to submit the manuscript based on the focus of the particular journal. Guidelines for publication, also known as "Information for Authors," are journal-specific and provide information regarding style, citations, and formatting. Typically research articles include the following:

- Abstract
- Introduction
- Background and significance

- Literature review (sometimes includes theoretical framework)
- Methodology
- Results
- Discussion
- Conclusions

Critical appraisal is the process of identifying the methodological flaws or omissions that may lead the reader to question the outcome(s) of the study or, conversely, to document the strengths and limitations. It is a process for objectively judging that the study is sound and provides consistent, quality evidence that supports applicability to practice. Such judgments are the hallmark of promoting a sound evidence base for quality nursing practice.

CRITIQUE OF A QUANTITATIVE RESEARCH STUDY

THE RESEARCH STUDY

The study "Telephone Assessment and Skill-Building Kit for Stroke Caregivers: A Randomized Controlled Clinical Trial," by Tamilyn Bakas and colleagues, published in *Stroke*, is critiqued. The article is presented in its entirety and followed by the critique.

TELEPHONE ASSESSMENT AND SKILL-BUILDING KIT FOR STROKE CAREGIVERS

A Randomized Controlled Clinical Trial

Tamilyn Bakas, PhD, RN; Joan K. Austin, PhD, RN; Barbara Habermann, PhD, RN; Nenette M. Jessup, MPH, CCRP; Susan M. McLennon, PhD, RN; Pamela H. Mitchell, PhD, RN; Gwendolyn Morrison, PhD; Ziyi Yang, MS; Timothy E. Stump, MA; Michael T. Weaver, PhD, RN

Background and Purpose—There are few evidence-based programs for stroke family caregivers postdischarge. The purpose of this study was to evaluate efficacy of the Telephone Assessment and Skill-Building Kit (TASK II), a nurse-led intervention enabling caregivers to build skills based on assessment of their own needs.

Methods—A total of 254 stroke caregivers (primarily female TASK II/information, support, and referral 78.0%/78.6%; white 70.7%/72.1%; about half spouses 48.4%/46.6%) were randomized to the TASK II intervention (n=123) or to an information, support, and referral group (n=131). Both groups received 8 weekly telephone sessions, with a booster at 12 weeks. General linear models with repeated measures tested efficacy, controlling for patient hospital days and call minutes. Prespecified 8-week primary outcomes were depressive symptoms (with Patient Health Questionnaire Depressive Symptom Scale PHQ-9 ≥5), life changes, and unhealthy days.

Results—Among caregivers with baseline PHQ-9 ≥5, those randomized to the TASK II intervention had a greater reduction in depressive symptoms from baseline to 8, 24, and

52 weeks and greater improvement in life changes from baseline to 12 weeks compared with the information, support, and referral group ($P<0.05$); but not found for the total sample. Although not sustained at 12, 24, or 52 weeks, caregivers randomized to the TASK II intervention had a relatively greater reduction in unhealthy days from baseline to 8 weeks ($P<0.05$).

Conclusions—The TASK II intervention reduced depressive symptoms and improved life changes for caregivers with mild to severe depressive symptoms. The TASK II intervention reduced unhealthy days for the total sample, although not sustained over the long term.

Clinical Trial Registration—URL: https://www.clinicaltrials.gov. Unique identifier: NCT01275495.

Despite decline in stroke mortality in past decades, stroke remains a leading cause of disability, with ≈45% of stroke survivors being discharged home, 24% to inpatient rehabilitation facilities, and 31% to skilled nursing facilities.[1] Most stroke survivors eventually return home, although many family members are unprepared for the caregiving role and have many unmet needs during the early discharge period.[2-4] Despite this, caregivers commonly receive little attention from healthcare providers.[5,6]

Caregiver depressive symptoms, negative life changes, and unhealthy days (UD) often result from unmet caregiver needs. Many caregivers (30%-52%) have depression,[7-10] with a study reporting higher rates in the caregivers than in the stroke survivors.[7] Studies show that family caregivers are at risk for negative life changes, psychosocial impairments, poor health, and even mortality as a result of providing care.[8,9,11-13] Furthermore, the caregiver's emotional well-being can influence the stroke survivor's depressive symptoms.[14-16] In addition, the caregiver's depressive symptoms can affect the stroke survivor's recovery,[15] communication, social participation, and mood.[16] Finally, caregiver stress is a leading cause of institutionalization for stroke survivors and other older adults.[9,17,18]

Recommendations for stroke family caregiver education and support include: (1) assessment of caregiver needs and concerns, (2) counseling focused on problem solving and social support, (3) information on stroke-related care, and (4) attention to caregivers' emotional and physical health.[19] Scientific statements and practice guidelines on stroke family caregiving recommend individualized caregiver interventions that combine skill building (eg, problem solving, stress management, and goal setting) with psychoeducational

---

Received August 6, 2015; final revision received September 24, 2015; accepted October 13, 2015.

From the Indiana University School of Nursing, Indianapolis (T.B., J.K.A., S.M.M.); University of Cincinnati College of Nursing, OH (T.B.); College of Health Sciences, University of Delaware, Newark (B.H.); Indiana University Melvin and Bren Simon Cancer Center, Indianapolis (N.M.J.); School of Nursing, University of Washington, Seattle (P.H.M.); Indianapolis Economics Department, Indiana University Purdue University (G.M.); Richard M. Fairbanks School of Public Health, Indianapolis, IN (Z.Y., T.E.S.); and College of Nursing, University of Florida, Gainesville (M.T.W.).

Guest Editor for this article was Eric E. Smith, MD.

Presented in part at the American Heart Association Scientific Sessions, Orlando, FL, November 7–11, 2015.

Correspondence to Tamilyn Bakas, PhD, RN, College of Nursing, University of Cincinnati, 3110 Vine St, Procter Hall No. 231, PO Box 210038, Cincinnati, OH 45221. E-mail tamilyn.bakas@uc.edu

strategies to improve caregiver outcomes.[20-23] There are few evidence-based, easy-to-deliver programs for family caregivers of stroke survivors postdischarge that incorporate these recommendations. The revised Telephone Assessment and Skill-Building Kit (TASK II) clinical trial addressed these recommendations by offering a comprehensive, multicomponent program that enables caregivers to assess their needs, build skills in providing care, deal with personal responses to caregiving, and incorporate skill-building strategies into their daily lives.

METHODS

Design

A prospective randomized controlled clinical trial design, with outcome data collectors blinded to treatment assignment, was used to evaluate the efficacy of the revised TASK II relative to an information, support, and referral (ISR) comparison group. Both the groups received written materials, 8 weekly calls from a nurse, and a booster session 1 month later. The study was approved by the Indiana University Office of Research Compliance Human Subjects Office (Institutional Review Board) for protection of human subjects and by each facility where recruitment occurred. Recruitment occurred May 1, 2011 through October 7, 2013. Enrolled subjects gave informed consent.

The primary aim was to examine the short-term (immediately postintervention at 8 weeks) and long-term, sustained (12, 24, and 52 weeks) efficacy of the TASK II intervention relative to the ISR comparison group for improving caregivers' depressive symptoms, caregiving-related life changes, and UD. For depressive symptoms, primary analyses were performed for the subgroup with mild to severe depressive symptoms at baseline; secondary analyses for depressive symptoms used the entire cohort. Selected covariates were included in the analyses to adjust for group differences in potential confounders.

Participants

A total of 254 stroke family caregivers were randomized either to the TASK II group (n=123) or to the ISR comparison group (n=131). Family caregivers were recruited from 2 rehabilitation hospitals and 6 acute care hospitals in the Midwest. Participants were screened within 8 weeks after the survivor was discharged home. Caregivers were included if the following criteria were met: was the primary caregiver (unpaid family member or significant other), 21 or more years of age, fluent in the English language, had access to a telephone, had no difficulties hearing or talking on the telephone, planned to be providing care for ≥1 year, and were willing to participate in 9 calls from a nurse, and 5 data collection interviews. Caregivers were excluded if: the patient had not had a stroke, did not need help from the caregiver, or was going to reside in a nursing home or long-term care facility; the caregiver scored <16 on the Oberst Caregiving Burden Scale Task Difficulty Subscale[24] or <4 on a 6-item cognitive impairment screener.[25] In addition, caregivers and stroke survivors were excluded if either was pregnant; a prisoner or on house arrest; had a terminal illness (eg, cancer, end-of-life condition, and renal failure requiring dialysis); had a history of Alzheimer, dementia, or severe mental illness (eg, suicidal tendencies, severe untreated depression or manic depressive disorder, and schizophrenia); or had been hospitalized for alcohol or drug abuse.

Study Protocol

Study Instruments

The Patient Health Questionnaire Depressive Symptom Scale (PHQ-9), measuring 9 depressive indicators from the Diagnostic and Statistical Manual of Mental Disorders (DSM-IV), has been widely used in clinical and research settings.[26] Depressive symptom severity are categorized as: no depressive symptoms (0−4), mild (5−9), moderate (10−14), moderately severe (15−19), or severe (20−27).[26] Evidence of internal consistency reliability has been documented in primary care[26] and with stroke caregivers.[11,12] The Cronbach α for the PHQ-9 for this study was 0.82.

The 15-item Bakas Caregiving Outcomes Scale (BCOS) was used to measure life changes (ie, changes in social functioning, subjective well-being, and physical health), specifically as a result of providing care.[11] Content, construct, and criterion-related validity have been documented, as well as internal consistency reliability in stroke caregivers.[11] Cronbach α for the BCOS for this study was 0.87.

UD were measured by summing 2 items asking caregivers to estimate the number of days in the past 30 days that their own physical or mental health had not been good, with a cap of 30 days.[27] The UD measure has been used to track population health status as part of the Behavioral Risk Factor Surveillance System used across states and communities in support of Healthy People 2010.[27] Strong evidence of construct, concurrent, and predictive validity has been documented, as well as reliability and responsiveness.[27]

Caregiver and survivor characteristics were measured using a demographic form, along with the Chronic Conditions Index,[28] Cognitive Status Scale,[29] and the Stroke-Specific Quality of Life Proxy (SS SSQOL proxy)[30]; all instruments have acceptable psychometric properties and have been used in the context of stroke.

TASK II Intervention Arm

Stroke caregivers randomized to the TASK II intervention group received the TASK II Resource Guide and a pamphlet from the American Heart Association entitled Caring for Stroke Survivors.[31] The TASK II Resource guide included the caregiver needs and concerns checklist[2] addressing 5 areas of needs: (1) finding information about stroke, (2) managing the survivor's emotions and behaviors, (3) providing physical care; (4) providing instrumental care, and (5) dealing with personal responses to providing care, along with corresponding tip sheets addressing each of the items on the caregiver needs and concerns checklist.[32] Five skill-building tip sheets were included that respectively addressed strengthening existing skills, screening for depressive symptoms, maintaining realistic expectations, communicating with healthcare providers, and problem solving, as well as a stress management workbook for the caregiver and stroke survivor.[32] The TASK II intervention added the use of the BCOS at the fifth call for caregivers to further assess their life changes and to select corresponding tip sheets.[33] Calls to caregivers in the TASK II group focused on training caregivers how to identify and prioritize their needs and concerns, find corresponding tip sheets, and address their priority needs and concerns using innovative skill-building strategies.

ISR Comparison Arm

Stroke caregivers randomized to the ISR group received only the American Heart Association pamphlet.[31] Calls to caregivers in the ISR group focused on providing support through the use of active listening strategies.[32,33] Both the groups received 8 weekly calls from a nurse with a booster call at 12 weeks. Caregivers in both the groups were encouraged to seek additional information from the American Stroke Association or from their healthcare providers.

Treatment Fidelity and Training

The treatment fidelity checklist[34] addressing design, training, delivery, receipt, and enactment was used to maintain and track treatment fidelity for both the TASK II intervention and ISR procedures.[35] Training included the use of detailed training manuals and podcasts, training booster sessions, self-evaluation of audio recordings, evaluation by supervisors, quality checklists, and frequent team meetings.[35] Protocol adherence was excellent at 80% for the TASK II and 92% for the ISR.[35] Focus groups with nurses yielded further evidence for treatment fidelity.[35]

Study Timetable and Assessments

Baseline data collection occurred within 8 weeks after the stroke survivor was discharged home because the early discharge period is a time when caregivers need the most information and skills related to providing care.[2,3,6,36,37] Follow-up data were collected at 8 weeks (immediately postintervention), with longer term follow-up data collected at 12 weeks (after the booster session) and at 24 and 52 weeks to explore sustainability of the intervention. Enrollment occurred from January 21, 2011 to July 10, 2013, with follow-up data collection at 52 weeks completed on July 9, 2014.

Randomization and Masking

After baseline, caregivers were assigned to groups using a block randomized approach with stratification by recruitment site, type of relationship (spouse versus adult child/other), and baseline depressive symptoms (PHQ-9 <5 no depressive symptoms; PHQ-9 ≥ 5 mild to severe depressive symptoms). Random allocation sequence was generated using SAS PROC PLAN[38] to create the randomized blocks within strata to obtain, as closely as possible, similar numbers and composition (balance) between the groups, and facilitate maintenance of blinding of data collectors. After baseline data collection, the project manager informed the biostatistician of the caregiver's recruitment site, type of relationship, and depressive symptoms (PHQ-9 score). The biostatistician then notified the project manager of the group assignment, who mailed the appropriate materials to the caregiver and assigned a nurse. Separate nurses were used for TASK II and ISR groups to prevent treatment diffusion. Data collectors were blinded to the caregiver's randomization status at subsequent data collection points. Separate team meetings were held with outcome data collectors to maintain blinding.

Sample Size and Statistical Analysis

The participant flow diagram is provided in Figure 1. Of the 2742 stroke caregivers assessed for eligibility, 254 were randomized to the TASK II intervention (n=123) or to the ISR comparison group (n=131). The refusal rate was minimal at 17.1%; 29.8% caregivers were unable to contact; and 43.8% were ineligible, primarily because the survivor did not need help from a family caregiver, or the survivor was residing in a nursing home or long-term care facility. Attrition rates ranged from 8.1% at 8 weeks to 32.5% at 52 weeks for the TASK II

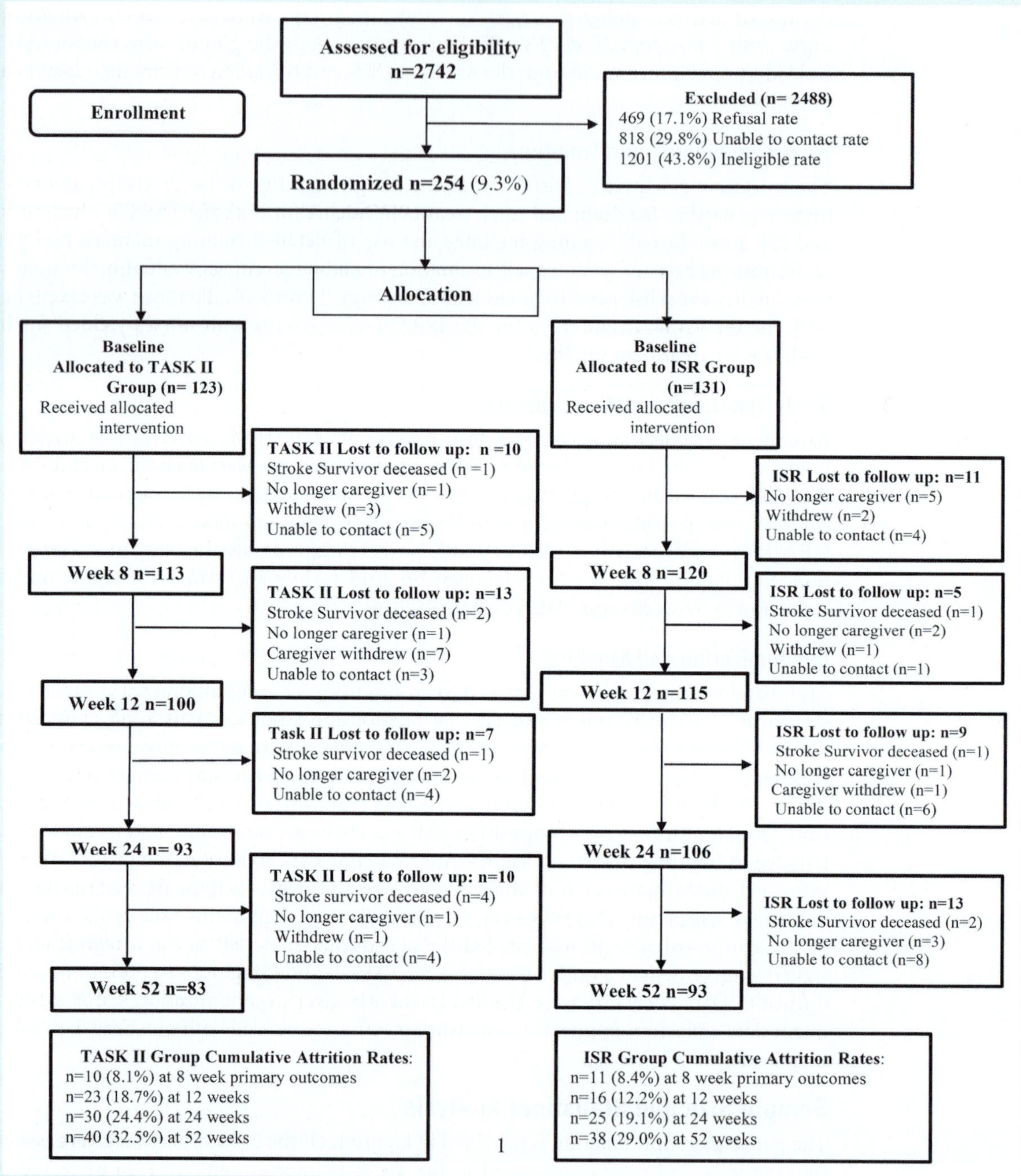

FIG 1 Participant flow diagram. ISR indicates information, support, and referral; and TASK, Telephone Assessment and Skill-Building Kit.

group and 8.4% at 8 weeks to 29.0% at 52 weeks for the ISR group. The sample size was determined based on pilot data anticipating a 10% attrition rate for the 8-week time point for the primary outcomes, using power estimates. Given the full sample of 100 subjects per group, a 0.20 effect size provided a power of 0.81 to detect the treatment by time interactions. Given the 10% attrition rate, a sample of 220 caregivers would be needed. To complete those being assessed for eligibility, enrollment exceeded the projected 220 caregivers by an additional 34 caregivers (total, 254 caregivers). On the basis of pilot data of 38% screening positive for depressive symptoms (PHQ-9 $\geq$5), it was estimated that there would be a total of 76 caregivers (38 per group), which would provide a power of 0.81 to detect an effect size of 0.33 for the treatment by time interaction using a 5% type I error rate. The sample consisted of a total of 111 caregivers (49 TASK II and 62 ISR) who screened positive for depressive symptoms.

Study data were collected and managed using REDCap electronic data capture tools hosted at Indiana University.[39] All analyses were conducted using SAS version 9.4.[38] Baseline equivalence in demographic characteristics and outcome measures between TASK II and ISR groups was tested using independent samples t (continuous variables) or χ^2 (categorical variables). Variables with significant differences between the 2 groups were selected as covariates. Using an intent-to-treat approach, dependent variables consisting of change relative to baseline value for depressive symptoms, life changes, and UD were entered into general linear models.[40] These models incorporated covariates and took into account the correlation among repeated measures on the same individual.[41]

RESULTS

Caregivers in TASK II and ISR groups were similar across all demographic characteristics (Table 1). Caregivers were primarily female (78.0%, TASK II; 78.6% ISR), about half spouses (48.4%, TASK II; 46.6%, ISR), predominantly white (70.7%, TASK II; 72.1%, ISR), and ranged in age from 22 to 87 years. Stroke survivors were similar across demographic characteristics, except that survivors whose caregivers were in the ISR group had spent relatively more days in the hospital (TASK II mean [SD]=17.8 [15.7]; ISR mean [SD]=23.1 [23.4]; P=0.037; Table 2). Although stroke severity was not directly measured, caregiver perceptions of the survivor's functioning as measured by the SSQOL Proxy[30] were similar for both the groups (Table 2). As expected, the number of minutes across all calls with the nurse (ie, intervention dosage) differed between groups and was used as a covariate in the models (TASK II mean [SD]=215.2 [100.8]; ISR mean [SD]=128.1 [85.8], $t=-7.38$; $P<0.001$).[35] Primary outcome means were similar between caregivers in the 2 groups at baseline (Table 3).

Primary End Point (8 Weeks)

At baseline, 47.2% of caregivers in the TASK II group and 50.4% in the ISR group reported mild to severe depressive symptoms (PHQ-9 $\geq$5; Table 3). Among these caregivers, those in the TASK II group reported a greater reduction in depressive symptoms from baseline to 8 weeks than those in the ISR group (mean difference [SE]=−2.6 [1.1]; P=0.013; Table 4). This represented a statistically significant interaction between time and treatment. Secondary analyses for depressive symptoms were not significant using the total sample. Groups were similar from baseline to 8 weeks for life changes. Caregivers in the TASK II group reported a greater reduction in UD from baseline to 8 weeks than those in

TABLE 1 Caregiver Characteristics With Group Equivalence

Caregiver Characteristics	TASK II	ISR	*P* Value
CG age, y, mean (SD, range)	54.0 (12.5, 26-83)	54.7 (11.4, 22-87)	0.627
CG sex, n (%)			
Male	27 (22.0)	28 (21.4)	0.911
Female	96 (78.0)	103 (78.6)	
CG race, n (%)			
White	87 (70.7)	93 (72.1)	0.877
Black	30 (24.4)	33 (25.6)	
American Indian/Alaskan Native	1 (0.8)	0	
Asian	2 (1.6)	1 (0.8)	
>1 Race	3 (2.4)	2 (1.6)	
Ethnicity, n (%)			
Hispanic/Latino	3 (2.5)	0	0.110
Non-Hispanic/Non-Latino	116 (97.5)	128 (100.0)	
CG education years, mean (SD, range)	13.8 (2.8, 8–21)	13.5 (2.5, 7–22)	0.357
CG perceived income, n (%)			
Just have enough to make ends meet	51 (41.8)	55 (42.3)	0.807
Comfortable	35 (28.7)	41 (31.5)	
Not enough to make ends meet	36 (29.5)	34 (26.2)	
CG employment, n (%)			
Employed full time	39 (32.2)	46 (35.1)	0.594
Employed part time	14 (11.6)	12 (9.2)	
Unemployed	15 (12.4)	25 (19.1)	
Retired	27 (22.3)	28 (21.4)	
Homemaker	10 (8.3)	7 (5.3)	
Other	16 (13.2)	13 (9.9)	
CG type of relationship, n (%)			
Spouse	59 (48.4)	61 (46.6)	0.810
Son or daughter (in law)	39 (32.0)	37 (28.2)	
Other relative	15 (12.3)	18 (13.7)	
Friend	2 (1.6)	4 (3.1)	
Other	7 (5.7)	11 (8.4)	
CG length of care months, mean (SD)	13.0 (63.5, 0–684)	18.5 (64.8, 0–492)	0.498
CG care days per week, n (%)			
Daily (7 d/wk)	100 (81.3)	107 (81.7)	0.369
5–6 d/wk	7 (5.7)	9 (6.9)	
3–4 d/wk	10 (8.1)	4 (3.1)	
1–2 d/wk	5 (4.1)	9 (6.9)	
<1 d/wk	1 (0.8)	2 (1.5)	
CG depression diagnosed, n (%)			
No	86 (70.5)	93 (71.0)	0.930
Yes	36 (29.5)	38 (29.0)	
CG antidepressants, n (%)			
No	80 (65.6)	85 (64.9)	0.909
Yes	42 (34.4)	46 (35.1)	
CG counseling depression, n (%)			
No	98 (81.7)	108 (83.7)	0.668
Yes	22 (18.3)	21 (16.3)	
CG no. of chronic conditions, mean (SD)	2.2 (1.9, 0–9)	2.2 (1.7, 0–7)	0.963

Independent samples *t* test (continuous variables) and χ^2 (categorical variables) were used to test equivalence. CG indicates caregiver; ISR, information, support, and referral; and TASK, Telephone Assessment and Skill-Building Kit.

TABLE 2 Survivor Characteristics With Group Equivalence

Stroke Survivor Characteristics	TASK II	ISR	*P* Value
SS age, y, mean (SD, range)	62.7 (14.5, 23–91)	63.4 (14.5, 25–94)	0.685
SS sex, n (%)			
Male	60 (49.6)	66 (50.8)	0.852
Female	61 (50.4)	64 (49.2)	
SS race, n (%)			
White	87 (71.3)	92 (71.3)	0.877
Black	32 (26.2)	36 (27.9)	
Asian	1 (0.8)	1 (0.8)	
Hawaiian/Pacific Islander	1 (0.8)	0	
Other or Unknown	1 (0.8)	0	
Ethnicity, n (%)			
Hispanic/Latino	1 (0.9)	0	0.478
Non-Hispanic/Non-Latino	116 (99.1)	128 (100.0)	
SS education years, mean (SD, range)	13.0 (2.7, 0–20)	12.7 (2.6, 7–23)	0.320
SS hospital days, mean (SD, range)	17.8 (15.7, 0–83)	23.1 (23.4, 0–103)	0.037*
SS no. of days discharge to study enrollment, mean (SD, range)	40.0 (39.2, 7–56)	37.5 (19.0, 4–56)	0.525
SS no. of strokes, n (%)			
1	82 (68.3)	77 (60.2)	0.519
2	21 (17.5)	28 (21.9)	
3	10 (8.3)	11 (8.6)	
≥ 4	7 (5.8)	12 (9.4)	
SS inpatient rehab, n (%)			
No	23 (18.9)	29 (22.5)	0.478
Yes	99 (81.1)	100 (77.5)	
SS no. of outpatient rehabilitation therapy visits past 3 mo, mean (SD, range)	9.7 (12.5, 0–75)	10.0 (12.7, 0–90)	0.853
SS depression diagnosed, n (%)			
No	77 (63.6)	74 (56.5)	0.247
Yes	44 (36.4)	57 (43.5)	
SS antidepressants, n (%)			
No	68 (56.2)	71 (54.2)	0.750
Yes	53 (43.8)	60 (45.8)	
SS counseling depression			
No	102 (85.0)	116 (88.5)	0.406
Yes	18 (15.0)	15 (11.5)	
SS no. of chronic conditions (proxy), mean (SD, range)	4.0 (1.6, 1–9)	4.1 (1.8, 0–9)	0.466
SS Cognitive Status Score (proxy), mean (SD, range)	34.0 (5.3, 16–40)	33.7 (5.4, 13–40)	0.596
SS SSQOL 7 domain scores (proxy), mean (SD, range)			
Thinking	2.7 (1.1)	2.7 (1.1)	0.764
Language	3.9 (1.0)	3.8 (1.1)	0.394
Vision	4.1 (1.0)	4.3 (0.9)	0.257
Energy	2.2 (1.2)	2.1 (1.1)	0.731
Physical function	3.3 (1.0)	3.2 (1.0)	0.554
Mental function	2.9 (1.0)	3.0 (1.1)	0.655
Role function	2.2 (1.0)	2.3 (1.0)	0.748
SS SSQOL 7 domain total (proxy)	3.3 (0.7)	3.2 (0.7)	0.576

Independent samples *t* test (continuous variables) and χ^2 (categorical variables) were used to test equivalence. ISR indicates information, support, and referral; SS, Status Scale; SSQOL, stroke-specific quality of life; and TASK, Telephone Assessment and Skill-Building Kit.
*$P<0.05$.

TABLE 3 Primary Outcomes at Baseline With Group Equivalence

Outcome Measures	TASK II (n=123)	ISR (n=131)	*P* Value
Depressive symptoms (PHQ-9), mean (SD, range)	5.4 (5.1, 0–25)	5.4 (4.6, 0–21)	0.991
Depressive symptoms (PHQ-9) ≥5, mean (SD, range)	9.4 (4.5, 5–25)	8.9 (3.8, 5–21)	0.465
CG depressive symptoms (PHQ-9 <5 vs ≥5), n (%)			
PHQ-9 score <5	65 (52.8)	65 (49.6)	0.607
PHQ-9 score ≥5	58 (47.2)	66 (50.4)	
Life changes (BCOS), mean (SD, range)	56.2 (11.2, 19–93)	55.9 (9.5, 27–89)	0.788
Unhealthy days, mean (SD, range)	9.7 (9.82, 0–30)	8.5 (9.83, 0–30)	0.340

Independent samples *t* test (continuous variables) was used to test equivalence. BCOS indicates Bakas Caregiving Outcomes Scale; CG, caregiver; ISR, information, support, and referral; PHQ, patient health questionnaire; and TASK, Telephone Assessment and Skill-Building Kit.

TABLE 4 Least Square Means of Change Scores From Baseline to Postbaseline for Primary Outcomes by Group

Outcome Measures	n, n TASK II, ISR	TASK II, Mean (SE)	ISR, Mean (SE)	Difference, Mean (SE)	95% CI	T	*P* Value
Depressive symptoms (PHQ-9)							
8 wk§	109, 117§	−1.0 (0.5)*§	0.1 (0.5)§	−1.0 (0.7)§	(−2.3 to 0.3)§	−1.6§	0.116§
12 wk	99, 112	−1.4 (0.5)†	−0.8 (0.5)	−0.6 (0.6)	(−1.8 to 0.7)	−0.9	0.359
24 wk	90, 103	−1.1 (0.4)*	−0.6 (0.4)	−0.5 (0.6)	(−1.7 to 0.7)	−0.9	0.398
52 wk	82, 92	−1.5 (0.5) †	−0.4 (0.5)	−1.1 (0.7)	(−2.4 to 0.3)	−1.6	0.122
Depressive symptoms (PHQ-9)ll							
8 wk§	49, 62§	−3.6 (0.8)‡§	−0.9 (0.7)§	−2.6 (1.1)*§	(−4.7 to −0.6)§	−2.5§	0.013§
12 wk	45, 60	−3.9 (0.8) ‡	−2.0 (0.7)†	−1.9 (1.1)	(−4.0 to −0.2)	−1.8	0.072
24 wk	43, 55	−3.6 (0.7) ‡	−1.6 (0.6)†	−1.9 (0.9)*	(−3.8 to −0.1)	−2.1	0.041
52 wk	39, 48	−4.0 (0.8) ‡	−1.1 (0.7)	−3.0 (1.1)†	(−5.2 to −0.8)	−2.7	0.008
Life changes (BCOS)							
8 wk§	109, 117§	2.9 (1.3)*§	1.2 (1.2)§	1.6 (1.8)§	(−1.9 to 5.1)§	0.9§	0.363§
12 wk¶	99, 112	3.9 (1.3)†	1.5 (1.2)	2.4 (1.8)	(−1.1 to 5.9)	1.4	0.178¶
24 wk	90, 103	3.1 (1.2)*	1.6 (1.2)	1.5 (1.7)	(−1.8 to 4.8)	0.9	0.384
52 wk	82, 92	3.5 (1.4)*	2.1 (1.3)	1.4 (1.9)	(−2.4 to 5.2)	0.7	0.465
Unhealthy days							
8 wk§	108, 116§	−1.1 (0.9)§	1.8 (0.9)§	−2.9 (1.3)*§	(−5.5 to −0.4)§	−2.3§	0.025§
12 wk	99, 111	−1.2 (1.0)	0.1 (1.0)	−1.2 (1.4)	(−4.1 to 1.6)	−0.9	0.395
24 wk	90, 103	−1.7 (1.0)	0.7 (1.0)	−2.4 (1.4)	(−5.3 to 0.4)	1.7	0.094
52 wk	82, 92	−0.8 (1.0)	0.5 (0.9)	−1.2 (1.3)	(−3.9 to 1.4)	−0.9	0.354

Change scores were calculated by subtracting baseline from postbaseline scores. BCOS indicates Bakas Caregiving Outcomes Scale; CI, confidence interval; ISR, information, support, and referral; PHQ, Patient Health Questionnaire; and TASK, Telephone Assessment and Skill-Building Kit.

**P*<0.05; †*P*<0.01; ‡*P*<0.001.

§Primary end point.

llSubgroup who had PHQ-9 ≥5 at baseline.

¶Further analyses of the BCOS using the PHQ-9 ≥5 subgroup showed a significant group difference from baseline to 12 weeks (difference mean [SE], 5.8 [2.9]; 95% CI, [0.1–11.6]; *t*=2.0; *P*=0.046).

the ISR group (mean difference [SE]=−2.9 [1.3]; P=0.025; Table 4). Caregivers within the TASK II group reported improvements in depressive symptoms in both the subgroup (P<0.001) and the entire cohort (P<0.05) and life changes (P<0.05) from baseline to 8 weeks (Table 4).

Secondary End Points (12, 24, and 52 Weeks)

Similar to results at the primary end point, caregivers with PHQ-9 ≥5 in the TASK II group reported a greater reduction in depressive symptoms than those in the ISR group from baseline to 24 weeks (mean difference [SE]=−1.9 [0.09]; P=0.041) and from baseline to 52 weeks (mean difference [SE]=−3.0 [1.1]; P=0.008); although these results were not significant using the entire cohort (Table 4). Although life changes were similar for the full sample from baseline to 12 weeks (P=0.178; Table 4), for caregivers with PHQ-9 ≥5 at baseline, TASK II participants had greater improvement in life changes than ISR participants from baseline to 12 weeks (mean difference [SE]=5.8 [2.9]; P=0.046). Moreover, caregivers within the TASK II group reported improvements in depressive symptoms for the PHQ-9 ≥5 subgroup (P<0.001) and the entire cohort (P<0.05) and life changes (P<0.05) from baseline to 12, 24, and 52 weeks (Table 4). Caregivers within the ISR group reported improvement in depressive symptoms in the PHQ ≥5 subgroup from baseline to 12 and 24 weeks (P<0.01; Table 4).

DISCUSSION

At 8 weeks, the TASK II intervention, compared with the ISR group, reduced UD, did not significantly affect life changes, and reduced depressive symptoms in the subgroup that had mild to severe baseline depressive symptoms. As expected, secondary analyses of depressive symptoms using the entire cohort from baseline to 8, 12, 24, and 52 weeks were not significant. Some caregivers who were not depressed at baseline may have developed depressive symptoms over time; however, TASK II within group differences showed improvement in depressive symptoms at each follow-up time point.

Fewer Depressive Symptoms

Nevertheless, the TASK II program for family caregivers of stroke survivors postdischarge successfully reduced depressive symptoms within a subgroup experiencing mild to severe depressive symptoms compared with those in the ISR group. These results were evident at our primary end point of 8 weeks and were sustained at both 24 and 52 weeks. Although other stroke caregiver intervention studies have reported improvements in caregiver depressive symptoms,[20] only one study reported sustainability at 52 weeks.[42] The study by Kalra et al[42] was a well-designed, randomized controlled clinical trial that tested the efficacy of a hands-on caregiver training program in a sample of 300 stroke caregivers. The intervention group received 3 to 5 inpatient sessions and 1 home visit focused on a variety of skills that included goal setting and tailored psychoeducation, although tailoring of the intervention was based on the needs of the stroke survivor rather than the caregiver. The TASK II intervention is unique in that it is delivered completely by telephone, trains caregivers how to assess and address their own needs, and is applicable to a wide variety of stroke caregivers (eg, spouses, adult children, and others). Screening for and addressing caregiver depressive symptoms, as in the TASK II program, not only have the potential to improve caregiver outcomes,[10,12,19,20] but may improve the survivors' recovery[15] and reduce the potential for their long-term institutionalization.[9,17,18]

Improvement in Life Changes

At 8, 12, 24, and 52 weeks, the TASK II intervention did not significantly affect life changes for the total sample. However, the TASK II program improved caregiver life changes in caregivers with mild to severe depressive symptoms compared with those randomized to the ISR group at 12 weeks. Although life changes were similar for both TASK II and ISR groups across the total sample, it is possible that caregivers with some depressive symptoms experienced more life changes as a result of providing care. Life changes and depressive symptoms have been found to be correlated.[10–12] Improvement in life changes in caregivers with some depressive symptoms builds on our previous work with the original TASK intervention, which had little effect on life changes.[33] For the TASK II intervention, we incorporated the BCOS into the intervention during the fifth call with the nurse as an additional assessment, encouraging caregivers to select priority needs that were targeted toward improving their own personal life changes. Further refinement of the TASK II intervention may be to use the BCOS earlier, (eg, second or third call) to allow caregivers more time to address their own life changes. Only one other intervention study has reported life changes as an outcome in stroke caregivers.[43] King et al[43] found that life changes improved for a group of caregivers who received a problem-solving intervention immediately postintervention; however, results were not sustained at 6 months or 1 year, and there were high attrition rates. Generalizability was limited to spousal caregivers. Other intervention studies have measured similar quality of life concepts with mixed results.[20] Caregivers commonly experience adverse life changes because they neglect their own needs while providing care, and they often need encouragement to care for themselves.[2,3,10–12,36] The TASK II intervention encourages caregivers to attend the needs of the survivor and their own changes in social functioning, subjective well-being, and physical health.

Reduction of UD

Most notably, UD were reduced for the caregivers in the TASK II group compared with those randomized to the ISR group at our primary end point of 8 weeks. A trend toward fewer UD was noted for the TASK II group at 12, 24, and 52 weeks (Figure 2). Future enhancements of the TASK II program may be warranted to include a stronger focus on referring caregivers to healthcare providers to address their own physical and mental health needs. Addressing health conditions as well as preventive healthcare measures is important for both stroke survivors and family caregivers. The stroke family caregiver intervention literature is limited with regard to caregiver health[20]; only 2 studies found improvement in general health of the caregiver.[43,44] Other studies had nonsignificant findings using the SF-36 general health subscale.[33,45] TASK II intervention having a significant impact on a global measure of UD[27] underscores the strength of the TASK II intervention and its potential to improve population health in general for family caregivers.

Limitations

The study used a convenience sample of stroke caregivers recruited from acute care and inpatient rehabilitation settings in the Midwest where most of the participants were white and Non-Hispanic. Caregivers were recruited within 8 weeks of the survivor's discharge to home, making findings less generalizable to long-term caregivers. Caregivers were older (mean age, 54–55 years), making findings less applicable to younger caregivers who were also parents of young children. Survivor characteristics were collected by caregiver proxy.

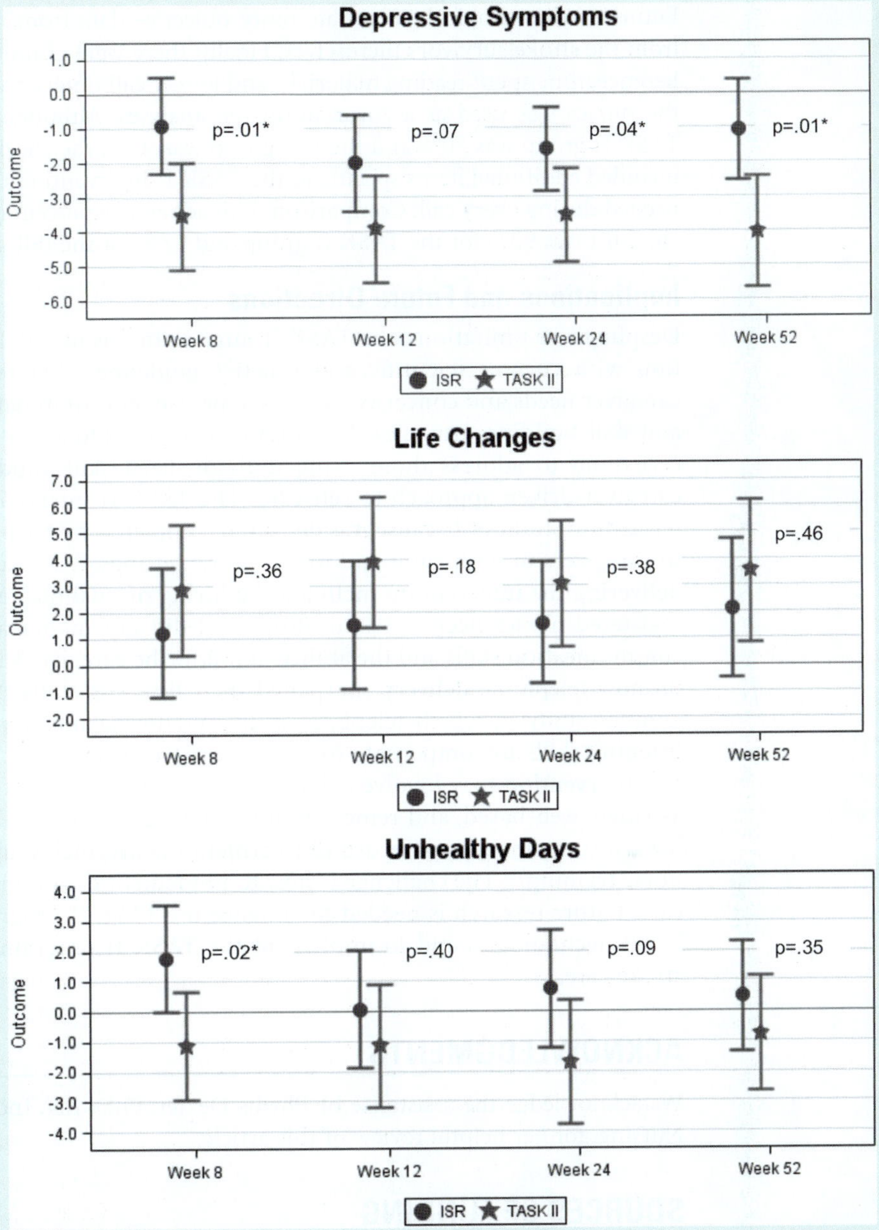

FIG 2 Change plots by treatment and by time for depressive symptoms, life changes, and unhealthy days. ISR indicates information, support, and referral; and TASK, Telephone Assessment and Skill-Building Kit.

Future studies should incorporate more objective data from medical records or directly from the stroke survivors themselves. Finally, there were group differences in protocol adherence, time spent reading materials, and longer call time; although, longer call time with the nurses was used as a covariate in the analyses. Although overall adherence for the TASK II group was 80% and the ISR group was 92%, the checklist for the TASK II group included additional items specific to the TASK II intervention that were repetitive and not needed during every call. Comparison with adherence percentages for shared items on the checklist was 90% for the TASK II group and 92% for the ISR group.[35]

Implications and Future Directions

Despite these limitations, the TASK II intervention is useful. It includes a close connection with current scientific and practice guidelines that recommend assessment of caregiver needs and concerns, as well as the use of a combination of psychoeducational and skill-building strategies.[19–22] Training caregivers to assess their own needs and concerns and to address those using individualized skill-building strategies provides a caregiver-driven approach to self-care. The TASK II intervention is unique among intervention studies[20] because it is delivered completely by telephone, making it accessible to caregivers in both rural and urban home settings.[32,33,35] Key attributes of the nurses delivering the intervention included the hiring of qualified, engaged nurses who had a registered nurses licence.[35] Education level did not matter as much as the quality of communication skills and the ability to follow the caregiver's lead.[35] Nurses commented on how telephone delivery sharpened their listening skills,[35] similar to findings from another study in which telephone delivery allowed interveners to develop enhanced listening skills to compensate for the absence of visual cues.[46] Future development of the intervention may involve enhanced use of other telehealth modes of delivery, such as video, web-based, and remote monitoring technologies.[47] The TASK II intervention has a documented track record of treatment fidelity, including structured protocols for nurse training.[35] The challenge is how to implement the program into stroke systems of care. Future research is needed to enhance the TASK II program using innovative telehealth technologies and to implement the TASK II program into ongoing systems of stroke care.

ACKNOWLEDGMENTS

We acknowledge the assistance of Phyllis Dexter, PhD, RN, Indiana University School of Nursing, for her helpful review of this article.

SOURCES OF FUNDING

This study was funded by the National Institutes of Health, National Institute of Nursing Research, R01NR010388, and registered with the clinical trials identifier NCT01275495 https://www.clinicaltrials.gov/ct2/show/NCT01275495?term=Bakas&rank=3.

DISCLOSURES

None.

REFERENCES

1. Mozaffarian, D., Benjamin, E. J., Go, A. S., Arnett, D. K., Blaha, M. J., Cushman, M., et al.; American Heart Association Statistics Committee and Stroke Statistics Subcommittee. (2015). Heart disease and stroke statistics-2015 update: a report from the American Heart Association. *Circulation, 131,* e29–e322. doi: 10.1161/CIR.0000000000000152.
2. Bakas, T., Austin, J. K., Okonkwo, K. F., Lewis, R. R., Chadwick, L. (2002). Needs, concerns, strategies, and advice of stroke caregivers the first 6 months after discharge. *J Neurosci Nurs, 34,* 242–251.
3. King, R. B., & Semik, P. E. (2006). Stroke caregiving: difficult times, resource use, and needs during the first 2 years. *J Gerontol Nurs, 32,* 37–44.
4. Quinn, K., Murray, C., & Malone, C. (2014). Spousal experiences of coping with and adapting to caregiving for a partner who has a stroke: a meta-synthesis of qualitative research. *Disabil Rehabil, 36,* 185–198. doi: 10.3109/09638288.2013.783630.
5. King, R. B., Hartke, R. J., Lee, J., & Raad, J. (2013). The stroke caregiver unmet resource needs scale: development and psychometric testing. *J Neurosci Nurs, 45,* 320–328. doi: 10.1097/JNN.0b013e3182a3ce40.
6. Ski, C., & O'Connell, B. (2007). Stroke: the increasing complexity of carer needs. *J Neurosci Nurs, 39,* 172–179.
7. Berg, A., Palomaki, H., Lonnqvist, J., Lehtihalmes, M., & Kaste, M. (2005). Depression among caregivers of stroke survivors. *Stroke, 36,* 639–643. doi: 10.1161/01.STR.0000155690.04697.c0.
8. Cameron, J. I., Cheung, A. M., Streiner, D. L., Coyte, P. C., & Stewart, D. E. (2011). Stroke survivor depressive symptoms are associated with family caregiver depression during the first 2 years poststroke. *Stroke, 42,* 302–306. doi: 10.1161/STROKEAHA.110.597963.
9. Han, B., & Haley, W. E. (1999). Family caregiving for patients with stroke. *Review and analysis. Stroke, 30,* 1478–1485.
10. Peyrovi, H., Mohammad-Saeid, D., Farahani-Nia, M., & Hoseini, F. (2012). The relationship between perceived life changes and depression in caregivers of stroke patients. *J Neurosci Nurs, 44,* 329–336. doi: 10.1097/ JNN.0b013e3182682f4c.
11. Bakas, T., Champion, V., Perkins, S. M., Farran, C. J., & Williams, L. S. (2006). Psychometric testing of the revised 15-item Bakas Caregiving Outcomes Scale. *Nurs Res, 55,* 346–355.
12. McLennon, S. M., Bakas, T., Jessup, N. M., Habermann, B., & Weaver, M. T. (2014). Task difficulty and life changes among stroke family caregivers: relationship to depressive symptoms. *Arch Phys Med Rehabil, 95,* 2484–2490. doi: 10.1016/j.apmr.2014.04.028.
13. Schulz, R., & Beach, S. R. (1999). Caregiving as a risk factor for mortality: the Caregiver Health Effects Study. *JAMA, 282,* 2215–2219.
14. Chung, M. L., Bakas, T., Plue, L. D., & Williams, L. S. (published online ahead of print February 5, 2015). Effects of self-esteem, optimism, and perceived control on depressive symptoms in stroke survivor-spouse dyads. *J Cardiovasc Nurs.* http://journals.lww.com/jcnjournal/pages/articleviewer.aspx?year=9000&issue=00000&article=99639&type=abstract. Accessed October 15, 2015.
15. Grant, J. S., Clay, O. J., Keltner, N. L., Haley, W. E., Wadley, V. G., Perkins, M. M., et al. (2013). Does caregiver well-being predict stroke survivor depressive symptoms? A mediation analysis. *Top Stroke Rehabil, 20,* 44–51. doi: 10.1310/tsr2001-44.
16. Klinedinst, N. J., Gebhardt, M. C., Aycock, D. M., Nichols-Larsen, D. S., Uswatte, G., Wolf, S. L., et al. (2009). Caregiver characteristics predict stroke survivor quality of life at 4 months and 1 year. *Res Nurs Health, 32,* 592–605. doi: 10.1002/nur.20348.
17. Gaugler, J. E., Duval, S., Anderson, K. A., & Kane, R. L. (2007). Predicting nursing home admission in the U.S: a meta-analysis. *BMC Geriatr, 7,* 13. doi: 10.1186/1471-2318-7-13.
18. Kao, H. F., & McHugh, M. L. (2004). The role of caregiver gender and caregiver burden in nursing home placements for elderly Taiwanese survivors of stroke. *Res Nurs Health, 27,* 121–134. doi: 10.1002/nur.20007.

19. Miller, E. L., Murray, L., Richards, L., Zorowitz, R. D., Bakas, T., Clark, P., et al; American Heart Association Council on Cardiovascular Nursing and the Stroke Council. (2010). Comprehensive overview of nursing and interdisciplinary rehabilitation care of the stroke patient: a scientific statement from the American Heart Association. *Stroke, 41*, 2402–2448. doi: 10.1161/STR.0b013e3181e7512b.
20. Bakas, T., Clark, P. C., Kelly-Hayes, M., King, R. B., Lutz, B. J., Miller, E. L.; American Heart Association Council on Cardiovascular and Stroke Nursing and the Stroke Council. (2014). Evidence for stroke family caregiver and dyad interventions: a statement for healthcare professionals from the American Heart Association and American Stroke Association. *Stroke, 45*, 2836–2852. doi: 10.1161/STR.0000000000000033.
21. Duncan, P. W., Zorowitz, R., Bates, B., Choi, J. Y., Glasberg, J. J., Graham, G. D., et al. (2005). Management of Adult Stroke Rehabilitation Care: a clinical practice guideline. *Stroke, 36*, e100–e143. doi: 10.1161/01. STR.0000180861.54180.FF.
22. Lindsay, P., Bayley, M., Hellings, C., Hill, M., Woodbury, E., Phillips, S.; on behalf of the Canadian Stroke Strategy, a joint initiative of the Canadian Stroke Network and the Heart and Stroke Foundation of Canada. (2008). Canadian best practice recommendations for stroke care: summary. *Can Med Assoc J, 179*, S1–S25.
23. van Heugten, C., Visser-Meily, A., Post, M., & Lindeman, E. (2006). Care for carers of stroke patients: evidence-based clinical practice guidelines. *J Rehabil Med, 38*, 153–158. doi: 10.1080/16501970500441898.
24. Bakas, T., Austin, J. K., Jessup, S. L., Williams, L. S., & Oberst, M. T. (2004). Time and difficulty of tasks provided by family caregivers of stroke survivors. *J Neurosci Nurs, 36*, 95–106.
25. Callahan, C. M., Unverzagt, F. W., Hui, S. L., Perkins, A. J., & Hendrie, H. C. (2002). Six- item screener to identify cognitive impairment among potential subjects for clinical research. *Med Care, 40*, 771–781. doi: 10.1097/01. MLR.0000024610.33213.C8.
26. Kroenke, K., Spitzer, R. L., & Williams, J. B. (2001). The PHQ-9: validity of a brief depression severity measure. *J Gen Intern Med, 16*, 606–613.
27. Centers for Disease Control and Prevention. (2000). *Measuring Healthy Days*. Atlanta, GA: CDC. http://www.cdc.gov/hrqol/pdfs/mhd.pdf. Accessed October 15, 2015.
28. Cornoni-Huntley, J., Brock, D. B., Ostfeld, A., Taylor, J. O., & Wallace, R. B. (1986). *Established Populations for Epidemiological Studies of the ELDERLY RESOURCE Data Book*. Washington, DC: U.S. Department of Health and Human Services. Rep. No. NIH Publication No. 86-2443.
29. Pearlin, L. I., Mullan, J. T., Semple, S. J., & Skaff, M. M. (1990). Caregiving and the stress process: an overview of concepts and their measures. *Gerontologist, 30*, 583–594.
30. Williams, L. S., Bakas, T., Brizendine, E., Plue, L., Tu, W., Hendrie, H., et al. (2006). How valid are family proxy assessments of stroke patients' health- related quality of life? *Stroke, 37*, 2081–2085. doi: 10.1161/01. STR.0000230583.10311.9f.
31. American Heart Association, American Stroke Association. (2010). *Caring for Stroke Survivors. Stroke Connection Special Edition*. Krames Patient Education No. 50–1682. Updated version No. 50-1699. https://www.kramesstore.com/0A_HTML/ibeSpringSearchResults_kra.jsp?q=50– 1682&ksw001_kswp=00MAL0WynM_RJgYPjj9waXrJ:S&ksw001_ kswp_pses=ZGEEE7D-8846BAA57167EE5F7FCF0C4DD8F67543AA 034625EC6715051EF6B60530E6640276CC8FB-89186C8762EFE1147 D01B552E4081BA583B8BCE548B405144C44. Accessed October 15, 2015.
32. Bakas, T., Farran, C. J., Austin, J. K., Given, B. A., Johnson, E. A., & Williams, L. S. (2009). Content validity and satisfaction with a stroke caregiver intervention program. *J Nurs Scholarsh, 41*, 368–375. doi: 10.1111/j.1547-5069.2009.01282.x.
33. Bakas, T., Farran, C. J., Austin, J. K., Given, B. A., Johnson, E. A., & Williams, L. S. (2009). Stroke caregiver outcomes from the Telephone Assessment and Skill-Building Kit (TASK). *Top Stroke Rehabil, 16*, 105–121. doi: 10.1310/tsr1602-105.
34. Borrelli, B., Sepinwall, D., Ernst, D., Bellg, A. J., Czajkowski, S., Breger, R., et al. (2005). A new tool to assess treatment fidelity and evaluation of treatment fidelity across 10 years of health behavior research. *J Consult Clin Psychol, 73*, 852–860. doi: 10.1037/0022-006X.73.5.852.

35. McLennon, S. M., Hancock, R. D., Redelman, K., Scarton, L. J., Riley, E., Sweeney, B., et al. (published online ahead of print May 7, 2015). Comparing treatment fidelity between study arms of a randomized controlled clinical trial for stroke family caregivers. *Clin Rehabil.* http://cre.sage-pub.com/content/early/2015/05/05/0269215515585134.full.pdf+html. Accessed October 15, 2015.
36. Cameron, J. I., Naglie, G., Silver, F. L., & Gignac, M. A. (2013). Stroke family caregivers' support needs change across the care continuum: a qualitative study using the timing it right framework. *Disabil Rehabil, 35,* 315–324. doi: 10.3109/09638288.2012.691937.
37. Cameron, J. I., Tsoi, C., & Marsella, A. (2008). Optimizing stroke systems of care by enhancing transitions across care environments. *Stroke, 39,* 2637–2643. doi: 10.1161/STROKEAHA.107.501064.
38. SAS Institute Inc. (2013). *What's New in SAS® 9.4.* Cary, NC: SAS Institute Inc.
39. Harris, P. A., Taylor, R., Thielke, R., Payne, J., Gonzalez, N., & Conde, J. G. (2009). Research electronic data capture (REDCap)–a metadata-driven methodology and workflow process for providing translational research informatics support. *J Biomed Inform, 42,* 377–381. doi: 10.1016/j. jbi.2008.08.010.
40. Allison, P. D. (1990). Change scores as dependent variables in regression analysis. *Sociological Methodology, 20,* 93–114.
41. Fitzmaurice, G. M., Laird, N. M., & Ware, J. H. (2004). *Applied Longitudinal Analysis.* 2nd ed. Hoboken, NJ: John Wiley & Sons.
42. Kalra, L., Evans, A., Perez, I., Melbourn, A., Patel, A., Knapp, M., et al. (2004). Training carers of stroke patients: randomised controlled trial. *BMJ, 328,* 1099. doi: 10.1136/bmj.328.7448.1099.
43. King, R. B., Hartke, R. J., Houle, T., Lee, J., Herring, G., Alexander-Peterson, B. S., et al. (2012). A problem-solving early intervention for stroke caregivers: one year follow-up. *Rehabil Nurs, 37,* 231–243. doi: 10.1002/rnj.039.
44. Mant, J., Carter, J., Wade, D. T., & Winner, S. (2000). Family support for stroke: a randomised controlled trial. *Lancet, 356,* 808–813. doi: 10.1016/ S0140-6736(00)02655-6.
45. Grant, J. S., Elliott, T. R., Weaver, M., Bartolucci, A. A., & Giger, J. N. (2002). Telephone intervention with family caregivers of stroke survivors after rehabilitation. *Stroke, 33,* 2060–2065.
46. Pettinari, C. J., & Jessopp, L. (2001). "Your ears become your eyes": managing the absence of visibility in NHS Direct. *J Adv Nurs, 36,* 668–675.
47. Chi, N. C., & Demiris, G. (2015). A systematic review of telehealth tools and interventions to support family caregivers. *J Telemed Telecare, 21,* 37–44. doi: 10.1177/1357633X14562734.

THE CRITIQUE

This is a critical appraisal of the article "Telephone Assessment and Skill-Building Kit for Stroke Caregivers: A Randomized Controlled Clinical Trial" (Bakas et al., 2015) to determine its usefulness and applicability for nursing practice.

Problem and Purpose

The purpose of this study, to evaluate the short-term and long-term efficacy of the Telephone Assessment and Skill-Building Kit (TASK II) intervention on caregivers' depressive symptoms, caregiving-related life changes, and unhealthy days, is concise and clearly stated. The purpose of the study is substantiated in the review of literature. The independent variable is the method of caregiver information and support (TASK II vs. information, support, and referral [ISR]), and the dependent variables are depressive symptoms, life changes, and unhealthy days. The population under study is clearly defined, and the results are important to assist caregivers of stroke survivors in dealing with their own unmet needs and build skills in providing care.

Review of the Literature

The authors provide a thorough summary of the literature related to the needs of caregivers of stroke survivors. They accurately describe literature that supports higher rates of depression, risks of negative life changes, and poor health of caregivers. Stress of caregivers is a leading cause of stroke survivor's institutionalization. Although recommendations and guidelines for education and support of stroke caregivers have been reported, few "easy-to-deliver" programs that incorporate all of the recommendations exist. Therefore this study helps to meet that identified gap in the literature.

Research Questions

The clearly stated primary purpose or aim of the study was to examine the short- and long-term effects of the TASK II intervention compared with the ISR comparison group on improving caregivers' depressive symptoms, caregiving-related life changes, and unhealthy days. Although a hypothesis was not explicitly stated, the information reported in the background, methods, and results provided imply the hypothesis of the study.

Sample

The convenience sample consisted of 254 stroke family caregivers recruited from rehabilitation and acute care hospitals in the Midwest. The sample size was appropriately justified by power analysis, as 100 subjects per group provided a power of 81%. The authors accounted for 10% attrition, which meant an additional 10 subjects per group would be needed. The effect size was determined by using analyses of pilot data to determine a difference in group means of the primary measures.

Inclusion and exclusion criteria were clearly specified. Screening and enrollment procedures were provided.

Although the sample was not randomly selected, there was appropriate random assignment to the TASK II intervention or ISR groups. There were no significant demographic differences between the two caregiver groups. Table 18.1 provides an overview of the group characteristics. Although there were no differences among the groups at baseline, a strength, the sample was predominantly female and predominantly white. This should be mentioned in the discussion section and considered when assessing external validity of the study. The stroke survivors were similar in demographics, with the exception that survivors whose caregivers were in the ISR group had spent significantly more days in the hospital compared with the TASK II group. The difference should be acknowledged when the study results are interpreted.

Research Design

The three required elements of an RCT are present in this study, which provides Level II evidence. After baseline, participants were randomly assigned to the TASK II intervention group or the ISR comparison group. A randomized block design with stratification by recruitment site, type of relationship of caregiver/survivor, and baseline depressive symptoms was appropriately used to allocate participants to groups. The stratified randomization after baseline strengthens the representativeness of the sample.

Threats to Internal Validity

Selection bias may be an issue in studies that use convenience sampling, and in this study all subjects were recruited from acute and inpatient rehabilitation facilities; a majority of the sample was non-Hispanic and white. The sample was also recruited within 8 weeks of discharge home, early in the start of caregiving. However, the randomization used in this study helped control for selection bias. In this study, there is also the risk of instrumentation bias as stroke survivor data was collected by caregiver proxy report. Self-report was also used as an instrument in this study. However, all of the instruments had appropriate reliability and validity, decreasing the risks of instrumentation bias.

Threats to External Validity

The investigators appropriately recognized and reported threats to external validity in the limitations section of the manuscript. As mentioned previously, subjects were randomized to each intervention group when enrolled in the study. However, the sample size was predominately white and non-Hispanic; therefore generalizability to other ethnic groups and races could be minimal. Also, all participants were enrolled in the same geographical area and facility types; therefore the ability to generalize to other geographical areas is a threat to external validity. The investigators used masking (blinding) and took efforts to maximize treatment fidelity. These factors minimize the threats to external validity.

Research Methodology

The research methodology is clearly described. Data collection occurred by telephone at baseline, 8, 12, 24, and 52 weeks post intervention. The procedures to maintain treatment fidelity were provided and indicate systematic and consistent data collection. Data collectors were blinded to caregiver treatment groups, which decreases the chance of differential treatment of the participants.

Legal-Ethical Issues

The study was reviewed and approved by the appropriate institutional review board, and informed consent was obtained from all participants before study initiation.

Instruments

Acceptable reliability and validity data were reported for the Patient Health Questionnaire Depressive Symptom Scale (PHG-9) and the Bakas Caregiving Outcomes Scale (BCOS). The authors provided references that describe the reliability and validity of the instruments for the two-item scale used to measure unhealthy days, and the instruments used to measure the caregiver and survivor characteristics.

Data Analysis

Demographic characteristics were appropriately summarized and analyzed for equivalence using descriptive statistics. The analysis used for both categorical and continuous variables is appropriate. These variables are presented clearly in Tables 1 and 2. General linear models with repeated measures were appropriately used to examine the effect of the intervention. Three tables are used to visually display the data.

Conclusions, Implications, and Recommendations

The authors reported that at 8 weeks the total TASK II intervention group experienced reduced depressive symptoms and greater reduction in unhealthy days compared with the ISR group: (P = .013). However, in a subgroup of caregivers experiencing mild to severe depressive symptoms, those in the TASK II intervention group had reduced depressive symptoms from baseline to 8 weeks (P = .001), 24 weeks (P = .041), and 52 weeks (P = .008) and larger improvement in life changes from baseline to 12 weeks ($P \leq .05$) than the ISR group.

The Level II RCT design, when including all required elements (i.e., randomization, intervention and control groups, and manipulation of the independent variable), is what allows the investigator to determine cause-and-effect relationships. In this case, minimizing threats to internal validity strengthens the study. By ensuring a relatively homogeneous sample, maintaining consistency in data collection, manipulating the independent variables, and randomly assigning patients to groups, the threat to external validity is minimized.

Limitations of the study, as clearly described by the investigator, included generalizability and differences in adherence to the protocol. However, overall protocol adherence is impressive at 80% for the TASK II group and 92% for the ISR group.

Implications for Nursing Practice

This is a well-designed and well-conducted RCT that provides Level II evidence. The interventions pose minimal risk and seem feasible to implement in larger studies of more heterogeneous populations. The strengths in the study design, data collection methods, and measures to minimize threats to internal and external validity make this strong Level II evidence that demonstrates that the TASK II intervention is useful in incorporating the assessment of caregivers' needs with delivery of education and skill-building training for caregivers of stroke survivors.

CRITIQUE OF A QUANTITATIVE RESEARCH STUDY

THE RESEARCH STUDY

The study "Symptoms as the Main Predictors of Caregivers' Perception of the Suffering of Patients with Primary Malignant Brain Tumors" by Renata Zelenikova and colleagues, published in *Cancer Nursing*, is critiqued. The article is presented in its entirety and followed by the critique.

Symptoms as the Main Predictors of Caregivers' Perception of The Suffering of Patients with Primary Malignant Brain Tumors

Renáta Zeleníková, PhD
Dianxu Ren, MD, PhD
Richard Schulz, PhD
Barbara Given, PhD
Paula R. Sherwood, PhD

Key Words
Brain neoplasms
Caregivers
Neurobehavioral manifestations

Background: The perception of suffering causes distress. Little is known about what predicts the perception of suffering in caregivers. **Objective:** The aims of this study were to determine the predictors of caregivers' perceptions of the suffering of patients with a primary malignant brain tumor and to find to what extent perceived suffering predicts the caregivers' burden and depression. **Methods:** Data were obtained as part of a descriptive longitudinal study of adult family caregivers of persons with a primary malignant brain tumor. Recruitment took place in outpatient neuro-oncology and neurosurgery clinics. Caregiver perception of care recipient suffering was measured by 1 item on a scale from 1 to 6. **Results:** The sample of caregiver interviews 4 months after recipients were diagnosed consisted of 86 dyads. While controlling for age, years of education, tumor type, being a spousal caregiver, spiritual well-being, and anxiety, perception of overall suffering was predicted by such symptoms as difficulty understanding, difficulty remembering, difficulty concentrating, feeling of distress, weakness, and pain. Caregivers' perception of the patient's degree of suffering was the main predictor of caregiver burden due to schedule 4 months following diagnosis. **Conclusions:** Care recipient symptoms play an important role in caregivers' perception of the care recipients' suffering. Perception of care recipient suffering may influence caregiver burden. **Implications for Practice:** Identifying specific predictors of overall suffering provides meaningful information for healthcare providers in the field of neuro-oncology and neurosurgery.

In the nursing and healthcare literature, suffering is commonly described in terms of an awareness of the impact of a deteriorating physical state on an individual[1]: the construction of events such as pain or loss as threats to the individual self[2]; a visceral awareness of the self's vulnerability to being broken or diminished at any time and in many ways[3]; and the experience of having to endure, undergo, or submit to an evil of some sort.[4] Suffering is an intensely personal experience[5] whose presence and extent can be known

---

Author Affiliations: Department of Nursing and Midwifery, Faculty of Medicine, University of Ostrava, Czech Republic (Dr Zeleníková); Department of Health and Community Systems, School of Nursing, University of Pittsburgh, Pennsylvania (Dr Ren); University Center for Social and Urban Research, University of Pittsburgh, Pennsylvania (Dr Schulz); College of Nursing, Michigan State University, East Lansing (Dr Given); and Department of Acute and Tertiary Care, School of Nursing, University of Pittsburgh, Pennsylvania (Dr Sherwood).

This study was funded by the National Cancer Institute (award R01 CA118711, principal investigator P.R.S.).

The authors have no conflicts of interest to disclose.

Correspondence: Renáta Zeleníková, PhD, Department of Nursing and Midwifery, Faculty of Medicine, University of Ostrava, Syllabova 19, Ostrava, 703 00 Czech Republic (renata.zelenikova@osu.cz).

Accepted for publication February 16, 2015.

DOI: 10.1097/NCC.0000000000000261

only to the sufferer,[1] something unsharable[6] that, paradoxically, involves asking the question "why."[5] Researchers in diverse settings consistently have concluded that suffering exists across dimensions of physical, psychological and emotional, social and interpersonal, and spiritual and existential well-being.[5] For our purposes, suffering is a broad construct defined as a state of severe distress associated with events that threaten the intactness of the person as a complex physical, social, psychological, and spiritual being and that is subjective and unique to the individual.[7,8]

Serious disease can result in serious suffering.[9] Analogous to the association of pain with suffering is the association of cancer with death. Another major factor in the association of cancer with suffering is the recognition of the drastic effects of cancer treatments. Even with a good prognosis, the effects of surgery, chemotherapy, and radiation therapy are distressing and can be devastating.[5] Suffering of patients with primary malignant brain tumors (PMBTs) can be particularly notable across the cancer trajectory encompassing initial diagnosis, treatment, remission, and even long-term survival. In addition, patients with PMBT can have cognitive deficits including difficulty speaking, difficulty remembering, or difficulty concentrating. These neurologic deficits can drastically interfere with daily life and function. Persons diagnosed with a PMBT are faced with a unique and challenging set of circumstances that affect not only them but also those close to them.[10] Caregivers of persons with a PMBT must deal with both oncological and neurologic issues. They are charged with caring for a person with a potentially terminal diagnosis who is undergoing active cancer treatment and may have cognitive and neuropsychiatric sequelae.[11] Suffering typically occurs in an interpersonal context and is shaped by and affects others exposed to it.[12] Predictors of caregivers' perceptions of suffering in persons diagnosed with PMBT are not established in part because of a lack of valid and reliable instruments to measure the caregiver's perception of the care recipient suffering.

The main purpose of this study was to determine the predictors of caregivers' perceptions of the suffering of patients with PMBT. We predicted that care recipients' symptoms would be the main predictors of caregivers' perceptions of the suffering while controlling for tumor type and caregivers' characteristics (age, years of education, being a spousal caregiver, spiritual well being, and anxiety).

THEORETICAL FRAMEWORK

The study framework was derived from the work of Schulz and colleagues[13] and reflected perceived suffering, caregiver compassion, and caregiver helping and health; this framework guided identifying potential predictors of caregivers' perceptions of the suffering of patients with PMBT and to find out to what extent caregivers' perceptions of the patients' suffering predicted the burden borne by caregivers and caregiver depression. Although the framework emphasizes the directional effects of perceived suffering on compassion, 1 of the framework components depicts perceived suffering as directly linked to psychiatric and physical morbidity. Therefore, we hypothesized that perceived suffering can impact caregiver burden and caregiver depression.

Being exposed to the suffering of others is an important and unique source of distress.[12] Research in dementia patient populations indicates that perceived suffering can contribute to care giver depression and caregiver burden.[7,12] Similarly, descriptive findings in a longitudinal study in 1330 older married couples enrolled in the Cardiovascular Health Study confirmed that exposure to spousal suffering is an independent and unique source of distress in couples and contributes to psychiatric and physical morbidity.[14]

Psychobehavioral responses of caregivers that include depression, burden, anxiety, and positive responses to care have been studied previously, mostly in patients' population with dementia or oncology disease. Caregiver burden and depression may be considered as a general distress response for caregivers.[15] Caregiver burden is a multidimensional concept and represents the impact of providing care on different areas of the caregiver's life (schedule, self-esteem, health, finances, feeling of abandonment), psychosocial reaction resulting from an imbalance of care demands relative to caregivers' personal time, social roles, physical and emotional states, financial resources, and on formal care resources given the other multiple roles they fulfill.[15]

Depression is 1 of the most important potential adverse consequences for caregivers because it is common, associated with poor quality of life, and is a risk factor for other adverse outcomes including functional decline and mortality.[16] Caregiver depression is a complex process, mediated by cultural factors (as measured by the ethnicity of the patient), patient characteristics, and caregiver characteristics.[16] Positive aspects of caregiving may decrease feelings of being burdened and subsequently lead to a more positive effect of health outcomes.

MEASURING SUFFERING

Research methods for approaching human suffering are often qualitative and are based on interviews with people who are assumed to have experienced suffering.[17] Some authors believe that attempting to measure suffering is reductionist and futile because of its personal and unsharable nature.[7] While suffering is personal and potentially ultimately incommunicable, from a practical standpoint, that is, in order to design suitable interventions to relieve suffering, measures that approximately capture a communicable core of suffering are needed. According to Monin and Schulz,[18] both the experience of suffering and the perception of suffering by others can be measured. Ultimately, measures of suffering should focus on the patient's experience, the patient's direct and indirect expressions of suffering, caregiver perceptions of the patient's degree of suffering, and caregiver perceptions of whether the patient's expression of suffering is an accurate reflection of his/her actual degree of suffering.[13]

Measuring suffering via caregiver perceptions of suffering is useful and important, especially for patients with impaired cognitive status because this patient population may not be able to report suffering. To better understand the perceived suffering, we examined caregivers' anxiety and spirituality. Caregivers can play a role in relieving the suffering of their loved one by sharing the experiences, or if the suffering cannot be relieved, then caregivers can help their loved one to bear it through their companionship and compassion. To help caregivers cope with caregiving distress, researchers need to identify how caregivers perceive the suffering of their patients and the predictors of these perceptions.

AIM

The main aim of this study was to determine the predictors of caregivers' perceptions of the suffering of patients with PMBTs. The secondary aim was to find out to what extent caregivers' perceptions of the care recipients' suffering predicted the care givers' burden and depression.

METHODS

Design and Setting

Data were obtained as part of a descriptive longitudinal study of adult family caregivers of persons with PMBT (R01 CA118711). Care recipient and caregiver dyads were recruited from suburban neurosurgery and neuro-oncology clinics in Western Pennsylvania. Recruitment took place in outpatient neuro-oncology and neurosurgery clinics from October 2005 through June 2011. Data were collected from persons with a PMBT and their family caregivers. Interviews with caregivers were conducted in person or via telephone. Data were collected at 3 timepoints over the disease trajectory—right after diagnosis and 4 and 8 months after diagnosis. Data for this analysis are from the second timepoint—4 months after diagnosis to focus on a time of illness progression. Approval from the institutional review board at the University of Pittsburgh and informed consent from participants were obtained prior to data collection. Both the patient and caregiver had to consent to enroll in the study.

Participants

Caregivers were queried regarding sociodemographic characteristics, personal characteristics, and psychological responses, and care recipients were queried regarding the tumor grade, functional and neurologic ability, and symptom status. Care recipients were required to be older than 21 years, newly diagnosed (within 1 month of recruitment) with a PMBT verified by a pathology report. After the death of the care recipient, the corresponding caregiver was given the option of continuing to participate in the study. Caregivers were required to be older than 21 years, nonprofessional (ie, not paid caregivers), not a primary caregiver for anyone else (excluding children aged <21 years), and English speaking and to have regular and reliable access to a phone.

Overall, 228 caregiver and care recipient dyads were approached, with 164 agreeing to participate (70%). The main reasons for declining participation (n = 64) were lack of interest (52%), feeling overwhelmed (33%), reason not given (11%), too busy (3%), and too ill (1%). Of 164 dyads who agreed to participate, 78 ended study participation (47.6%) for various reasons: care recipients died, caregivers were overwhelmed by caregiving duties and life changes, or caregivers were not interested anymore. As a result, the sample of caregivers at the 4-month data point consisted of 86 dyads.

Procedures

Dependent Variables

The primary outcome variable in this study was caregiver perception of the care recipient's suffering during the past week as measured by 1 item; caregivers were asked at the fourth month to rate the care recipient's suffering during the previous week on a scale of 1 (care recipient is not suffering) to 6 (care recipient is suffering terribly). This item was developed by the study investigators. A single-item was purposefully used for its simplicity and ease of use.

Secondary outcomes included caregiver burden and caregiver depression. Caregiver burden was measured using the Caregiver Reaction Assessment (CRA) scale. The CRA is a feasible, reliable, and valid instrument for assessing specific caregiver experiences, including both negative and positive experiences, in caregivers of cancer patients.[19] The CRA comprises 24 items forming 5 distinct unidimensional subscales: disrupted schedule (5 items), financial problems (3 items), lack of family support (5 items), health problems (4 items), and self-esteem (7 items).[20] Respondents were asked to indicate their level of agreement with statements about their feelings regarding caregiving over the previous month. Responses were scaled on a 5-point Likert-type format (5 = strongly agree to 1 = strongly disagree). This analysis focuses on 3 subscales: the self-esteem subscale, the abandonment subscale, and the schedule subscale (which measures the perception of burden on the caregiver's daily activities as a result of providing care). For the self-esteem subscale, a higher score indicates a lower burden related to self-esteem, that is, a positive reaction to caregiving. For abandonment and schedule subscales, a higher score indicates a higher burden, that is, negative reactions to caregiving. Reported reliability analyses[19] showed sufficient internal consistency based on standardized Cronbach's α (.62–.83).

Caregivers' depressive symptoms were measured using the Shortened Center for Epidemiologic Studies Depression Scale (CES-D). The original CES-D scale is a 20-item self-report scale designed to measure depressive symptoms in the general population. The items on the scale are symptoms associated with depression that were chosen from previously validated scales.[21] We used a shortened CES-D with 10 items.[22] Response categories indicate the frequency of occurrence of each item and are scored on a 4-point scale ranging from 0 (rarely or none of the time/$<$1 day) to 3 (most or all of the time/5–7 days). Scores for items 5 and 8 were reversed before summing up all items to yield a total score. Total scores can range from 0 to 30. Higher scores indicate more severe symptoms.[23] Validity for the CES-D has been well established in caregivers and well adults.[22]

Independent/Predictor Variables

Independent variables were chosen based on previous associations reported in the literature as well as hypotheses generated from clinical knowledge in neuro-oncology. Perceived severity of the care recipient's symptoms was measured using the M. D. Anderson Symptom Inventory–Brain Tumor (MDASI-BT). Caregivers were asked to rate the severity of the care recipient's difficulty understanding (speaking, remembering, concentrating) at its worst in the last 24 hours. The MDASI-BT questionnaire is a valid and reliable 22-item measure of the severity of cancer- and treatment-related symptoms based on 6 criteria: affective, cognitive, focal neurologic deficits, treatment-related symptoms, general disease status, and gastrointestinal symptoms.[24–26] Each of the care recipient's symptoms was rated on an 11-point scale (0–10) to indicate its severity, with 0 being "not present" to 10 being "symptom was as bad as you can imagine it could be."[24] This instrument can be used to identify symptom occurrence throughout the disease trajectory and to evaluate interventions designed for symptom management. The MDASI-BT has established validity and reliability. Reported internal consistency (reliability) of the instrument is .91.[24]

Positive aspects of caregiving were assessed using 11 items on the Positive Aspects of Care scale, phrased as statements about the caregiver's mental-affective state in relation to the caregiving experience. Each item began with the statement "Providing help to care recipient has . . . " followed by specific items such as "made me feel more useful."[27] Each item is rated on a scale from 0 (strongly disagree) to 4 (strongly agree). Higher scores indicate greater caregiver benefit. Reported reliability measured by Cronbach's α is .89.[27]

Caregivers' anxiety was measured using the Shortened Profile of Mood States (POMS)–Anxiety. The Shortened POMS-Anxiety consists of 3 items. Each item has 5 grading possibilities from 1 (never) to 5 (always). Caregivers were asked how often during the previous week they felt on edge, nervous, or tense. The original scale[28] incorporated 65 adjectives rated on a 5-point Likert scale ranging from 1 (not at all) to 5 (extremely).[29] Six subscales (depression, vigor, confusion, anxiety, anger, and fatigue) were derived. Our study used a shortened version of 3 items. A higher score indicates greater anxiety. Internal consistency reliability coefficients for the shortened 3-item version of Anxiety subscale were reported as .91 to .92.[30] Validity for the POMS has been established using several other measures.

Caregivers' spirituality was measured using the FACIT-Sp (The Functional Assessment of Chronic Illness Therapy–Spiritual Well-being Scale). FACIT-Sp (version 4) consists of 12 items. Each item has a rating scale score of 0 to 4 indicating the degree to which one agrees with the statements (0 = not at all, 1 = a little bit, 2 = somewhat, 3 = quite a bit, 4 = very much). The instrument comprises 2 subscales: one measuring a sense of meaning and peace and the other assessing the role of faith in illness.[31] The FACIT-Sp is 1 of the most validated instruments for the assessment of a person's perception of spirituality.[32] The reported α coefficients for the total scale and the 2 subscales range from .81 to .88.[31] Participants were required to indicate how true each statement had been for them during the previous 7 days.

Sociodemographic Characteristics. Several sociodemographic characteristics were included in the statistical analysis: age, gender, years of education, relationship of caregivers to the care recipients, and tumor type.

Statistical Analyses

Statistical analyses were conducted using SAS for Windows (version 9.3; SAS Institute Inc, Cary, North Carolina). First, descriptive analyses of the study sample were performed. Correlation between the dependent and independent variables were analyzed. The Spearman correlation coefficient was used to examine the correlation between the main outcome (caregivers' perceptions of care recipients' suffering) and each item of the MDASI-BT (severity of symptoms) as well as the correlation among items of the MDASI-BT. Univariate analyses of measures were then conducted to identify potential predictors of perception of care recipient suffering. Finally, a multivariable linear regression model was built, including all predictors significant at $P < .15$ in univariate analyses. The statistical significance of individual regression coefficients was tested using the Wald χ^2 statistic.

RESULTS

Sample

This analysis includes a total of 86 caregiver-care recipient dyads who completed follow-up assessment 4 months after diagnosis. The majority of caregivers were female (n = 59; 69%) and caring for spouses (n = 69; 80%). The average age of caregivers was 52.23 (SD, 12.7) years (range, 24–99 years); the average age of care recipients was 52.66 (SD, 14.6) years (range, 22–76 years). The caregivers had completed 14.55 (SD, 2.6) years of education on average (range, 8–23 years); the care recipients had completed 15.2 (SD, 3.0) years of education on average (range, 12–22 years). The majority of care recipients were diagnosed with a glioblastoma (n = 49; 57%) (Table 1). Other dyad characteristics are presented in Table 2.

Suffering at 4 months after diagnosis, 37% of caregivers reported that the patient was not suffering; 24% of caregivers rated the patient's suffering as moderate (score of 3), whereas only 4% of caregivers rated the patient's suffering as terrible (score of 6). The average score of perceived suffering was 2.63 (SD 1.56) (Table 3).

TABLE 1 Dyad Characteristics (n = 86)

	CAREGIVERS		CARE RECIPIENTS	
Characteristics	**n (%)**		**n (%)**	
Gender				
Female	59 (69)		50 (58)	
Male	27 (31)		36 (42)	
Relationship to the care recipient				
Spouse	69 (80)			
Other (parent, daughter, sibling)	17 (20)			
Tumor type				
GBM			49 (57)	
Astrocytoma III			20 (23)	
Astrocytoma II			7 (8)	
Oligodendroglioma			5 (6)	
Other			5 (6)	
	Mean (SD)	**Range**	**Mean (SD)**	**Range**
Mean age, y	52.23 (12.7)	24–99	52.66 (14.6)	22–76
Years of education	14.55 (2.6)	8–23	15.2 (3.0)	12–22

Abbreviation: GBM, glioblastoma multiforme.

TABLE 2 Others Selected Dyad Characteristics

	CAREGIVERS		CARE RECIPIENTS	
Characteristic	**Mean (SD)**	**Range**	**Mean (SD)**	**Range**
Anxiety (POMS total sum)	7.97 (2.6)	3–15	6.69 (2.3)	1–12
CRA				
Self-esteem	19.11 (3.3)	11–24		
Abandonment	10.97 (2.5)	6–20		
Schedule	14.76 (4.4)	5–22		
CES-D	6.95 (5.3)	0–26		
MDASI-BT	38.12 (26.7)	0–126		
Spiritual well-being (FACIT total score)	34.78 (7.9)	9–48		
PAC total score	31.56 (8.2)	10–44		

Abbreviations: CES-D, Center for Epidemiologic Studies Depression Scale; CRA, Caregiver Reaction Assessment; MDASI-BT, M. D. Anderson Symptom Inventory–Brain Tumor; FACIT, The Functional Assessment of Chronic Illness Therapy–Spiritual Well-being Scale; PAC, Positive Aspects of Care scale; POMS, Shortened Profile of Mood States.

TABLE 3 Perception of Overall Suffering

Overall Suffering	n (%)	Mean (SD)
1 (Not suffering)	32 (37)	2.63 (1.56)
2	9 (10)	
3	21 (24)	
4	10 (12)	
5	11 (13)	
6 (Suffering terribly)	3 (4)	

Preliminary Analysis

A strong correlation (Table 4) was found only between the perceived suffering of the care recipient and severity of weakness ($r_s = 0.67$). This suggests that care recipients' weakness is associated with caregiver reports of the care recipient's suffering. Moderate correlations were found between perceived suffering and 3 cognitive symptoms: difficulty understanding ($r_s = 0.41$), difficulty remembering ($r_s = 0.46$), and difficulty concentrating ($r_s = 0.42$); and between perceived suffering and a feeling of distress ($r_s = 0.4$) and pain ($r_s = 0.41$) (Table 4).

Correlations among symptoms that were strongly and moderately correlated (a correlation exceeding 0.4) with perceived suffering were examined. Strong correlations were found between difficulty understanding and difficulty remembering (0.69), difficulty

TABLE 4 Correlation of the Severity of Each Symptom With Caregiver Reports of Care Recipient's Overall Suffering at the 4-Month Point

Item of MDASI-BT	r_s	P
Strong correlation		
How severe was care recipient's weakness?	0.67343	<.0001
Moderate correlations		
How severe was care recipient's difficulty remembering?	0.45803	<.0001
How severe was care recipient's difficulty concentrating?	0.41597	.0001
How severe was care recipient's pain?	0.41068	.0001
How severe was care recipient's difficulty understanding?	0.40915	.0001
How severe were care recipient's feelings of distress?	0.40362	.0002
Weak or very weak correlations		
How severe was care recipient's fatigue (tiredness)?	0.38545	.0004
How severe was care recipient's disturbed sleep?	0.34661	.0015
How severe was care recipient's drowsiness (sleepy)?	0.31780	.0038
How severe was care recipient's difficulty speaking?	0.30383	.0058
How severe were care recipient's feelings of sadness?	0.26399	.0172
How severe was care recipient's numbness?	0.24600	.0278
How severe was care recipient's shortness of breath?	0.22094	.0475
How severe were changes in the care recipient's vision?	0.20204	.0705
How severe was care recipient's nausea?	0.20157	.0711
How severe was care recipient's irritability?	0.14288	.2032
How severe was care recipient's lack of appetite?	0.13284	.2371
How severe was care recipient's vomiting?	0.08530	.4490

Abbreviation: MDASI-BT, M. D. Anderson Symptom Inventory–Brain Tumor.

understanding and difficulty concentrating (0.7), and difficulty remembering and difficulty concentrating (0.74). Thus, caregivers giving higher ratings of the severity of the care recipient's difficulty understanding also provided higher ratings of the care recipient's difficulty concentrating and other cognitive symptoms. Moderate correlations were found among the symptoms difficulty concentrating and feelings of distress (0.59), difficulty remembering and feelings of distress (0.51), feelings of distress and pain (0.46), and difficulty concentrating and pain (0.4). Other correlations were weak.

A multivariate model was constructed to evaluate the relationship between the continuous outcome variable of perceived suffering and each of 6 individual symptoms that were correlated (with a correlation exceeding 0.4) with perceived suffering. Other variables—potentially important predictors of perception of suffering—were identified from the univariate analyses of the 4-month measures (all predictors significant at $P < .15$ in univariate analyses). The dependent variable was the caregiver's rating of the care recipient's suffering over the previous week.

In all the models tested (Table 5), the only variables that significantly affected perceived suffering were individual symptoms. While controlling for age, years of education, tumor type, being a spousal caregiver, spiritual well-being (FACIT), and anxiety (POMS), caregiver's perception of the care recipient's suffering at the 4-month point was predicted by such symptoms as difficulty understanding, difficulty remembering, difficulty concentrating, feeling of distress, weakness, and pain. Caregivers who reported perceiving higher levels of the previously mentioned symptoms tended to report higher levels of perceived suffering in the care recipient. In the models, the variables accounted for 22.8% to 43.71% of the variance of the outcome variable (suffering).

Four items (severity of seizures, severity of dry mouth, severity of change in appearance, severity of disruptions in bowel movement patterns) from the MDASI-BT were excluded, and the total score was considered as 1 of the predictors (designated "total symptoms").

TABLE 5 Association of Continuous Outcome Variable Overall Suffering With Each of 6 Individual Symptoms While Controlling for Age, Years of Education, Tumor Type, Being a Spousal Caregiver, Spiritual Well-being (FACIT-Sp), and Anxiety (POMS)

Variable	β	SE	t	P
Model 1: $R^2 = 0.2280$, $F = 2.40$ ($P = .0247$)				
Difficulty understanding	.16	0.06	2.55	.0132
Model 2: $R^2 = 0.2566$, $F = 2.80$ ($P = .0098$)				
Difficulty remembering	.19	0.06	3.04	.0034
Model 3: $R^2 = 0.2447$, $F = 2.63$ ($P = .0145$)				
Difficulty concentrating	.16	0.05	2.84	.0060
Model 4: $R^2 = 0.2517$, $F = 2.73$ ($P = .0116$)				
Feelings of distress	.17	0.05	2.96	.0043
Model 5: $R^2 = 0.4371$, $F = 6.31$ ($P \leq .0001$)				
Weakness	.28	0.04	5.75	<.0001
Model 6: $R^2 = 0.2439$, $F = 2.62$ ($P = .0149$)				
Pain	.19	0.06	2.83	.0062

Abbreviations: FACIT, Functional Assessment of Chronic Illness Therapy–Spiritual Well-being Scale; POMS, Shortened Profile of Mood States.

The 4 items were excluded on the basis of weak correlations, a low incidence rate, and expert panel discussion. Other regression models were developed to examine predictors of the continuous outcome variable caregivers' perceptions of the care recipients' suffering and predictors of the following psychological outcomes: depression and caregiver burden due to schedule at 4 months, while controlling for age, years of education, tumor type, being a spousal caregiver, spiritual well-being (FACIT), and anxiety (POMS).

Four months after the patient's diagnosis, total symptoms of MDASI-BT were the single predictor of perceived suffering ($P < .0001$). The total symptoms score (MDASI-BT) represents the severity of the symptoms. The higher the total score, the more severe the patient's symptoms. The model accounted for 36.56% ($F = 4.68$; $P = .0001$) of the variance in the outcome variable suffering (model A).

Caregiver depressive symptoms were predicted by the caregiver's age ($P = .0223$) and total symptoms ($P = .0067$) (model B). Caregivers who were younger had a tendency to report more depressive symptoms. Another predictor of caregiver depression was total symptoms; the higher the caregiver's perception of the severity of the care recipient's symptoms, the more depressive symptoms they tended to report.

Being a spousal caregiver ($P = .0054$) and caregiver perception of care recipient suffering ($P = .0052$) were the main predictors of burden related to schedule (model C). Caregivers who were a spouse to the care recipient and those who reported higher perception of the care recipient's suffering were more likely to report higher levels of burden due to schedule (Table 6).

DISCUSSION

Persons with PMBTs have a specific treatment and disease trajectory. Having a brain tumor subjects the person to the rigors of a cancer and its treatment (eg, adverse effects from chemotherapy and radiation) but often causes significant neurologic deficits that interfere with daily life and function.[33] The presence of complications in patients with advanced cancer as well as neuropsychological and neurologic dysfunction, such as memory problems, affects the family caregivers of persons with PMBT who are likely to perceive their loved one's suffering as quite distressing. The main purpose of this study was to determine

TABLE 6 Regression Models

Variable	β	SE	t	P
Model A: predictors of overall *suffering*, $R^2 = 0.3656$, $F = 4.68$ ($P = .0001$)				
Total symptoms	.02	0.00	4.69	<.0001
Model B: predictors of *depression;* $R^2 = 0.2163$, $F = 3.13$ ($P = .0091$)				
Caregiver's age	−.11	0.04	−2.34	.0223
Total symptoms	.06	0.02	2.79	.0067
Model C: predictors of *caregiver burden due to schedule;* $R^2 = 0.2778$, $F = 4.68$ ($P = .0004$)				
Being spousal caregivers	3.29	1.14	2.87	.0054
Overall suffering	.85	0.29	2.88	.0052

the predictors of caregivers' perceptions of the suffering of persons with PMBT and how perceived suffering relates to caregivers' burden and depression.

Care Recipient Symptoms as the Main Predictors of Caregiver Perception of Suffering

Our study contributes a number of interesting findings regarding the care recipient's symptoms and the caregiver's perception of suffering. Care recipients' symptoms are the main predictors of caregiver perception of care recipient suffering. The results of this study showed moderate correlations between caregiver perceptions of the care recipient's degree of suffering and 3 cognitive symptoms (difficulty understanding, difficulty remembering, and difficulty concentrating) and between perceived suffering and a feeling of distress and pain. Our results showed the dominance of the physical component of perceived suffering in persons with a PMBT.

Wilson et al[8] found that although suffering had a multidimensional character, the physical component was uppermost for many participants with advanced cancer at the end of life. Hebert et al[34] characterized patient suffering as a constellation of physical, psychosocial, and spiritual signs and symptoms. Little is known about what contributes to suffering in patients, about the variability in its display to caregivers, or about the factors that contribute to the accurate or inaccurate assessment of suffering by caregivers.[34] Of all care recipient symptoms in our study, neurologic symptoms seemed to be the most important in predicting caregiver perception of care recipient suffering. In addition to neurologic symptoms, pain and weakness were also important in predicting perceived suffering. Although symptoms are clearly an important component of patient suffering, they do not constitute the whole suffering.[34] A lower percentage of variance in all our models indicates that there are other variables that can affect and predict suffering of patients with PMBT.

Perceived Suffering and Caregivers' Burden and Depression

The perception of suffering causes distress.[35] Our results confirm that caregivers' perception of the patient's degree of suffering is the main predictor of caregiver burden at 4 months following diagnosis. Another predictor of caregivers' burden was being a spousal caregiver. Given the relationship between patient suffering and caregiver well-being, it is reasonable to expect that, to the extent that these symptoms are successfully treated, caregiver well-being should improve.[34]

The hypothesis that caregivers' perception of the patient's degree of suffering is the main predictor of caregiver depression was not confirmed. The caregiver's age and total symptoms (MDASI-BT) were the main predictors of caregiver depression. Neurologic dysfunction in the care recipient forces caregivers of persons with a PMBT to face stressors similar to those of caregivers of persons with dementia, a subset of caregivers who have been shown to suffer from negative psychobehavioral responses such as depressive symptoms, anxiety, and difficulty sleeping.[10] According to Covinsky et al,[16] there is strong evidence that difficult patient behaviors such as anger and aggressiveness influence caregiver depression, and behavioral manifestations of dementia may be more influential than the degree of cognitive impairment. Schulz et al[7] assessed the relationship between suffering in persons with dementia, caregiver depression, and antidepressant medication use in 1222 dementia patients and their caregivers and assessed the prevalence of 2 types of patient suffering, emotional and existential distress. Each aspect of perceived suffering independently contributed to caregiver depression. Their study was the first using a large sample to show that perceived patient suffering independently contributed to caregiver depression and medication use.[7] The variance in results in our study suggests that analyses should be conducted using a larger sample. Furthermore, Schulz et al,[12] in their study of older individuals, showed that perceived care recipient suffering is associated with caregiver depression and burden, after controlling for the physical and cognitive functioning of the care recipient. They reported that caregivers may overestimate the magnitude of suffering of their care recipient.[12] In a study of 109 caregivers of patients with heart failure, caregivers' poor functional status, overall perception of caregiving distress, and perceived control were associated with depressive symptoms.[36]

Our study provides evidence that the perception of suffering may influence caregiver burden due to schedule. Suffering evokes compassion and respect for someone who bears it with dignity—and intimidates as well.[4] While being able to recognize and respond to the outward signs of a person's distress, we cannot actually enter into the realm of their personal experience of suffering.[6] We need to better understand moderating variables such as the level of contact, intimacy, and attachment between patient and caregiver that likely contribute to patient suffering and caregiver well-being. Most important are studies that seek to identify methods for diminishing or eliminating suffering.

Counseling interventions that empower the caregiver to address the suffering of the patient and/or help caregivers appraise their care recipients' suffering as less threatening should be beneficial. Clinicians can play an important role in the process by monitoring the suffering of the patient, observing its impact on the caregiver, and intervening to address patient suffering and/or caregiver's concerns about patient suffering.[7]

Limitations

The study has several limitations. The first is its small sample size, which limits generalizability. The second limitation arises from the use of proxy accounts of suffering, given the care recipients' neurologic dysfunction. It is possible that caregivers overestimate the magnitude of suffering of their care recipients.[12] The third limitation is associated with rating the care recipients' suffering during the week prior to data collection, which opens up the possibility of faulty recall. The fourth limitation of the study is that caregivers' perception of care recipients' suffering was measured by a single item. Internal consistency cannot be computed for a single-item measure. A single-item instrument provides clinicians with limited information about caregivers' perception of care recipients' suffering, but it can serve as a screening tool. Future research should focus on developing a multi-item instrument measuring perception of suffering in patients with PMBT.

CONCLUSION

In summary, our study provides initial evidence of the role of care recipients' symptoms in perceived suffering. These results suggest that care recipient symptoms (mostly cognitive symptoms) play an important role in caregivers' perception of the care recipients' suffering. Identifying specific predictors such as these provides meaningful information for healthcare providers in the field of neuro-oncology and neurosurgery. Specifically targeted interventions can relieve symptoms of patients with PMBT as well as their caregivers' distress. Interventions that focus on the relief of patients' cognitive symptoms can be seen as a way to improve caregiver well-being.

REFERENCES

1. Cassell, E.J. (2004). *The Nature of Suffering and the Goals of Medicine*. Oxford: University Press.
2. Kahn, D. L., & Steeves, R. H. (1996). An understanding of suffering grounded in clinical practice and research. In B. R. Ferrel (Ed.), *Suffering* (pp. 3–28). Sudbury, MA: The Oncology Nursing Society.
3. Black, H. K., & Rubenstein, R. L. (2004). Themes of suffering in later life. *J Gerontol B Psychol Sci Soc Sci, 59*(1), S17–S24.
4. Harris, I. (2007). The gift of suffering. In N. E. Johnston, A. Scholler-Jaquish (Eds.), *Meaning in Suffering. Caring Practices in the Health Professions* (pp. 60–97). Madison, WI: The University of Wisconsin Press.
5. Ferrell, B. R., & Coyle, N. (2008). The nature of suffering and the goals of nursing. *Oncol Nurs Forum, 35*(2), 217–247.
6. Wilkinson, I. (2005). *Suffering: A Sociological Introduction*. Cambridge: Polity Press.
7. Schulz, R., McGinnis, K. A., Zhang, S., et al. (2008). Dementia patient suffering and caregiver depression. *Alzheimer Dis Assoc Disord, 22*(2), 170–176.
8. Wilson, K. G., Chochinov, H. M., McPherson, C. J., et al. (2007). Suffering with advanced cancer. *J Clin Oncol, 25*(13), 1691–1697.
9. Ruijs, K. D. M., Onwuteaka-Philipsen, B. D., der Wal, G., Kerkhof, A. J. F. M. (2009). Unbearability of suffering at the end of life: the development of a new measuring device, the SOS-V. *BMJ Palliat Care, 8,* 16.
10. Bradley, S. E., Sherwood, P. R., Kuo, J., et al. (2009). Perceptions of economic hardship and emotional health in a pilot sample of family caregivers. *J Neurooncol, 93*(3), 333–342.
11. Sherwood, P. R., Given, B. A., Given, Ch., W., et al. (2006). Predictors of distress in caregivers of persons with a primary malignant brain tumor. *Res Nurs Health, 29,* 105–120.
12. Schulz, R., Monin, J. K., Czaja, S. J., et al. (2010). Measuring the experience and perception of suffering. *Gerontologist, 50*(6), 774–784.
13. Schulz, R., Hebert, R. S., Dew, M. A., et al. (2007). Patient suffering and caregiver compassion: new opportunities for research, practice, and policy. *Gerontologist, 47*(1), 4–13.
14. Schulz, R., Beach, S.R., Hebert, R. S., et al. (2009). Spousal suffering and partner's depression and cardiovascular disease: the cardiovascular health study. *Am J Geriatr Psychiatry, 17*(3), 246–254.
15. Given, B., Wyatt, G., Given, Ch., et al. (2004). Burden and depression among caregivers of patients with cancer at the end of life. *Oncol Nurs Forum, 31*(6), 1105–1117.
16. Covinsky, K. E., Newcomer, R., Fox, P., et al. (2003). Patient and caregiver characteristics associated with depression in caregivers of patients with dementia. *J Gen Intern Med, 18*(12), 1006–1014.
17. Arman, M. (2006). How can we research human suffering? *Scand J Caring Sci,* 20(3), 239–240.
18. Monin, J. K., & Schulz, R. (2009). Interpersonal effects of suffering in older adult caregiving relationships. *Psychol Aging, 24*(3), 681–695.
19. Njiboer, Ch., Triemstra, M., Tempelaar, R., et al. (1999). Measuring both negative and positive reactions to giving care to cancer patients: psychometric qualities of the Caregiver Reaction Assessment (CRA). *Soc Sci Med, 48,* 1259–1269.
20. Given, C. W., Given, B., Stommel, M., et al. (1992). The caregiver reaction assessment (CRA) for caregivers to persons with chronic physical and mental impairments. *Res Nurs Health, 15*(4), 271–283.
21. Radloff, L. S. (1991). The use of the center for epidemiologic studies depression scale in adolescents and young adults. *J Youth Adolesc, 20*(2), 149–166.
22. Andresen, E. M., Malmgren, J. A., Carter, W. B., & Patrick, D. L. (1994). Screening for depression in well older adults: evaluation of a short-form of the CES-D. *Am J Prev Med, 10*(2), 77–84.
23. Wisniewski, S. R., Belle, S. H., Coon, D. W., et al. (2003). The Resources for Enhancing Alzheimer's Caregiver Health (REACH): project design and baseline characteristics. *Psychol Aging, 18*(3), 375–384.

24. Armstrong, T. S., Mendoza, T., Gning, I., et al. (2006). Validation of the M.D. Anderson Symptom Inventory Brain Tumor Module (MDASI-BT). *J Neurooncol, 80*(1), 27–35.
25. Armstrong, T. S., Gning, I., Mendoza, T. R., et al. (2009). Clinical utility of the MDASI-BT in patients with brain metastases. *J Pain Symptom Manage, 37*(3), 331–340.
26. Armstrong T. S., Wefel JS, Gning I, et al. (2012). Congruence of primary brain tumor patient and caregiver symptom report. *Cancer, 118*(50), 1–12.
27. Tarlow, B. J., Wisniewski, S. R., Belle, S. H., et al. (2004). Positive aspects of caregiving, contributions of the REACH project to the development of a new measure for Alzheimer's caregiving. *Res Aging, 26*(4), 429–453.
28. McNair, D. M., & Lorr, M. (1964). An analysis of mood in neurotics. *J Abnorm Psychol, 69*(6), 620–627.
29. Nyenhuis, D. L., Yamamoto, Ch., Luchetta, T., et al. (1999). Adult and geriatric normative data and validation of the profile of mood states. *J Clin Psychol, 55*(1), 79–86.
30. Norcross, J. C., Guadagnoli, E., & Prochaska, J. (1984). Factor structure of the Profile of Mood States (POMS): two partial replications. *J Clin Psychol, 40*(5), 1270–1277.
31. Peterman, A. H., Fitchett, G., Brady, M.J., et al. (2002). Measuring spiritual wellbeing in people with cancer: the Functional Assessment of Chronic Illness Therapy–Spiritual Well-Being Scale (FACIT-Sp). *Ann Behav Med, 24*(1), 49–58.
32. Monod, S., Brennan, M., Theologian Rochat, E., et al. (2011). Instruments measuring spirituality in clinical research – systematic review. *J Gen Intern Med, 26*(11), 1345–1357.
33. Hricik, A., Donovan, H., Bradley, S. E., et al. (2011). Changes in caregiver perceptions over time in response to providing care for a loved one with a primary malignant brain tumor. *Oncol Nurs Forum, 38*(2), 149–155.
34. Hebert, R. S., Arnold, R. M., & Schulz, R. (2007). Improving well-being in caregivers of terminally ill patients. *Making the case for patient suffering as a focus for intervention research. J Pain Symptom Manage, 34*(5), 539–546.
35. Monin, J. K., Schulz, R., Feeney, B. C., & Cook, T. B. (2010). Attachment insecurity and perceived partner suffering as predictors of personal distress. *J Exp Soc Psychol, 46*(6), 1143–1147.
36. Chung, M. L., Pressler, S. J., Dunbar, S. B., et al. (2010). Predictors of depressive symptoms in caregivers of patients with heart failure. *J Cardiovasc Nurs, 25*(5), 411–419.

THE CRITIQUE

This is a critical appraisal of the article, "Symptoms as the Main Predictors of Caregivers' Perception of the Suffering of Patients with Primary Malignant Brain Tumors" (Zelenikova et al., 2016) to determine its usefulness and applicability for nursing practice.

Problem and Purpose

Patients with primary malignant brain tumors (PMBTs) experience a unique cancer trajectory that can affect their daily life and function. Suffering of patients with PMBTs not only affects the patient but also their caregivers. The purpose of this study is clearly stated as follows: "To determine the predictors of caregivers' perceptions of the suffering of patients with PMBT."

Review of the Literature

The introduction of the article explains that suffering is a state of severe distress, is subjective, and is unique to the individual. Any threat to the intactness of a person, like serious disease, can result in suffering. Patients with PMBTs are unique in the course of their treatment and the effects of the cancer and treatment on their neurological and physical functioning. Caregivers of patients with PMBT experience suffering related to caring for the patient faced with terminal diagnosis who is also undergoing treatment and may be exhibiting cognitive deficits.

The authors describe the lack of literature related to predictors of caregivers' perceptions of suffering in persons with PMBT. The authors clearly describe the theoretical framework and gaps in the literature that support the need for the current study. Although published studies have explored caregivers' perceived suffering and responses to the suffering, most of this work has been done in populations with dementia or general oncology disease. The current study will fill the gap in the literature related specifically to predictors of caregiver suffering and the effect on caregiver burden and depression in patients with PMBTs.

Research Questions

The objective of this study is to determine the predictors of caregivers' perceptions of the suffering of patients with PMBTs, and determine the extent caregivers' perceptions of the care recipient's suffering predicted the caregivers' burden and depression. Although this is a descriptive study, the authors hypothesized that the care recipient's main symptoms would predict the caregiver' perceptions of suffering, and the perceived suffering would impact caregiver burden and depression.

Sample

A convenience sample of 164 care recipient and caregiver dyads were enrolled in the study. Of the 164 who consented to the study, 86 dyads remained enrolled in the study at the 4-month data period. The authors clearly described the recruitment and enrollment process and the inclusion criteria. The sample size was not justified with use of power analysis. Given the exploratory nature of the study, the sampling procedure is adequate, but the results must be interpreted cautiously because of limited generalizability.

Research Design

A descriptive, correlational longitudinal design was used, providing Level IV evidence. Data were collected at three time points. This is a nonexperimental study because no randomization was done and there is no manipulation of the independent variables, nor is there a control group. The relationship of the variables can be explored, but no causality can be inferred. It is important to note that although this study provides a lower level of evidence than an RCT, as long as the design is sound and appropriate for the research questions, it may provide preliminary data to support future intervention studies. Since there is a gap in the literature, the findings of this study may provide the best available evidence.

Threats to Internal Validity

No threats from history, mortality (or attrition), or maturation affect this study. Selection bias is a common threat when a convenience sample is used. Psychometric properties of the instrument used to measure the primary outcome variable, caregiver perception, are not reported, which is acknowledged by the authors in the limitation section. Validity is not reported for the Caregiver Reaction Assessment (CRA) or Center for Epidemiologic Studies Depression Scale (CES-D); however, the authors cite the original reference of the tool, which reports adequate validity. The threat of testing is also apparent in this study, with the time of rating the care recipient's suffering during the week prior to data collection.

Threats to External Validity

As this is a convenience sample, potential bias may unknowingly be introduced, limiting generalizability of the results. The sample is predominantly female and caregivers are predominantly spouses. All participants were recruited from a suburban area, which also limits generalizability.

Research Methods

Interviews of caregivers were conducted in person or via telephone. It appears that data collection methods were carried out consistently with each participant, although there was no mention of the specific data collection process, including training or supervision of data collectors, thereby posing questions about fidelity.

Legal-Ethical Issues

The protocol was approved by the appropriate institutional review board. Both caregivers and care recipients completed the informed consent prior to enrolling in the study.

Instruments

The primary outcome of caregiver perception of the care recipient's suffering was measured by a single-item scale that was developed by the study investigators for this protocol. Reliability and validity data are not reported on this scale. The CRA scale was used to measure caregiver burden. Reliability of the 24-item scale is acceptable with Cronbach's alpha .62 to .83. Validity was not reported. The shortened CES-D was used to measure caregivers' depression. Reliability is not reported; however, the authors cite other studies in support of validity of the scale.

Several instruments were used to measure the predictor variables. The authors report an acceptable reliability for each of those instruments.

Reliability and Validity

All of the instruments used in this study do not demonstrate adequate psychometric properties, or the authors do not present the reliability and validity of the instrument. This is a weakness and leads to questions about the accuracy with which the tools measure the variables of interest.

Data Analysis

To assess the relationship between the dependent and independent variables, Spearman's correlation was appropriately used to assess the relationship between the caregivers' perceptions of care recipients' suffering, and the severity of symptoms measured by the M. D. Anderson Symptom Inventory-Brain Tumor (MDASI-BT). Potential predictors of perception of care recipients' suffering were analyzed using a univariate analysis of measures and multivariable linear regression model. Six tables appropriately were used to visually display the data.

Conclusions, Implications, and Recommendations

Conclusions and implications for practice are clearly stated and are consistent with the reported results. Recommendations for future research are implied in the discussion. Care recipient symptoms are found to be the main predictors of caregivers' perception of the care recipients' suffering. Specifically, difficulty understanding, difficulty remembering, difficult concentrating, feeling distress, and pain showed moderate correlations with the caregivers' perception of the care recipients' suffering. In addition, the findings indicated that the caregivers' perception of the care recipients' degree of suffering and the relationship as a spousal caregiver were the main predictors of caregivers' burden. The age of the caregiver and the total symptoms of the care recipient were the main predictors of caregiver depression.

Application to Nursing Practice

This nonexperimental, correlational study provides data that may eventually lead to an intervention study. The findings support the association between caregivers' perceptions of care recipients' suffering and care recipients' symptoms. Knowing predictors of the perception and how this relates to the caregivers' burden and depression can lead to targeted interventions to relieve symptoms and caregiver distress. The strengths outweigh the weaknesses, although the results must be interpreted with caution because of limited generalizability. The risks are minimal, and there are no potential benefits for the individual subjects, but there may be a benefit to the greater society by the dissemination of findings in the literature and applicability to future studies. Further studies with larger sample size would be useful to confirm this.

CRITICAL THINKING CHALLENGES

- Discuss how the stylistic considerations of a journal affect the researcher's ability to present the research findings of a quantitative report.
- Discuss how the limitations of a research study affect generalizability of the findings.
- Discuss how you differentiate the "critical appraisal" process from simply "criticizing" a research report.
- Analyze how threats to internal and external validity affect the strength and quality of evidence provided by the findings of a research study.
- How would a staff nurse who has just critically appraised the study by Bakas and colleagues determine whether the findings of this study were applicable to practice?

REFERENCES

Bakas, T., Austin, J. K., Habermann, B., et al. (2015). Telephone assessment and skill-building kit for stroke caregivers: A randomized controlled clinical trial. *Stroke, 46*, 3478–3487.

Zelenikova, R., Dianxu, R. Schulz, R., et al. (2016). Symptoms as the main predictors of caregivers' perception of the suffering of patients with primary malignant brain tumors. *Cancer Nursing, 39*(2), 97–105.

Go to Evolve at **http://evolve.elsevier.com/LoBiondo/** for review questions, critiquing exercises, and additional research articles for practice in reviewing and critiquing.

PART IV

Application of Research: Evidence-Based Practice

RESEARCH VIGNETTE

LYMPHEDEMA SYMPTOM SCIENCE: SYNERGY BETWEEN BIOLOGICAL UNDERPINNINGS OF SYMPTOMOLOGY AND TECHNOLOGY-DRIVEN SELF-CARE INTERVENTIONS

Mei R. Fu, PhD, RN, FAAN
Associate Professor
NYU Rory Meyers College of Nursing
New York University

Each year, millions of women worldwide are diagnosed with breast cancer. Lymphedema, an abnormal accumulation of lymph fluid in the ipsilateral body area or upper limb, remains an ongoing major health problem affecting more than 40% of 3.1 million breast cancer survivors in the United States (Fu, 2014). Many breast cancer survivors suffer from daily distressing symptoms related to lymphedema, including arm swelling, breast swelling, chest wall swelling, heaviness, firmness, tightness, stiffness, pain, aching, soreness, tenderness, numbness, burning, stabbing, tingling, arm fatigue, arm weakness, and limited movement in the shoulder, arm, elbow, wrist, and fingers (Fu & Rosedale, 2009; Fu, Axelrod, Cleland, et al., 2015). The experience of lymphedema symptoms has been linked to clinically relevant and detrimental outcomes, such as disability and psychological distress, both of which are known risk factors for breast cancer survivors' poor quality of life (QOL).

My program of research on lymphedema symptom science grew out of my passion and desire to understand how patients manage lymphedema in their daily lives. Being a nurse who witnessed patients' daily suffering from lymphedema, I felt it imperative to help patients relieve their symptoms. I was determined to pursue doctoral studies so I could systematically and scientifically investigate the phenomenon of managing lymphedema from a patient's perspective.

During my doctoral program, I received funding from the National Institute of Health (NIH) to complete three descriptive phenomenology studies about the phenomenon of managing lymphedema in different ethnic groups, including white, Chinese American, and African American breast cancer survivors. These studies provide important evidence: (1) breast cancer survivors were distressed that no or limited education was given to them about lymphedema (Fu, 2005); (2) they described the lymphedema symptom experience as living with "a plethora of perpetual discomfort"; and (3) feasible self-care behaviors that were easy to integrate into a daily routine were central to lymphedema management in breast cancer survivors' daily lives (Fu, 2010).

From my early research, I have purposefully built my research in two related lines of scientific inquiry: (1) lymphedema symptom science to discover the biological underpinnings of lymphedema symptomology; and (2) technology-driven interventions to develop pragmatic symptom assessment and self-care mobile health (mHealth) interventions to reduce the risk of lymphedema and optimize lymphedema management through symptom assessment and management. Starting with qualitative inquiry to understand patients' daily symptom experience, I have developed and tested instruments to effectively assess symptoms (Fu et al., 2007; Fu, Axelrod, et al., 2008), pushed the boundaries of using cutting-edge technology for quantifying lymphedema (Fu, Axelrod, Guth, et al., 2015a), and conducted prospective studies to discover the biological pathway of lymphedema symptomology using a genomic approach (Fu, Conley, Axelrod, et al., 2016). My research has documented evidence that lymphedema symptoms are strongly associated with increased limb volume; symptoms alone can accurately detect lymphedema defined by greater than 200 mL limb volume difference, as well as evidence for patterns of obesity and lymph fluid level. Supported by NIH, my research findings reveal that lymphedema symptoms do have inflammatory biological mechanisms, evidenced by significant relationships with several inflammatory genes. This important study provides a foundation for precision assessment of heterogeneity of lymphedema phenotype and understanding the biological mechanism of each phenotype through the exploration of inherited genetic susceptibility, which is essential for finding a cure. Further exploration of investigative intervention in the context of genotype and gene expressions will advance our understanding of heterogeneity of lymphedema phenotype.

I also played a leadership role by conducting two studies supported by the Oncology Nursing Society and the International American Lymphedema Framework Project, documenting the need for oncology nurses to enhance their lymphedema knowledge and identify predictors for effective lymphedema care. This work identifies (1) the critical need for patient and clinician education about the importance of managing lymphedema symptoms, and (2) the critical need to manage lymphedema symptoms among breast cancer survivors through self-care behavioral interventions addressing physiological personal factors such as a compromised lymphatic system and body mass index (BMI). Based on the identified research gap, my team and I developed the Optimal Lymph Flow intervention, a face-to-face-nurse-delivery, patient-centered, feasible, and safe self-care program for managing lymphedema symptoms and reducing the risk of lymphedema (Fu, 2014). Grounded in research-driven self-care strategies, The Optimal Lymph Flow self-care program focuses on innovative self-care to promote lymph flow by empowering, rather than inhibiting, how breast cancer survivors live their lives. It features a safe, feasible 5-minute lymphatic exercise program that is easily integrated into the daily routine and easy to follow nutrition guidance. This program is effective in enhancing lymphedema risk reduction. The study provides initial evidence that translates research findings to support an emerging change in lymphedema care from a treatment-focus to a proactive risk reduction approach.

Advancing lymphedema self-management using the Internet, a venue that offers universal access to web-based programs, was the next evidence-based innovation. Patient requests inspired my team to develop and pilot test a web-based mHealth system for lymphedema symptom assessment and management (Fu, Axelrod, Guth, et al., 2016a, 2016b). The Optimal Lymph Flow mHealth system (TOLF) is a technologically driven delivery model featuring patient-centered, web- and mobile-based educational and behavioral interventions focusing on safe, innovative, and pragmatic electronic assessment and self-care strategies for lymphedema management. Based on principles fostering accessibility, convenience, and efficiency of an mHealth system to enhance training and motivating assessment of and self-care for lymphedema symptoms, the TOLF innovation includes self-care skills to promote symptom management among breast cancer survivors at risk for lymphedema. TOLF is guided by the Model of Self-Care for Lymphedema Symptom Management program. Avatar video simulations provide a novel and standardized training system to assist in building self-care skills by visually showing how lymph fluid drains in the lymphatic system when performing lymphatic exercises. Patients can use the TOLF mHealth system to monitor and evaluate their lymphedema symptoms virtually anytime and anywhere. Upon the submission of their symptom report, patients immediately receive a symptom evaluation in terms of fluid accumulation and recommended self-care strategies.

Currently, I am the principal investigator for a web- and mobile-based pilot clinical trial funded by Pfizer to evaluate the effectiveness of TOLF mHealth intervention in managing chronic pain and symptoms related to lymph fluid accumulation (Fu, Axelrod, Guth, et al., 2016c). Collaborating with engineering expert Dr. Yao Wang, I am also the principal investigator for an R01 technology innovation research award from National Cancer Institute to develop a precision assessment of lymphedema risk from patient self-reported symptoms through machine learning, as well as to develop a Kinect-enhanced intervention training system, which can track patients' movement and provide instant audio-visual feedback to patients, to enable them to follow prescribed movements more accurately, thereby making self-care interventions more effective. The innovation of precision risk prediction and intervention will be hosted in TOLF. This project has the potential to enhance lymphedema risk assessment and risk reduction for patients worldwide to achieve automated precision symptom assessment, detection, and prediction of lymphedema based on lymphedema symptom evaluation.

For more than a decade, my research has advanced symptom science, an important focus that has contributed to building an evidence-based applicable for nursing practice. The sustained funding for my research has allowed me to pioneer research innovation in genomics, biomarkers, and technology in symptom science research and to seamlessly build a program of research. From early on in my career, I have been building a global research network for symptom science, significant in today's global health network world. The international funding for my research, in collaboration with researchers from China, South Korea, and Brazil has allowed me and my international team to build a global platform in symptom science research by translating and testing culturally appropriate symptom assessment instruments and interventions to relieve patients' distressful symptoms (Fu et al., 2002; Fu, Xu, et al., 2008; Li et al., 2016; Paim et al., 2008; Ryu et al., 2013; Shi et al., 2016). The multidisciplinary nature of my work is an important key to success. I have worked collaboratively as a nurse scientist with researchers from many other fields, including medicine, surgery, radiation, pathology, engineering, molecular biology, biostatistics and physical therapy, front-line clinicians, hospital administrators, and patients. The findings derived from my research have informed policy related to development of national practice standards, the National Lymphedema Network position paper on screening and measurement for early detection of breast cancer related lymphedema, and the American Cancer Society guideline for breast cancer survivorship care. Cancer centers in the United States and China have implemented digital technology for patients to report lymphedema symptoms and lymphedema risk reduction programs to automate referrals for early detection and treatment of lymphedema. My ongoing research on mHealth will continue to impact health care delivery and future policy for cancer survivorship and lymphedema care.

REFERENCES

Fu, M. R. (2005). Breast cancer survivors' intentions of managing lymphedema. *Cancer Nursing*, *28*(6), 446–457. PMID: 16330966.

Fu, M. R. (2010). Cancer Survivors' views of lymphoedema management. *Journal of Lymphoedema*, *5*(2), 39–48.

Fu, M. R. (2014). Breast cancer-related lymphedema: symptoms, diagnosis, risk reduction, and management. *World Journal of Clinical Oncology*, *5*(3), 241–247. doi: 10.5306/wjco.v5.i3.241. PMID: 25114841.

Fu, M. R., & Rosedale, M. (2009). Breast cancer survivors' experience of lymphedema related symptoms. *Journal of Pain and Symptom Management*, *38*(6), 849–859. PMID: 19819668.

Fu, M. R., Rhodes, V. A., & Xu, B. (2002). The Chinese translation: The index of nausea, vomiting, and retching (INVR). *Cancer Nursing*, *25*(2), 134–140. PMID: 11984101.

Fu M. R., McDaniel R. W., & Rhodes V. A. (2007). Measuring symptom occurrence and symptom distress: Development of the symptom experience index. *Journal of Advanced Nursing*, *59*(6), 623–634. PMID: 17672849.

Fu, M. R., Axelrod, D., & Haber, J. (2008). Breast cancer-related lymphedema: Information, symptoms, and risk reduction behaviors. *Journal of Nursing Scholarship*, *40*(4), 341–348. PMID: 19094149.

Fu, M. R., Xu, B., Liu, Y., et al. (2008). "Making the best of it": Chinese women's experiences of adjusting to breast cancer diagnosis and treatment. *Journal of Advanced Nursing*, *63*(2), 155–165. PMID: 18537844.

Fu, M. R., Axelrod, D., Cleland, C.M., et al. (2015). Symptom reporting in detecting breast cancer-related lymphedema. *Breast Cancer: Targets and Therapy*, *7*, *345*–352 (#1825502). doi: 10.2147/BCTT.S87854. PMID: 26527899.

Fu, M. R., Axelrod, D., Guth, A., et al. (2015a). Patterns of obesity and lymph fluid level during the first year of breast cancer treatment: a prospective study. *Journal of Personalized Medicine*, *5*(3), 326–340. doi: 10.3390/jpm5030326. PMID: 26404383.

Fu, M. R., Axelrod, D., Guth, A. A., et al. (2016a). Usability and feasibility of health IT interventions to enhance self-care for lymphedema symptom management in breast cancer survivors. *Internet Interventions*, *5*, 56–64.

Fu, M. R., Axelrod, D., Guth, A. A., et al. (2016b). mHealth self-care interventions: managing symptoms following breast cancer treatment. *mHealth*, *2*, 28. doi: 10.21037/mhealth.2016.07.03. PMID: 27493951.

Fu, M. R., Axelrod, D., Guth, A. A., et al. (2016c). A web- and mobile-based intervention for women treated for breast cancer to manage chronic pain and symptoms related to lymphedema: Randomized clinical trial rationale and protocol. *JMIR Research Protocol*, *5*(1), e7. <http://www.researchprotocols.org/2017/1/e7/>. doi: 10.2196/resprot.5104.

Fu, M. R., Conley, Y. P., Axelrod, D., et al. (2016). Precision assessment of heterogeneity of lymphedema phenotype, genotypes and risk prediction. *The Breast*, doi: 10.1016/j.breast.2016.06.023. PMID: 27460425 (Epub ahead print).

Li, K., Fu, M.R., Zhao, Q., et al. (2016). Translation and evaluation of Chinese version of the symptom experience index. *International Journal of Nursing Practice*, *22*, 556–564. doi: 10.1111/ijn.12464. PMIC: 27560042.

Paim, C. R., de Paula Lima, E. D., Fu, M. R., et al. (2008). Post lymphadenectomy complications and quality of life among breast cancer patients in Brazil. *Cancer Nursing*, *31*(4), 302–309; quiz 310–311. PMID: 18600117.

Ryu, E., Kim, K., Choi, S. Y., et al. (2013). The Korean version of the symptom experience index: A psychometric study. *International Journal of Nursing Studies*, *50*(8), 1098–1107. doi: 10.1016/j.ijnurstu.2012.12.008. PMID: 23290258 (Epub 2013 Jan 3).

Shi, S., Lu, Q., Fu, M. R., et al. (2015). Psychometric properties of the breast cancer and lymphedema symptom experience index: The Chinese version. *European Journal of Oncology Nursing*, *20*, 10–16. pii: S1462-3889(15)00076-9. doi: 10.1016/j.ejon.2015.05.002. PMID: 26071198 (Epub ahead print).

19

Strategies and Tools for Developing an Evidence-Based Practice

Carl A. Kirton

Go to Evolve at **http://evolve.elsevier.com/LoBiondo/** for review questions, critiquing exercises, and additional research articles for practice in reviewing and critiquing.

LEARNING OUTCOMES

After reading this chapter, you should be able to do the following:

- Identify the key elements of a focused clinical question.
- Discuss the use of databases to search the literature.
- Screen a research article for relevance and validity.
- Critically appraise study results and apply the findings to practice.
- Make clinical decisions based on evidence from the literature combined with clinical expertise and patient preferences.

KEY TERMS

confidence interval
electronic index
information literacy
likelihood ratio
negative likelihood ratio
negative predictive value
null value
number needed to treat
odds ratio
positive likelihood ratio
positive predictive value
prefiltered evidence
relative risk
relative risk reduction
sensitivity
specificity

In today's environment of knowledge explosion, new investigations that potentially impact maintaining a practice that is based on evidence can be challenging. However, the development of an evidence-based nursing practice is contingent on applying new and important evidence to clinical practice. A few simple strategies will help you move to a practice that is evidence oriented. This chapter will assist you in becoming a more efficient and effective reader of the literature. Through a few important tools and a crisp understanding of the important components of a study, you will be able to use an evidence base to determine the merits of a study for your practice and for your patients.

Consider the case of a nurse who uses evidence from the literature to support her practice: Sheila Tavares is a staff registered nurse who works in the prenatal clinic. She is teaching a class to pregnant women. Sheila teaches the future mothers that they should avoid sugar-sweetened beverages during pregnancy because it causes weight gain in the infant. The mothers want to know if artificially sweetened beverages (diet drinks) can be consumed. Sheila is not sure about the effect on infant weight and decides to consult the literature to answer this question.

EVIDENCE-BASED STRATEGY #1: ASKING A FOCUSED CLINICAL QUESTION

Developing a focused clinical question will help Sheila focus on the relevant issue and prepare her for subsequent steps in the evidence-based practice process (see Chapters 1, 2, and 3). A focused clinical question using the PICO format (see Chapters 2 and 3) is developed by answering the following four questions:

1. What is the *population* I am interested in?
2. What is the *intervention* I am interested in?
3. What will this intervention be *compared* with? (Note: Depending on the study design, this step may or may not apply.)
4. How will I know if the intervention makes things better or worse (thus identifying an *outcome* that is measurable)?

As you recall from Chapters 2 and 3, the simple mnemonic PICO is used to develop a well-designed clinical question (Table 19.1). Using this format Sheila develops the following clinical question: *Does consumption of artificially sweetened beverages [intervention] among pregnant women [population] affect infant body weight [outcome]?*

Once a clinical question has been framed, it is useful to assign the question to a clinical category. These categories are predominately based on study designs that you read about in previous chapters. These categories help you search for the correct type of study to answer the clinical question. Being able to critique research is an important skill in evidence-based practice. Because clinicians may feel they lack the skills to critique published research, clinical category worksheets are available to guide your assessment of the extent to which the author implemented a well-designed study. It also helps you answer the important question of whether or not the study finding applies to your specific patient or group.

- **Therapy category:** When you want to answer a question about the effectiveness of a particular treatment or intervention, you will select studies that have the following characteristics:
  - An experimental or quasi-experimental study design (see Chapter 9)
  - Outcome known or of probable clinical importance observed over a clinically significant period of time
  - For studies in this category, you use a therapy appraisal tool to evaluate the study. A therapy tool can be accessed at http://www.cebm.net/critical-appraisal/.

TABLE 19.1 Using PICO to Formulate Clinical Questions

Patient population	What group do you want information on?	Pregnant mothers
Intervention (or exposure)	What event do you want to study the effect of?	Artificially sweetened beverages
Comparison	Compared with what? Is it better or worse than no intervention at all, or than another intervention?	No artificially sweetened beverages
Outcomes	What is the effect of the intervention?	Infant body weight

- **Diagnosis category:** When you want to answer a question about the usefulness, accuracy, selection, or interpretation of a particular measurement instrument or laboratory test, you will select studies that have the following characteristics:
  - Cross-sectional/case control/retrospective study design (see Chapter 10) with people suspected to have the condition of interest
  - Administration to the patient of both the new instrument or diagnostic test and the accepted "gold standard" measure
  - Comparison of the results of the new instrument or test and the "gold standard"
  - When studies are in this category, you use a diagnostic test appraisal tool to evaluate the article. A diagnostic tool can be accessed at http://www.cebm.net/critical-appraisal/.
- **Prognosis category:** When you want to answer a question about a patient's likely course for a particular disease state or identify factors that may alter the patient's prognosis, you will select studies that have the following characteristics:
  - Nonexperimental, usually a longitudinal/cohort/prospective study of a particular group for a specific outcome or disease (see Chapter 10)
  - Follow-up for a clinically relevant period of time (time is the exposure)
  - Determination of factors in those who do and do not develop a particular outcome
  - For studies in this category, you use a prognosis appraisal tool (sometimes called a cohort tool) to evaluate the study. A prognosis tool can be accessed at http://www.cebm.net/critical-appraisal/.
- **Harm category:** When you want to determine the cause(s) of a particular symptom, problem, or disorder, you will select studies that have the following characteristics:
  - Nonexperimental, usually longitudinal or retrospective (ex post facto/case control study designs over a clinically relevant period of time; see Chapter 10)
  - Assessment of whether or not the patient has been exposed to the independent variable
  - For studies in this category, you use a harm appraisal tool (sometimes called a case-control tool) to evaluate the study. A harm tool can be accessed at http://www.cebm.net/critical-appraisal/.

EVIDENCE-BASED STRATEGY #2: SEARCHING THE LITERATURE

All the skills that Sheila needs to consult the literature and answer a clinical question are conceptually defined as **information literacy**. Your librarian is the best person to help you develop the necessary skills to become information literate. Part of being information literate is having the skills necessary to electronically search the literature to obtain the best evidence for answering your clinical question.

The literature is organized into **electronic indexes** or *databases*. Chapter 3 discusses the differences among databases and how to use these databases to search the literature. You can also learn how to effectively search databases through a web-based tutorial located at https://www.nlm.nih.gov/bsd/disted/nurses/cover.html.

Using the PubMed database (www.pubmed.gov), Sheila uses the search function and enters the term "artificial sweeteners AND pregnancy." This strategy provides her with 6069 articles. Of course, there are too many articles for Sheila to review, and she does a quick scan and realizes that many of the articles do not answer her clinical question. Many are not research studies, and some articles have nothing to do with artificial sweeteners consumed by pregnant women. She recalls that the PubMed database has a filter option that helps her find citations that correspond to a specific clinical category. A careful perusal of the list of articles and a well-designed clinical question help Sheila select the key articles.

QSEN EVIDENCE-BASED PRACTICE TIP

Prefiltered sources of evidence can be found in journals and electronic format. **Prefiltered evidence** is evidence in which an editorial team has already read and summarized articles on a topic and appraised its relevance to clinical care. Prefiltered sources include *Clinical Evidence,* available online at http://clinicalevidence.com/x/index.html and in print; *Evidence-based Nursing,* available online at http://ebn.bmj.com/ and in print; and *The Joanna Briggs Institute,* available online at http://joannabriggs.org.

EVIDENCE-BASED STRATEGY #3: SCREENING YOUR FINDINGS

Once you have searched and selected the potential articles, how do you know which articles are appropriate to answer your clinical question? This is accomplished by screening the articles for quality, relevance, and credibility by answering the following questions (Munn et al., 2015; Warren, 2015):

1. Is each study from a peer-reviewed journal? Studies published in peer-reviewed journals have had an extensive review and editing process (see Chapter 3).
2. Are the setting and sample of each study similar to mine so that results, if valid, would apply to my practice or to my patient population (see Chapter 12)?
3. Are any of the studies sponsored by an organization that may influence the study design or results (see Chapter 13)?

Your responses to these questions can help you decide to what extent you want to appraise each article. **Example:** ➤ If the study population is markedly different from the one to which you will apply the results, you may want to consider selecting a more appropriate study. If an article is worth evaluating, you should use the category-specific tool identified in evidence-based strategy 1 to critically appraise the article.

Sheila reviews the abstract of the articles retrieved from her PubMed citation lists and selects the following article: "Association Between Artificially Sweetened Beverage Consumption During Pregnancy and Infant Body Mass Index" (Azad et al., 2016). This study was published in 2016 in *JAMA Pediatrics*, a peer-reviewed journal. This is an observational study that has a longitudinal/cohort design and is a prognosis clinical category study. Sheila reads the abstract and finds that the objective of the study was to observe maternal consumption of artificial sweeteners during pregnancy and evaluate its influence on infant body mass index, measured at 1 year of age. The population and setting of the study were mothers from Canada. The study authors received funding for this investigation from the Children's Hospital Research Institute of Manitoba and supported by the Canadian Institute of Health Research and the Allergy, Genes and Environment Network of Centres of Excellence. Sheila finds that there were no funding or conflict of interest issues noted; she decides that this study is worth evaluating and selects the prognosis category tool.

HELPFUL HINT

If you are selecting a therapy study, consider both studies with significant findings (treatment is better) and studies with nonsignificant findings (treatment is worse or there is no difference). Studies reporting nonsignificant findings are more difficult to find but are equally important.

EVIDENCE-BASED STRATEGY #4: APPRAISE EACH ARTICLE'S FINDINGS

Applying study results to individual patients or to a specific patient population and communicating study findings to patients in a meaningful way are the hallmark of evidence-based practice. Common evidence-based practice conventions that researchers and research consumers use to appraise and report study results are identified by four different types of clinical categories: therapy, diagnosis (sensitivity and specificity), prognosis, and harm. The language common to meta-analysis was discussed in Chapter 11. An appraisal tool for a meta-analysis (systematic review) can be found at http://www.cebm.net/critical-appraisal/. Familiarity with these evidence-based practice clinical categories will help Sheila search for, screen, select, and appraise articles appropriate for answering clinical questions.

Therapy Category

In articles that belong to the therapy category (experimental, randomized controlled trials [RCTs], or intervention studies), investigators attempt to determine if a difference exists between two or more interventions. The evidence-based language used in a therapy article depends on whether the numerical values of the study variables are *continuous* (a variable that measures a degree of change or a difference on a range, such as blood pressure) or *discrete,* also known as dichotomous (measuring whether or not an event did or did not occur, such as the number of people diagnosed with type 2 diabetes) (Table 19.2).

Generally speaking, therapy studies measure outcomes using discrete variables and present results as measures of association as relative risk (RR), relative risk reduction, or odds ratio (OR), as illustrated in Table 19.3. Understanding these measures is challenging but particularly important because they are used by all health care providers to communicate with each other and to patients the risks and benefits or lack of benefits of a treatment (or treatments). They are particularly useful to nurses, as they inform decision making that validates current practice or provides evidence that supports the need for a clinical practice change.

Example: ➤ Haas and colleagues (2015) examined a smoking cessation intervention among individuals of lower socioeconomic status (low-SES). Investigators randomized the smokers to usual care from their health care team or to an intervention group that received care from a tobacco treatment specialist along with other resources. Abstinence was measured 9 months after randomization. The data revealed that smokers in the intervention group were more likely to report quitting than individuals in the control group (OR, 2.5;

TABLE 19.2 **Difference Between Continuous and Discrete Variables**

Researcher Objective	Variable	How the Outcome Is Described in the Research Article
Continuous Variables		
Researcher is interested in degree of change after exposure to an intervention	Pain score, levels of psychological distress, blood pressure, weight	Measures of central tendency (e.g., mean, median, or standard deviation)
Discrete Variables		
Researcher is interested in whether or not an "event" occurred or did not occur	Death, diarrhea, pressure ulcer, pregnancy: "Yes" or "No"	Measures of event probability (e.g., relative risk or odds ratio)

TABLE 19.3 Measures of Association for Trials That Report Discrete Outcomes

Measure of Association	Definition	Comment
Relative risk, also called risk ratio	Compares the probability of the outcome in each group.	The RR is calculated by dividing the EER/CER. If CER and EER are the same, the RR = 1 (this means there is no difference between the experimental and control group outcomes). If the risk of the event is reduced in EER compared with CER, RR < 1. *The further to the left of 1 the RR is, the greater the event, the less likely the event is to occur.* If the risk of an event is greater in EER compared with CER, RR > 1. *The further to the right of 1 the RR is, the greater the event is likely to occur.*
Relative risk reduction	This value tells us the reduction in risk in relative terms. The RRR is an estimate of the percentage of baseline risk that is removed as a result of the therapy; it is calculated as the ARR between the treatment and control groups divided by the absolute risk among patients in the control group.	Percent reduction in risk that is removed after considering the percent of risk that would occur anyway (the control group's risk), calculated as EER − CER/CER
OR	Estimates the odds of an event occurring. The OR is usually the measure of choice in the analysis of nonexperimental design studies. It is the probability of a given event occurring to the probability of the event not occurring.	If the OR = 1.0, this means there is no difference in the probability of an event occurring between the experimental and control group outcomes. If the probability of the event is reduced between groups, the OR is < 1.0 (i.e., the event is less likely in the treatment group than the control group). If the odds of an event is increased between groups, the OR > 1.0 (i.e., the event is more likely to occur in the treatment group than the control group).

CER, Control group event rate; *EER,* experimental group event rate; *OR,* odds ratio; *RR,* relative risk; *RRR,* relative risk reduction.
Note: When the experimental treatment *increases* the probability of a *good outcome* (e.g., satisfactory hemoglobin A_{1c} levels), there is a **benefit increase** rather than a risk reduction. The calculations remain the same.

95% CI, and 1.5 to 4.0) (Haas et al., 2015). This means that those receiving care from a tobacco treatment specialist and other resources were two and a half times more likely to quit smoking than those who received usual care.

Two other measures can help you determine if the reported or calculated measures are clinically meaningful. They are the **number needed to treat** (NNT) and the **confidence interval** (CI). These measures allow you to make inferences about how realistically the results about the effectiveness of an intervention can be generalized to individual patients and to a population of patients with similar characteristics.

The NNT is a useful measure for determining intervention effectiveness and its application to individual patients. It is defined as the number of people who need to receive a treatment (or the intervention) in order for one patient to receive any benefit. The NNT may or may not be reported by the study researchers but is easily calculated. Interventions with a high NNT require considerable expense and human resources to provide any benefit or to prevent a single episode of the outcome, whereas a low NNT is desirable because it means that more individuals will benefit from the intervention. In the Haas and colleagues (2015) study that studied smoking cessation interventions, the NNT = 10. The interpretation for the NNT is that we would have to provide 10 patients with the study intervention for one of them to benefit from the intervention. In other words, 1 in 10 patients will quit smoking. This gives us a very different and clinically useful perspective of the intervention; obviously the lower the NNT, the better the intervention.

The second clinically useful measure is the CI. The CI is a range of values, based on a random sample of the population that often accompanies measures of central tendency and measures of association and provides you with a measure of precision or uncertainty about the sample findings. Typically investigators record their CI results as a 95% degree of certainty; at times you may also see the degree of certainty recorded as 99%. Journals often include CIs as one of the statistical methods used to interpret study findings. Even when CIs are not reported, they can be easily calculated from study data. The method for performing these calculations is widely available in statistical texts.

Returning to the Haas and colleagues (2015) study, it was found that the OR for smoking cessation for study participants who received the intervention was 2.5. The authors accompanied this data with a 95% CI so that the OR with CI is reported as 2.5 (1.5 to 4.0). The CI, the number in parentheses, helps us place the study results in context for all patients similar to those in the study (generalizability).

As a result of the calculated CI for the Haas and colleagues (2015) study, it can be stated that in adults who smoke (the study population) we can be 95% certain that when they receive counseling, nicotine replacement therapy, and community based resources, the odds of abstinence are between 1.5 and 4.0; this is the range of effectiveness of the intervention. Recall that the odds of something happening is the ratio between success and failure (or something happening or not happening). Thus, at a minimum, you can expect that with the intervention treatment the odds of smoking cessation are one and half times greater than the odds of continued smoking. At best, you can expect that with the intervention the odds of smoking cessation are four times greater than the odds of continued smoking.

Another unique feature of the CI is that it can tell us whether or not the study results are statistically significant. When an experimental value is obtained that indicates there is no difference between the treatment and control groups (e.g., no difference in the abstinence rates in smokers who received the intervention and those who didn't), we label that value "the value of no effect," or the **null value**. The value of no effect varies according to the outcome measure.

When examining a CI, if the interval *does not* include the null value, the effect is said to be statistically significant. When the CI *does* contain the null value, the results are said to be nonsignificant because the null value represents the value of no difference—that is, there is no difference between the treatment and control groups. In studies of equivalence (e.g., a study to determine if two treatments are similar) this is a desired finding, but in studies of superiority or inferiority (e.g., a study to determine if one treatment is better than the other), this is not the case.

The null value varies depending on the outcome measure. For numerical values determined by proportions/ratio (e.g., RR, OR), the null value is "1." That is, if the CI does not include the value "1," the finding is statistically significant. If the CI does include the value "1," the finding is not statistically significant. If we examine an actual result from Table 3 in Appendix A, we can see an excellent demonstration of this concept; the authors report the factors associated with noncompletion of a vaccination series. The factors are accompanied by ORs and CIs. Can you identify which factors are significant and which are not by examining the CIs? For numerical values determined by a mean difference between the score in the intervention group and the control group (usually with continuous measures), the null value is zero. In this case if the CI includes the null value of zero, the result is not statistically significant. If the CI does not include the null value of zero, the result is statistically significant, as illustrated in Fig. 19.1A–D.

Diagnosis Articles

In studies that answer clinical questions of diagnosis, investigators study the ability of screening or diagnostic tests, or components of the clinical examination to detect (or not detect) disease when the patient has (or does not have) the particular disease of

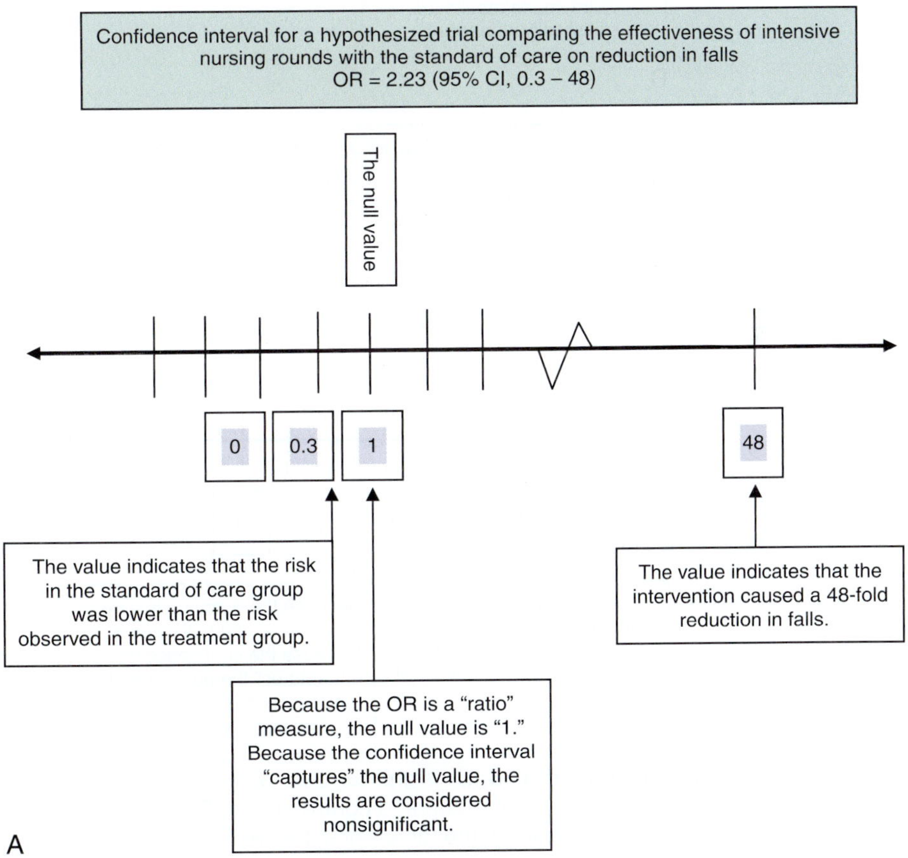

FIG 19.1 A, Confidence interval (CI) (nonsignificant) for a hypothesized trial comparing the ratio of events in the experimental group and control group. *Continued*

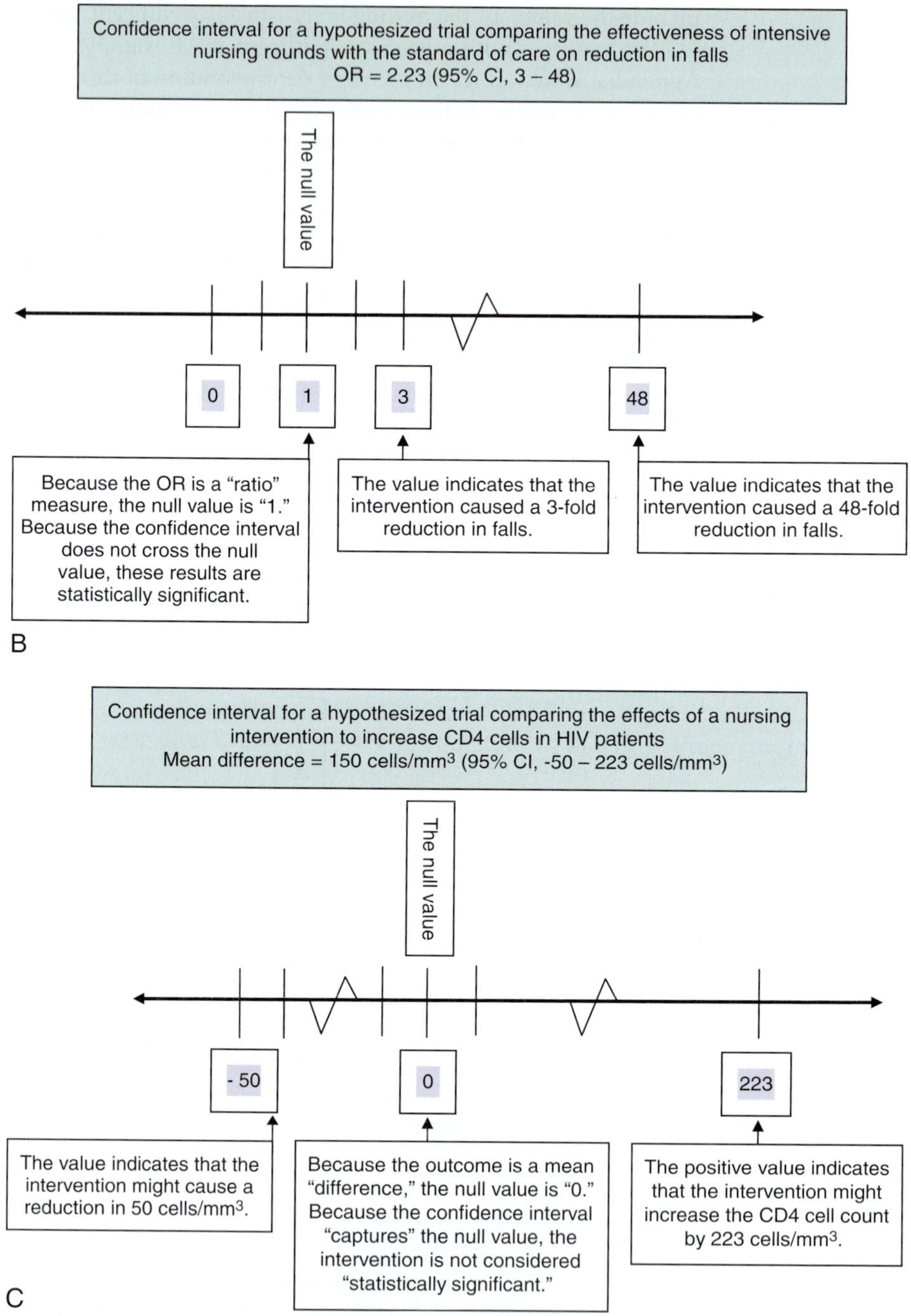

FIG 19.1, cont'd B, CI (significant) for a hypothesized trial comparing the ratio of events in the experimental group and control group. **C,** CI (nonsignificant) for a hypothesized control trial comparing the difference between two treatments.

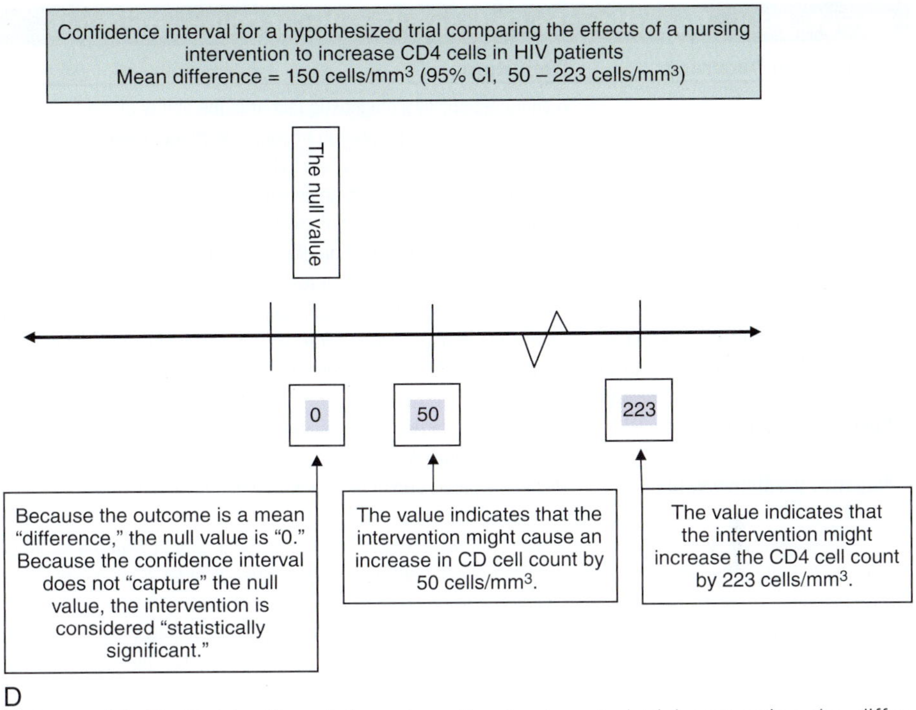

FIG 19.1, cont'd D, CI (significant) for a hypothesized control trial comparing the difference between two treatments.

interest. The accuracy of a test, or technique, is measured by its sensitivity and specificity (Table 19.4).

Sensitivity is the proportion of those with disease who test positive; that is, sensitivity is a measure of how well the test detects disease when it is really there—a highly sensitive test has few false negatives. **Specificity** is the proportion of those without disease who test negative. It measures how well the test rules out disease when it is really absent; a specific test has few false positives. Sensitivity and specificity have some deficiencies in clinical use, primarily because sensitivity and specificity are merely characteristics of the performance of the test.

Describing diagnostic tests in this way tells us how good the test is, but what is more useful is how well the test performs in a particular population with a particular disease prevalence. This is important because in a population in which a disease is quite prevalent, there are fewer incorrect test results (false positives) as compared with populations with low disease prevalence, for which a positive test may truly be a false positive. Predictive values are a measure of accuracy that accounts for the prevalence of a disease. As illustrated in Table 19.4, a **positive predictive value** (PPV) expresses the proportion of those with positive test results who truly have disease, and a **negative predictive value** (NPV) expresses the proportion of those with negative test results who truly do not have disease. Let us observe how these characteristics of diagnostic tests are used in nursing practice.

TABLE 19.4 Reporting the Outcome Results of Diagnostic Trials

Measure of Accuracy	Definition	Comments
Sensitivity	A characteristic of a diagnostic test. It is the ability of the test to detect the proportion of people with the disease or disorder of interest. For a test to be useful in ruling out a disease, it must have a high sensitivity.	Formula for sensitivity: TP/(TP + FN), where TP and FN are number of true positive and false negative results, respectively.
Specificity	A characteristic of a diagnostic test. It is the ability of the test to detect the proportion of people without the disease or disorder of interest. For a test to be useful at confirming a disease, it must have a high specificity.	Formula for specificity: TN/(TN + FP), where TN and FP are number of true negative and false positive results, respectively.
PPV and NPV are closely related to sensitivity and specificity (how well the test performs) but differ in that sensitivity and specificity are fixed characteristics of a diagnostic test, whereas PPV and NPV consider how well the test performs in populations with difference prevalence of the disease it is testing.		
Positive predictive value	This is the proportion of people with a positive test who have the target disorder.	Formula for PPV: PPV = TP/(TP + FP)
Negative predictive value	This is the proportion of people with a negative test who do not have the target disorder.	Formula for NPV: NPV = TN/(TN + FN)
LR: A likelihood ratio is a measure that a given test result would be expected in a patient with the target disorder compared with the likelihood that the same result would be expected in a patient without the target disorder. It measures the power of a test to change the pretest into the posttest probability of a disease being present.		
Positive likelihood ratio	The LR of a positive test tells us how well a positive test result does by comparing its performance when the disease is present to that when it is absent. The best test to use for ruling in a disease is the one with the largest likelihood ratio of a positive test.	Formula for positive likelihood ratio: Sensitivity/(1 − Specificity)
Negative likelihood ratio	The LR of a negative test tells us how well a negative test result does by comparing its performance when the disease is absent to that when it is present. The better test to use to rule out disease is the one with the smaller likelihood ratio of a negative test.	Formula for negative likelihood ratio: (1 − Sensitivity)/Specificity

FN, False negative; *FP*, false positive; *LR*, likelihood ratio; *NPV*, negative predictive value; *PPV*, positive predictive value; *TN*, true negative; *TP*, true positive.

Nurses developed a four-step tool to screen stroke patients for dysphagia (difficulty swallowing) (Cummings et al., 2015). A total of 49 patients were evaluated following their stroke. An experienced speech language therapist evaluated all patients for dysphagia using standard objective methods and determined if dysphagia was present or absent. Nurses used the four-step dysphagia tool (the new test) to evaluate whether or not dysphagia was present or absent. The nurse's dysphagia tool had a sensitivity of 89% and a specificity of 90%. Table 19.5 shows how sensitivity and specificity are easily calculated and how these numbers are interpreted. Sensitivity and specificity apply to the diagnostic test and tell what portion of the people will have a positive or negative test. Clinicians and patients often want to know when a test is negative or positive what the probability is of actually having the disease. The PPV and NPV answer these question. Table 19.5 shows how the PPV and NPV are calculated. In the study, the probability of having dysphagia when screened positive on the dysphagia tool is 84%, and the probability of not having dysphagia when screened negative on the dysphagia tool is 93%.

TABLE 19.5 Results for Dysphagia Screen With a Standardized Speech and Language Pathology Screen and Nurse Dysphagia Screen

		SLP SCREEN: DYSPHAGIA PRESENT? (GOLD STANDARD)		
Method	**Test Result**	**Yes**	**No**	**Totals**
Nurse screen: Dysphagia present?	Yes	16 TP	3 FP	19
	No	2 FN	28 TN	30
Totals	—	18	31	49

Calculations Made from Study Results

Sensitivity = TP/(TP + FN)	16/18 = 0.89 or 89% *Interpretation:* The nurse's tool is 89% accurate in identifying patients with dysphagia.
Specificity = TN/(TN + FP)	28/31 = 0.90 or 90% *Interpretation:* The nurse's tool is 90% accurate in identifying patients without dysphagia.
Prevalence of dysphagia = (TP + FN)/Total population	18/49 = 0.367 or 37% *Interpretation:* The prevalence of dysphagia in stroke patients on this unit is 37%.
Positive predictive value = TP/(TP + FP)	16/19 = 84.2% *Interpretation:* The probability of having dysphagia is 84.2% when the screen is positive.
Negative predictive value = TN/(TN + FN)	28/30 = 93.3% *Interpretation:* The probability of not having dysphagia is 93.3% when the screen is negative.
Positive LR = Sensitivity/(1 − Specificity)	0.89/(1 − 0.90) = 0.89/0.1 = 8.9 *Interpretation:* Here are some general guidelines when interpreting likelihood ratios: The first thing to realize about LRs is that an LR greater than 1 increases the probability that the target disorder is present, and an LR less than 1 decreases the probability that the target disorder is present. See Table 19.6, which describes how much likelihood ratio changes the probability of disease.
Negative LR = (1 − Sensitivity)/Specificity	1 − 0.89/0.90 = 0.122 *Interpretation:* See above

FN, False negative; *FP,* false positive; *LR,* likelihood ratio; *TN,* true negative; *TP,* true positive.

Combining sensitivity, specificity, PPV, NPV, and prevalence to make clinical decisions based on the results of testing is cumbersome and complex. Fortunately, all of these measures can be described by one number, the **likelihood ratio** (LR). This value takes a pretest probability, and when the test is applied (either a positive test or a negative test) gives us a new probability. In other words, it tells us how much more we are certain the patient has the disease as a result of the test. As you can see from Table 19.5, the LR is calculated from the test's sensitivity and specificity, and with more training in determining disease prevalence (or pretest probability), you could actually state the numerical probability that a patient might have a disease based on the test's LR.

As illustrated in Table 19.6, a test with a large **positive likelihood ratio** (e.g., greater than 10), when applied, provides the clinician with a high degree of certainty that the patient has the suspected disorder. Conversely, tests with a very low positive likelihood ratio (e.g., less than 2), when applied, provide you with little to no change in the degree of certainty that the patient has the suspected disorder.

TABLE 19.6 How Much Do Likelihood Ratio Changes Affect Probability of Disease?

Likelihood Ratio Positive	Likelihood Ratio Negative	Probability That Patient Has (LR) or Does Not Have (LR)
LR > 10	LR < 0.1	Large
LR 5–10	LR 0.1–0.2	Moderate
LR 2–5	LR 0.2–0.5	Small
LR < 2	LR > 0.5	Tiny
LR = 1.0	—	Test provides no useful information

LR, Likelihood ratio.

When a test has a LR of 1 (the null value), the test will not contribute to decision making in any meaningful way and should not be used. A test with a large **negative likelihood ratio** provides the clinician with a high degree of certainty that the patient does not have the disease. The further away from 1 the negative LR is, the better the test will be for its use in ruling out disease (i.e., there will be few false negatives). More and more journal articles require authors to provide test LRs; they may also be available in secondary sources.

Prognosis Articles

In studies that answer clinical questions of prognosis, investigators conduct studies in which they want to determine the outcome of a particular disease or condition. Prognosis studies can often be identified by their longitudinal cohort design (see Chapter 10). At the conclusion of a longitudinal study, investigators statistically analyze data to determine which factors are strongly associated with the study outcomes, usually through a technique called multivariate regression analysis or simply multiple regression (see Chapter 16).

From this advanced statistical analysis, several factors are usually identified that predict the probability of developing the outcome or a particular disease. The probability is called an **odds ratio**. The OR (see Table 19.3) indicates how much more likely certain independent variables (factors) predict the probability of developing the dependent variable (outcome or disease).

Returning to our case, Sheila reviews a prospective cohort, longitudinal study of pregnant mothers. The authors collected data on maternal consumption of artificially sweetened beverages during pregnancy. At 1 year of age infants were weighed; 5% of the infants were overweight. Daily consumption of artificially sweetened beverages was significantly associated with having an infant overweight at 1 year of age (OR, 2.19; 95% CI, 1.23 to 3.88). The interpretation of the ORs is described in Table 19.7. A higher OR indicates a greater probability of the development of the outcome. An OR below 1 indicates that the probability of developing the outcome is reduced. Also recall from our discussion that whenever we are appraising CIs (to determine statistical significance) we have to examine the CI for the presence of the null value. Because we are evaluating a "ratio," the null value is equal to 1. Thus any OR CI interval that contains a null value of 1 is not a significant finding. Looking at the CI given previously, we can see that all of the values are above 1 and this does not include the null value; as such, this is a statistically significant finding.

Using prognostic information with an evidence-based lens helps the nurse and patient focus on reducing factors that may lead to disease or disability. It also helps the nurse with providing education and information to patients and their families regarding the course of the condition.

TABLE 19.7 Measures of Association for Trials That Report Discrete Outcomes

Measure of Association	Definition	Comment
Reporting Events in Terms of the Probability of It Occurring (Good or Bad)		
Odds ratio (OR)	We could estimate the odds of an event occurring. The OR is usually the measure of choice in the analysis of nonexperimental design studies. It is the probability of a given event occurring to the probability of the event not occurring.	If the OR = 1.0, this means there is no difference in the probability of an event occurring between the experimental and control group outcomes. If the probability of the event is reduced between groups, the OR is < 1.0 (i.e., the event is less likely in the treatment group than the control group). If the odds of an event is increased between groups, the OR > 1.0 (i.e., the event is more likely to occur in the treatment group than the control group).

IPE HIGHLIGHT

It is important that all members of your team understand the importance of being able to read tables included in research reports. The information you need to answer your clinical question should be contained in one or more of the tables.

Harm Articles

In studies that answer clinical questions of harm, investigators want to determine if an individual has been harmed by being exposed to a particular event. Harm studies can be identified by their case-control design (see Chapter 10). In this type of study, investigators select the outcome they are interested in (e.g., pressure ulcers), and they examine if any one factor explains those who have and do not have the outcome of interest. The measure of association that best describes the analyzed data in case-control studies is the OR.

Tomlinson and colleagues (2016) used a case-control study design to identify factors that contribute to delirium in hospitalized patients (incident delirium). Table 19.8 presents data examining factors that might be associated with incident delirium.

The interpretation of the data is relatively straightforward. You can see from the table that most of the ORs are greater than 1. Examining the table, you can see being >80 years of age, having anemia, having chronic obstructive airway disease, and many other factors are associated with the development of incident delirium while hospitalized. Based on the previous discussion of CIs you know that the CI indicates how well the study findings can be generalized. A quick review of the CIs demonstrates that some of these factors are not statistically significant findings; for example, having anemia and cancer are not statistically significant findings.

Harm data, with its measure of probabilities, help you identify factors that may or may not contribute to an adverse or beneficial outcome. This information will be useful for the nursing plan of care, program planning, or patient and family education.

Meta-Analysis

Meta-analysis statistically combines the results of multiple studies (usually RCTs) to answer a focused clinical question through an objective appraisal of carefully synthesized

TABLE 19.8 **Comparisons of Predisposing Risk Factors for Incident Delirium**

Predisposing Factor Present	Case (N = 161) N (%)	Control (N = 321) N (%)	Odds Ratio (95 % CI)
Age > 80 years	124 (77.0)	178 (55.5)	2.69 (1.75 – 4.13)
Anemia	6 (3.7)	13 (4.0)	1.09 (0.41 – 2.92)
Cancer	21 (13.0)	44 (13.7)	0.94 (0.54 – 1.65)
COAD	27 (16.8)	77 (24.0)	1.57 (0.96 – 2.55)
Cognitive impairment	61 (37.9)	54 (16.8)	3.01 (1.96 – 4.65)
Depression	35 (21.7)	53 (16.5)	1.41 (0.87 – 2.26)
Dementia	26 (16.1)	20 (6.2)	2.90 (1.56 – 5.37)
Diabetes	40 (24.8)	72 (22.4)	0.86 (0.56 – 1.36)
Functional impairment	71 (44.1)	66 (20.6)	3.05 (2.02 – 4.60)
Fall on admission	51 (31.7)	53 (16.5)	2.34 (1.50 – 3.65)
Fracture on admission	29 (18.0)	31 (9.7)	2.06 (1.19 – 3.55)
Male gender	67 (41.6)	149 (46.4)	0.82 (0.56 – 1.21)
Hearing impairment	30 (18.6)	48 (15.0)	1.30 (0.79 – 2.15)
Hypertension	92 (57.1)	185 (57.6)	1.02 (0.70 – 1.49)
Hypercholesterolemia	54 (33.5)	76 (23.7)	1.61 (1.08 – 2.44)
Ischemic heart disease	28 (17.4)	51 (15.9)	0.90 (0.54 – 1.49)
Joint replacement	22 (13.7)	27 (8.4)	1.72 (0.95 – 3.13)

From Tomlinson, E. J., Phillips, N., Mohebbi, M., & Hutchinson, A. M. (2016). Risk factors for incident delirium in an acute general medical setting: a retrospective case-control study. *Journal of Clinical Nursing.* doi:10.1111/jocn.13529.

research evidence. The strength of a meta-analysis lies in its use of statistical analysis to summarize studies. As discussed in Chapter 11:

- A clinical question is used to guide the process.
- All relevant studies, published and unpublished, on the question are gathered using pre-established inclusion and exclusion criteria to determine the studies to be used in the meta-analysis.
- At least two individuals independently assess the quality of each study based on pre-established criteria.
- Statistically combine the results of individual studies and present a balanced and impartial quantitative and narrative evidence summary of the findings that represents a "state-of-the-science" conclusion about the strength, quality, and consistency of evidence supporting benefits and risks of a given health care practice (García-Perdomo, 2016).

A methodologically sound meta-analysis is more likely than an individual study to be successful in identifying the true effect of an intervention because it limits bias. An RR or, more commonly, the OR is the statistic of choice for use in a meta-analysis (see Tables 19.3 and 19.7). Meta-analysis can also report on continuous data; typically the mean difference in outcomes will be reported.

The typical manner of displaying data in a meta-analysis is by a pictorial representation known as a *blobbogram,* accompanied by a summary measure of effect size in RR, OR, or mean difference (see Chapter 11). Let us see how blobbograms (sometimes called forest plots) and ORs are used to summarize the studies in a systematic review by practicing with the data from the article in Appendix E. Box A lists nine studies that looked at all-cause mortality. The next four columns list the number of deaths in the nursing group and the nonnursing group (control group). The next column assigns a weight to each study based on the number of subject participants. The larger the sample size, the greater the weight assigned to the study for analysis purposes. In the next column you will note the OR for each of the studies along with its CI. At the end of the table you see a horizontal line represents each trial in the analysis. The findings from each individual study are represented as a blob or square (the measured effect) on the horizontal line. You may also note that each blob or square is a bit different in size. This size reflects the weight the study has on the overall analysis. This is determined by the sample size and the quality of the study. The width of the horizontal line represents the 95% CI. The vertical line is the line of no effect (i.e., the null value), and we know that when the statistic is the OR, the null value is 1.

HELPFUL HINT

When appraising the different review types, it is important to be able to distinguish a meta-analysis that analytically assesses studies, from a systematic review that appraises the literature with or without an analytic approach, to an integrative review that also appraises and synthesizes the literature but without an analytic process (see Chapter 11).

When the CI of the result (horizontal line) touches or crosses the line of no effect (vertical line), we can say that the study findings did not reach statistical significance. If the CI does not cross the vertical line, we can say that the study results reached statistical significance. Can you tell which studies are significant and which ones are not? (Hint: There are only two significant studies.)

You will also notice other important information and additional statistical analyses that may accompany the blobbogram table, such as a test to determine how well the results of each of the individual trials are mathematically compatible (heterogeneity) and a test for overall effect. The reader is referred to a book of advanced research methods for discussion of these topics.

A diamond represents the summary ratio for all studies combined. There is a subtotal diamond for the effect of a nurse led clinic on all-cause mortality. In this case, after statistically pooling the results of each of the controlled trials, it shows that these studies, statistically combined, overall favor the treatment (the nurse led clinic). You will note that the diamond does not touch the line of no effect and as such is a statistically significant finding. The overall interpretation is that a nurse led clinic reduces all-cause mortality in patients with cardiovascular disease. If this is a methodologically sound review, it can be used to support or change nursing practice or specific nursing interventions. A simple tool to help determine whether or not a systematic review is methodologically sound can be found at http://www.cebm.net/critical-appraisal/.

QSEN EVIDENCE-BASED PRACTICE TIP

When answering a clinical question, check to see if a Cochrane review has been performed. This will save you time searching the literature. A Cochrane review is a systematic review that primarily uses meta-analysis to investigate the effects of interventions for prevention, treatment, and rehabilitation in a health care setting or on health-related disorders. Most Cochrane reviews are based on RCTs, but other types of evidence may also be taken into account, if appropriate. If the data collected in a review are of sufficient quality and similar enough, they are summarized statistically in a meta-analysis. You should always check the Cochrane website, www.cochrane.org, to see if a review has been published on the topic of interest.

EVIDENCE-BASED STRATEGY #5: APPLYING THE FINDINGS

Evidence-based practice is about integrating individual clinical expertise and patient preferences with the best external evidence to guide clinical decision making (Sackett et al., 1996). With a few simple tools (see the links listed earlier in this chapter) and some practice, your day-to-day practice can be more evidence based. We know that using evidence in clinical decision making by nurses and all other health care professionals interested in matters associated with the care of individuals, communities, and health systems is increasingly important to achieving quality patient outcomes and cannot be ignored. Let us see how Sheila uses evidence to answer the expectant mothers' question.

Sheila critically appraises the article. This was a cohort study of mother–infant dyads in Canada. Women in the study completed dietary assessments during pregnancy, and their infants' weights were measured at 1 year of age. Twenty-six percent of the women consumed artificially sweetened beverages; 5% of the women drank these beverages daily. Compared with no consumption, daily consumers have a twofold higher risk of having an overweight infant at 1 year of age (OR, 2.19; 95% CI 1.23 to 3.88). Sheila knows that an OR greater than 1 means that there was an increase in the number of overweight babies in the consumers of artificially sweetened beverages relative to the control group (nonconsumers). She also examines the CIs and notes that the range does not include the null value of 1, making this finding statistically significant. Sheila is surprised by the study's findings and plans to examine other studies on this subject. She will report back to the mothers that they should avoid drinking artificially sweetened beverages, as this is associated with weight gain in their baby at 1 year. She will be sure to tell the mothers that this effect was measured at 1 year; she does not know if this effect remains beyond the first year of life. She will also tell the mothers that although the findings are statistically significant there could be other factors that were not examined that could have influenced study results, such as smoking, diet quality, and breastfeeding duration.

SUMMARY

Clinical questions about nursing practice occur frequently; these questions come from nursing assessments, planning, and interventions; from patients; and from questions about the effectiveness of care. Nurses need to think about how they can effectively review the literature for research evidence to answer a clinical question. It is important for nurses and all health care providers and the teams they are part of to be competent at using critical appraisal tools as a resource to evaluate clinical studies that can be used to inform clinical decision making about whether research findings are applicable to clinical practice. Nurses should understand and be able to interpret common measures of association, such as the OR and CIs, and apply this understanding to how data can be used to support current "best practices" or recommend changes in clinical care.

KEY POINTS

- Asking a focused clinical question using the PICO approach is an important evidence-based practice tool.
- Several types of evidence-based practice clinical categories used for evaluating research studies are therapy, diagnosis, prognosis, and harm. These categories focus on development of the clinical question, the literature search, and critical appraisal of research.

- An efficient and effective literature search, using information literacy skills, is critical in locating evidence to answer the clinical question.
- Sources of evidence (e.g., articles, evidence-based practice guidelines, evidence-based practice protocols) must be screened for relevance and credibility.
- Appraising the evidence generated by a study using an accepted critiquing tool is essential in determining the strength, quality, and consistency of evidence offered by a study.
- Studies that belong to the therapy category are designed to determine if a difference exists between two or more treatments.
- Studies that belong to the diagnosis category are designed to investigate the ability of screening or diagnostic tests, tools, or components of the clinical examination to detect whether or not the patient has a particular disease using LRs.
- Studies in the prognosis category are designed to determine the outcomes of a particular disease or condition.
- Studies in the harm category are designed to determine if an individual has been harmed by being exposed to a particular event.
- Meta-analysis is a research method that statistically combines the results of multiple studies (usually RCTs) and is designed to answer a focused clinical question through objective appraisal of synthesized evidence.

CRITICAL THINKING CHALLENGES

- How would you use the PICO format to formulate a clinical question? Provide a clinical example.
- How can the nurse determine if reported or calculated measures in a research study are clinically significant enough to inform evidence-based clinical decisions?
- How can a nurse in clinical practice determine whether the strength and quality of evidence provided by a diagnostic tool is sufficient to justify ordering it as a diagnostic test? Provide an example of a diagnostic test used to diagnose a specific illness.
- IPE How could your interprofessional QI team use the PICO format to formulate a clinical question? Provide a clinical example from the QI data from your unit.
- Choose a meta-analysis from a peer-reviewed journal and describe how you as a nurse would use the findings of this meta-analysis in making a clinical decision about the applicability of a nursing intervention for your specific patient population and clinical setting.

REFERENCES

Azad, M. B., Sharma, A. K., de Souza, R. J., et al. (2016). Association between artificially sweetened beverage consumption during pregnancy and infant body mass index. *JAMA Pediatrics, 170*(7), 662–670. doi:10.1001/jamapediatrics.2016.0301.

Cummings, J., Soomans, D., O'Laughlin, J., et al. (2015). Sensitivity and specificity of a nurse dysphagia screen in stroke patients. *Medsurg Nursing, 24*(4), 219–222, 263.

García-Perdomo, H. A. (2016). Evidence synthesis and meta-analysis: a practical approach. *International Journal of Urological Nursing, 10*(1), 30–36. doi:10.1111/ijun.12087.

Haas, J. S., Linder, J. A., Park, E. R., et al. (2015). Proactive tobacco cessation outreach to smokers of low socioeconomic status: a randomized clinical trial. *JAMA Internal Medicine, 175*(2), 218–226. doi:10.1001/jamainternmed.2014.6674.

Munn, Z., Lockwood, C., & Moola, S. (2015). The development and use of evidence summaries for point of care information systems: a streamlined rapid review approach. *Worldviews on Evidence Based Nursing, 12*(3), 131–138.

Sackett, D. L., Rosenberg, W. M. C., Gray, J. A. M., et al. (1996). Evidence based medicine: what it is and what it isn't. *British Medical Journal, 312,* 71–72.

Tomlinson, E. J., Phillips, N., Mohebbi, M., et al. (2016). Risk factors for incident delirium in an acute general medical setting: a retrospective case-control study. *Journal of Clinical Nursing.* doi:10.1111/jocn.13529.

Warren, E. (2015). Evidence-based practice. *Practice Nurse, 45*(12), 27–32.

Go to Evolve at **http://evolve.elsevier.com/LoBiondo/** for review questions, critiquing exercises, and additional research articles for practice in reviewing and critiquing.

20

Developing an Evidence-Based Practice

Marita Titler

Go to Evolve at **http://evolve.elsevier.com/LoBiondo/** for review questions, critiquing exercises, and additional research articles for practice in reviewing and critiquing.

LEARNING OUTCOMES

After reading this chapter, you should be able to do the following:

- Differentiate among conduct of nursing research, evidence-based practice, and translation science.
- Describe the steps of evidence-based practice.
- Describe strategies for implementing evidence-based practice changes.
- Identify steps for evaluating an evidence-based change in practice.
- Use research findings and other forms of evidence to improve the quality of care.

KEY TERMS

conduct of research
dissemination
evaluation
evidence-based practice
evidence-based practice guidelines
knowledge-focused triggers
opinion leaders
problem-focused triggers
translation science

Evidence-based health care practices are available for a number of conditions. However, these practices are not always implemented in care delivery settings. Variation in practices abounds, and availability of high-quality research does not ensure that the findings will be used to affect patient outcomes (Agency for Healthcare Research and Quality [AHRQ], 2015; Titler et al., 2011, 2013). The use of evidence-based practices (EBPs) is now an expected standard, as demonstrated by regulations from the Centers for Medicare and Medicaid Services (CMS) regarding nonpayment for hospital acquired events such as injury from falls, Foley catheter-associated urinary tract infections, and stage 3 and 4 pressure ulcers. These practices all have a strong evidence base and, when enacted, can prevent these events. However, implementing such evidence-based safety practices is a challenge and requires the use of strategies that address the systems of care, individual practitioners, and senior leadership, and ultimately change health care cultures to be EBP environments (Dockham et al., 2016; Moore et al., 2014; Newhouse et al., 2013; Titler et al., 2016).

Translation of research into practice (TRIP) is a multifaceted, systemic process of promoting adoption of EBPs in delivery of health care services that goes beyond dissemination of evidence-based guidelines (Berwick, 2003; Rogers, 2003). **Dissemination** activities take many forms, including publications, conferences, consultations, and training programs, but promoting knowledge uptake and changing practitioner behavior requires active interchange with those in direct care (Titler et al., 2013, 2016). This chapter presents an overview of EBP and the process of applying evidence in practice to improve patient outcomes.

OVERVIEW OF EVIDENCE-BASED PRACTICE

The relationships among conduct, dissemination, and use of research are illustrated in Fig. 20.1. **Conduct of research** is the analysis of data collected from subjects who meet study inclusion and exclusion criteria for the purpose of answering research questions or testing hypotheses. The conduct of research includes dissemination of findings via research reports in journals and at scientific conferences.

Evidence-based practice is the conscientious and judicious use of current best evidence in conjunction with clinical expertise and patient values and circumstances to guide health care decisions (Straus et al., 2011; Titler, 2014). Best evidence includes findings from randomized controlled trials, evidence from other scientific methods such as descriptive and qualitative research, as well as information from case reports and scientific principles. When adequate research evidence is available, practice should be guided by research evidence in conjunction with clinical expertise and patient values. In some cases, however, a sufficient research base may not be available, and health care decision making is derived principally from evidence sources such as scientific principles, case reports, and quality improvement projects. As illustrated in Fig. 20.1, the application of research findings in

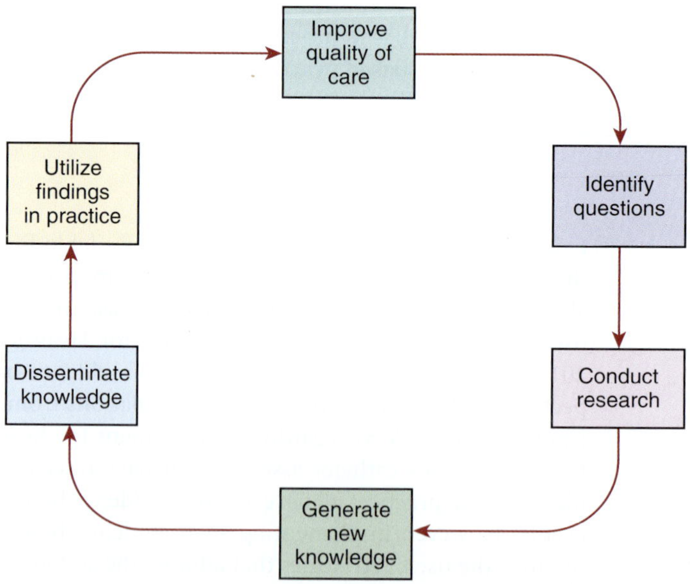

FIG 20.1 The model of the relationship among conduct, dissemination, and use of research. (From Weiler, K., Buckwalter, K., & Titler, M. [1994]. Debate: Is nursing research used in practice? In J. McCloskey, & H. Grace [Eds.], *Current issues in nursing* [4th ed.]. St Louis, MO: Mosby.)

practice may not only improve quality care but also create new and exciting questions to be addressed via conduct of research.

In contrast, **translation science** focuses on testing implementation interventions to improve uptake and use of evidence to improve patient outcomes and population health, as well as to explicate what implementation strategies work for whom, in what settings, and why (Titler, 2014). An emerging body of knowledge in translation science provides an empirical base for guiding the selection of implementation strategies to promote adoption of EBPs in real-world settings (Dobbins et al., 2009; Titler et al., 2016). Thus EBP and translation science, though related, are not interchangeable terms; EBP is the actual application of evidence in practice (the "doing of" EBP), whereas translation science is the study of implementation interventions, factors, and contextual variables that effect knowledge uptake and use in practices and communities.

Models of Evidence-Based Practice

Multiple models of EBP and translation science are available (Milat et al., 2015; Rycroft-Malone & Bucknall, 2010; Schaffer et al., 2013; Wilson et al., 2010). Common elements of these models are:

- Syntheses of evidence
- Implementation
- Evaluation of the impact on patient care
- Consideration of the context/setting in which the evidence is implemented.

Although review of these models is beyond the scope of this chapter, implementing evidence in practice must be guided by a conceptual model to organize the strategies being used and to clarify extraneous variables (e.g., behaviors, facilitators) that may influence adoption of EBPs (e.g., organizational size, characteristics of users).

The Iowa Model of Evidence-Based Practice

An overview of the Iowa Model of Evidence-Based Practice as an **example** ➤ of an EBP model is illustrated in Fig. 20.2. This model has been widely disseminated and adopted in academic and clinical settings (Titler et al., 2001).

In this model, knowledge- and problem-focused "triggers" lead staff members to question current nursing practices and whether patient care can be improved through the use of research findings. If through the process of literature review and critique of studies, it is found that there is not a sufficient number of scientifically sound studies to use as a base for practice, consideration is given to conducting a study. Findings from such studies are then combined with findings from existing scientific knowledge to develop and implement these practices. If there is insufficient research to guide practice and conducting a study is not feasible, other types of evidence (e.g., case reports, scientific principles, theory) are used and/or combined with available research evidence to guide practice. Priority is given to projects in which a high proportion of practice is guided by research evidence. Practice guidelines usually reflect research and nonresearch evidence and therefore are called **evidence-based practice guidelines** (NAM, formally Institute of Medicine [IOM], 2011; see Chapter 11).

Recommendations for practice are developed based on evidence synthesis. The recommended practices, based on evidence, are compared with current practice, and a decision is made about the necessity for a practice change. If a practice change is warranted, changes are implemented using a planned change process. The practice is first implemented with a small group of patients, and a pilot evaluation is conducted. The EBP is then refined based

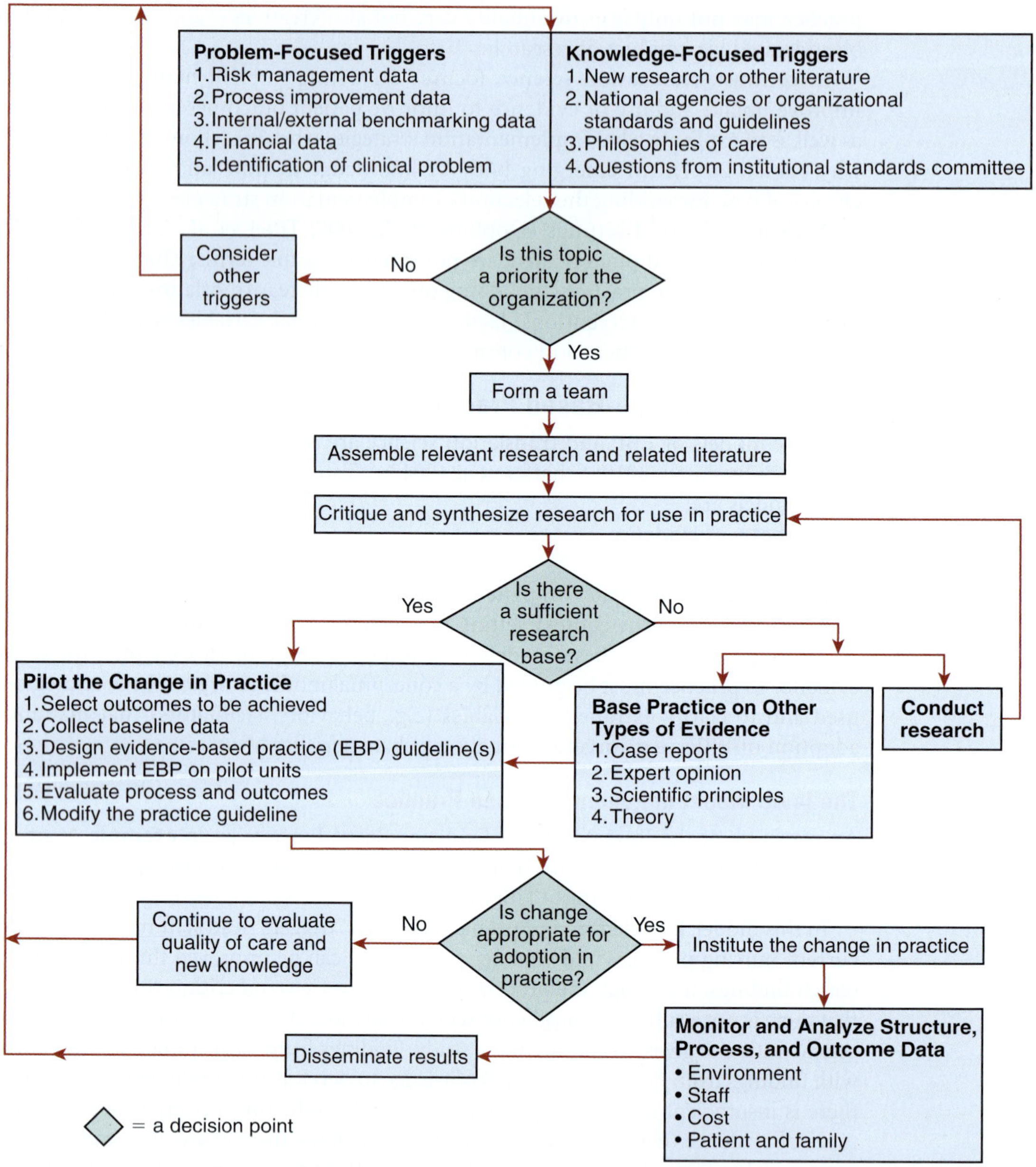

FIG 20.2 The Iowa model of evidence-based practice to promote quality care. (From Titler, M. G., Kleiber, C., Steelman, V. J., et al. [2001]. The Iowa model of evidence-based practice to promote quality care. *Critical Care Nursing Clinics of North America, 13*[4]:497–509.)

on evaluation data, and the change is implemented with additional patient populations for which it is appropriate. Patient/family, staff, and fiscal outcomes are monitored.

STEPS OF EVIDENCE-BASED PRACTICE

The Iowa Model of Evidence-Based Practice to Promote Quality Care (Titler et al., 2001; see Fig. 20.2), in conjunction with Rogers's diffusion of innovations model (Rogers, 2003), provides steps for actualizing EBP. A team approach is most helpful in fostering a specific EBP.

Selection of a Topic

The first step is to select a topic. Ideas for EBP come from several sources categorized as problem- and knowledge-focused triggers. **Problem-focused triggers** are those identified by staff through quality improvement, risk surveillance, benchmarking data, financial data, or recurrent clinical problems. An example of a problem-focused trigger is increased incidence of central line occlusion in pediatric oncology patients.

Knowledge-focused triggers are ideas generated when staff read research, listen to scientific papers at conferences, or encounter EBP guidelines published by federal agencies or specialty organizations. This includes those EBPs that CMS expects are implemented in practice, and CMS now bases reimbursement of care on adherence to indicators of the EBPs. Examples include treatment of heart failure, community-acquired pneumonia, and prevention of nosocomial pressure ulcers. Each of these topics includes a nursing component, such as discharge teaching, instructions for patient self-care, or pain management. Sometimes topics arise from a combination of problem- and knowledge-focused triggers, such as the length of bed rest time after femoral artery catheterization. In selecting a topic, it is essential to consider how the topic fits with organization, department, and unit priorities to garner support from leaders within the organization and the necessary resources to successfully complete the project. Criteria to consider when selecting a topic are outlined in Box 20.1.

IPE HIGHLIGHT

Regardless of which approach is used to select an evidence-based practice topic, it is critical that your team who will implement the potential practice change are involved in selecting the topic, developing the clinical question, and viewing it as contributing significantly to the quality of care for your patient population.

BOX 20.1 Selection Criteria for an Evidence-Based Practice Project

1. Priority of the topic for nursing and for the organization
2. Magnitude of the problem (small, medium, large)
3. Applicability to several or few clinical areas
4. Likelihood of the change to improve quality of care, decrease length of stay, contain costs, or improve patient satisfaction
5. Potential "land mines" associated with the topic and capability to diffuse them
6. Availability of baseline quality improvement or risk data that will be helpful during evaluation
7. Multidisciplinary nature of the topic and ability to create collaborative relationships to effect the needed changes
8. Interest and commitment of staff to the potential topic
9. Availability of a sound body of evidence, preferably research evidence

Forming a Team

A team is responsible for development, implementation, and evaluation of the EBP. A task force approach also may be used, in which a group is appointed to address a practice issue. The composition of the team is directed by the topic selected and should include interested stakeholders. **Example:** ➤ A team working on evidence-based pain management should be interdisciplinary and include pharmacists, nurses, physicians, and psychologists. In contrast, a team working on the EBP of bathing might include a nurse expert in skin care, assistive nursing personnel, and staff nurses. Although not traditionally included in the team, the engagement of patients, family members, and consumers as team members is receiving more attention in EBP (Moore et al., 2014, 2015; Shuman et al., 2016). Consideration should be given to including a layperson team who has experience with the topic. **Example:** ➤ A team focusing on prevention of **necrotizing enterocolitis** (NEC) in premature neonates may invite a parent to participate on the team because feeding breast milk (instead of formula) is one strategy to prevent NEC.

In addition to forming a team, key stakeholders who can facilitate the EBP project or put up barriers against successful implementation should be identified. A **stakeholder** is a key individual or group of individuals who will be directly or indirectly affected by the implementation of the EBP. Some of these stakeholders are likely to be members of the team. Others may not be team members but are key individuals within the organization or unit who can adversely or positively influence the adoption of the practice. Questions to consider in identification of key stakeholders include the following:

- How are decisions made in the areas where the EBP will be implemented?
- What types of system changes will be needed?
- Who is involved in decision making?
- Who is likely to lead and champion implementation of the EBP?
- Who can influence the decision to proceed with implementation of the practice?
- What type of cooperation is needed from stakeholders for the project to be successful?

Failure to involve or keep supportive stakeholders informed may place the success of the project at risk because they are unable to anticipate and/or defend the rationale for changing practice, particularly with resistors (e.g., nonsupportive stakeholders) who have a great deal of influence among their peer group.

An important early task for the EBP team is to formulate the PICO question. This helps set boundaries around the project and assists in evidence retrieval. This approach is illustrated in Table 20.1 (see Chapters 1 to 3, and 19).

Evidence Retrieval

Once a topic is selected, relevant research and related literature need to be retrieved (see Chapters 3 and 11). AHRQ (www.AHRQ.gov) sponsors the Evidenced-Based Practice Centers and a National Guideline Clearinghouse, where abstracts of EBP guidelines are available. Current best evidence from specific studies of clinical problems can be found in an increasing number of electronic databases such as the Cochrane Library (www.thecochranelibrary.com), the Centers for Health Evidence (www.cche.net), and Best Evidence (www.acponline.org) (see Chapters 3 and 11). Once the literature is located, it

TABLE 20.1 Using PICO to Formulate the Evidence-Based Practice Question

	Patient/Population/ Problem	Intervention/ Treatment	Comparison Intervention	Outcome(s)
Tips for building the question	How would we describe a group of patients similar to ours?	Which main intervention are we considering?	What is the main alternative to compare with the intervention?	What can we hope to accomplish?
Example 1	Pain management for elders admitted to a hospital with a hip fracture	Pain assessment—pain tool Patient-controlled analgesia	Standard of care Nurse-administered analgesic	Regular (e.g., q4hr) pain assessment Less pain intensity Earlier mobility Decreased length of stay
Example 2	Pain assessment of cognitively impaired elders	Pain assessment tool designed for assessing pain in cognitively impaired elders in long-term care setting	Not assess pain Yes/no question	Regular pain assessment with treatment of pain Fewer residents in pain

From University of Illinois at Chicago, P.I.C.O. Model for Clinical Questions, www.uic.edu/depts/lib/lhsp/resources/pico.shtml.

is helpful to classify the articles as clinical (nonresearch), theory, research, systematic reviews, and EBP guidelines. Before reading and critiquing the research, it is useful to read background articles to have a broad view of the topic and related concepts, and to then critique the existing EBP guidelines. It is helpful to read/critique articles in the following order:

1. Clinical articles to understand the state of the practice
2. Theory articles to understand the theoretical perspectives and concepts that may be encountered in critiquing studies
3. Systematic reviews and synthesis reports to understand the state of the science
4. EBP guidelines and evidence reports
5. Research articles, including meta-analyses

Schemas for Grading the Evidence

There is no consensus among professional organizations or across health care disciplines regarding the best system to use for denoting the type and quality of evidence, or the grading schemas to denote the strength of the body of evidence (Balshem et al., 2011; NAM, formally IOM, 2011). See Tables 20.2 and 20.3 for grading and assessing quality of research studies. The information posted on the GRADE website (www.gradeworkinggroup.org) is important information to understand the challenges and approaches for assessing the quality of evidence and strength of recommendations. The important domains and elements to include in grading the strength of the evidence are defined in Table 20.4.

In grading the evidence, two important areas are essential to address: (1) the quality of the evidence (e.g., individual studies, systematic reviews, meta-analyses), and (2) the strength of the body of evidence. Important domains and elements of any system used to rate quality of individual studies are listed in Table 20.3 by type of study. The domains and elements to include in grading the strength of the evidence are defined in Table 20.4.

TABLE 20.2 **Examples of Evidence Rating Systems**

Grade Working Group (www.gradeworkinggroup.org)	US Preventative Services Task Force (USPSTF) (www.uspreventiveservicestaskforce.org/)
Quality of the Evidence (Balshem et al., 2011; Guyatt et al., 2011, 2013) **High:** Very confident that the true effect lies close to that of the estimate of the effect. Scientific evidence provided by well-designed, well-conducted, controlled trials (randomized and nonrandomized) with statistically significant results that consistently support the recommendation. **Moderate:** Moderately confident in the effect estimate: The true effect is likely to be close to the estimate of the effect, but there is a possibility that it is substantially different. **Low:** Confidence in the effect estimate is limited: The true effect may be substantially different from the estimate of the effect. **Very low:** Very little confidence in the effect estimate: The true effect is likely to be substantially different from the estimate of effect. **Note:** The type of evidence is first ranked as follows: Randomized trial = High Observational study = Low Any other evidence = Very low **Quality may be downgraded due to** design flaws/threats to internal validity (risk of bias), important inconsistency of results, uncertainty about the directness of the evidence, imprecise or sparse data, and high probability of publication bias can lower the evidence grade. **Factors that may increase quality of evidence of observational studies:** 1. Large magnitude of effect (direct evidence, relative risk [RR] = 2-5 or RR=0.5-0.2 with no plausible confounders); very large with RR > 5 or RR < 0.2 and no serious problems with risk of bias or precision (sufficiently narrow confidence intervals); more likely to rate up if the effect is rapid and out of keeping with prior trajectory; usually supported by indirect evidence. 2. Dose-response gradient 3. All plausible residual confounders or biases would reduce a demonstrated effect, or suggest a spurious effect when results show no effect.	**Levels of Certainty Regarding Net Benefit (Quality of Evidence) (USPSTF, 2015)** **High:** Available evidence usually includes consistent results from a multitude of well-designed, well-conducted studies in representative primary care populations. These studies assess effects of the preventive service on health outcomes. This conclusion is therefore unlikely to be strongly affected by the results of future studies. **Moderate:** The available evidence is sufficient to determine the effects of the preventive service on health outcomes, but confidence in the estimate is constrained by such factors as: • The number, size, or quality of individual studies • Some heterogeneity of outcome findings or intervention models across the body of studies • Mild to moderate generalizability of findings to routine primary care practice As more information becomes available, the magnitude or direction of the observed effect could change, and this change may be large enough to alter the conclusion. **Low:** The available evidence is insufficient to assess effects on health outcomes. Evidence is insufficient because of one or more of the following: • The very limited number or size of studies • Inconsistency of direction or magnitude of findings across the body of evidence • Critical gaps in the chain of evidence • Findings are not generalizable to routine primary care practice. • A lack of information on prespecified health outcomes • Lack of coherence across the linkages in the chain of evidence • More information may allow estimation of effects on health outcomes.

TABLE 20.2 Examples of Evidence Rating Systems—cont'd

Grade Working Group (www.gradeworkinggroup.org)	US Preventative Services Task Force (USPSTF) (www.uspreventiveservicestaskforce.org/)
Strength of Recommendations (Andrews et al., 2013) **Strong:** Confident that desirable effects of adherence to a recommendation outweigh undesirable effects. **Weak:** Desirable effects of adherence to a recommendation probably outweigh the undesirable effects, but developers are less confident. **Note:** Strength of recommendation is determined by the balance between desirable and undesirable consequences of alternative management strategies, quality of evidence, variability in values and preferences (trade-offs), and resource use.	**Recommendation Grades (USPSTF, 2015)** A. USPSTF recommends the service. There is high certainty that the net benefit is substantial. B. USPSTF recommends the service. There is high certainty that the net benefit is moderate or there is moderate certainty that the net benefit is moderate to substantial. C. USPSTF recommends selectively offering or providing this service to individual patients based on professional judgment and patient preferences. There is at least moderate certainty that the net benefit is small. D. USPSTF recommends against the service. There is moderate or high certainty that the service has no net benefit or that the harms outweigh the benefits. E. The USPSTF concludes that the current evidence is insufficient to assess the balance of benefits and harms of the service. Evidence is lacking, of poor quality, or conflicting, and the balance of benefits and harms cannot be determined.

TABLE 20.3 Important Domains and Elements for Systems to Rate Quality of Individual Articles

Systematic Reviews	Randomized Clinical Trials	Observational Studies	Diagnostic Test Studies
Study question	Study question	Study question	*Study population*
Search strategy	*Study population*	Study population	Adequate description of test
Inclusion and exclusion criteria	Randomization	*Comparability of subjects*	Appropriate reference standard
Interventions	Blinding	*Exposure or intervention*	Blinded comparison of test and reference
Outcomes	Interventions	*Outcome measurement*	Avoidance of verification bias
Data extraction	Outcomes	*Statistical analysis*	
Study quality and validity	Statistical analysis	Results	
Data synthesis and analysis	Results	Discussion	
Results	Discussion	*Funding or sponsorship*	
Discussion	*Funding or sponsorship*		
Funding or sponsorship			

From Agency for Healthcare Research and Quality (AHRQ). (2002). *Systems to rate the strength of scientific evidence: evidence report/technology assessment number 47*. Rockville, MD: Agency for Healthcare Research and Quality, U.S. Department of Health and Human Services.
Key domains are in ***italics***.

TABLE 20.4 Important Domains and Elements for Systems to Grade the Strength of Evidence

Quality	The aggregate of quality ratings for individual studies, predicated on the extent to which bias was minimized
Quantity	Magnitude of effect, numbers of studies, and sample size or power
Consistency	For any given topic, the extent to which similar findings are reported using similar and different study designs
Relevance	Relevance of findings to characteristics of individual groups
Benefits and harms	The overall benefits and harms. Net benefits. Do the benefits outweigh the harms?

Modified from Institute of Medicine (IOM). (2011). *Clinical practice guidelines we can trust*. Washington, DC: The National Academies Press.

In Chapter 1, Fig. 1.1 provides an evidence hierarchy used for grading evidence that is an adaptation similar to the evidence hierarchies that appear in Table 20.2.

Critique and Synthesis of Research

Critique of evidence-based guidelines (see Chapter 11) and studies (see Chapters 8 to 10) should use the same methodology, and the critique process should be a shared responsibility. It is helpful, however, to have one individual provide leadership for the project and design strategies for completing critiques. A group approach to critiques is recommended because it distributes the workload, helps those responsible for implementing the changes understand the scientific base for the practice change, arms nurses with citations and research-based language to use in advocating for changes with peers and other disciplines, and provides novices an environment to learn critique and application of research findings. Methods to make the critique process fun and interesting include the following:

- Using a journal club to discuss critiques done by each member of the group
- Pairing a novice and expert to do critiques
- Eliciting assistance from students who may be interested in the topic and want experience doing critiques
- Assigning the critique process to graduate students interested in the topic
- Making a class project of critique and synthesis of research for a given topic
- Using the critique criteria at the end of each chapter and the critique criteria summary tables in Chapters 6 and 18

> **HELPFUL HINT**
>
> Keep critique processes simple, and encourage participation by staff members who are providing direct patient care.

Once studies are critiqued, a decision is made regarding the use of each study in the synthesis of the evidence for application in practice. Factors that should be considered for inclusion of studies in the synthesis of findings are (1) overall scientific merit; (2) type of subjects enrolled (e.g., age, gender, pathology) and the similarity to the patient population to which the findings will be applied; and (3) relevance of the study to the topic of question. **Example:** ➤ If the practice area is prevention of deep venous thrombosis in postoperative patients, a descriptive study using a heterogeneous population of medical patients is not appropriate for inclusion in the synthesis of findings.

To synthesize the findings from research critiques, it is helpful to use a summary table in which critical information from studies can be documented. Essential information to include in such a summary is as follows:

- Research questions/hypotheses
- Independent and dependent variables studied
- Description of the study sample and setting
- Type of research design
- Methods used to measure each variable and outcome
- Study findings

An **example** ➤ of a summary form is illustrated in Table 20.5.

TABLE 20.5 **Example of a Summary Table for Research Critiques**

Citation	Research Question	Study Design	Sample	Independent Variables and Measures	Dependent Variables and Measures	Results	General Strengths	General Weaknesses	Overall Quality of Study[a]	Summary Statements for Practice

[a]Use a consistent rating system (e.g., good, fair, poor).

HELPFUL HINT

Use of a summary form helps identify commonalities across studies with regard to study findings and the types of patients to which findings can be applied. It also helps in synthesizing the overall strengths and weakness of the studies as a group.

Setting Forth Evidence-Based Practice Recommendations

Based on the critique of practice guidelines and synthesis of research, recommendations for practice are set forth. The type and strength of evidence used to support the practice needs to be clearly delineated in your evidence table. Box 20.2 is another useful tool to assist with this activity.

Decision to Change Practice

After studies are critiqued and synthesized, the next step is to decide if the findings are appropriate for use in practice. Criteria to consider include:

- Relevance of evidence for practice
- Consistency in findings across studies and/or guidelines
- A significant number of studies and/or EBP guidelines with sample characteristics similar to those to which the findings will be used
- Consistency among evidence from research and other nonresearch evidence
- Feasibility for use in practice
- The risk/benefit ratio (risk of harm versus the potential benefit for the patient)

Synthesis of study findings and other evidence may result in supporting current practice, making minor practice modifications, undertaking major practice changes, or developing a new area of practice.

Development of Evidence-Based Practice

The next step is to document the evidence base of the practice using the agreed-upon grading schema. When critique results and synthesis of evidence support practice or suggest a practice change, a written EBP standard (e.g., policy, standard of practice protocol,

BOX 20.2 Consistency of Evidence from Critiqued Research, Appraisals of Evidence-Based Practice Guidelines, Critiqued Systematic Reviews, and Nonresearch Literature

1. Are there replication of studies with consistent results?
2. Are the studies well designed?
3. Are recommendations consistent among systematic reviews, evidence-based practice guidelines, and critiqued research?
4. Are there identified risks to the patient by applying evidence-based practice recommendations?
5. Are there identified benefits to the patient?
6. Have cost analysis studies been conducted on the recommended action, intervention, or treatment?
7. Summary recommendations about assessments, actions, interventions/treatments from the research, systematic reviews, evidence-based guidelines with an assigned evidence grade.

From Titler, M. G. (2002). *Toolkit for promoting evidence-based practice.* Iowa City, IA: Department of Nursing Services and Patient Care, University of Iowa Hospitals and Clinics.

BOX 20.3 Key Questions for Focus Groups

1. What is needed by staff (e.g., nurses, physicians) to use the evidence-based practice in your setting?
2. In your opinion, how will this standard improve patient care in your unit/practice?
3. What modifications would you suggest in the evidence-based practice standard before using it in your practice?
4. What content in the evidence-based practice standard is unclear? What needs revision?
5. What would you change about the format of the evidence-based practice standard?
6. What part of this evidence-based practice change do you view as most challenging?
7. Do you have any other suggestions?

guideline) is warranted. This is necessary so that individuals know (1) that the practices are based on evidence and (2) the type of evidence (e.g., randomized controlled trial, expert opinion) used in development of the practice.

It is imperative that once the EBP standard is written, key stakeholders have an opportunity to review it and provide feedback to the individual(s) responsible for developing it. Focus groups are a useful way to provide discussion about the EBP and to identify key areas that may be potentially troublesome during the implementation phase. Key questions that can be used in focus groups are in Box 20.3.

HELPFUL HINT

Use a consistent approach to developing EBP standards and referencing the research and related literature.

Implementing the Practice Change

If a practice change is warranted, the next steps are to make the changes. This goes beyond writing a policy or procedure that is evidence based; it requires interaction among direct care providers to champion and foster evidence adoption, leadership support, and system changes. The diffusion of innovations model (Rogers, 2003) is extremely useful in selecting strategies for promoting the adoption of EBPs. According to this model, the adoption of EBP innovations is influenced by the nature of the innovation (e.g., the type and strength of evidence, the clinical topic) and the manner in which it is communicated (disseminated) to care providers of a social system (organization, health care professions). Strategies for promoting EBP adoption must address these areas within a context of participative, planned change.

Nature of the Innovation/Evidence-Based Practice

Characteristics of an innovation or EBP that affect adoption include the relative advantage of the EBP (e.g., effectiveness, relevance to the task, social prestige); the compatibility with values, norms, work, and perceived needs of users; and complexity of the EBP topic (Rogers, 2003). **Example:** ➤ EBP topics that are perceived by users as relatively simple (e.g., influenza vaccines for older adults) are more easily adopted in less time than those that are more complex (e.g., acute pain management for hospitalized older adults).

A key principle to remember when planning implementation of an EBP is that the attributes of the practice topic as perceived by users and stakeholders (e.g., ease of use, valued part of practice) are neither stable features nor sure determinants of their adoption. Rather, it is the interaction among the characteristics of the EBP topic, the intended users, and a particular context of practice that determines the rate and extent of adoption (Dogherty et al., 2012).

Practitioner review and "reinvention" of EBP recommendations to fit the local context, along with the use of clinical reminders, decision aids, and quick reference guides (QRGs), are implementation strategies to educate and promote the nature of the EBP topic (Berwick, 2003; IOM, 2011; Titler et al., 2016; Wilson et al., 2016). An example of a quick reference guide is shown in Fig. 20.3.

Empirical support for evidence-based electronic clinical decision support interventions is mixed (IOM, 2011). Electronic reminders have small to modest effects on clinician behavior and appear to be more effective than alerts alone when included as a part of multifaceted implementation strategies (Arditi et al., 2012; Kahn et al., 2013).

Methods of Communication

Interpersonal communication and influence among social networks of users affect adoption of EBPs (Rogers, 2003). Education, use of opinion leaders, change champions, and educational outreach are tested strategies that promote adoption of EBPs. Education is necessary but not sufficient to change practice, and didactic continuing education alone does little to change practice behavior (Flodgren et al., 2013; Giguère et al., 2012). It is important that

Risk factor
Compromised mobility, gait instability, or lower limb weakness

Indicators	Interventions	Hints and tips
• Unsteady/veering during transfers or walking • Reaching for walls or other supports while walking • Overbalancing, especially when reaching, bending, straightening, or turning • Unable to rise from chair without assistance	• Ambulate 3-4 times per day with assistance unless contraindicated • Refer patient to PT for assessment, gait, and strength training • Active or passive range of motion three times daily • Minimize use of immobilizing equipment (e.g., indwelling urinary catheters) • Assure proper assist equipment is readily available	• Seek advice from PT about safe exercises and activities the patient can perform on their own or with supervision • Ask patient's family and friends to assist with mobility interventions as appropriate • Without contraction muscle strength decreases by as much as 5% per day

FIG 20.3 Quick reference guide fall prevention: interventions to mitigate mobility risk factors. (From Titler, M. G., Conlon, P., Reynolds, M. A., et al. [2016]. The effect of translating research into practice intervention to promote use of evidence-based fall prevention interventions in hospitalized adults: a prospective pre-post implementation study in the U.S. *Applied Nursing Research, 31*, 52–59.)

staff know the scientific basis for improvements in quality of care anticipated by the changes. Disseminating information to staff needs to be done creatively. A staff in-service may not be the most effective method nor reach the majority of the staff. Although it is unrealistic for all staff to have participated in the critique process or to have read all studies used, it is important that they know the myths and realities of the EBP. Staff education must also ensure competence in the skills necessary to carry out the new practice.

One method of communicating information to staff is through use of colorful posters that identify myths and realities or describe the essence of the change in practice (Titler et al., 2016). Visibly identifying those who have learned the information and are using the EBP (e.g., via buttons, ribbons, pins) stimulates interest in others who may not have internalized the change. As a result, the "new" learner may begin asking questions about the practice and be more open to learning. Other educational strategies such as train-the-trainer programs, computer-assisted instruction, and competency testing are helpful in education of staff (Titler et al., 2016). Several studies have demonstrated that opinion leaders are effective in changing behaviors of health care practitioners (Dagenais et al., 2015; Flodgren et al., 2011), especially in combination with educational outreach or performance feedback. **Opinion leaders** are from the local peer group, viewed as a respected source of influence, considered by associates as technically competent, and trusted to judge the fit between the EBPs and the local situation (Dobbins et al., 2009; Flodgren et al., 2011). The key characteristic of an opinion leader is a trusted ability to evaluate new information in the context of group norms. To do this, an opinion leader must be considered by associates as technically competent and a full and dedicated member of the local group (Rogers, 2003).

Opinion leadership is multifaceted and complex, with role functions varying by the circumstances, but few successful projects that have implemented EBPs have managed without the input of identifiable opinion leaders. Social interactions such as "hallway chats," one-on-one discussions, and addressing questions are important yet often overlooked components of translation (Jordan et al., 2009). If the EBP that is being implemented is interdisciplinary, discipline-specific opinion leaders should be used to promote the practice change. Role expectations of an opinion leader are listed in Box 20.4.

Change champions are also helpful for implementing innovations (Dogherty et al., 2012). They are practitioners within the local group setting (e.g., clinic, patient care unit) who are expert clinicians, are passionate about the innovation, are committed to improving quality of care, and have a positive working relationship with other health professionals (Rogers, 2003). They circulate information, encourage peers to adopt the innovation, arrange demonstrations, and orient staff to the innovation (Titler et al., 2016). The change champion believes in an idea; will not take "no" for an answer; is undaunted by insults and rebuffs; and above all, persists.

BOX 20.4 Role Expectations of an Opinion Leader

1. Be/become an expert in the evidence-based practice.
2. Provide organizational/unit leadership for adopting the evidence-based practice.
3. Implement various strategies to educate peers about the evidence-based practice.
4. Work with peers, other disciplines, and leadership staff to incorporate key information about the evidence-based practice into organizational/unit standards, policies, procedures, and documentation systems.
5. Promote initial and ongoing use of the evidence-based practice by peers.

From Titler, M. G., Herr, K., Everett, L. Q., et al. (2006). *Book to bedside: Promoting and sustaining EBPs in elders.* Iowa City, IA: University of Iowa College of Nursing.

Multiple studies have demonstrated the effectiveness of educational outreach, also known as academic detailing, in improving the practice behaviors of clinicians (Avorn, 2010; NAM, formally IOM, 2011; Wilson et al., 2016). Educational outreach involves interactive face-to-face education of practitioners in their practice setting by an individual (usually a clinician) with expertise in a particular topic (e.g., cancer pain management). Academic detailers are able to explain the research foundations of the EBP recommendations and respond convincingly to specific questions, concerns, or challenges that a practitioner might raise. An academic detailer also might deliver feedback on provider or team performance with respect to an EBP recommendation (e.g., frequency of pain assessment).

Users of the Innovation/Evidence-Based Practice

Members of a social system (e.g., nurses, physicians, clerical staff) influence how quickly and widely EBPs are adopted (Rogers, 2003). Audit and feedback, performance gap assessment (PGA), and trying the EBP are strategies that have demonstrated effectiveness in improving EBP behaviors (Hysong et al., 2012; Ivers et al., 2012; Titler et al., 2016).

PGA (baseline practice performance) provides information of current practices relative to recommended EBPs at the beginning of a practice change. This implementation strategy is used to engage clinicians in discussions of practice issues and formulation strategies to promote alignment of their practices with EBP recommendations. Specific practice indicators selected for PGA are derived from the EBP recommendations for the specified topic such as every-4-hour pain assessment for acute pain management. Studies have demonstrated improvements in performance when PGA is part of multifaceted implementation strategies (see Chapters 19 and 21) (Titler et al., 2016; Yano, 2008).

Audit and feedback is ongoing auditing of performance indicators, aggregating data into reports, and discussing the findings with practitioners during the practice change (Ivers et al., 2012; Hysong et al., 2012; Wilson et al., 2016). This strategy helps staff know and see how their efforts to improve care and patient outcomes are progressing throughout the implementation process (Ivers et al., 2014).

Users of an innovation usually try it for a period of time before adopting it in their practice. When "trying an evidence-based practice" (i.e., piloting a change) is incorporated as part of the implementation process, users have an opportunity to use it, provide feedback to those in charge of implementation, and modify the practice if necessary. Piloting the practice as part of implementation has a positive influence on the extent of adoption of the new practice (Rogers, 2003).

Social System

Clearly, the social system or context of care delivery matters when implementing EBPs (Rogers, 2003; Squires et al., 2015; Titler, 2010; Yousefi-Nooraie et al., 2014). **Example:** ➤ Investigators demonstrated the effectiveness of a prompted voiding intervention for urinary incontinence in nursing homes, but sustaining the intervention in day-to-day practice was limited when the responsibility of carrying out the intervention was shifted to nursing home staff (rather than the investigative team) and required staffing levels in excess of a majority of nursing home settings (Engberg et al., 2004). This illustrates the importance of embedding interventions into ongoing care processes.

As part of the work of implementing EBPs, it is important that the social system (e.g., unit, service line, clinic) ensure that policies, procedures, standards, clinical pathways, and documentation systems support the use of the EBPs (Titler, 2010). Documentation forms or clinical information systems may need revision to support practice changes; documentation systems that fail to readily support the new practice thwart change. **Example:** ➤ If staff members are expected to reassess and document pain intensity within 30 minutes after administration of an analgesic agent, documentation forms must reflect this practice standard. It is the role of leadership to ensure that organizational documents and systems are flexible and supportive of the EBPs.

A learning organizational culture and proactive leadership that promotes knowledge sharing are important components for building an EBP (Duckers et al., 2009; Stetler et al., 2009). Components of a receptive context for EBP include the following:

- Strong leadership
- Clear strategic vision
- Good managerial relations
- Visionary staff in key positions
- A climate conducive to experimentation and risk taking
- Effective data-capture systems

An organization may be generally amenable to innovations, but not ready or willing to assimilate a particular EBP. Elements of system readiness include the following (French et al., 2009; Litaker et al., 2008):

- Tension for change
- EBP practice–system fit
- Assessment of implications
- Support and advocacy for the EBP
- Dedicated time and resources
- Capacity to evaluate the impact of the EBP during and following implementation

Leadership support is critical for promoting the use of EBPs (French et al., 2009), and is expressed verbally and by providing necessary resources, materials, and time to fulfill responsibilities (Stetler et al., 2009). Senior leadership needs to create an organizational mission, vision, and strategic plan that incorporates EBP, implements performance expectations for staff that include EBP work, integrates the work of EBP into the governance structure of the health care system, demonstrates the value of EBPs through administrative behaviors, and establishes explicit expectations that nurse leaders will create microsystems that value and support clinical inquiry (see Chapter 21).

In summary, making an evidence-based change in practice involves a series of action steps in a complex, nonlinear process. Implementing the change takes time to integrate, depending on the nature of the practice change. Merely increasing staff knowledge about an EBP and passive dissemination strategies are unlikely to work, particularly in complex health care settings. Strategies that seem to have a positive effect on promoting use of EBPs include audit and feedback, use of clinical reminders and practice prompts, opinion leaders, change champions, interactive education, educational outreach/academic detailing, and the context of care delivery (e.g., leadership, learning, questioning). It is important that senior leadership and those leading EBP improvements are aware of change as a process and continue to encourage and teach peers about the change in practice. The new practice must be continually reinforced and sustained or the practice change will be intermittent and soon fade, allowing more traditional methods of care to return.

Evaluation

Evaluation provides an opportunity to collect and analyze data with regard to the use of new EBPs and then to modify the practice as necessary. It is important that the evidence-based change is evaluated, both at the pilot testing phase and when the practice is changed in additional settings or sites of care. The importance of the evaluation cannot be overemphasized; it provides information for performance gap assessment, audit, and feedback, and provides information necessary to determine if the EBP should be retained, modified, or eliminated.

An outcome achieved in a controlled environment (as when a researcher is implementing a study protocol for a homogeneous group of study patients) may not result in the same outcome when the practice is implemented in the clinical setting by several caregivers to a more heterogeneous patient population. Steps of the evaluation process are summarized in Box 20.5.

Evaluation should include both process and outcome measures (Titler et al., 2016). The process component focuses on how the practice change is being implemented. It is important to know if staff are using the practice and implementing the practice as noted in the EBP guideline. Evaluation of the process also should note (1) barriers that staff encounter in carrying out the practice (e.g., lack of information, skills, or necessary equipment), (2) differences in opinions among health care providers, and (3) difficulty in carrying out the steps of the practice as originally designed (e.g., shutting off tube feedings 1 hour before aspirating contents for checking placement of nasointestinal tubes). Process data can be collected from staff and/or patient self-reports, medical record audits, or observation of clinical practice. Examples of process and outcome questions are shown in Table 20.6.

Outcome data are an equally important part of evaluation. The purpose of outcome evaluation is to assess whether the patient, staff, and/or fiscal outcomes expected are achieved. Therefore it is important that baseline data be used for a preintervention/postintervention comparison (Titler et al., 2016). The outcome variables measured should

BOX 20.5 Steps of Evaluation for Evidence-Based Projects

1. Identify process and outcome variables of interest.
   Example: Process variable—Patients > 65 years will have a Braden scale completed on admission.
   Outcome variable—Presence/absence of nosocomial pressure ulcer; if present, determine stage as I, II, III, IV.
2. Determine methods and frequency of data collection.
   Example: Process variable—Chart audit of all patients > 65 years, 1 day a month.
   Outcome variable—Patient assessment of all patients > 65 years, 1 day a month.
3. Determine baseline and follow-up sample sizes.
4. Design data collection forms.
   Example: Process chart audit abstraction form.
   Outcome variable—pressure ulcer assessment form.
5. Establish content validity of data collection forms.
6. Train data collectors.
7. Assess interrater reliability of data collectors.
8. Collect data at specified intervals.
9. Provide "on-site" feedback to staff regarding the progress in achieving the practice change.
10. Provide feedback of analyzed data to staff.
11. Use data to assist staff in modifying or integrating the evidence-based practice change.

TABLE 20.6 Examples of Evaluation Measures

	NURSES' SELF-RATING				
Example Process Questions	**SD**	**D**	**NA/D**	**A**	**SA**
I feel well prepared to use the Braden scale with older patients.	1	2	3	4	5
Malnutrition increases patient risk for pressure ulcer development.	1	2	3	4	5
Example Outcome Question	**Patient**				
On a scale of 0 (no pain) to 10 (worst possible pain), how much pain have you experienced over the past 24 hours?					

A, Agree; *D*, disagree; *NA/D*, neither agree nor disagree; *SA*, strongly agree; *SD*, strongly disagree.

be those that are projected to change as a result of changing practice. **Example:** ➤ Research demonstrates that less restricted family visiting practices in critical care units result in improved satisfaction with care. Thus patient and family member satisfaction should be an outcome measure that is evaluated as part of changing visiting practices in adult critical care units. Outcome measures should be assessed before the change in practice is implemented, after implementation, and every 6 to 12 months thereafter. Findings must be provided to clinicians to reinforce the impact of the change and to ensure that they are incorporated into quality improvement programs. When collecting process and outcome data for evaluation of a practice change, it is important that the data collection tools are user-friendly, short, concise, easy to complete, and have content validity. Focus must be on collecting the most essential data. Those responsible for collecting evaluative data must be trained on data collection methods and be assessed for interrater reliability (see Chapters 14 and 15). It is our experience that those individuals who have participated in implementing the protocol can be very helpful in evaluation by collecting data, providing timely feedback to staff, and assisting staff to overcome barriers encountered when implementing the changes in practice (see Chapter 21).

One question that often arises is how much data are needed to evaluate this change. The preferred number of patients (*N*) is somewhat dependent on the size of the patient population affected by the practice change. **Example:** ➤ If the practice change is for families of critically ill adult patients and the organization has 1000 adult critical care patients annually, 50 to 100 satisfaction responses preimplementation, and 25 to 50 responses postimplementation, 3 and 6 months should be adequate to look for trends in satisfaction and possible areas that need to be addressed in continuing this practice (e.g., more bedside chairs in patient rooms). The rule of thumb is to keep the evaluation simple, because data often are collected by busy clinicians who may lose interest if the data collection, analysis, and feedback are too long and tedious. It is also important to check with your institution's guidelines for collecting data related to practice changes, because institutional approval may be needed.

The evaluation process includes planned feedback to staff who are making the change. The feedback includes verbal and/or written appreciation for the work and visual demonstration of progress in implementation and improvement in patient outcomes. The key to effective evaluation is to ensure that the evidence-based change in practice is warranted (e.g., will improve quality of care) and that the intervention does not bring harm to patients.

HELPFUL HINT

Include patient outcome measures (e.g., pressure ulcer prevalence) and cost (e.g., cost savings, cost avoidance) in evaluation practice projects.

FUTURE DIRECTIONS

Education must include knowledge and skills in the use of research evidence in practice. Nurses are increasingly being held accountable for practices based on scientific evidence. Thus we must communicate and integrate into our profession the expectation that it is the professional responsibility of all nurses to read and use research in their practice, and to communicate with nurse scientists the many and varied clinical problems for which we do not yet have a scientific base.

KEY POINTS

- EBP and translation science, though related, are not interchangeable terms; EBP is the actual application of evidence in practice (the "doing of" EBP), whereas translation science is the study of implementation interventions, factors, and contextual variables that effect knowledge uptake and use in practices and communities.
- There are several models of EBP. A key feature of all models is the judicious review and synthesis of research and other types of evidence to develop an EBP standard.
- The steps of EBP using the Iowa Model of Evidence-Based Practice are as follows: (1) selecting a topic, (2) forming a team, (3) retrieving the evidence, (4) grading the evidence, (5) developing an EBP standard, (6) implementing the EBP, and (7) evaluating the effect on staff, patient, and fiscal outcomes.
- Adoption of EBPs requires education of staff, as well as the use of change strategies such as opinion leaders, change champions, educational outreach, performance gap assessment, and audit and feedback.
- It is important to evaluate the change. Evaluation provides data for performance gap assessment, audit, and feedback, and provides information necessary to determine if the practice should be retained.
- Evaluation includes both process and outcome measures.
- It is important for organizations to create a culture of EBP. Creating this culture requires an interactive process. Organizations need to provide access to information, access to individuals who have skills necessary for EBP, and a written and verbal commitment to EBP in the organization's operations.

CRITICAL THINKING CHALLENGES

- Discuss the differences among nursing research, EBP, and translation science. Support your discussion with examples.
- Why would it be important to use an EBP model, such as the Iowa Model of Evidence-Based Practice, to guide a practice project focused on justifying and implementing a change in clinical practice?
- IPE You are a staff nurse working on a cardiac step-down unit. You are asked to join an interprofessional QI team for the cardiac division. You find that many of your

colleagues from other disciplines do not understand evidence-based practice. How would you help your colleagues to understand the relevance of evidence-based practice to providing care that addresses the Triple Aim for this patient population?

- What barriers do you see to applying EBP in your clinical setting? Discuss strategies to use in overcoming these barriers.

REFERENCES

Agency for Healthcare Research and Quality (AHRQ). (2002). *Systems to rate the strength of scientific evidence: Evidence report/technology assessment number 47*. Rockville, MD: Agency for Healthcare Research and Quality, U.S. Department of Health and Human Services.

Agency for Healthcare Research and Quality (AHRQ). (2015). *2014 national healthcare quality and disparities report* (AHRQ publication no. 15-0007). Rockville, MD: U.S. Department of Health and Human Services. Retrieved from http://www.ahrq.gov/research/findings/nhqrdr/nhqdr14/index.html.

Andrews, J., Guyatt, G., Oxman, A. D., et al. (2013). GRADE guidelines: 14. Going from evidence to recommendations: the significance and presentation of recommendations. *Journal of Clinical Epidemiology*, 66, 719–725. doi:10.1016/j.jclinepi.2012.03.013, PMID: 23312392.

Arditi, C., Rege-Walther, M., Wyatt, J. C., et al. (2012). Computer-generated reminders delivered on paper to healthcare professionals: effects on professional practice and health care outcomes. *Cochrane Database of Systematic Reviews*, 12. doi:10.1002/14651858.CD001175.pub3.

Avorn, J. (2010). Transforming trial results into practice change: the final translational hurdle: comment on "Impact of the ALLHAT/JNC7 Dissemination Project on thiazide-type diuretic use." *Archives of Internal Medicine*, 170(10), 858–860. doi:10.1001/archinternmed.2010.125.

Balshem, H., Helfand, M., Schunemann, H. J., et al. (2011). GRADE guidelines: 3. Rating the quality of evidence. *Journal of Clinical Epidemiology*, 64(4), 401–406. doi:10.1016/j.jclinepi.2010.07.015.

Berwick, D. M. (2003). Disseminating innovations in health care. *Journal of the American Medical Association*, 289(15), 1969–1975. doi:10.1001/jama.289.15.1969, PMID: 12697800.

Dagenais, C., Laurendeau, M.-C., & Briand-Lamarche, M. (2015). Knowledge brokering in public health: a critical analysis of the results of a qualitative evaluation. *Evaluation and Program Planning*, 53, 10–17. doi:10.1016/j.evalprogplan.2015.07.003.

Dobbins, M., Robeson, P., Ciliska, D., et al. (2009). A description of a knowledge broker role implemented as part of a randomized controlled trial evaluating three knowledge translation strategies. *Implementation Science*, 4, 23. doi:10.1186/1748-5908-4-23.

Dockham, B., Schafenacker, A., Yoon, H., et al. (2016). Implementation of a psychoeducational program for cancer survivors and family caregivers at a cancer support community affiliate: a pilot effectiveness study. *Cancer Nursing*, 39(3), 169–180. doi:10.1097/NCC.0000000000000311.

Dogherty, E. J., Harrison, M. B., Baker, C., & Graham, I. D. (2012). Following a natural experiment of guideline adaptation and early implementation: a mixed methods study of facilitation. *Implementation Science*, 7, 9. doi:10.1186/1748-5908-7-9.

Duckers, M. L. A., Spreeuwenberg, P., Wagner, C., & Groenewegen, P. P. (2009). Exploring the black box of quality improvement collaboratives: modelling relations between conditions, applied changes and outcomes. *Implementation Science*, 4, 74. doi:10.1186/1748-5908-4-74.

Engberg, S., Kincade, J., & Thompson, D. (2004). Future directions for incontinence research with frail elders. *Nursing Research*, 53(Suppl 6), S22–S29. PMID: 15586144.

Flodgren, G., Conterno, L. O., Mayhew, A., et al. (2013). Interventions to improve professional adherence to guidelines for prevention of device-related infections. *Cochrane Database of Systematic Reviews*, 3. doi:10.1002/14651858.CD006559.pub2, PMID: 23543545.

Flodgren, G., Parmelli, E., Doumit, G., et al. (2011). Local opinion leaders: effects on professional practice and health care outcomes. *Cochrane Database of Systematic Reviews*, 8, Article No. CD000125. doi:10.1002/14651858.CD000125.pub4, PMID: 21833939, PMCID: PMC4172331.

French, B., Thomas, L., Baker, B., et al. (2009). What can management theories offer evidence-based practice? A comparative analysis of measurement tools for organizational context. *Implementation Science*, 4, 28. doi:10.1186/1748-5908-4-28.

Giguère, A., Légaré, F., Grimshaw, J., et al. (2012). Printed educational materials: effects on professional practice and healthcare outcomes. *Cochrane Database of Systematic Reviews*, 10, Article No. CD004398. doi:10.1002/14651858.CD004398.pub3, PMID: 23076904.

Guyatt, G. H., Oxman, A. D., Sultan, S., et al. (2013). GRADE guidelines: 11. Making an overall rating of confidence in effect estimates for a single outcome and for all outcomes. *Journal of Clinical Epidemiology*, 66(2), 151–157. doi:10.1016/j.jclinepi.2012.01.006.

Guyatt, G. H., Oxman, A. D., Sultan, S., et al. (2011). GRADE guidelines: 9. Rating up the quality of evidence. *Journal of Clinical Epidemiology*, 64(12), 1311–1316. doi:10.1016/j.jclinepi.2011.06.004.

Hysong, S. J., Teal, C. R., Khan, M. J., & Haidet, P. (2012). Improving quality of care through improved audit and feedback. *Implementation Science*, 7, 45. doi:10.1186/1748-5908-7-45, PMID: 22607640, PMCID: PMC3462705.

Institute of Medicine (IOM). (2011). *Clinical practice guidelines we can trust*. Washington, DC: The National Academies Press. doi:10.17226/13058, PMID: 24983061.

Ivers, N., Jamtvedt, G., Flottorp, S., et al. (2012). Audit and feedback: effects on professional practice and healthcare outcomes. *Cochrane Database of Systematic Reviews*, 6, Article No. CD000259. doi:10.1002/14651858.CD000259.pub3, PMID: 22696318.

Ivers, N. M., Sales, A., Colquhoun, H., et al. (2014). No more "business as usual" with audit and feedback interventions: towards an agenda for a reinvigorated intervention. *Implementation Science*, 9, 14. doi:10.1186/1748-5908-9-14.

Jordan, M. E., Lanham, H. J., Crabtree, B. F., et al. (2009). The role of conversation in health care interventions: enabling sensemaking and learning. *Implementation Science*, 4, 15. doi:10.1186/1748-5908-4-15, PMID: 19284660, PMCID: PMC2663543.

Kahn, S. R., Morrison, D. R., Cohen, J. M., et al. (2013). Interventions for implementation of thromboprophylaxis in hospitalized medical and surgical patients at risk for venous thromboembolism. *Cochrane Database of Systematic Reviews*, 7. doi:10.1002/14651858.CD008201.pub2, PMID: 23861035.

Litaker, D., Ruhe, M., Weyer, S., & Stange, K. C. (2008). Association of intervention outcomes with practice capacity for change: subgroup analysis from a group randomized trial. *Implementation Science*, 3, 25. doi:10.1186/1748-5908-3-25.

Milat, A. J., Bauman, A., & Redman, S. (2015). Narrative review of models and success factors for scaling up public health interventions. *Implementation Science*, 10, 113. doi:10.1186/s13012-015-0301-6, PMID: 26264351, PMCID: PMC4533941.

Moore, J. E., Kane-Low, L., Titler, M. G., et al. (2014). Moving towards patient centered care: Women's decisions, perceptions, and experiences of the induction of labor process. *Birth*, 41(2), 138–146. doi:10.1111/birt.12080, PMID: 24702312.

Moore, J. E., Titler, M. G., Kane-Low, L., et al. (2015). Transforming patient-centered care: development of the evidence-informed decision-making through engagement model. *Women's Health Issues*, 25(3), 276–282. doi:10.1016/j.whi.2015.02.002, PMID: 25864022.

Newhouse, R., Bobay, K., Dykes, P. C., et al. (2013). Methodology issues in implementation science. *Medical Care*, 51(4 Suppl 2), 32–40. doi:10.1097/MLR.0b013e31827feeca, PMID: 23502915.

Rogers, E. M. (2003). *Diffusion of innovations* (5th ed.). New York, NY: Free Press.

Rycroft-Malone, J., & Bucknall, T. (2010). *Models and frameworks for implementing evidence-based practice*. Hoboken, NJ: Wiley-Blackwell.

Schaffer, M. A., Sandau, K. E., & Diedrick, L. (2013). Evidence-based practice models for organizational change: Overview and practical applications. *Journal of Advanced Nursing*, 69(5), 1197–1209. doi:10.1111/j.1365-2648.2012.06122.x, PMID: 22882410.

Shuman, C. J., Liu, J., Montie, M., et al. (2016). Patient perception and experiences with falls during hospitalization and after discharge. *Applied Nursing Research*, 31, 79–85. doi:10.1016/j.apnr.2016.01.009, PMID: 27397823.

Squires, J. E., Graham, I. D., Hutchinson, A. M., et al. (2015). Identifying the domains of context important to implementation science: a study protocol. *Implementation Science*, 10(1), 135. doi:10.1186/s13012-015-0325-y, PMID: 26416206, PMCID: PMC4584460.

Stetler, C. B., Ritchie, J. A., Rycroft-Malone, J., et al. (2009). Institutionalizing evidence-based practice: an organizational case study using a model of strategic change. *Implementation Science*, 4, 78. doi:10.1186/1748-5908-4-78, PMID: 19948064, PMCID: PMC2795741.

Straus, E., Richardson, R. B., Glasziou, P., et al. (2011). *Evidence-based medicine: How to practice and teach* (4th ed.). New York, NY: Elsevier.

Titler, M. G. (2002). *Toolkit for promoting evidence-based practice*. Iowa City, IA: Department of Nursing Services and Patient Care, University of Iowa Hospitals and Clinics.

Titler, M. G. (2014). Overview of evidence-based practice and translation science. *Nursing Clinics of North America*, 49(3), 269–274. doi:10.1016/j.cnur.2014.05.001, PMID: 25155527.

Titler, M. G., Conlon, P., Reynolds, M. A., et al. (2016). The effect of translating research into practice intervention to promote use of evidence-based fall prevention interventions in hospitalized adults: a prospective pre-post implementation study in the U.S. *Applied Nursing Research*, 31, 52–59. doi:10.1016/j.apnr.2015.12.004.

Titler, M. G., Herr, K., Everett, L. Q., et al. (2006). *Book to bedside: Promoting and sustaining EBPs in elders* (Final Progress Report to AHRQ, Grant No. 2R01 HS010482-04). Iowa City, IA: University of Iowa College of Nursing.

Titler, M. G., Kleiber, C., Steelman, V. J., et al. (2001). The Iowa model of evidence-based practice to promote quality care. *Critical Care Nursing Clinics of North America*, 13(4), 497–509. PMID: 11778337.

Titler, M. G., Shever, L. L., Kanak, F., et al. (2011). Factors associated with falls during hospitalization in an older adult population. *Research and Theory for Nursing Practice*, 25(2), 127–152. doi:10.1891/1541-6577.25.2.127, PMID: 21696092.

Titler, M. G., Wilson, D. S., Resnick, B., & Shever, L. L. (2013). Dissemination and implementation: INQRI's potential impact. *Medical Care*, 51(4 Suppl 2), S41–S46. doi:10.1097/MLR.0b013e3182802fb5, PMID: 23502916.

USPSTF. (2015). U.S. Preventative Services Task Force procedure manual. U.S. Preventative Services Task Force, December 2015. Retrieved August 2016 from http://www.uspreventiveservicestaskforce.org/Page/Name/methods-and-processes.

Weiler, K., Buckwalter, K., & Titler, M. (1994). Debate: is nursing research used in practice? In J. McCloskey, & H. Grace (Eds.), *Current issues in nursing* (4th ed.). St Louis, MO: Mosby.

Wilson, D. S., Montie, M., Conlon, P., et al. (2016). Nurses' perceptions of implementing fall prevention interventions to mitigate patient-specific fall risk factors. *Western Journal of Nursing Research*, 38(8), 1012–1034. doi:10.1177/0193945916644995, PMID: 27106881.

Wilson, P. M., Petticrew, M., Calnan, M. W., & Nazareth, I. (2010). Disseminating research findings: what should researchers do? A systematic scoping review of conceptual frameworks. *Implementation Science*, 5, 91. doi:10.1186/1748-5908-5-91, PMID: 21092164, PMCID: PMC2994786.

Yano, E. M. (2008). The role of organizational research in implementing evidence-based practice: QUERI series. *Implementation Science*, 3, 29. doi:10.1186/1748-5908-3-29, PMID: 18510749, PMCID: PMC2481253.

Yousefi-Nooraie, R., Dobbins, M., & Marin, A. (2014). Social and organizational factors affecting implementation of evidence-informed practice in a public health department in Ontario: a network modeling approach. *Implementation Science, 9*, 29. doi:10.1186/1748-5908-9-29.

Go to Evolve at **http://evolve.elsevier.com/LoBiondo/** for review questions, critiquing exercises, and additional research articles for practice in reviewing and critiquing.

21

Quality Improvement

Maja Djukic and Mattia J. Gilmartin

Go to Evolve at **http://evolve.elsevier.com/LoBiondo/** for review questions, critiquing exercises, and additional research articles for practice in reviewing and critiquing.

LEARNING OUTCOMES

After reading this chapter, you should be able to do the following:

- Discuss the characteristics of quality health care defined by the Institute of Medicine.
- Compare the characteristics of the major quality improvement (QI) models used in health care.
- Identify two databases used to report health care organizations' performance to promote consumer choice and guide clinical QI activities.
- Describe the relationship between nursing-sensitive quality indicators and patient outcomes.
- Describe the steps in the improvement process, and determine appropriate QI tools to use in each phase of the improvement process.
- List four themes for improvement to apply to the unit where you work.
- Describe ways that nurses can lead QI projects in clinical settings.
- Use the SQUIRE Guidelines to critique a journal article reporting the results of a QI project.

KEY TERMS

accreditation
benchmarking
Clinical Microsystems
common cause and special cause variation
control chart
flowchart
Lean
nursing-sensitive quality indicators
Plan-Do-Study-Act Improvement Cycle
public reporting
quality health care
quality improvement
root cause analysis
run chart
Six Sigma
SQUIRE Guidelines

TOTAL QUALITY MANAGEMENT/CONTINUOUS QUALITY IMPROVEMENT

The Institute of Medicine (IOM, 2001) defines **quality health care** as care that is safe, effective, patient-centered, timely, efficient, and equitable (Box 21.1). The quality of the health care system was brought to the forefront of national attention in several important reports (IOM, 1999, 2001), including *Crossing the Quality Chasm*, which concluded that

BOX 21.1 Six Dimensions and Definitions of Health Care Quality

1. **Safe:** Avoiding injuries to patients from the care that is intended to help them.
2. **Effective:** Providing services based on scientific knowledge to all who could benefit, and refraining from providing services to those not likely to benefit.
3. **Patient-centered:** Providing care that is respectful of and responsive to individual patient preferences, needs, and values, and ensuring that patient values guide all clinical decisions.
4. **Timely:** Reducing waits and sometimes harmful delays for both those who receive and those who give care.
5. **Efficient**: Avoiding waste, including waste of equipment, supplies, ideas, and energy.
6. **Equitable:** Providing care that does not vary in quality because of personal characteristics such as gender, ethnicity, geographic location, and socioeconomic status.

From Institute of Medicine (IOM). (2001). *Crossing the quality chasm: A new health system for the 21st century. Executive summary*. Washington, DC: The National Academies Press.

"between the health care we have and the care we could have lies not just a gap, but a chasm" (IOM, 2001, p. 1). The report notes that "the performance of the health care system varies considerably. It may be exemplary, but often is not, and millions of Americans fail to receive effective care" (IOM, 2001, p. 3).

Since the IOM (2001) report was published, quality of care has improved for some conditions (Nuti et al., 2015). Based on data from over 4000 US hospitals, core composite quality process measures for acute myocardial infarction (e.g., aspiring on arrival), heart failure (e.g., smoking cessation advice), and pneumonia (e.g., influenza vaccine) improved from 96% to 99%, 85% to 98%, and 83% to 97%, respectively, from 2006 to 2011 (Nuti et al., 2015). Also, overall positive improvement trends across more than 200 quality measures are noted, led by 17% reduction of hospital-acquired conditions from 2010 to 2014 (Agency for Healthcare Research and Quality [AHRQ], 2016). Improvements are, however, needed for about 20% of measures in person-and-family-centered care, such as receiving care as soon as needed, and for about 40% of measures of healthy living, such as getting prompt smoking cessation help for people trying to quit (AHRQ, 2016). Further, disparities in quality based on earnings, race, and ethnicity continue to persist. For example, "people from poor households compared to those from high-income households received worse care for about 60% of quality measures; Blacks, Hispanics, American Indians, and Alaska Natives compared to Whites received worse care for about 40% of quality measures" (AHRQ, 2016, p. 11). Despite these quality issues, the United States spends twice as much on health care per capita per year at $8508, compared with other developed nations, while ranking last in health care quality in comparison with 10 other countries (Davis et al., 2014).

The purpose of this chapter is to introduce you to the principles of **quality improvement** (QI) and provide examples of how to apply these principles in your practice so you can effectively contribute to needed health care improvements. QI "uses data to monitor the outcomes of care processes and improvement methods to design and test changes to continuously improve the quality and safety of health care systems" (Cronenwett et al., 2007, p. 127).

NURSES' ROLE IN HEALTH CARE QUALITY IMPROVEMENT

Florence Nightingale championed QI by systematically documenting high rates of morbidity and mortality resulting from poor sanitary conditions among soldiers serving in the

Crimean War of 1854 (Henry et al., 1992). She used statistics to document changes in soldiers' health, including reductions in mortality resulting from a number of nursing interventions such as hand hygiene, instrument sterilization, changing of bed linens, ward sanitation, ventilation, and proper nutrition (Henry et al., 1992). Today, nurses continue to be vital to health system improvement efforts (IOM, 2015). One main initiative developed to bolster nurses' education in health system improvements is *Quality and Safety Education for Nurses* (QSEN) (Cronenwett et al., 2007). The overall goal of this project is to help build nurses' competence in the areas of QI, patient-centered care, teamwork and collaboration, patient safety, informatics, and evidence-based practice (EBP). Other initiatives, such as the *Care Innovation and Transformation Program* (American Organization of Nurse Executives, 2016), have been developed to increase nurses' engagement in QI. To effectively influence improvements in the work setting and ensure that all patients consistently receive excellent care, it is important to:

- Align national, organizational, and unit level goals for QI.
- Recognize external drivers of quality, such as accreditation, payment, and performance measurement.
- Develop skills to apply QI models and tools.

NATIONAL GOALS AND STRATEGIES FOR HEALTH CARE QUALITY IMPROVEMENT

The National Quality Strategy, first published in 2011 and established by the Affordable Care Act to pursue the triple health care improvement aim of better care, affordable care, and healthy people/healthy communities (US Department of Health and Human Services [USDHHS], 2016a), set aims and priorities for QI (Box 21.2). Achieving these national quality targets requires major redesign of the health care system. One way you can contribute to this redesign is to familiarize yourself with the national priorities, corresponding improvement goals, and national initiatives (Table 21.1) and use them to guide improvements in your work setting.

BOX 21.2 National Quality Aims and Priorities

National Quality Aims	National Quality Priorities for Achieving the Aims
• **Better Care:** Improve the overall quality of care by making health care more patient-centered, reliable, accessible, and safe.	• Make care safer by reducing harm caused in the delivery of care. • Ensure all people and families are engaged as partners in their care.
• **Healthy People/Healthy Communities:** Improve the health of the US population by supporting proven interventions to address behavioral, social, and environmental determinants of health in addition to delivering higher-quality care.	• Promote effective communication and care coordination. • Promote the most effective prevention and treatment practices for the leading causes of mortality, starting with cardiovascular disease. • Work with communities to promote wide use of best practices to enable healthy living.
• **Affordable Care:** Reduce the cost of quality health care for individuals, families, employers, and government.	• Make quality care more affordable for individuals, families, employers, and governments by developing and spreading new health care delivery models.

From 2015 National Healthcare Quality and Disparities Report and 5th Anniversary Update on the National Quality Strategy. Agency of Healthcare Research and Quality, Rockville, MD. http://www.ahrq.gov/research/findings/nhqrdr/nhqdr15/index.html.

TABLE 21.1 National Quality Strategy Priorities, Improvement Goals, and Related Initiatives

National Quality Strategy Priority	Long-Term Goals	Related National Initiatives
Patient safety	1. Reduce preventable hospital admissions and readmissions. 2. Reduce the incidence of adverse health care-associated conditions. 3. Reduce harm from inappropriate or unnecessary care.	Partnership for Patients, Hospital Readmission Reduction Program, Children's Hospital of Pittsburgh of UPMC
Person- and family-centered care	1. Improve patient, family, and caregiver experience of care related to quality, safety, and access across settings. 2. In partnership with patients, families, and caregivers—and using a shared decision-making process—develop culturally sensitive and understandable care plans. 3. Enable patients and their families and caregivers to navigate, coordinate, and manage their care appropriately and effectively.	Consumer Assessment of Healthcare Providers and Systems, National Partnership for Women and Families, Colorado Coalition for the Homeless
Effective communication and care coordination	1. Improve the quality of care transitions and communications across care settings. 2. Improve the quality of life for patients with chronic illness and disability by following a current care plan that anticipates and addresses pain and symptom management, psychosocial needs, and functional status. 3. Establish shared accountability and integration of communities and health care systems to improve quality of care and reduce health disparities.	Argonaut Project, Boston Children's Hospital Community Asthma Initiative
Prevention and treatment of leading causes of morbidity and mortality	1. Promote cardiovascular health through community interventions that result in improvement of social, economic, and environmental factors. 2. Promote cardiovascular health through interventions that result in adoption of the most healthy lifestyle behaviors across the life span. 3. Promote cardiovascular health through receipt of effective clinical preventive services across the life span in clinical and community settings.	The Million Hearts Campaign, Wind River Reservation
Health and well-being of communities	1. Promote healthy living and well-being through community interventions that result in improvement of social, economic, and environmental factors. 2. Promote healthy living and well-being through interventions that result in adoption of the most important healthy lifestyle behaviors across the life span. 3. Promote healthy living and well-being through receipt of effective clinical preventive services across the life span in clinical and community settings.	Let's Move!, Health Leads
Making quality care more affordable	1. Ensure affordable and accessible high-quality health care for people, families, employers, and governments. 2. Support and enable communities to ensure accessible, high-quality care while reducing waste and fraud.	Blue Cross Blue Shield Massachusetts Alternative Quality Contract, Medicare Shared Savings Program, Pioneer Accountable Care Organization Model Arkansas Center for Health Improvement

From the US Department of Health and Human Services. (2016a). *National quality strategy overview.* Retrieved from http://www.ahrq.gov/workingforquality/nqs/overview.pdf.

QUALITY STRATEGY LEVERS

QI relies on aligning institutional priorities with several strategy levers that drive QI. The National Quality Strategy encourages multiple members of the health care community, including individuals, family members, payers, providers, and employers, to collaborate on using one or more of the nine strategy levers (USDHHS, 2016a, p. 8); we describe briefly how each lever is used for QI:

1. **Measurement and feedback**—Provide performance feedback to plans and providers to improve care. National health care performance standards are developed using a consensus process in which stakeholder groups, representing the interests of the public, health professionals, payers, employers, and government, identify priorities, measures, and reporting requirements to document and manage the quality of care (National Quality Forum [NQF], 2004). See Box 21.3 for examples of groups responsible for developing measurement standards.
2. **Public reporting**—Compare treatment results, costs, and patient experience for the consumer. Several major public reporting systems are described in Box 21.4.
3. **Learning and technical assistance**—Foster learning environments that offer training, resources, tools, and guidance to help organizations achieve quality improvement goals.
4. **Certification, accreditation, regulation**—Adopt or adhere to approaches to meet safety and quality standards. Several accrediting bodies are listed in Box 21.5.
5. **Consumer incentives and benefits designs**—Help consumers adopt healthy behaviors and make informed decisions.
6. **Payment**—Reward and incentivize providers to deliver high-quality, patient-centered care. Box 21.6 shows examples of payment incentives.
7. **Health information technology**—Improve communications, transparency, and efficiency for better coordinated health and health care.

BOX 21.3 Performance Measurement Standard Setting Groups

Introduction to Performance Measurement Standards

National Quality Forum (NQF) is a nonprofit organization that seeks to measure and improve the quality of health care in the United States by establishing national healthcare quality and safety goals and priorities. The NQF's evidence-based measure endorsement process is the gold standard for healthcare quality measurement. The NQF endorsement process is a transparent, consensus-based model that brings together stakeholders from the private and public sectors to foster quality improvement. Approximately 300 NQF-endorsed measures are used by federal public and private pay-for-performance programs, as well as, in private-sector and state healthcare quality programs.[a]

Agency for Healthcare Research and Quality, Quality Indicators (AHRQ). The AHRQ Quality Indicators are standardized, evidence-based measures of the quality of hospital care that are readily available using hospital administrative data. There are 101 Quality Indicators organized into the four main categories of inpatient quality for adult and pediatric patients; preventative quality indicators for ambulatory care and avoidable complications. Approximately half of the AHRQ quality indicators are endorsed by the National Quality Forum and used to support hospital quality improvement, health system planning and pay for performance initiatives.[b]

[a]National Quality Forum. (2015). *National Quality Forum, What We Do.* Retrieved from http://www.qualityforum.org/what_we_do.aspx.

[b]Agency for Healthcare Research and Quality. (2015). *About AHRQ Quality Indicators.* Retrieved from: http://qualityindicators.ahrq.gov/FAQs_Support/FAQ_QI_Overview.aspx.

BOX 21.4 Public Reporting Systems

- **Hospital Compare** allows consumers to compare information on hospitals. The database includes performance measures on timely and efficient care, readmissions and deaths, complications, use of medical imaging, survey of patients' experiences, and payment and value of care. For more information, visit www.hospitalcompare.hhs.gov/.
- **Nursing Home Compare** allows consumers to compare information about nursing homes. It contains quality of care information on every Medicare and Medicaid-certified nursing home in the country. The database includes performance measures on health inspections, staffing, and clinical quality. For more information, visit www.medicare.gov/NursingHomeCompare/.
- **Home Health Compare** has information about the quality of care provided by Medicare-certified home health agencies that meet federal health and safety requirements throughout the nation. For more information, visit www.medicare.gov/homehealthcompare.
- **Hospital Consumer Assessment of Healthcare Providers and Systems (HCAHPS)**. Developed by the Agency for Healthcare Research and Quality, the HCAHPS is a standardized survey and data collection method for measuring patients' perspectives on hospital care. The HCAHPS survey contains 32 questions about patient perspectives on care for eight key topics: communication with doctors; communication with nurses; responsiveness of hospital staff; pain management; communication about medicines; discharge information; cleanliness of the hospital environment; and quietness of the hospital environment, posthospital transitions, admissions through the emergency room, and mental and emotional health. HCAHPS performance is used to calculate incentive payments in the Hospital Value-Based Purchasing program for hospital discharges beginning in October 2012. For more information, visit http://www.hcahpsonline.org/Files/HCAHPS_Fact_Sheet_June_2015.pdf.
- **Physician Quality Reporting Initiative** is a program administered by the CMS that collects performance data at the physician/provider clinical level in the ambulatory and primary care sectors. For more information, visit www.cms.gov/Medicare/Quality-Initiatives-Patient-Assessment-Instruments/PQRS/index.html.
- **The Leapfrog Group** is an initiative of organizations that buy health care who are working to improve the safety, quality, and affordability of health care for Americans. The Leapfrog Group conducts a survey for comparing hospitals' performance on the national standards of safety, quality, and efficiency that are most relevant to consumers and purchasers of care. For more information, visit www.leapfroggroup.org/.

CMS, Center for Medicare and Medicaid Services.

BOX 21.5 Quality Improvement Accrediting Organizations

- **Joint Commission:** Responsible for ensuring a minimum standard of structures, processes, and outcomes for patient care. Accreditation by the Joint Commission is voluntary, but it is required to receive reimbursement for patient care services. For more information, see www.jointcommission.org/.
- **National Committee for Quality Assurance Accreditation for Health Plans (NCQA):** A private not-for-profit organization dedicated to improving health care quality. The NCQA is responsible for accrediting health insurance programs. Accredited health insurance programs are exempt from many or all elements associated with annual state audits. The NCQA developed and maintains the Healthcare Effectiveness Data and Information Set (HEDIS).
- **The Healthcare Effectiveness Data and Information Set (HEDIS):** A tool used by the majority of America's health plans to measure performance on important dimensions of care and service. HEDIS allows for comparison of performance across health plans. For more information, see http://www.ncqa.org/HEDISQualityMeasurement.aspx.
- **American Nurses' Credentialing Center Magnet Recognition Program** recognizes health care organizations that provide the very best in nursing care and uphold the tradition of professional nursing practice. For more information, see www.nursecredentialing.org/Magnet.aspx.

BOX 21.6 Financial Incentives to Promote Quality in the Health Care Sector

Capitation: A payment arrangement for health care services. Pays a provider (physician or nurse practitioner) or provider group a set amount for each enrolled person assigned to them, per period of time, whether or not that person seeks care. These providers generally are contracted with a type of health maintenance organization (HMO). Payment levels are based on average expected health care use of a particular patient, with greater payment for patients with significant medical history.[a]

Bundled Payments Initiative: Links payments for multiple services that patients receive during an episode of care. Payments seek to align incentives for hospitals, post acute care providers, doctors, and other practitioners to improve the patient's care experience during a hospital stay in an acute care hospital through postdischarge recovery.[b]

Pay for Performance: An emerging movement in health insurance where providers are rewarded for meeting pre-established targets for health care delivery services. This model rewards physicians, hospitals, medical groups, and other health care providers for meeting certain performance measures for quality and efficiency.[c]

Value-Based Health Care Purchasing: A project of participating health plans, including the CMS, where buyers hold providers of health care accountable for both cost and quality of care. Value-based purchasing brings together information on health care quality, patient outcomes, and health status, with data on the dollar outlays going toward health. The focus is on managing health care system use to reduce inappropriate care and to identify and reward the best-performing providers.[d]

Accountable Care Organization (ACO): A payment and care delivery model that seeks to tie provider reimbursements to quality metrics and reductions in the total cost of care for an assigned population of patients. A group of coordinated health care providers form an ACO, which then provides care to a group of patients. The ACO may use a range of payment models (e.g., capitation, fee-for-service). The ACO is accountable to the patients and the third-party payer for the quality, appropriateness, and efficiency of the health care provided.[e]

CMS, Center for Medicare and Medicaid Services.

[a]American Medical Association. (2012). *Capitation.* Retrieved from http://www.ama-assn.org/ama/pub/advocacy/state-advocacy-arc/state-advocacy-campaigns/private-payer-reform/state-based-payment-reform/evaluating-payment-options/capitation.page.

[b]Centers for Medicare and Medicaid Services. (2016). *Bundled payments for care improvement initiative: General information.* Retrieved from https://innovation.cms.gov/initiatives/Bundled-Payments/index.html.

[c]Integrated Healthcare Association. (2013). *National pay for performance issue brief.* Retrieved from http://www.iha.org/sites/default/files/resources/issue-brief-value-based-p4p-2013.pdf.

[d]Damberg, C. L., Sorbero, M. E., Lovejoy, S. L., et al. (2014). *Measuring success in health care value-based purchasing programs: Summary and recommendations.* Santa Monica, CA: RAND Corporation, RR-306/1-ASPE, Retrieved from http://www.rand.org/pubs/research_reports/RR306z1.html.

[e]American Hospital Association. (2014). *Accountable care organizations: Findings from the survey of care systems and payment.* Retrieved from http://www.aha.org/content/14/14aug-acocharts.pdf.

8. **Innovation and diffusion**—Foster innovation in health care quality improvement, and facilitate rapid adoption within and across organizations and communities.
9. **Workforce development**—Invest in people to prepare the next generation of health care professionals and support lifelong learning for providers.

Measuring Nursing Care Quality

Nurses deliver the majority of health care and therefore have a substantial influence on its overall quality (IOM, 2015). However, nursing's contribution to the overall quality of health care has been difficult to quantify, owing in part to insufficient standardized measurement systems capable of capturing nursing care contribution to patient outcomes. The Robert Wood Johnson Foundation has funded the NQF to recommend nursing-sensitive consensus standards to be used to set standards for public accountability and QI. The work of the NQF (2004) resulted in the endorsement of **15 nursing-sensitive quality indicators** (Table 21.2). Since the endorsement of "NQF 15," several data reporting mechanisms have been established for performance sharing internally among providers to identify areas in need of improvement, externally for purposes of accreditation and payment, and with

TABLE 21.2 National Voluntary Standards for Nursing-Sensitive Care

Framework Category	Measure	Description
Patient-centered outcome measures	Death among surgical inpatients with treatable serious complications (failure to rescue)	Percent of major surgical inpatients who experience hospital-acquired complications (e.g., sepsis, pneumonia, gastrointestinal bleeding, shock/cardiac arrest, deep vein thrombosis/pulmonary embolism) that result in death.
	Pressure ulcer prevalence[a]	Percent of inpatients who have hospital-acquired pressure ulcers (Stage 2 or greater).
	Falls prevalence[a]	Number of inpatient falls per inpatient days.
	Falls with injury	Number of inpatient falls with injuries per inpatient days.
	Restraint prevalence (vest and limb only)	Percent of patients who have a vest or limb restraint.
	Urinary catheter–associated UTI for ICU patients[a]	Rate of UTI associated with use of urinary catheters for ICU patients.
	Central line catheter-associated blood stream infection rate for ICU and HRN patients[a]	Rate of bloodstream infections associated with use of central line catheters for ICU or HRN patients.
	Ventilator-associated pneumonia for ICU and HRN patients[a]	Rate of pneumonia associated with use of ventilators for ICU and HRN patients.
Nursing-centered intervention measures	Smoking cessation counseling for AMI[a]	Percent of AMI inpatients with smoking history in the past year who received smoking cessation advice or counseling during hospitalization.
	Smoking cessation counseling for HF[a]	Percent of HF inpatients with smoking history within the past year who received smoking cessation advice or counseling during hospitalization.
	Smoking cessation counseling for pneumonia[a]	Percent of pneumonia inpatients with smoking history within the past year who received smoking cessation advice or counseling during hospitalization.
System-centered measures	Skill mix (RN, LVN/LPN, UAP and contract)	• Percent of RN care hours to total nursing care hours. • Percent of LVN/LPN care hours to total nursing care hours. • Percent of UAP care hours to total nursing care hours. • Percent of contract hours (RN, LVN/LPN, and UAP) to total nursing care hours.
	Nursing care hours per inpatient day (RN, LVN/LPN, and UAP)	• Number of RN care hours per patient day. • Number of nursing staff hours (RN, LVN, LPN, UAP).
	PES-NWI (composite and five subscales)	Composite score and mean presence scores for each of the following subscales derived from PES-NWI: • Nurse participation in hospital affairs. • Nursing foundations for quality of care. • Nurse manager ability, leadership, and support of nurses. • Staffing and resource adequacy. • Collegial nurse–physician relations.
	Voluntary turnover	Number of voluntary uncontrolled separations during the month for RNs and advanced practice nurses, LVN/LPNs, and nurse assistant/aides.

AMI, Acute myocardial infarction; *HF,* heart failure; *HRN,* high-risk nursery; *ICU,* intensive care unit; *LVP/LPN,* licensed vocational/practical nurse; *PES-NWI,* practice environment scale-nursing work index; *RN,* registered nurse; *UAP,* unlicensed assistive personnel; *UTI,* urinary tract infection.

From National Quality Forum. (2012). *Measuring performance.* Retrieved from www.qualityforum.org/Measuring_Performance/ABCs_of_Measurement.aspx.

[a]NQF-endorsed national voluntary consensus standard for hospital care.

health care consumers so that they can choose providers based on the quality of services provided. Examples include *Hospital Compare* (USDHHS, 2016b) and the nursing-specific databases described by Alexander (2007):

- **The National Database of Nursing Quality Indicators** is a proprietary database of the Press Ganey. The database collects and evaluates unit-specific nurse-sensitive data from hospitals in the United States. Participating facilities receive unit-level comparative data reports to use for QI purposes. For more information, visit http://www.pressganey.com/solutions/clinical-quality/nursing-quality.
- **California Nursing Outcomes Coalition (CalNOC)** is a data repository of hospital-generated, unit-level, acute nurse staffing and workforce characteristics and processes of care, as well as key NQF-endorsed, nursing-sensitive outcome measures, submitted electronically via the web. For more information, visit http://www.calnoc.org.
- **Veterans Affairs Nursing Outcomes Database** was originally modeled after CalNOC. Data are collected at the unit and hospital levels to facilitate the evaluation of quality and enable benchmarking within and among Veterans Affairs facilities.

HELPFUL HINT

To find out how your hospital compares in nursing-sensitive quality indicators such as pressure ulcers, infections, and falls with another hospital in your area, go to https://www.medicare.gov/hospitalcompare/search.html. Identify high-performing organizations in your area from which you can learn.

Benchmarking

The measurement of quality indicators must be done methodically using standardized tools. Standardized measurement allows for **benchmarking**, which is "a systematic approach for gathering information about process or product performance and then analyzing why and how performance differs between business units" (Massoud et al., 2001, p. 74). Benchmarking is critical for QI because it helps identify when performance is below an agreed-upon standard and signals the need for improvement. For example, when you record assessment of your patient's risk for falls using one of the standardized assessment tools such as the Hendrich II Fall Risk Model or Morse Fall Scale and newly identified risk factors such as use of antidepressants, hypnotics, diuretics, antidiabetic medications, and polypharmacy (Callis, 2016), it allows for comparison of your assessment to those of providers in other organizations who provide care to a similar patient population and who use the same tools to document assessments. Tracking changes in the overall fall risk score over time allows you to intervene if the score falls below a set standard, indicating high risk for falls. Equally, after you implement needed interventions focused on altered elimination, mental status, or musculoskeletal weakness, you can track changes in the fall risk score to determine whether the interventions were effective in reducing risk for falls. Therefore standardized measurement can tell you when changes in care are needed and whether implemented interventions have resulted in the actual improvement of patient outcomes.

When all clinical units document care in the same way, it is possible to document pressure ulcer care across units. These performance data are useful for benchmarking efforts where clinical teams learn from each other how to apply best practices from high-performing units to the care processes of lower-performing units. Benchmarking (Massoud et al., 2001, p. 75) can be used to:

- Develop plans to address improvement needs.
- Borrow and adapt successful ideas from others.
- Understand what has already been tried.

COMMON QUALITY IMPROVEMENT PERSPECTIVES AND MODELS

QI as a management model is both a philosophy of organizational functioning and a set of statistical analysis tools and change techniques used to reduce variations in the quality of goods or services that an organization produces (Nelson et al., 2007). The QI model emphasizes customer satisfaction, teams and teamwork, and the continuous improvement of work processes. Other defining features of QI include the use of transformational leadership by leaders at all levels to set performance goals and expectations, use of data to make decisions, and standardization of work processes to reduce variation across providers and service encounters (Nelson et al., 2007). The key principles associated with QI are shown in Table 21.3.

Although QI has its roots in the manufacturing sector, many of the ideas, tools, and techniques used to measure and manage quality have been applied in health care organizations to improve clinical outcomes and reduce waste (McConnell et al., 2016). The major QI models used in health care include:

- Total Quality Management/Continuous Quality Improvement (TQM/CQI)
- Six Sigma
- Lean
- Clinical Microsystems

The key characteristics of each of these models are described in Table 21.4. Because QI uses a holistic approach, leaders often select one quality model that is used to guide the organization's overarching improvement agenda.

It is important to note that health care organizations have adopted principles and practices associated with the industrial QI approach relatively recently. Historically, the quality of health care was assessed retrospectively using the quality assurance (QA) model. The QA model uses chart audits to compare care against a predetermined standard. Corrective actions associated with QA focus on assigning individual blame and correcting deficiencies in operations. Another model commonly associated with health care QI is the *Structure-Process-Outcome Framework* (Donabedian, 1966). This framework is used to examine the resources that make up health care delivery services, clinicians' work practices, and the outcomes associated with the structure and processes. The evolution of the key perspectives used to understand and manage QI in health care organizations is summarized in Table 21.5.

QUALITY IMPROVEMENT STEPS AND TOOLS

Similar to the nursing process, which you use to guide your assessment, diagnoses, and treatment of patient problems, you can use the QI process steps (Massoud et al., 2001) for the following:

1. Assessing health system performance by collecting and monitoring data
2. Analyzing data to identify a problem in need of improvement
3. Developing a plan to treat the identified problem
4. Testing and implementing the improvement plan

TABLE 21.3 Principles of Quality Improvement

Improvement Principle	Key Benefits
Principle 1—Customer focus/Patient focus Health care organizations rely on patients and therefore should understand current and future patient needs, should meet patient requirements, and strive to exceed patient expectations.	• Increased customer value • Increased revenue and market share obtained through flexible and fast responses to market opportunities • Increased effectiveness in the organization's resources use to enhance patient satisfaction • Improved patient loyalty leading to repeat business
Principle 2—Leadership Leaders establish unity of purpose, and the organization's direction should create and maintain an internal environment in which people can become fully involved in organization's objectives achievement.	• People understand and are motivated toward the organization's goals and objectives • Activities are evaluated, aligned and implemented in a unified way • Miscommunication between organization levels are minimized
Principle 3—Engagement of people People at all levels are the essence of an organization and are essential to enhance organizational capability to create and deliver value.	• Motivated, committed, and involved people within the organization • Innovation and creativity further the organization's objectives • People are accountable for own performance • Enhanced involvement of people in improvement activities
Principle 4—Process approach Consistent results are achieved with more efficiently and effectively when activities are understood and managed as a system of interrelated processes.	• Lower costs and shorter cycle times through effective use of resources • Improved, consistent, and predictable results through a system of aligned processes • Focused and prioritized improvement opportunities
Principle 5—Improvement Successful organizations have an ongoing focus on improvement. Continual improvement is essential creating new opportunities.	• Performance advantage through improved organizational capabilities • Focus on root-cause analysis, followed by prevention and corrective action • Consideration of incremental and breakthrough improvements
Principle 6—Evidence-based decision making Effective decisions are based on the analysis and evaluation of data and information are more likely to produce desired results.	• Improved decision-making processes • Increased ability to demonstrate effectiveness of past decisions • Increased ability to review, challenge, and change opinions and decisions
Principle 7—Relationship Management An organization and its suppliers are interdependent and a mutually beneficial relationship enhances ability of both to create value.	• Increased capability to create value for both parties by sharing resources and managing quality-related risks • A well-managed supply chain that provides a stable flow of goods and services • Optimization of costs and resources

From International Organization for Standardization. (2015). *ISO 9001 quality management principles*. Retrieved from http://www.iso.org/iso/home/standards/management-standards/iso_9000.htm.

Several tools facilitate each step of the QI process (Table 21.6). You can use these tools to assist with collecting and analyzing data and to identify and test improvement ideas. A case example, *Nurse Response Time to Patient Call Light Requests* (Box 21.7), is presented to introduce the steps of the improvement process and apply several basic QI tools used to measure and manage system performance.

Forming a Lead Quality Improvement Team

QI is inherently an interprofessional team process and requires contributions from various perspectives to assess the potential causes of system malfunction and improvement ideas (Nelson et al., 2007). A lead QI team should be composed of representatives from multiple

TABLE 21.4 Overview of Quality Improvement Models Used in Health Care

Model	Main Characteristics	Related Resources
TQM/CQI (Langley et al., 2009)	• A holistic management approach used to improve organizational performance • Seeks to understand and manage variation in service delivery • Emphasizes customer satisfaction as an important performance measure • Relies on team work and collaboration among workers to deliver technically excellent and customer/patient-centered services • Quality management science uses tools and techniques from statistics, engineering, operations research, management, market research and psychology • TQM/CQI tools and techniques are applied to specific performance problems in the form of improvement projects • The extent to which unit-level QI projects align with larger organizational quality goals, is related to their success and sustainability	Institute for Healthcare Improvement: http://www.ihi.org/resources/Pages/default.aspx
Six Sigma (DelliFraine et al., 2010)	• Developed at Motorola in the 1980s • Six Sigma takes its name from the statistical notation of sigma (σ) used to measure variation from the mean • Emphasizes meeting customer requirements and eliminating errors or rework with the goal of reducing process variation • Focuses on tightly controlling variations in production processes with the goal of reducing the number of defects to 3.4 units per 1 million units produced • Process control achieved by applying DMAIC improvement model • DMAIC includes defining, measuring, analyzing, improving, and controlling • Practitioners achieve mastery levels using statistical tools to measure and manage process variation (e.g., yellow-belt, green-belt, black-belt)	AHRQ Innovations Exchange: www.innovations.ahrq.gov https://innovations.ahrq.gov/qualitytools/lean-hospitals-six-sigma-and-lean-healthcare-forms
Lean (DelliFraine et al., 2010)	• Sometimes referred to as the Toyota Quality Model • Focus: Eliminating waste from the production system by designing the most efficient and effective system • Production controlled through standardization and placing the right person and materials at each step of the process • Uses the PDSA improvement cycle • Statistical tools include value stream mapping and Kanban, or a visual cue, used to warn clinicians that there is a process problem • Performance measures vary from project to project and may inform the creation of new performance measures • Uses a master teacher ("Sensei") to spread the practices of Lean though the organizational culture	Institute for Healthcare Improvement: www.ihi.org/knowledge/Pages/IHIWhitePapers/GoingLeaninHealthCare.aspx
Clinical Microsystems (Nelson et al., 2007)	• Model of service excellence developed specifically for health care • Clinical microsystem is considered the building block of any health care system and is the smallest replicable unit in an organization • Members of a clinical microsystem are interdependent and work together toward a common aim	Clinical Microsystems: www.clinicalmicrosystem.org

AHRQ, Agency for Healthcare Research and Quality; *CQI,* continuous quality improvement; *PDSA,* plan-do-study-act; *QI,* quality improvement; *TQM,* total quality management.

TABLE 21.5 Evolution of Quality Improvement Perspectives in Health Care

Model	Key Features	Quality Monitoring Mechanisms	Representative Research Questions
1920s–1980s QA Used to correct differences between what should be and what actually is (Chassin & Loeb, 2011)	• Uses external standards to guide quality • Quality assessed after the fact • Corrective action is punitive • The focus is on symptoms, individual failures, and compliance with standards	• Accreditation • Chart audit • Morbidity and mortality rounds	What is the effect of the Race program, led by clinical nurse specialist in partnership with nurse leaders to engage front line staff in process improvement and quality assurance programs to improve nurses' impact on patient safety? Adapted from Tidwell et al. (2016).
1960s–2010s Structure-Process-Outcome Framework examines system components that lead to health care quality (Donabedian, 1966)	• Stresses professional responsibility for evaluating care quality • *Structure* focuses on provider and organizational characteristics • *Process* focuses on how care is delivered • *Outcome* focuses on the end results of medical care	• Accreditation • Work redesign • Benchmarking • Professional education and credentialing	What is the predictive power of measures representing patient characteristics, nurse workload, nurse expertise, and HAPU preventative processes of care on HAPU prevalence? Adapted from Aydin et al. (2015).
1990s–2010s TQM/CQI Model used to continually improve services and organizational performance (Bigelow & Arndt, 1995)	• Systems approach to improve efficiency • Incorporates clinical, financial, administrative, and patient satisfaction perspectives • Focuses on meeting actual and unanticipated patient needs • Uses statistical analysis to reduce variation in service processes • Relies on team work and data-based decisions	• Accreditation • Benchmarking (HCAHPS) • Clinical practice guidelines • PDSA cycles • Process redesign • Lean • Six Sigma	How do P-D-S-A cycles of change that incorporate peer-reviewed evidence improve patient-centeredness, teamwork, communication, and safety in a 16-bed medical and surgical pediatric intensive care unit? Adapted from Tripathi et al. (2015).
2000s–2010s Patient Safety Systems approach to reduce harm to patients (Chassin & Loeb, 2011)	• Applies safety science methods to design health care delivery systems • Focuses on reducing or avoiding adverse events • Domains include patients; providers; care routines; system design	• Accreditation • Sentinel event reporting; • National Patient Safety Goals • High reliability organization model • Root cause analysis	What is the relationship between employee engagement and the dimensions of patient safety culture in critical care units? Adapted from Collier et al. (2016).

CQI, Continuous quality improvement; *HAPU,* hospital-acquired pressure ulcers; *HCAHPS*, Hospital consumer assessment of health care providers and systems; PDSA, plan-do-study-act; *QA,* quality assurance; *TQM,* total quality management.

TABLE 21.6 Quality Improvement Tools and Activities

Basic Tools and Activities	Step 1 Assess	Step 2 Analyze	Step 3 Plan and Implement	Step 4 Test and Evaluate
Data collection	X	X	X	X
Flowcharts	X	X	X	X
Cause-and-effect analysis	—	X	—	—
Bar and pie charts	X	X	—	X
Run charts	X	X	—	X
Control charts	X	X	—	X
Histograms	X	X	—	X
Pareto charts	X	X	—	X
Benchmarking	X	—	—	X
Gantt charts	—	X	—	X

From Massoud R, Askov K, Reinke J, et al. (2001). A modern paradigm for improving healthcare quality. *QA Monograph Series 1*(1). Bethesda, MD: Published for the US Agency for International Development by the Quality Assurance Project.

BOX 21.7 Applying the Quality Improvement Steps to a Clinical Performance Problem

A Case Study of a Call Bell Response Time Improvement Project

Case Study Background

After reviewing a year of HCAHPS patient satisfaction data, the QI team on the 6 East orthopedic unit noticed that the unit's scores were consistently below the hospital average on the call bell response time. In addition to the somewhat mediocre patient satisfaction scores, the nurses were also frustrated with the way that the unit staff responded to patient calls. Using the patient and staff satisfaction HCAHPS data as a starting point, the QI team selected call bell response time as an opportunity for improvement.

Improvement Step 1: Assessment

The goal of the 6 East QI project was to understand and manage system variation associated with patient's satisfaction with call bell response times. The QI team began the improvement project by asking the broad questions:

- What time of day is associated with a higher frequency of call bell use?
- What is the average time that it takes a staff member to answer a call bell?
- Are there variations in call bell response time based on the location of the patient's room in relation to the central nursing station?

The QI team designed a ***check sheet*** to collect data on the number of call bell requests each hour by patient room number. The charge nurse and unit clerk took turns recording call bell requests during a 24-h period. The QI team downloaded data from the call bell system to gain information on the average response time as well as information about unit staffing patterns and patient's admitting diagnoses.

Improvement Step 2: Analysis

To begin, the QI team tallied the call response time with a histogram using 5-min intervals. In graphing the data, a clear pattern emerged. The patient wait times fell into three groups:

- One group waited an average of 8 min.
- The second group waited an average of 12 min.
- A third group waited an average of 20 min for a member of staff to respond to the call bell request.

Upon further analysis of the data, the QI team discovered that the patients with the longest waiting times were in rooms that are the furthest from the central nursing station. The QI team constructed a ***Pareto diagram*** to understand the nature and frequency of the patients' requests. This analysis revealed that the three most frequently occurring patient requests were:

- Pain medication
- Assistance with repositioning
- Assistance with opening and positioning food on the tray table during meal time

Finally, the team constructed a ***fishbone diagram*** to identify the factors associated with the 20-min response delays. Using these data, the QI team was able to identify the likely cause of the problem and its symptoms.

Improvement Step 3: Develop a Plan for Improvement

The QI team worked with the hospital librarian to identify relevant studies to develop their improvement project plan. The QI team reviewed a number of research studies about patient requests and response rates from both the patient and nurse perspectives. The team also reviewed studies about work redesign to involve the food service team more directly into the unit's workflow. Based on a critical appraisal of the evidence, the QI team decided to try two interventions for the improvement project:

1. Hourly nurse rounding to improve responsiveness for patient's pain medication requests, and
2. Role redesign for the dietary staff to reduce patient's request for meal assistance.

The QI team agreed on the ***specific aim statements*** to guide the project:

1. In 30 days, we aim to reduce the number of call bell requests for pain medication from 15 per hour to 3 per 8-h shift.
2. In 30 days, we aim to decrease average wait time for pain medication from 12 min to 5 min.

Improvement Step 4: Test and Implement the Improvement Plan

Case Study Continues: The QI team tested the two change ideas using ***PDSA cycles*** over two successive weeks. Hourly nurse rounding was tested using three nurses on the day and evening shift with patients admitted to three randomly assigned rooms for a 3-day period. During the hourly rounds, the nurses conducted pain assessments and administered medication and other pain management interventions. The nurses recorded their interventions on a data collection sheet in each patient's bedside chart. The unit clerk collected the call bell frequency

Continued

BOX 21.7 Applying the Quality Improvement Steps to a Clinical Performance Problem

A Case Study of a Call Bell Response Time Improvement Project—cont'd

and response time from the central system for the patients in the randomly assigned rooms during the PDSA testing period. During the testing period, the improvement team reviewed the data at the end of each shift to assess changes in performance.

During the next week, the improvement team piloted the change in the dietary aid's work responsibilities to include opening the food trays at the bedside, positioning patients to eat, and filling the water pitchers at the time the meals were served. The change in the dietary aid job responsibilities required training in infection control, body mechanics, and the creating of a new sign system to alert the dietary staff about the patients' dietary restrictions. This ***change idea*** was piloted using the same number of staff members, duration, patient rooms, and unit clerk documentation responsibilities as the PDSA cycle for the hourly nurse rounds. Staff feedback about the strengths and drawbacks of the hourly rounding and expanded food preparation responsibilities for the dietary aids, including suggestions for improving the practice changes, were collected.

Finally, to evaluate the effectiveness of the change ideas, the QI team used a ***run chart*** to track performance for the unit's call bell response time. The run chart was annotated to include the days that the team implemented the PDSA cycles to refine the process used for hourly nurse rounding and the change in the dietary aid's responsibilities to set up patients' meal trays. At the end of a month of experimentation, the QI team was able to reduce the number of call bell requests for pain medication from a high of 15 per hour at the beginning of the project, to three per shift. Similarly, the average time that patients waited for their pain medication dropped from 12 to 5 min. The team was able to achieve similar reductions in the call bell requests at meal time by expanding the role of the dietary aid to include meal setup. Based on the performance data, the QI team recommended that hourly nurse rounding and meal setup by the dietary aids become the standard of practice on the unit.

To embed the new practices into the unit routines, the QI team supervised PDSA cycles until the entire unit reached the performance goal in the specific aim statement. The run chart data suggested that the call bell response process was mostly stable with some variation attributed to new staff hired for the weekend day shift who were not fully oriented to the new routines for hourly nurse rounding and meal tray setup.

professions involved in patient care, support staff, patients, and families. While all professional staff, support staff, and patients should be involved throughout the improvement process, members of the lead team are responsible for planning, coordinating, implementing, and evaluating improvement efforts. To maintain a productive lead team, it is important to set a meeting schedule and use effective meeting tools such as the following (Nelson et al., 2007):

- Meeting agenda
- Meeting roles
- Ground rules
- Brainstorming
- Multivoting

Other tools that can help with project management to keep team and activities organized and focused include action plans and Gantt charts (Nelson et al., 2007). To download templates of meeting agendas, meeting role cards, action plans, and Gantt charts, go to the Clinical Microsystems website at https://clinicalmicrosystem.org and select the Materials/Worksheets tabs. After the lead team is assembled and team processes established, the team can begin assessment of the health system. To access resources on how to best facilitate interprofessional teamwork, visit The National Center for Interprofessional Education and Practice at https://nexusipe.org.

IPE HIGHLIGHT

To keep the interprofessional QI lead team engaged and on schedule, hold team meetings at least weekly and display a timeline of QI activities such as data collection, analysis, and results of PDSA cycles, with completion progress for each activity where all team members can see it.

Improvement Process Step 1: Assessment

In the assessment phase, the first step is to complete a structured assessment to understand more about performance patterns. The improvement team typically begins with a series of broad questions that are used to guide data collection. Common methods used to collect system performance data include *check sheets* and *data sheets* to understand performance patterns and *surveys, focus groups*, and *interviews* to gather information about patient and staff perceptions of system performance. Commonly collected data elements include information about the following (Nelson et al., 2007):

- Patients: What are the average age, gender, top diagnoses, and satisfaction scores?
- Professionals: What is the level of staff satisfaction? What is their skill set?
- Processes and patterns: What are the processes for admitting and discharging patients?
- Common performance metrics: What are the rates of pressure ulcers and falls with injury?

For useful data collection templates, select the Tools tab at https://clinicalmicrosystem.org/.

HELPFUL HINT

To reduce data collection burden related to QI projects, when starting the assessment phase of the QI process, first identify what performance data already exist in your organization. For example, find out if your organization is participating in the National Database of Nursing Care Quality Indicators program, which collects quarterly data on pressure ulcers, infections, falls, staff satisfaction, and other quality indicators.

Improvement Step 2: Analysis

The next phase of the improvement process focuses on data analysis. Because QI uses a team problem-solving approach, data are displayed in graphic form so all team members can see how the system is performing and generate ideas for what to improve. Several tools exist to help display and analyze performance data.

Trending Variation in System Performance With Run and Control Charts

If quality health care means that the right care is delivered to the right people, in the right way, at the right time, for every person, during each clinical encounter, it is important to learn when criteria are not met and why (IOM, 2001). One method is to track performance over time and understand sources of variation in system performance, which can guide improvement activities to design a better-functioning health system. Minimizing performance variation is one of the main QI goals. There are two main types of system variation (Nelson et al., 2007, p. 346):

- **Common cause variation** occurs at random and is considered a characteristic of the system. For example, you might never leave your house in time for prompt arrival to class. In this case, you must work on better managing multiple random causes of tardiness, such as getting up late or taking too long to shower, dress, and eat to improve your overall punctuality record.
- **Special cause variation** arises from a special situation that disrupts the causal system beyond what can be accounted for by random variation. An example might be that you usually leave your house on time for a prompt arrival to class, but special circumstances such as road construction or a broken elevator delay your arrival to class. Once these special causes of tardiness are resolved, you will arrive to class on time.

Variations in system performance over time are commonly displayed with run charts and control charts. A **run chart** is a graphical data display that shows trends in a measure of interest; trends reveal what is occurring over time (Nelson et al., 2007). The vertical axis of the run chart depicts the value of measure of interest, and the horizontal axis depicts the value of each measure running over time. A run chart shows whether the outcome of interest is running in a targeted area of performance, and how much variation there is from point to point and over time. For example, a patient newly diagnosed as having diabetes can record her blood glucose levels over a month using a run chart. By regularly charting blood glucose levels, the patient is able to reveal when blood glucose runs higher or lower than the target level of less than 100 mg/dL for fasting plasma glucose (FPG) test. The run chart in Fig. 21.1 shows that FPG levels are consistently higher than the target, with a median FPG of 130 mg/dL; the trend of FPG readings in the first 19 days of the month is indicative of common cause variation. These random variations in FPG readings are likely caused by a confluence of several factors such as diet, exercise, and medication adherence. To correct the undesirable variation, the patient can assess which factors might be influencing the higher FPG values and then work with her primary care provider to develop necessary interventions to better control her blood glucose by better managing multiple causal factors. To determine whether interventions were successful, the patient and her provider should continue to document blood glucose levels and then compare the median FPG values before and after interventions are implemented.

In addition, special cause variation in FPG is evident on days 19 to 28, where nine consecutive FPG readings are above the median line. It turns out that on these days, the patient had run out of her glucose-lowering medication; this special circumstance caused increased FPG. Although various rules exist for accurately determining the presence of special cause variation, generally special cause variation is present if the following are true (Nelson et al., 2007, p. 349):

- Eight data points in a row are above or below the median or mean.
- Six data points in a row are going up.
- Six data points in a row are going down.

Determining common and special causes of variation is important because treatment strategies for eliminating each type of variation will vary.

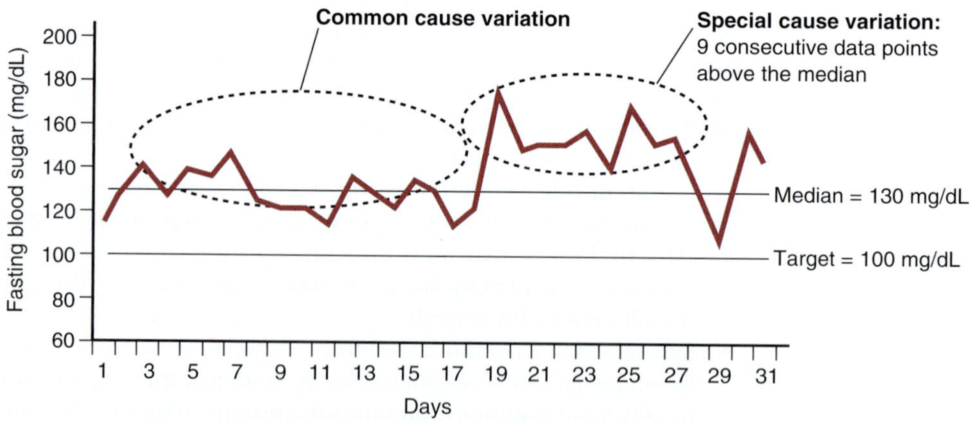

FIG 21.1 Run chart of daily fasting plasma glucose levels.

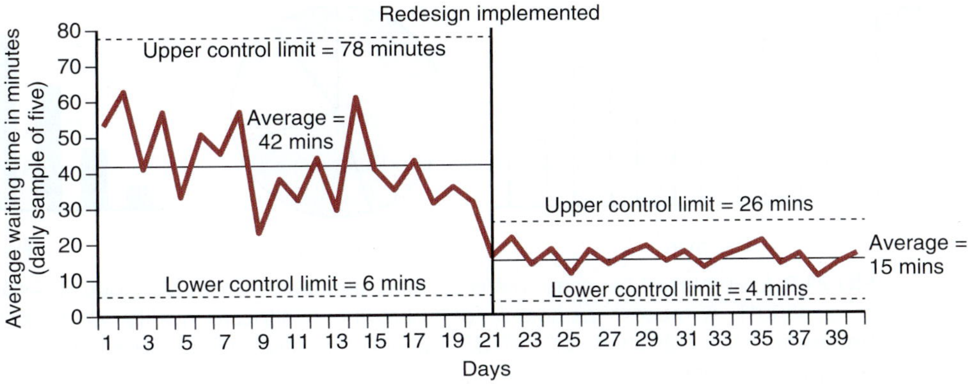

FIG 21.2 Control chart of average wait time before and after a redesign. (From Massoud R, Askov K, Reinke J, et al. [2001]. A modern paradigm for improving healthcare quality. *QA Monograph Series 1*[1]. Bethesda, MD: Published for the US Agency for International Development by the Quality Assurance Project.)

A **control chart** (Fig. 21.2) is also used to track system performance over time, but it is a more sophisticated data tool than a run chart (Nelson et al., 2007). A control chart includes information on the average performance level for the system depicted by a center line displaying the system's average performance (the mean value), and the upper and lower limits depicting one to three standard deviations from average performance level. The rules to detect special cause variation are the same for run and control charts, except that for control charts the upper and lower limits are additional tools used to detect special cause variation. Any point that falls outside the control limit is considered an outlier that merits further examination.

HELPFUL HINT

Use a run chart in step two of the QI process to analyze causes of variation in fasting plasma glucose (FPG) levels from the target level of 100 mg/dL and in step four of the QI process to evaluate if changes in diet, exercise, and medication adherence helped the patient achieve the targeted FPG.

Graphs

Graphs commonly used to understand system performance, displayed in Fig. 21.3, include **pie charts**, **bar charts**, and **histograms**. Selecting the appropriate chart depends on the type of data collected and the performance pattern the improvement team is trying to understand. A bar chart is used to display categorical-level data. A Pareto diagram is a special type of bar chart used to understand the frequency of factors that contribute to a common effect. It is used to display the Pareto Principle, sometimes referred to as the **80-20 Rule**, or the Law of the Few (Massoud et al., 2001), which states that 80% of variation in a problem originates with 20% of cases. In a Pareto diagram, the bars are displayed in descending order of frequency. A histogram is another type of bar chart used for continuous-level data to show the distribution of the data around the mean, commonly called the *bell curve* (Massoud et al., 2001).

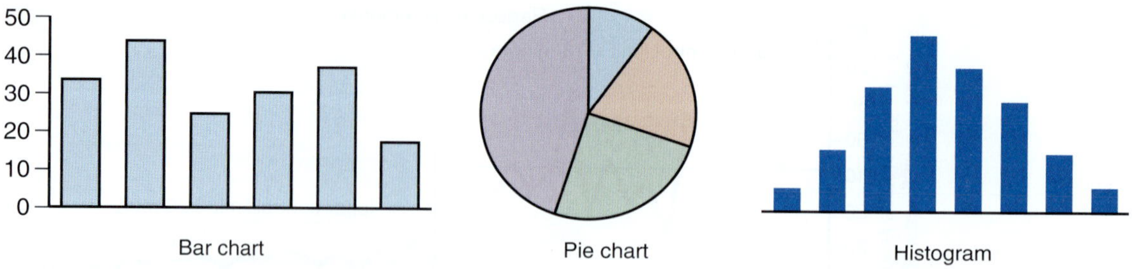

FIG 21.3 Examples of bar chart, pie chart, and histogram. (From Massoud R, Askov K, Reinke J, et al. [2001]. A modern paradigm for improving healthcare quality. *QA Monograph Series 1*[1]. Bethesda, MD: Published for the US Agency for International Development by the Quality Assurance Project.)

Cause and Effect Diagrams

More sophisticated visual data displays include **cause and effect diagrams** used to identify and treat the causes of performance problems. Two common tools in this category are a fishbone or Ishikawa diagram and a tree diagram (Massoud et al., 2001). The **fishbone diagram** facilitates brainstorming about potential causes of a problem by grouping potential causes into the categories of environment, people, materials, and process (Fig. 21.4). Fishbone diagrams can be used proactively to prevent quality defects, including errors, and retrospectively to identify factors that potentially contributed to quality defect or an error that has already occurred. An example of when a fishbone diagram is used retrospectively is during **root cause analyses** (RCAs) to identify system design failures that caused errors.

An RCA is a structured method used to understand sources of system variation that lead to errors or mistakes, including sentinel events, with the goal of learning from mistakes and mitigating hazards that arise as a characteristic of the system design (Zastrow, 2015). An RCA is conducted by a team that includes representatives from nursing, medicine, management, QI, or risk management and the individual(s) involved in the incident (sometimes including the patient or family members in the discovery process), and it emphasizes system failures while avoiding individual blame (Zastrow, 2015). An RCA seeks to answer three questions to learn from mistakes:

- What happened?
- Why did it happen?
- What can be done to prevent it from happening again?

Because the RCA is viewed as an opportunity for organizational learning and improvement, the most effective RCAs include a change in practice or work system design to lessen the chances of similar errors occurring in the future.

A **tree diagram** is particularly useful for identifying the chain of causes, with the goal of identifying the root cause of a problem. For example, consider medication errors. The improvement team could use the **Five Whys** method to establish the chain of causes leading to the medication error:

- Question 1: Why did the patient get the incorrect medicine?
  Answer 1: Because the prescription was wrong.
- Question 2: Why was the prescription wrong?
  Answer 2: Because the doctor made the wrong decision.

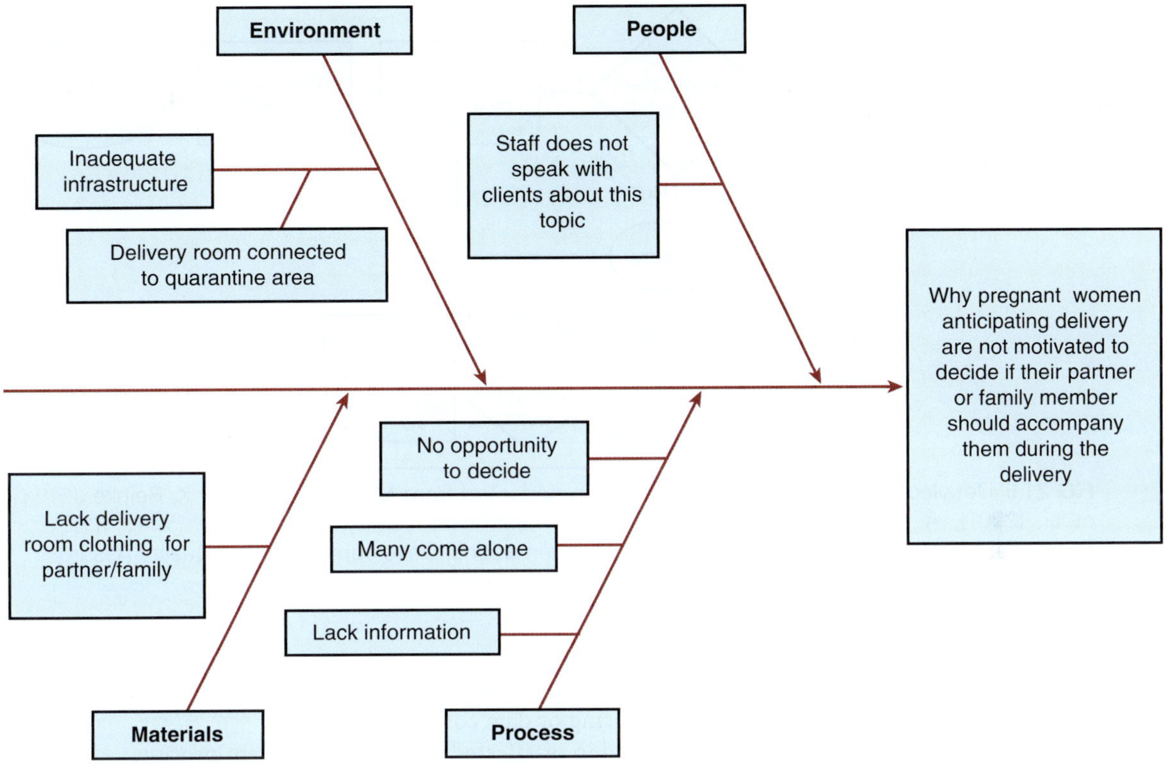

FIG 21.4 Fishbone diagram. (Adapted from Massoud R, Askov K, Reinke J, et al. [2001]. A modern paradigm for improving healthcare quality. *QA Monograph Series 1*[1]. Bethesda, MD: Published for the US Agency for International Development by the Quality Assurance Project.)

- Question 3: Why did the doctor make the wrong decision?
  Answer 3: Because he did not have complete information in the patient's chart.
- Question 4: Why wasn't the patient's chart complete?
  Answer 4: Because the doctor's assistant had not entered the latest laboratory report.
- Question 5: Why hadn't the doctor's assistant charted the latest laboratory report?
  Answer 5: Because the lab technician telephoned the results to the receptionist, who forgot to tell the assistant.

In this case, using the Five Whys technique suggests that a potential solution for avoiding wrong prescriptions in the future might be to develop a system for tracking lab reports (Massoud et al., 2001).

Flowcharting

A **flowchart** depicts how a process works, detailing the sequence of steps from the beginning to the end of a process (Massoud et al., 2001). Several types of flowcharts exist, including the most simple *(high level)*, a detailed version *(detailed)*, and one that also indicates the people involved in the steps *(deployment or matrix)*. Fig. 21.5 shows an example of a detailed flowchart. Massoud and colleagues (2001, p. 59) suggest using flowcharts to:

- Understand processes.
- Consider ways to simplify processes.

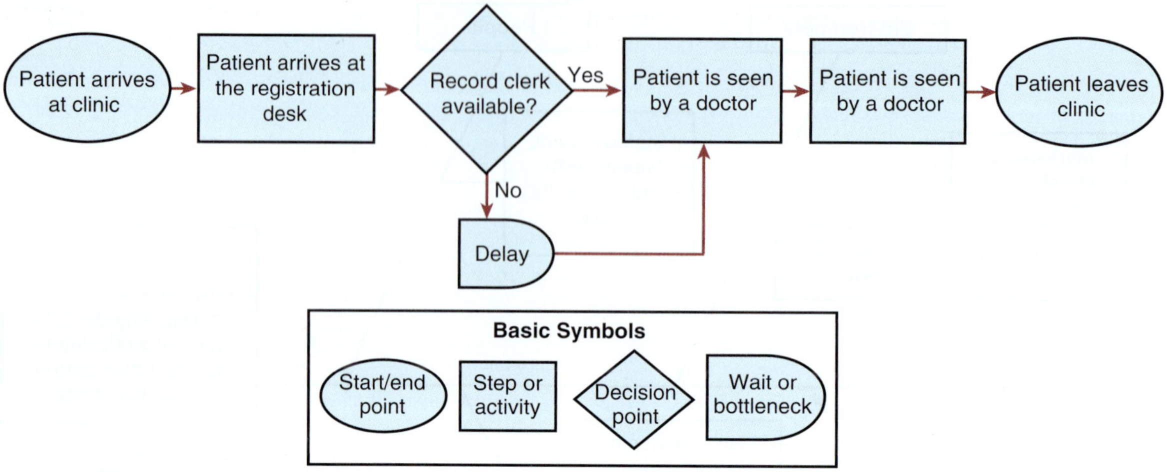

FIG 21.5 Detailed flowchart of patient registration. (Adapted from Massoud R, Askov K, Reinke J, et al. [2001]. A modern paradigm for improving healthcare quality. *QA Monograph Series 1*[1]. Bethesda, MD: Published for the US Agency for International Development by the Quality Assurance Project.)

- Recognize unnecessary steps in a process.
- Determine areas for monitoring or data collection.
- Identify who will be involved in or affected by the improvement process.
- Formulate questions for further research.

When flowcharting, it is important to identify a start and an end point of a process, then make a record of the actual, not the ideal, process. To obtain an accurate picture of the process, perform direct observation of the process steps and communicate with people who are directly part of the process to clarify all the steps.

Improvement Step 3: Develop a Plan for Improvement

By identifying potential sources of variation, the improvement team can pinpoint the problem areas in need of improvement. The next phase is to treat the performance problem. This phase involves developing and testing a plan for improvement. A simple yet powerful model for developing and testing improvements is the **Model for Improvement** (Langley et al., 2009). It begins with three questions to guide the change process and focus the improvement work (Langley et al., 2009):

1. **Aim**. What are we trying to accomplish? Set a clear aim with specific measurable targets.
2. **Measures**. How will we know that the change is an improvement? Use qualitative and quantitative measures to support real improvement work to guide change progress toward the stated goal.
3. **Changes**. What changes can we make that will result in an improvement? Develop a statement about what the team believes they can change to cause improvement.

The **change ideas** reflect the team's hypotheses about what could improve system performance. There are several ways in which change ideas can be generated. The change ideas can be identified from the root causes of the performance problems that are identified during cause and effect and process analyses using fishbone diagram, the Five Whys, and flowcharting tools in the analysis step of the improvement process. Another approach is to select common areas for change associated with the goals and philosophy of QI. Common **change topics**, also referred to as **themes for improvement**, include (Langley et al., 2009, p. 359):

- Eliminating waste
- Improving work flow
- Optimizing inventory
- Changing the work environment
- Managing time more effectively
- Managing variation
- Designing systems to avoid mistakes
- Focusing on products or services

Change ideas can also come from the evidence provided by your review of the available literature. This is where your EBP skills will be most helpful. You will need to critically appraise both research studies and QI studies of interventions that can be applied to remedy the identified problem. To help you decide whether a journal article is a research study or a QI study, see the *critical decision tree* in Fig. 21.6. Because QI studies capture the experiences of a particular organization or unit, the results of these studies are usually not generalizable. In an effort to promote knowledge transfer and learning from others' improvement experiences, the *Standards for Quality Improvement Reporting Excellence,* or the **SQUIRE Guidelines** (Ogrinc et al., 2015), were developed to promote the publication and interpretation of this type of applied research. The SQUIRE Guidelines are presented in Table 21.7; you should use them to evaluate QI studies.

Improvement Step 4: Test and Implement the Improvement Plan

The improvement changes that are identified in the planning phase are tested using the **Plan-Do-Study-Act (PDSA) Improvement Cycle**, which is the last step of the Improvement Model (Langley et al., 2009; Massoud et al., 2001) depicted in Fig. 21.7. The focus of PDSA is experimentation using small and rapid tests of change. Actions involved in each phase of the PDSA cycle are detailed in Fig. 21.7. In this step, you evaluate the success of the intervention in bringing about improvement. It is important for the team to monitor the intended and unintended changes in system performance, the patient and staff perceptions of the change, and ideally, the costs of the change. Also, in this phase of the improvement process, it is useful to track the stability and sustainability of the new work process by monitoring system performance over time. Results data should be presented in graphic data displays (explained earlier in the chapter) and compared with the baseline performance.

TAKING ON THE QUALITY IMPROVEMENT CHALLENGE AND LEADING THE WAY

Hospital leaders and other key stakeholders agree that enabling nurses to lead and participate in QI is vital for strengthening our health system's capacity to provide high-quality

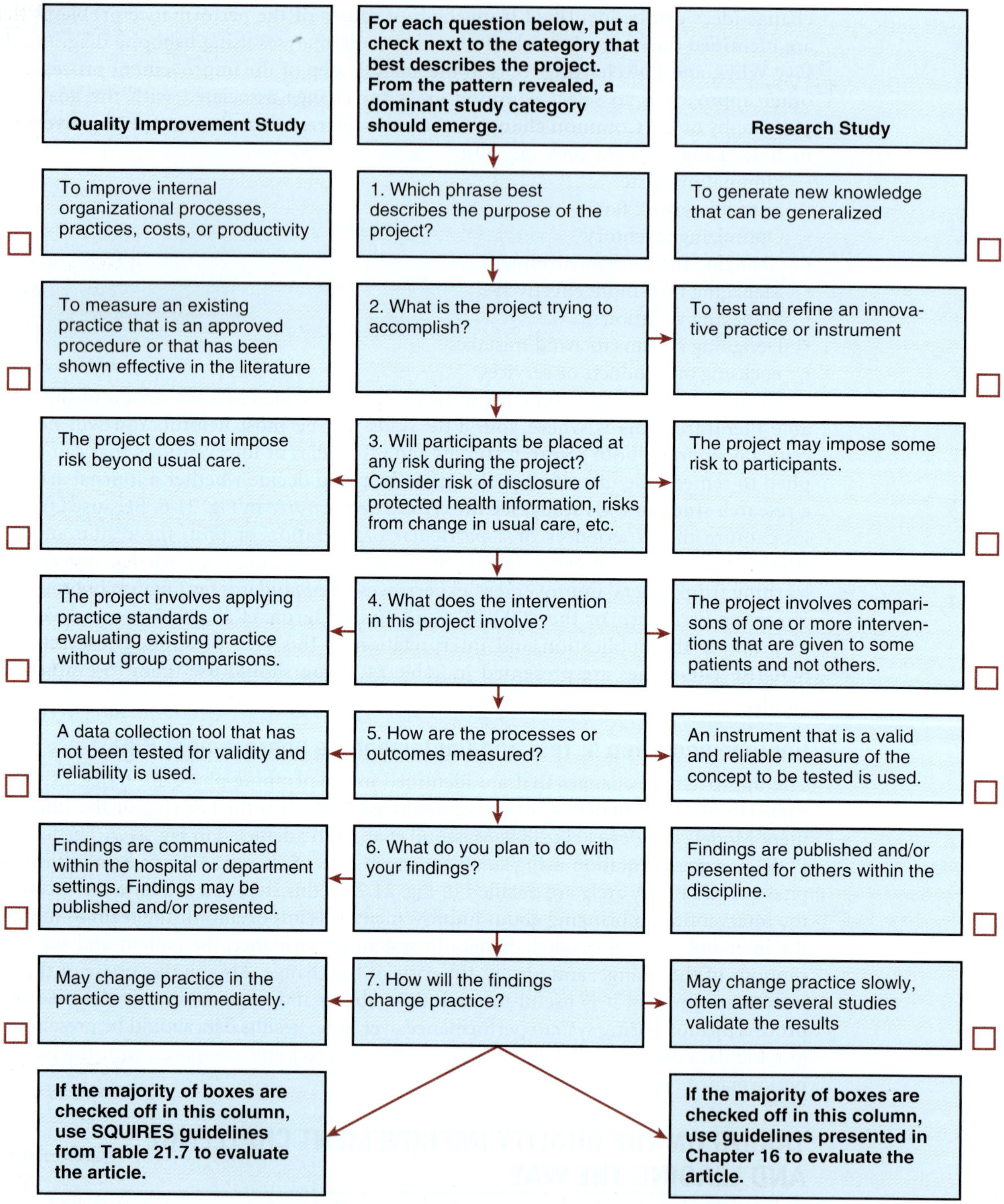

FIG 21.6 Differentiating QI from research projects. *SQUIRE,* Standards for Quality Improvement Reporting Excellence. (Adapted with permission from King, D. L. [2008]. Research and quality improvement: Different processes, different evidence. *Medsurg Nursing, 17*[3], 167.)

TABLE 21.7 Revised Squire Guidelines Standards for Quality Improvement Reporting Excellence (Squires 2.0)

Section	Description
Title and Abstract	
Title	Indicate that the manuscript concerns an initiative to improve health care (broadly defined to include the quality, safety, effectiveness, patient-centeredness, timeliness, cost, efficiency, and equity of health care).
Abstract	a. Provide adequate information to aid in searching and indexing b. Summarize all key information from various sections of the text using the abstract format of the intended publication or a structured summary such as background, local problem, methods, interventions, results, conclusions
Introduction—Why did you start?	
Problem description	Nature and significance of the local problem.
Available knowledge	Summary of what is currently known about the problem, including relevant previous studies.
Rationale	Informal or formal frameworks, models, concepts and/or theories used to explain the problem, any reasons or assumptions that were used to develop the intervention(s), and reasons why the intervention(s) was expected to work.
Specific aims	Purpose of the project and of this report.
Methods—What did you do?	
Context	Contextual elements considered important at the outset of introducing the intervention(s).
Intervention(s)	a. Description of the intervention(s) in sufficient detail that others could reproduce it b. Specifics of the team involved in the work
Study of intervention(s)	a. Approach chosen for assessing the impact of the intervention(s) b. Approach used to establish whether the observed outcomes were due to the intervention(s)
Measures	a. Measures chosen for studying processes and outcomes of the intervention(s), including rationale for choosing them, their operational definitions, and their validity and reliability b. Description of the approach to the ongoing assessment of contextual elements that contributed to the success, failure, efficiency, and cost c. Methods employed for assessing completeness and accuracy of data
Analysis	a. Qualitative and quantitative methods used to draw inferences from the data b. Methods for understanding variation within the data, including the effects of time as a variable
Ethical considerations	Ethical aspects of implementing and studying the intervention(s) and how they were addressed, including, but not limited to, formal ethics review and potential conflict(s) of interest.
Results—What did you find?	
Results	a. Initial steps of the intervention(s) and their evolution over time (e.g., timeline diagram, flowchart, or table), including modifications made to the intervention during the project b. Details of the process measures and outcomes c. Contextual elements that interacted with the intervention(s) d. Observed associations between outcomes, interventions, and relevant contextual elements e. Unintended consequences such as unexpected benefits, problems, failures, or costs associated with the intervention(s) f. Details about missing data
Discussion—What does it mean?	
Summary	a. Key findings, including relevance to the rationale and specific aims b. Particular strengths of the project
Interpretation	a. Nature of the association between the intervention(s) and the outcomes b. Comparison of results with findings from other publications c. Impact of the project on people and systems d. Reasons for any differences between observed and anticipated outcomes, including the influence of context e. Costs and strategic trade-offs, including opportunity costs

Continued

TABLE 21.7 Revised Squire Guidelines Standards for Quality Improvement Reporting Excellence (Squires 2.0)—cont'd

Limitations	a. Limits to the generalizability of the work b. Factors that might have limited internal validity such as confounding, bias, or imprecision in the design, methods, measurement, or analysis c. Efforts made to minimize and adjust for limitations
Conclusions	a. Usefulness of the work b. Sustainability c. Potential for spread to other contexts d. Implications for practice and for further study in the field e. Suggested next steps
Other Information	
Funding	Sources of funding that supported this work and role, if any, of the funding organization in the design, implementation, interpretation, and reporting.

From Ogrinc G, Davies L, Goodman D, et al. (2015). SQUIRE 2.0 (Standards for Quality Improvement Reporting Excellence): revised publication guidelines from a detailed consensus process. *BMJ Quality and Safety, 0,* 1–7. doi:10.1136/bmjqs-2015-004411.
Note: See www.squire-statement.org/ for more information on publishing QI studies.

patient care (Draper et al., 2008; IOM, 2015). Nurses are on the front lines of delivering care, and they offer unique perspectives on the root causes of dysfunctional care, as well as what interventions might work reliably and sustainably in everyday clinical practice to achieve best care. However, multiple barriers to nurses' participation in QI exist, including insufficient staffing, lack of leadership support and resources for nurses' participation in QI, and not enough educational preparation for knowledgeable and meaningful QI involvement (Draper et al., 2008). For nurses to contribute their knowledge and expertise to patient care delivery and the organization's quality enterprise, nursing leadership must engage in (Berwick, 2011, p. 326):

- Setting aims and building the will to improve
- Measurement and transparency
- Finding better systems
- Supporting PDSA activities, risk, and change
- Providing resources

Several common elements that make improvement work possible are captured in two bodies of knowledge (Berwick, 2011). One is **professional knowledge** that includes knowledge of one's discipline, subject matter, and values of the discipline. The other is **knowledge of improvement**, which includes knowledge of complex systems functioning through dynamic interplay among various technical and human elements; knowledge of how to detect and manage variation in system performance; knowledge of managing group processes through effective conflict resolution and communication; and knowledge of how to gain further knowledge by continual experimentation in local settings through rapid tests of change. Linking these two knowledge systems promotes continuous improvement in health care. This chapter provides a starting point for you to develop basic knowledge and skills for the improvement work, so you can better meet the challenges and expectations of a contemporary nursing practice.

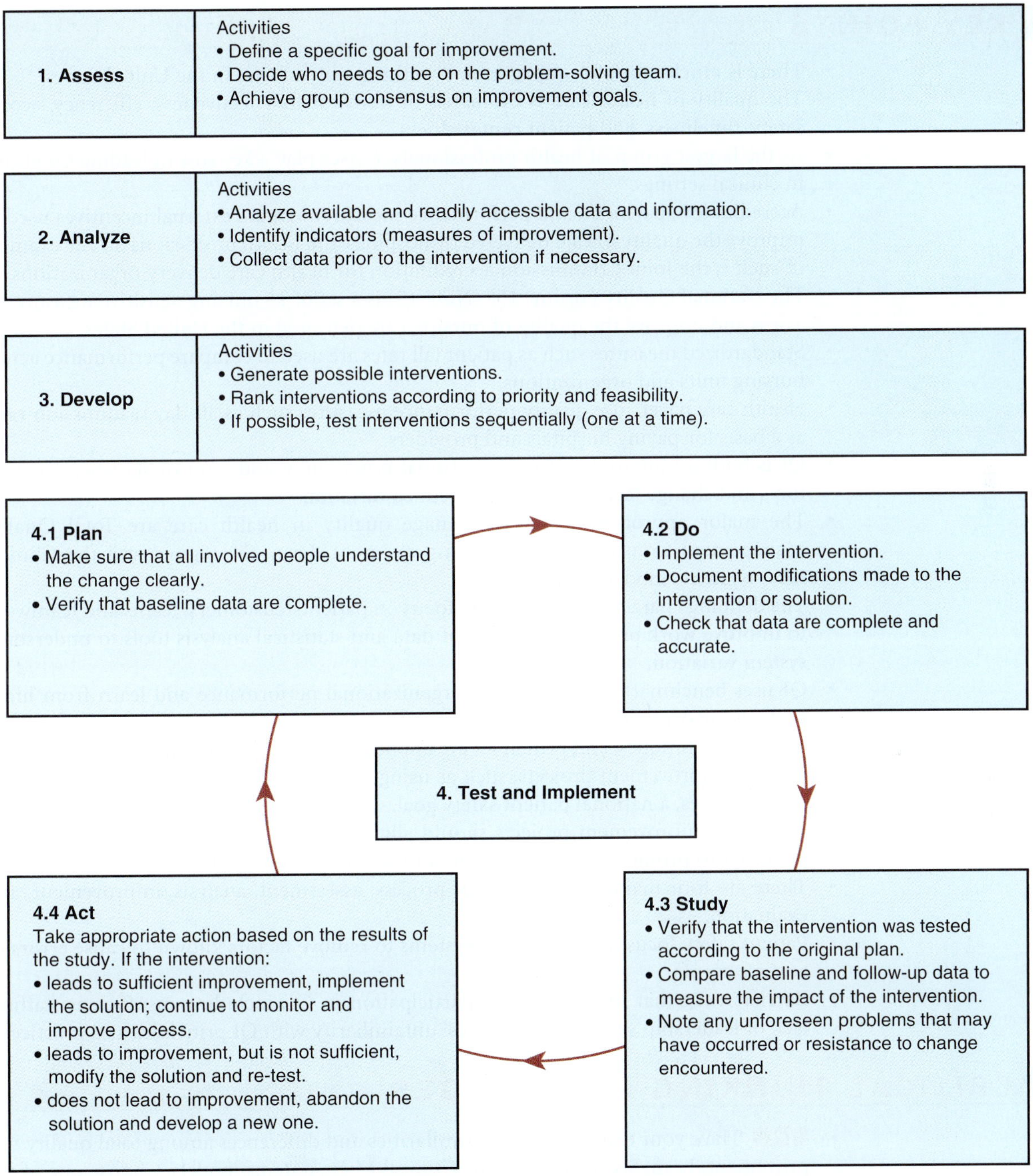

FIG 21.7 Summary of the QI process. (Adapted from Massoud R, Askov K, Reinke J, et al. [2001]. A modern paradigm for improving healthcare quality. *QA Monograph Series 1*[1]. Bethesda, MD: Published for the US Agency for International Development by the Quality Assurance Project.)

KEY POINTS

- There is much room for improvement in the quality of care in the United States.
- The quality of health care is evaluated in terms of its effectiveness, efficiency, access, safety, timeliness, and patient centeredness.
- As the largest group of health professionals, nurses play a key role in leading QI efforts in clinical settings.
- Accreditation, payment, and performance measurement are external incentives used to improve the quality of care delivered by hospitals and health professionals. One example of such is the Joint Commission accreditation for health care delivery organizations.
- The National Quality Forum "15" (NQF 15) is a set of 15 nursing-sensitive measures to assess and improve the quality of nursing care delivered in the United States.
- Standardized measures such as patient fall rates are used to compare performance across nursing units and organizations.
- Health care payers use quality performance measures such as 30-day readmission rates as a basis for paying hospitals and providers.
- QI is both a philosophy of organizational functioning and a set of statistical analysis tools and change techniques used to reduce variation.
- The major approaches used to manage quality in health care are Total Quality Management/Continuous Quality Improvement, Lean, Six Sigma, and the Clinical Microsystems model.
- The defining characteristics of QI are focus on patients/customers; teams and teamwork to improve work processes; and use of data and statistical analysis tools to understand system variation.
- QI uses benchmarking to compare organizational performance and learn from high-performing organizations.
- QI tools, techniques, and principles are applied to clinical performance problems in the form of improvement projects, such as using a presurgical checklist to prevent wrong-side surgeries, a national patient safety goal.
- Unit-level improvement projects should align with organizational-level improvement priorities to promote the sustainability of the unit-level projects.
- There are four major steps in the QI process: assessment, analysis, improvement, and evaluation.
- Patient safety focuses on designing systems to remove factors known to cause errors or adverse events.
- Barriers exist that impede nurses' participation in QI, including insufficient staffing, lack of leadership support, and nurses' unfamiliarity with QI principles and practices.

CRITICAL THINKING CHALLENGES

- IPE Have your team discuss the similarities and differences among total quality improvement, Lean, Six Sigma, and the Clinical Microsystems models. Choose one of the models for your team to use to guide your improvement project.
- Consider your unit's performance on the HCAHPS *(Hospital Consumer Assessment of Healthcare Providers and Systems)* Survey. What suggestions do you have for applying QI principles to improve your unit's score on these key performance indicators?

- Why is it important to document nurse-sensitive care outcomes using standardized performance measurement systems? How does performance measurement relate to QI activities?
- What barriers do you see for participating in unit-level quality improvement initiatives? What suggestions do you have for overcoming these barriers?
- In what ways do QI studies differ from research studies? How would you use the results of a QI study to inform a change in practice on your unit?

REFERENCES

Agency for Healthcare Research and Quality (AHRQ). (2016). *2015* National *healthcare quality and disparities report and 5th anniversary update on the National Quality Strategy*. (AHRQ Pub. No. 16-0015). Retrieved from http://www.ahrq.gov/sites/default/files/wysiwyg/research/findings/nhqrdr/nhqdr15/2015nhqdr.pdf.

Alexander, G. R. (2007). Nursing sensitivity databases: Their existence, challenges, and importance. *Medical Care Research and Review*, *64*(2), 44S–63S. doi:10.1177/558707299244.

American Organization of Nurse Executives. (2016). *Care innovation and transformation program*. Retrieved from http://www.aone.org/education/cit.shtml.

Aydin, C., Donaldson, N., Stotts, N. A., et al. (2015). Modeling hospital-acquired pressure ulcer prevalence on medical-surgical units: Nurse workload, expertise, and clinical processes of care. *Health Services Research*, *50*(2), 351–373.

Berwick, D. M. (2011). Preparing nurses for participation in and leadership of continual improvement. *Journal of Nursing Education*, *50*(6), 322–327.

Bigelow, B., & Arndt, M. (1995). Total quality management: Field of dreams? *Health Care Management Review*, *20*(4), 15–25.

Callis, N. (2016). Falls prevention: Identification of predictive fall risk factors. *Applied Nursing Research*, *29*, 53–58. doi:10.1016/j.apnr.2015.05.007.

Chassin, M. R., & Loeb, J. M. (2011). The ongoing quality improvement journey: Next stop, high reliability. *Health Affairs*, *30*(4), 559–568. doi:10.1377/hlthaff.2011.0076.

Cronenwett, L., Sherwood, G., Barnsteiner, J., et al. (2007). Quality and safety education for nurses. *Nursing Outlook*, *55*(3), 122–131. doi:10.1016/j.outlook.2007.02.006.

Davis, K., Stremikis, K., Squires, D., & Schoen, C. (2014). *Mirror, mirror on the wall: How the performance of the U.S. health care system compares internationally*. Retrieved from http://www.commonwealthfund.org/publications/fund-reports/2014/jun/mirror-mirror.

DelliFraine, J. L., Langabeer, J. R. II, & Nembhard, I. M. (2010). Assessing the evidence of Six Sigma and Lean in the health care industry. *Quality Management in Health Care*, *19*(3), 211–225. doi:10.1097/QMH.0b013e3181eb140e.

Donabedian, A. (1966). Evaluating the quality of medical care. *The Milbank Memorial Fund Quarterly*, *44*(3), 166–206.

Draper, D. A., Felland, L. E., et al. (2008). *The role of nurses in hospital quality improvement (CSHSC Report no. 3)*. Retrieved from http://www.hschange.org/CONTENT/972/.

Henry, B., Wood, S., & Nagelkerk, J. (1992). Nightingale's perspective of nursing administration. *Sogo Kango: Comprehensive Nursing Quarterly*, *27*, 16–26.

Institute of Medicine (IOM). (1999). *To err is human: Building a safer health system: executive summary*. Washington, DC: The National Academies Press. Retrieved from http://books.nap.edu/openbook.php?record_id=9728.

Institute of Medicine (IOM). (2001). *Crossing the quality chasm: A new health system for the 21st century: executive summary*. Washington, DC: The National Academies Press. Retrieved from http://books.nap.edu/catalog/10027.html.

Institute of Medicine (IOM). (2015). *Assessing progress on the IOM report The Future of Nursing.* Washington, DC: The National Academies Press.

Langley, G. J., Moen, R. D., Nolan, K. M., et al. (2009). *The improvement guide: A practical approach to enhancing organizational performance* (2nd ed.). San Francisco, CA: Jossey-Bass.

Massoud, R., Askov, K., Reinke, J., et al. (2001). A modern paradigm for improving healthcare quality. *QA Monograph Series 1*(1). Bethesda, MD: The Quality Assurance Project.

McConnell, J. K., Lindrooth, R. C., Wholey, D. R., et al. (2016). Modern management practices and hospital admissions. *Health Economics, 25*, 470–485. doi:10.1002/hec.3171.

National Quality Forum (NQF). (2004). *National voluntary consensus standard for nursing-sensitive care: an initial performance measure set.* Retrieved from http://www.qualityforum.org/Publications/2004/10/National_Voluntary_Consensus_Standards_for_Nursing-Sensitive_Care__An_Initial_Performance_Measure_Set.aspx.

Nelson, E. C., Batalden, P. B., & Godfrey, M. M. (2007). *Quality by design: A clinical microsystems approach.* San Francisco, CA: Jossey-Bass.

Nuti, S. V., Wang, Y., Masoudi, F. A., et al. (2015). Improvements in the distribution of hospital performance for the care of patients with acute myocardial infarction, heart failure, and pneumonia, 2006–2011. *Medical Care, 53*(6), 485–491.

Ogrinc, G., Davies, L., Goodman, D., et al. (2015). SQUIRE 2.0 (Standards for Quality Improvement Reporting Excellence): Revised publication guidelines from a detailed consensus process. *BMJ Quality and Safety, 0*, 1–7. doi:10.1136/bmjqs-2015-004411.

Tidwell, J., Busby, R., Lewis, B., et al. (2016). The race: Quality assurance performance improvement project aimed at achieving superior patient outcomes. *Journal of Nursing Care Quality, 31*(2), 99–104.

Tripathi, S., Arteaga, G., Rohlik, G., et al. (2015). Implementation of patient-centered bedside rounds in the pediatric intensive care unit. *Journal of Nursing Care Quality, 30*(2), 160–166.

US Department of Health and Human Services (USDHHS). (2016a). *National quality strategy overview.* Retrieved from http://www.ahrq.gov/workingforquality/nqs/overview.pdf.

US Department of Health and Human Services (USDHHS). (2016b). *Hospital Compare.* Retrieved from https://www.medicare.gov/hospitalcompare/search.html.

Zastrow, R. L. (2015). Root cause analysis in infusion nursing: Applying quality improvement tools for adverse events. *Journal of Infusion Nursing, 38*(3), 225–231. doi:10.1097/NAN.0000000000000104.

Go to Evolve at **http://evolve.elsevier.com/LoBiondo/** for review questions, critiquing exercises, and additional research articles for practice in reviewing and critiquing.

Example of a Randomized Clinical Trial (Nyamathi et al., 2015)

Nursing Case Management, Peer Coaching, and Hepatitis A and B Vaccine Completion Among Homeless Men Recently Released on Parole

Adeline Nyamathi, Benissa E. Salem, Sheldon Zhang, David Farabee, Betsy Hall, Farinaz Khalilifard, Barbara Leake

Background: Although hepatitis A virus (HAV) and hepatitis B virus (HBV) infections are vaccine-preventable diseases, few homeless parolees coming out of prisons and jails have received the hepatitis A and B vaccination series.

Objectives: The study focused on completion of the HAV and HBV vaccine series among homeless men on parole. The efficacy of three levels of peer coaching (PC) and nurse-delivered interventions was compared at 12-month follow-up: (a) intensive peer coaching and nurse case management (PC-NCM); (b) intensive PC intervention condition, with minimal nurse involvement; and (c) usual care (UC) intervention condition, which included minimal PC and nurse involvement. Furthermore, we assessed predictors of vaccine completion among this targeted sample.

Methods: A randomized control trial was conducted with 600 recently paroled men to assess the impact of the three intervention conditions (PC-NCM vs. PC vs. UC) on reducing drug use and recidivism; of these, 345 seronegative, vaccine-eligible subjects were included in this analysis of completion of the Twinrix HAV/HBV vaccine. Logistic regression was added to assess predictors of completion of the HAV/HBV vaccine series and chi-square analysis to compare completion rates across the three levels of intervention.

Results: Vaccine completion rate for the intervention conditions were 75.4% (PC-NCM), 71.8% (PC), and 71.9% (UC; $p = .78$). Predictors of vaccine noncompletion included being Asian and Pacific Islander, experiencing high levels of hostility, positive social support, reporting a history of injection drug use, being released early from California prisons, and being admitted for psychiatric illness. Predictors of vaccine series completion included reporting having six or more friends, recent cocaine use, and staying in drug treatment for at least 90 days.

Discussion: Findings allow greater understanding of factors affecting vaccination completion in order to design more effective programs among the high-risk population of men recently released from prison and on parole.

Key Words: accelerated Twinrix hepatitis A/B vaccine; ex-offenders; homelessness; parolees; prisoners; substance abuse

Nursing Research, May/June 2015, Vol 64, No 3, 177-189

With 1.6 million men and women behind bars, the United States has one of the largest numbers of incarcerated persons when compared to other nations (Pew Charitable Trusts, 2008). In California, over 130,000 are in custody and over 54,000 are on parole (California Department of Corrections and Rehabilitation, 2013b). Incarcerated populations are at significant risk for homelessness. When compared to the general population, those who were in jail were more likely to be homeless (Greenberg & Rosenheck, 2008). In one study, homeless inmates were more likely to have past criminal justice system involvement for both nonviolent and violent offenses, mental health and substance abuse problems, and lack of personal assets (Greenberg & Rosenheck, 2008).

Globally, incarcerated populations encounter a host of public healthcare issues; two such issues—hepatitis A virus (HAV) and hepatitis B virus (HBV) diseases—are vaccine preventable. In addition, viral hepatitis disproportionately impacts the homeless because of increased risky sexual behaviors and drug use (Stein, Andersen, Robertson, & Gelberg, 2012), along with substandard living conditions (Hennessey, Bangsberg, Weinbaum, & Hahn, 2009). Other risk factors include, but are not limited to, injection drug use (IDU), alcohol use, and older age, which place the population at risk for being seropositive (Stein et al., 2012).

INCARCERATED POPULATIONS ARE AT SIGNIFICANT RISK FOR HOMELESSNESS.

As a member of the hepatovirus family, HAV is primarily transmitted via the fecal-oral route (Zuckerman, 1996). The rate of acute hepatitis in the United States is 0.5 per 100,000 (Centers for Disease Control and Prevention, 2010). Although the rate among paroled populations is hard to ascertain, data suggest that HAV infection is related to unsanitary living conditions, that is, poor water sanitation (World Health Organization, 2014), for which homeless populations are at risk.

A member of the Hepadnavirus family, HBV (Immunization Action Coalition, 2013; Zuckerman, 1996) disproportionately burdens homeless (Nyamathi, Liu, et al., 2009; Nyamathi, Sinha, Greengold, Cohen, & Marfisee, 2010) and incarcerated populations (Immunization Action Coalition, 2013; Khan et al., 2005), leading to fulminant liver failure, chronic liver disease, hepatocellular carcinoma, and death (Rich et al., 2003). HBV can be transmitted through unprotected sexual activity, needle sharing, IDU (Diamond et al., 2003; Maher, Chant, Jalaludin, & Sargent, 2004), and percutaneous blood exposure. National prevalence statistics indicate that HBV affects between 13% and 47% of U.S. prison inmates (Centers for Disease Control and Prevention, 2004). Illicit drug use is a major contributor to incarceration and homelessness among ex-offenders (McNeil & Guirguis-Younger, 2012; Tsai, Kasprow, & Rosenheck, 2014), placing ex-offenders who use drugs at high risk for HBV infection.

Despite the availability of the HBV vaccine, there has been a low rate of completion for the three-dose core of the accelerated vaccine series (Centers for Disease Control and Prevention, 2012). Among incarcerated populations, HBV vaccine coverage is low; in a study among jail inmates, 19% had past HBV infection, and 12% completed the HBV vaccination series (Hennessey, Kim, et al., 2009). Although HBV vaccination is well accepted behind bars—because of a lack of funding and focus on prevention as a core in the prison system—few inmates may complete the series (Weinbaum, Sabin, & Santibanez, 2005).

In addition, prevention may not be a priority for those who are struggling with managing mental health, drug use, and dependency issues, along with the need to meet basic necessities (Nyamathi, Shoptaw, et al., 2010). Authors contend that, although the HBV vaccine is cost-effective, it is underutilized among high-risk (Rich et al., 2003) and incarcerated populations (Hunt & Saab, 2009).

For homeless men on parole, vaccination completion may be affected by level of custody; generally, the higher the level of custody, the higher the risk an inmate poses. In addition, various contract types, such as drug treatment related, and length of time in residential drug treatment (RDT)—for those with drug histories—may also affect completion of the vaccine series. For those transitioning into the community, stress, family reunification issues, and the potential for relapse and recidivism may represent real challenges (Seiter & Kadela, 2003) and may influence vaccine completion.

Until 1981, the HBV vaccine was not licensed in the U.S. (Centers for Disease Control and Prevention, 2012). Twenty years later, in 2001, a combination of the HAV and HBV vaccine, *Twinrix*, was developed by GlaxoSmithKline and approved by the Food and Drug Administration (Centers for Disease Control and Prevention, 2012). The standard dosing for this regimen is 0, 1, and 6 months. An alternative dosing schedule (core doses at 0, 7, and 21–31 days and a booster dose 12 months) was approved by the Food and Drug Administration in 2007 (Centers for Disease Control and Prevention, 2012). Thus, many individuals, particularly older individuals, may not have been vaccinated.

One strategy to improve vaccination for HAV and HBV among high-risk populations has been to utilize the accelerated Twinrix HAV/HBV vaccination, which provides the core doses at 0, 7, and 21–30 days (Nyamathi, Liu, et al., 2009). The Twinrix recombinant vaccination is administered intramuscularly (GlaxoSmithKline, 2011) by a licensed nurse. In a randomized controlled trial (RCT) comparing vaccination completion among incarcerated IDUs in Denmark—using the accelerated versus a standard vaccine schedule (0,1, and 6 months)—63% completed the three accelerated dose series compared to 20% of those who received the nonaccelerated series (Christensen et al., 2004). In another RCT conducted among 297 homeless adults with a history of incarceration, findings revealed that 50% completed the Twinrix vaccine series. Logistic regression analysis revealed that those who were more likely to complete the HBV vaccination were over 40 years of age (p = .02), partnered (p = .02), homeless for more than 1 year (p = .025), recent binge drinkers (p = .03), and had attended recent alcohol anonymous or narcotic anonymous meetings (p = .006; Nyamathi, Marlow, Branson, Marfisee, & Nandy, 2012). In another RCT focused on improving HAV/HBV vaccine completion among 256 homeless adults who were on methadone maintenance, a greater percentage of participants who completed the vaccine series also reduced their alcohol consumption by 50% as compared to those who were unsuccessful in reducing their alcohol consumption (74.4% vs. 64.1%; Nyamathi, Shoptaw, et al., 2010).

Finally, in a larger, three-group RCT with 865 homeless adults in shelters located in Los Angeles, individuals were randomly assigned to one of three groups: (a) nurse case-managed sessions plus hepatitis education, incentives, and tracking; (b) standard hepatitis education plus incentives and tracking; and (c) standard hepatitis education and incentives only. Findings reveal that those who were in the nurse case management education, incentives, and tracking program were significantly more likely to complete a standard three-series Twinrix vaccination or core of the accelerated dosing schedule (68% vs. 61% vs. 54%, respectively; p = .01) compared to those who were in the other two programs (Nyamathi, Liu, et al., 2009). Although accelerated vaccination programs have shown success in RCT studies, including those utilizing nurse case management, little is known about vaccine completion among an ex-offender population using varying intensities of nurse case management and peer coaches.

Theoretical Framework

The comprehensive health seeking and coping paradigm (Nyamathi, 1989), adapted from a coping model (Lazarus & Folkman, 1984), and the health seeking and coping paradigm (Schlotfeldt, 1981) guided this study and the variables selected (see Figure 1). The comprehensive health seeking and coping paradigm has been successfully applied by our team to improve our understanding of HIV and HBV/hepatitis C virus (HCV) protective behaviors and health outcomes among homeless adults (Nyamathi, Liu, et al., 2009)—many of whom had been incarcerated (Nyamathi et al., 2012).

In this model, a number of factors are thought to relate to the outcome variable, completion of the HAV/HBV vaccine series. These factors include sociodemographic factors, situational factors, personal factors, social factors, and health seeking and coping responses. Sociodemographic factors that might relate to completion of the vaccine series among incarcerated populations include age, education, race/ethnicity, and marital and parental status (Hennessey, Kim, et al., 2009; Salem et al., 2013). Situational factors such as being homeless (Nyamathi et al., 2012), history of criminal activities, and severity of criminal history (level of custody and contract type) may likewise influence interest in completing a vaccination series. Similarly personal factors, such as history of psychiatric and drug use problems (Hennessey, Kim, et al., 2009; Salem et al., 2013), having hostile tendencies (Nyamathi et al., 2014), or dealing with physical and mental health problems (Nyamathi et al., 2011), may interfere with health protective strategies, whereas having social factors present,

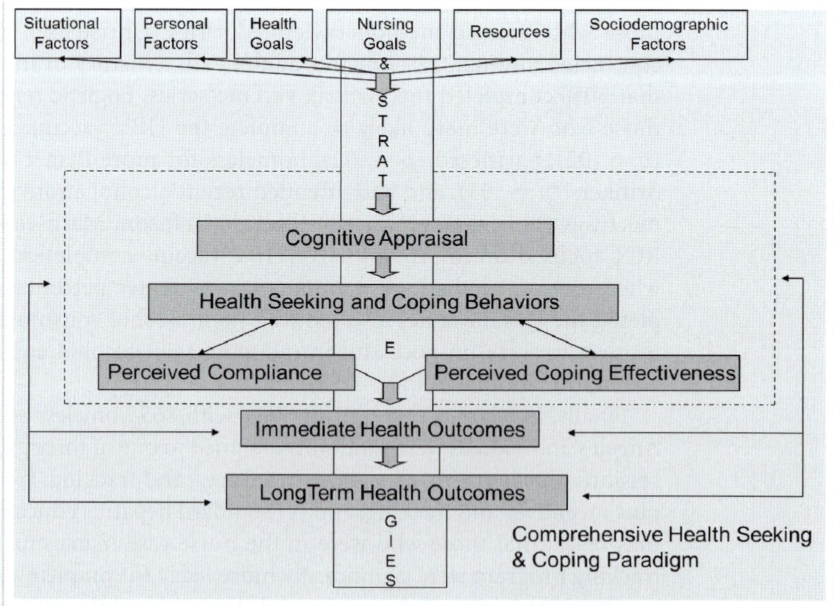

FIG 1 Comprehensive health seeking and coping paradigm.

such as social support, may facilitate health promotion. Finally, health seeking and coping strategies may also be known to impact health promotion (Nyamathi, Stein, Dixon, Longshore, & Galaif, 2003) and compliance with hepatitis vaccine completion.

Purpose

Despite knowledge of awareness of risk factors for HBV infection, intervention programs designed to enhance completion of the three-series Twinrix HAV/HBV vaccine and identification of prognostic factors for vaccine completion have not been widely studied. The purpose of this study was to first assess whether seronegative parolees previously randomized to any one of three intervention conditions were more likely to complete the vaccine series as well as to identify the predictors of HAV/HBV vaccine completion.

METHODS

Design

An RCT where 600 male parolees from prison or jail and participating in an RDT program were randomized into one of three intervention conditions aimed at assessing program efficacy on reducing drug use and recidivism at 6 and 12 months as well as vaccine completion in eligible subjects: (a) a 6-month intensive peer coaching and nurse case management (PC-NCM) intervention condition; (b) an intensive peer coaching (PC) intervention condition, with minimal nurse involvement; and (c) the usual care (UC) intervention condition, which had minimal PC and nurse involvement. Of these 600, 345 were eligible for the vaccine (seronegative) and constitute the sample for this report. Data were collected from February 2010 to January 2013. The study was approved by the University of California, Los Angeles Institutional Review Board and registered with Clinical Trials.gov (NCT01844414).

Sample and Site

There were four inclusion criteria for recruitment purposes in assessing program efficacy on reducing drug use and recidivism: (a) history of drug use prior to their latest incarceration, (b) between ages of 18 and 60, (c) residing in the participating RDT program, and (d) designated as homeless as noted on the prison or jail discharge form. A homeless individual was defined as one who does not have a fixed, regular, and adequate nighttime residence (National Health Care for the Homeless Council, 2014). Exclusion criteria included (a) monolingual speakers of languages other than English or Spanish and (b) persons judged to be cognitively impaired by the research staff. A total of 42 men were screened out because of the following reasons: age, not being on parole, had not been released from jail or prison within 6 months prior to entering the study, or had not used drugs 12 months prior to their most recent incarceration. Eligibility for receiving the HAV/HBV vaccine series was not considered an inclusion criterion regarding drug use and recidivism. Among those eligible and interested, urn randomization (Stout, Wirtz, Carbonari, & Del Boca, 1994) was used to allocate participants. The variables used in the urn randomization included age (18–29 and 30 and over), level of custody (1–2 vs. 3–4), HBV vaccine eligibility (HBV seronegative or seropositive), and level of substance use prior to prison time (low vs. moderate/high severity). For the present analysis, only vaccine-eligible subjects were included.

Amistad De Los Angeles (Amity) served as the main research site. For the last three decades, Amity, a nonprofit organization located in California, Arizona, and New Mexico, has been focused on substance abuse treatment and works with individuals and families (Amity Foundation, 2014) utilizing a therapeutic environment.

The State of California Assembly passed a criminal justice realignment legislation (Assem. Bill 109, 2011) on October 1, 2011, allowing low-level offenders (nonviolent, nonserious, and nonsex offenders) to serve their sentence in county jails instead of state prisons (California Department of Corrections and Rehabilitation, 2011). Postrealignment offenders were more likely to be convicted of a felony for drug and property crimes (California Department of Corrections and Rehabilitation, 2013a).

Power Analysis

With at least 114 men in each intervention condition, there was 80% power to detect differences of 15–20 percentage points (e.g., 50% vs. 70%, 75% vs. 90%) for vaccine completion between either of the two intervention conditions and the UC intervention condition at $p = .05$.

Vaccine Eligibility

Vaccine eligibility included being HBV seronegative and no absolute contraindications (having an allergy to yeast or neomycin, history of neurological disease [e.g., Guillian-Barre]), prior anaphylactic reaction to HAV/HBV vaccine, a fever of over 100.5°F, and reporting any moderate or severe acute illness beyond mild cold symptoms (e.g., nonproductive cough, rhinorrhea, or other upper respiratory symptoms). Of the total sample of 600 study participants, 345 men were eligible for the HAV/HBV vaccine. Figure 2 (CONSORT diagram) reflects both the larger sample and the subsample of vaccine-eligible participants.

Interventions

Building upon previous studies, we developed varying levels of peer-coached and nurse-led programs designed to improve HAV/HBV vaccine receptivity at 12-month follow-up among homeless offenders recently released to parole.

Peer Coaching-Nurse Case Management

The peer coach interacted weekly for about 45 minutes with their assigned participants in person, and for those who left the facility (interaction was by phone). Their focus was on building effective coping skills, personal assertiveness, self-management, therapeutic nonviolent communication, and self-esteem building. Attention was given to supporting avoidance of health-risk behaviors, increasing access to medical and psychiatric treatment, and improving compliance with medications, skill-building, and personal empowerment. Discussions also centered on strategies to assist in seeking support and assistance from community agencies as parolees prepare for completion of the drug treatment program. Integrated throughout, skill building in communication and negotiation and issues of empowerment were highlighted.

Peer coaches were also trained to deliver nonviolent communication, the goal of which was to increase participants' mastery of empathic communication skills via a specific process. The intervention comprised a series of interactive exercises and role-playing based on conflict in social situations, as identified by the participants. In our study, peer coaches were former parolees who successfully completed a similar RDT program; as paraprofessionals, they were positive role models with whom the parolees could identify and have successfully reintegrated into society. The peer coachers were selected based on

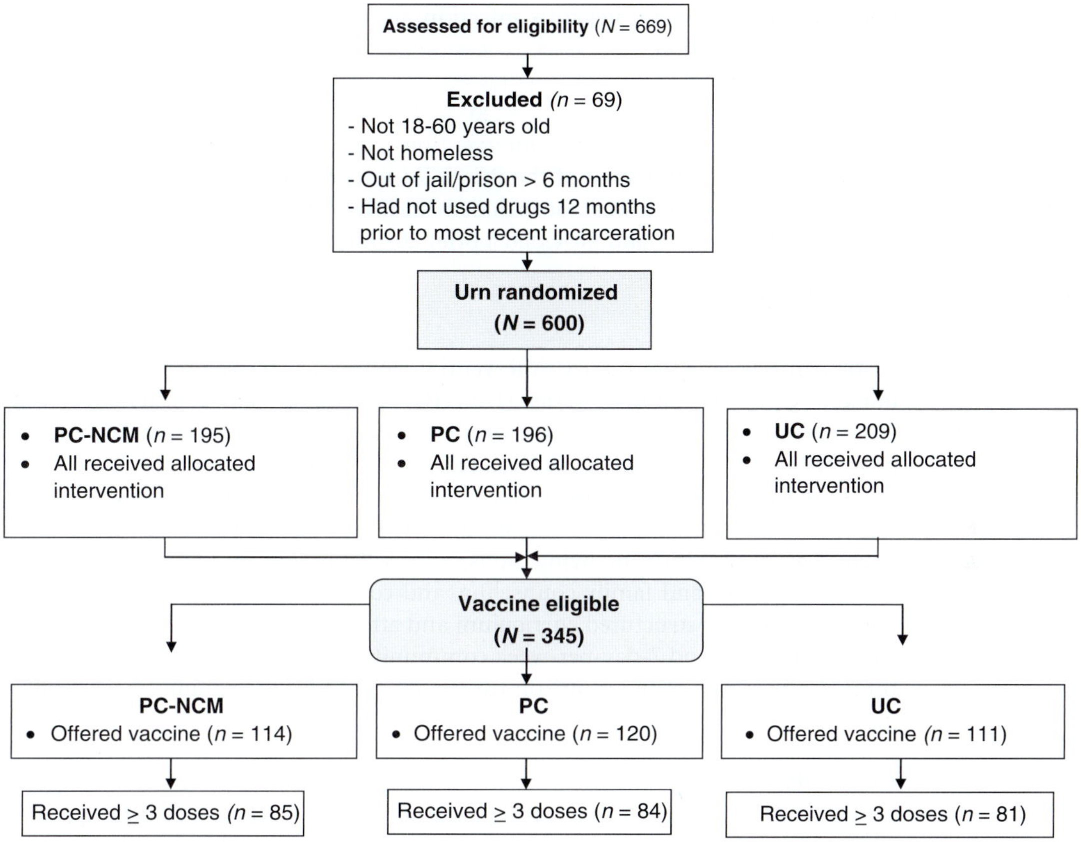

FIG 2 CONSORT diagram. PC = peer coaching; PC-NCM = peer coaching-nursing case management; UC = usual care.

having excellent social skills and found joy helping recent parolees to be successful. The assigned coach worked with up to 15 parolees at any given time. The coaches in the PC-NCM and PC intervention conditions were trained in (a) understanding the needs and challenges faced by parolees discharged to the community; (b) gaining information about the resources that are available in the community; and (c) normalizing parolee experiences, setting realistic expectations, and helping the parolee to problem solve with day-to-day events and build on strengths. The training period for coaches took about 1 month and consisted mock role-plays of coaching sessions—with many simulations of problematic and challenging participants and situations.

Case management, provided by a dedicated nurse (about 20 minutes), was delivered in a culturally competent manner weekly over eight consecutive weeks. Case management focused on health promotion, completion of drug treatment, vaccination compliance, and reduction of risky drug and sexual behaviors. Furthermore, the nurse engaged participants in role-playing exercises to help them identify potential barriers to appointment keeping and asked them to identify personal risk triggers that may hinder vaccine series completion and successful HAV, HBV, HCV, and HIV risk reduction. Nurses were trained by experts in nurse case management, hepatitis infection and transmission, and barriers that impede HAV/HBV vaccination.

Peer Coaching

Participants assigned to the PC intervention condition received weekly PC interaction similar to the PC component of the PC-NCM intervention condition. However, although nurse case management was not included, an intervention-specific nurse encouraged the HAV/HBV vaccination and provided a brief 20-minute education session on hepatitis and HIV risk reduction.

Usual Care

Participants assigned to the UC intervention condition received the encouragement by a nurse to complete the three-series HAV/HBV vaccine. In addition, they received a brief 20-minute session by a peer counselor about health promotion. They did not receive any intensive PC sessions or nurse case management sessions.

At the RDT site, all participants received recovery and rehabilitation services traditionally delivered for the parolee population, such as residential substance abuse services, assistance with independent living skills, job skills assistance, literacy, individual, group (small and large) and family counseling, and coordinated discharge planning. Residents also receive highly structured curriculum and aftercare services in this generally 6-month, 24-hour-per-day, and 7-day-per-week community. All coordination for services took place through the efforts of the in-prison treatment staff, RDT community-based staff, and the parole office.

Procedure

This RCT was conducted in a setting close to the one participating RDT program from which all participants were enrolled. Posted flyers announced the study to all incoming residents, and research staff visited the RDT frequently to respond to questions and provide information in group sessions and individually to those interested in a private location in the RDT setting. Among interested participants, an informed consent was signed that allowed the research staff to administer a brief screening questionnaire to assess eligibility criteria. Among participants who met eligibility criteria, a second informed consent allowed administration of a baseline questionnaire; a detailed locator guide allows participants to fill out contact information, addresses, and phone numbers for research staff to follow-up.

Vaccine Administration

Alter pretest counseling, the research nurses collected serum for testing HBV, HCV, and HIV (hepatitis B core antibody, hepatitis B surface antibody, hepatitis C antibody, and human immunodeficiency virus antibodies) and provided test results 1 week later. On the basis of the HBV test result, participants were educated regarding the timeline for the HAV/HBV vaccine series, provided consent regarding administration, were inoculated intramuscularly using three doses of the Standard Twinrix (hepatitis A inactivated and hepatitis B recombinant vaccines) for the accelerated dosing schedule of 0, 7, and 21–30 days. The recommended series of three intramuscular injections of 1.0 ml of Twinrix was administered in the deltoid muscle of the nondominant arm. All eligible study participants were encouraged to accept the HAV/HBV vaccine; however, this was not coercive. The nurse documented refusal for vaccination.

Vaccine Tracking

On a weekly basis, the research nurse or peer coach reviewed the vaccine dosing and tracked progress. To encourage participants to complete the vaccine series, participants were reminded regarding their next dose by the nurse or peer coach and provided appointment cards. Furthermore, they were called if not present any longer at the RDT facility as a reminder. A detailed locator guide, completed by the participant and interviewer, supported follow-up to be successful. Information included contact information to be used by the research staff for vaccine scheduling as well as administration of structured questionnaires at 6- and12-month follow-up.

Measures

Vaccine Completion

Receipt of three core doses on the accelerated schedule was considered completion. This was assessed by the vaccine tracking system.

Sociodemographics

Sociodemographic information was collected by a structured questionnaire assessing age, education, race/ethnicity, marital status, and parental status.

Situational Factors

Situational factors included being homeless, history of criminal activity, and severity of criminal history such as level of custody and contract type. Contract type was measured by asking participants whether they were in-custody drug treatment program, residential multiservice center, or parolee substance abuse program. Time in RDT was assessed by the total time participants resided at the RDT study site after discharge from jail/prison to RDT placement. RDT site was dichotomized at the median of 90 days for analysis.

Personal Factors

Personal factors included drug, alcohol, and tobacco use. A modified version of the Texas Christian University Drug History form (Simpson & Chatham, 1995) was used to measure use 6 months preceding the latest incarceration. Information regarding the frequency of use of alcohol, tobacco, and seven other drugs was collected, allowing us to review the use of these drugs and selected combinations of these drugs in terms of use by injection and orally, as well as to extract information about lifetime drug and alcohol use. Anglin et al. (1996) have verified the reliability and validity of this format. History of hospitalization for psychiatric and substance use problems and past treatment for alcohol or drug problems (number of times in formal treatment for alcohol and for drugs) was also obtained.

General health was assessed by a single item, which asked participants to rate their overall health on a 5-point scale (Stewart, Hays, & Ware, 1988). Responses included poor, fair, good, very good, and excellent—with a higher score indicating better perceived health. General health was dichotomized at fair/poor versus good/very good/excellent.

Hostility was measured by the five-item hostility subscale of the Brief Symptom Inventory (Derogatis & Melisaratos, 1983), in which participants rated the extent to which they have been bothered (0 = *not at all* to 4 = *extremely*) by selected issues. Cronbach's alpha for the hostility scale in this sample was .81. The cut-point for hostility was the upper quartile of 2. Depressive symptoms were assessed by the 10-item, short form of the Center for Epidemiological Studies Depression Scale (Radloff, 1977), which was previously used to assess depressive symptoms in homeless populations (Nyamathi, Christiani, Nahid, Gregerson, & Leake, 2006; Nyamathi et al., 2008). The 10-item, self-report Center for Epidemiological Studies Depression questionnaire measures the frequency of 10 depressive symptoms in the past week on a 4-point response scale, from 0 = *rarely* or *none of the time (less than 1 day)* to 3 = *all of the time (5–7days)*. Scale scores range from 0 to 30, with higher scores indicating greater severity of depressive symptoms. Reliability in this sample was .80.

Social Factors

Social factors included ever having been removed from their parents as children and having spent time in juvenile hall. In addition, social support was measured by the Medical Outcomes Study Social Support Survey (Sherbourne & Stewart, 1991). This 18-item scale includes four subscales: emotional support (eight items, reliability in this sample = .95), tangible support (three items, reliability = .88), positive support (three items, reliability = .89), and affective support (three items, reliability = .90). Items had 5-point, Likert-type response options ranging from 1 = *none of the time* to 5 = *all of the time*. Responses were summed for subscale formation with higher scores indicating more support. Respondents were also asked how many close friends they had outside of prison, which was dichotomized at the upper quartile of 6 for analysis.

Health seeking and coping were captured by history of drug use and treatment style, as well as coping. The Carver Brief Cope instrument (Carver, 1997) was used to measure six dimensions. Coping was assessed with two items for each; planning, instrumental support, religious, disengagement, denial, and self-blame. Item responses ranged from 1 = *I do not do this at all* to 4 = *I do this a lot*. Coping subscales were dichotomized at their medians for analysis.

Data Analysis

Sample characteristics were described with frequencies and percentages or means, and standard deviations and continuous variables were evaluated for normality. Because of highly skewed distributions that were not resolved by transformations, some variables had to be categorized for analysis. Associations of sample characteristics with intervention condition and vaccine noncompletion were assessed with chi-square tests or analysis of variance and two-sample tests. Because IDU may have confounded the relationship between intervention condition and vaccine noncompletion, we examined the impact of intervention condition on vaccine noncompletion controlling for IDU using multiple logistic regression analysis. The model contained IDU and dummy variables for each intervention condition; the only significant predictor of noncompletion was IDU (p values for the PC-NCM and PC intervention conditions were .70 and .79, respectively).

In examining other potential predictors of vaccine noncompletion, we emphasized noncompletion because individuals who did not complete the vaccine series are the ones who need to be targeted for future interventions. Variables that were related to vaccine noncompletion at the .10 level in unadjusted analyses were used as predictors in multiple logistic regression modeling of noncompliance. Although the overall significance level for race/ethnicity did not meet this inclusion criterion, it was included in the modeling because subgroupings (African American, "'other' race/ethnicity") did so. Predictors that were not significant at the .10 level were removed one by one in descending order of significance. The final model was checked for multicollinearity, and the Hosmer-Lemeshow test was used to assess model goodness of fit.

RESULTS

In terms of sociodemographic characteristics, the 345 participants who were eligible for the HAV/HBV vaccine reported a mean age of 42.0 (*SD* = 9 5) and were predominantly African American (51%) or Latino (31%), as shown in Table 1. The small subsample of men from "other" ethnicities comprised mostly Asian Americans and Pacific Islanders.

TABLE 1 Demographic, Social, Situational, Coping, and Personal Characteristics by Intervention Condition

		All (*N* = 345)		PC-NCM (*N* = 114)		PC (*N* = 120)		UC (*N* = 111)		
Type	**Characteristic**	***M***	***(SD)***	***M***	***(SD)***	***M***	***(SD)***	***M***	***(SD)***	***P***
Demographic	Age	42.0	(9.5)	41.3	(10.1)	42.3	(9.4)	42.6	(8.9)	.57
		n	**(%)**	***n***	**(%)**	***n***	**(%)**	***n***	**(%)**	
	Race/ethnicity									.30
	African American	175	(50.7)	51	(44.7)	70	(59.8)	54	(47.4)	
	Latino	107	(31.0)	40	(35.1)	29	(24.8)	38	(33.3)	
	Asian/Pacific Islander	16	(4.6)	6	(5.3)	3	(2.6)	7	(6.1)	
	White	47	(13.6)	17	(14.9)	15	(12.8)	15	(13.2)	
	Marital status (never)	204	(59.1)	66	(57.9)	71	(60.7)	67	(59.3)	.91
Social	Partners (≥2 = yes)	199	(57.7)	64	(56.1)	76	(65.0)	59	(51.8)	.12
	Removed from parents (yes)	189	(54.8)	64	(56.1)	69	(59.0)	56	(49.1)	.30
	Childhood sexual abuse (yes)	56	(16.2)	14	(12.3)	22	(18.8)	20	(17.5)	.36
	Childhood physical abuse (yes)	120	(34.8)	38	(33.3)	44	(37.6)	38	(33.3)	.73
	Friends (≥6 = yes)[a]	101	(29.3)	33	(29.0)	41	(35.0)	27	(23.7)	.17
	Instrumental coping (high)[b]	112	(32.5)	42	(36.8)	40	(34.2)	30	(26.3)	.21
	Religious coping (high)[b]	138	(40.0)	45	(39.5)	55	(47.0)	38	(33.3)	.10
	Juvenile hall (any time)	192	(55.7)	67	(58.8)	69	(59.0)	56	(49.2)	.23
Situational	Discharged from jail	193	(55.9)	59	(52.2)	64	(54.7)	70	(61.4)	.35
	Discharged from prison	151	(43.8)	54	(47.8)	53	(45.3)	44	(38.6)	
	Contract									.49
	ICDTP	105	(30.4)	32	(28.1)	31	(26.5)	42	(36.8)	
	RMSC	203	(58.8)	71	(62.3)	72	(61.5)	60	(52.6)	
	SAP	35	(10.1)	11	(9.7)	12	(10.3)	12	(10.5)	
	Pre/postrealignment (yes)	158	(45.8)	52	(45.6)	55	(47.0)	51	(44.7)	.94
	RDT time (days)									.67
	1–49	86	(24.9)	30	(26.3)	34	(29.1)	22	(19.3)	
	50–89	93	(27.0)	27	(23.7)	31	(26.5)	35	(30.7)	
	90–178	67	(19.4)	23	(20.2)	20	(17.1)	24	(21.1)	
	≥179	99	(28.7)	34	(29.8)	32	(27.4)	33	(29.0)	
Coping	Alcohol treatment (any)	103	(29.9)	31	(27.2)	38	(32.5)	34	(29.8)	.68
	Drug treatment (any)	290	(84.1)	94	(82.5)	101	(86.3)	95	(83.3)	.70
	Crack use (recent)[c]	153	(44.4)	44	(38.6)	54	(46.2)	55	(48.3)	.30
	Cocaine use (recent)[c]	94	(27.3)	26	(22.8)	35	(29.9)	33	(29.0)	.42
	Binge drinking (recent)[c]	132	(38.3)	43	(37.7)	48	(41.0)	41	(36.0)	.72

Continued

TABLE 1 Demographic, Social, Situational, Coping, and Personal Characteristics by Intervention Condition—cont'd

		All (*N* = 345)		PC-NCM (*N* = 114)		PC (*N* = 120)		UC (*N* = 111)		
Type	**Characteristic**	*n*	(%)	*n*	(%)	*n*	(%)	*n*	(%)	*P*
Personal	Health (fair/poor)	99	(28.7)	34	(29.8)	23	(20.0)	42	(37.2)	.01
	Hostility (high)[a]	67	(19.4)	28	(24.6)	21	(18.0)	18	(15.8)	.22
	Injection drug use (ever)	112	(32.5)	33	(29.0)	33	(28.2)	46	(40.4)	.09
	Methamphetamine use (ever)	171	(49.6)	61	(54.0)	53	(45.7)	57	(50.4)	.45
	Psychiatric hospitalization (ever)	63	(18.3)	18	(15.8)	27	(23.1)	18	(15.8)	.25
	HIV (positive)	7	(2.0)	0	(0)	4	(3.9)	3	(3.2)	.15
	HCV (yes)	97	(28.1)	32	(8.1)	30	(25.6)	35	(30.7)	.69
		M	*(SD)*	*M*	*(SD)*	*M*	*(SD)*	*M*	*(SD)*	
	CES-D (total)	20.8	(14.2)	9.0	(6.6)	8.7	(5.4)	9.2	(6.5)	.85
	Positive social support	24.2	(14.3)	10.5	(9.6)	10.5	(3.6)	9.7	(3.6)	.12

Note. *N* = 345. CES-D = Center for Epidemiological Studies-Depression; HCV = hepatitis C virus; HIV = human immuno-deficiency virus; ICDTP = in-custody drug treatment program; PC = peer coaching; PC-NCM = peer coachingnursing case management; RDT = residential drug treatment; RMSC = residential multiservice service center; SAP = substance abuse program; UC = usual care. [a]Upper quartile. [b]Score above median. [c]Within 6 months prior to most recent incarceration.

The mean education was 11.6 (*SD* = 1.4). Over half of the participants had never been married (59%). The distribution of participant characteristics was similar across the three intervention conditions.

Vaccine Completion Rates by Intervention Condition

In total, there were 345 individuals who were eligible for the Twinrix recombinant vaccine (PC-NCM: $n = 114$; PC: $n = 117$; and UC: $n = 114$). The vaccine completion rate for three or more doses was 73% among all three intervention conditions. Using chi-square tests (Group x Vaccine completion), findings revealed no differences in vaccine completion across groups ($p = .780$): PC-NCM, $n = 86$ (75.4%); PC, $n = 84$ (71.8%); and UC, $n = 82$ (71.9%).

Associations With Vaccine Noncompletion

A number of social, personal, coping, and situational factors were found to be related to vaccine noncompletion (Table 2). In particular, having six or more friends and high instrumental coping were related to vaccine completion, whereas having been taken away from parents or spending time in juvenile hall were related to noncompletion. A history of alcohol treatment was associated with vaccine completion while having been hospitalized for mental health problems was related to noncompletion. In terms of drug use, cocaine use within 6 months prior to the last incarceration was associated with vaccine completion, whereas the opposite was true for IDU ever. Being HCV positive was also associated with not completing the vaccine series. No association was found between vaccine noncompletion and childhood physical abuse, whereas a very weak association was found with childhood sexual abuse.

Finally, those who were released following prison realignment and those tested positive for HCV at baseline were both related to vaccine noncompletion. Those who spent 90 days or more in RDT facilities following release were more likely to complete the vaccine series.

TABLE 2 Associations Between Hepatitis A Virus/Hepatitis B Virus Vaccine Completion Status and Selected Variables

Type	Characteristic	NONCOMPLETERS (n = 93)		COMPLETERS (n = 252)		
		M	(SD)	M	(SD)	P
Demographic	Age	40.8	(9.9)	42.5	(9.3)	.13
	Education	11.4	(1.4)	11.7	(1.4)	.09
		n	(%)	n	(%)	
	Race/Ethnicity					.16
	African American	39	(41.9)	136	(54.0)	
	Latino	33	(35.5)	74	(29.4)	
	White	14	(15.1)	33	(13.1)	
	Asian/Pacific Islander	7	(7.5)	9	(3.6)	
Intervention	Peer coach-nurse case management	28	(30.1)	86	(34.1)	.78
	Peer coach	33	(35.5)	84	(33.3)	
	Usual care	32	(34.4)	82	(32.5)	
Social	Partners (≥2 or <2)	46	(49.5)	153	(60.7)	.06
	Removed from parents (yes or no)	59	(63.4)	130	(51.6)	.05
	Juvenile hall (any time or never)	60	(64.5)	132	(52.4)	.04
	Friends (≥6 or <6)	18	(19.4)	83	(32.9)	.01
	Instrumental coping (high or low)	19	(20.4)	88	(34.9)	.01
	Religious coping (high or low)	27	(29.0)	101	(40.1)	.06
Situational	Discharged from jail	59	(63.4)	133	(53.2)	.09
	Discharged from prison Contract type	34	(22.5)	117	(77.5)	.38
	ICDTP	30	(32.3)	76	(30.4)	
	RMSC	57	(61.3)	145	(58.0)	
	SAP	6	(6.5)	29	(11.6)	
	Post realignment[a]	60	(64.5)	97	(38.8)	.001
	RDT time ≥ 90[b]	10	(10.8)	155	(62.0)	.001
	HCV (positive)	34	(36.6)	63	(25.2)	.03
	HIV (positive)[c]	1	(1.2)	6	(2.8)	.68[d]
Coping	Alcohol treatment (any or none)	19	(20.4)	84	(33.3)	.02
	Drug treatment (any or none)	80	(86.0)	210	(83.3)	.55
	Crack use (recent or not)	34	(36.6)	119	(47.2)	.08
	Cocaine use (recent or not)	15	(16.1)	79	(31.4)	.005
	Binge drinking (recent or not)	41	(44.1)	91	(36.1)	.18
Personal	Hostility (high)	27	(29.0)	51	(20.2)	.08
	Injection drug use (ever or never)	39	(41.9)	73	(29.0)	.02
	Methamphetamine use (ever or never)	51	(54.8)	120	(48.2)	.27
	Psychiatric hospitalization (yes)	25	(26.9)	38	(15.1)	.01
		M	(SD)	M	(SD)	
	CES-D (total)	9.87	(6.4)	8.62	(6.1)	.09
	Positive social support	10.82	(3.3)	10.01	(3.6)	.06

Note. CES-D = Center for Epidemiological Studies-Depression; HCV= hepatitis C virus; HIV = human immunodeficiency virus; ICDTP = in-custody drug treatment program; RDT = residential drug treatment; RMSC = residential multiservice center; SAP = substance abuse program. [a]October 1, 2011. [b]Time in RDT program (days). [c]Based on 298 men. [d]Fishers exact test.

TABLE 3 Logistic Regression Model for Noncompletion of Hepatitis A Virus/Hepatitis B Virus Vaccine Series

Type	Predictor	Adjusted *OR*	95% CI	*P*
Intervention[a]	PC-NCM	0.59	[0.27, 1.28]	.18
	PC	0.83	[0.39, 1.76]	.63
Demographics	Race[b]			
	African American	1.80	[0.68, 4.78]	.24
	Latino	2.33	[0.87, 6.21]	.09
	Asian/Pacific Islander	5.86	[1.23, 27.92]	.03
Social	Friends (≥6 = yes)	0.46	[0.22, 0.95]	.04
Situational	Postrealignment (yes)	2.21	[1.19, 4.09]	.01
	RDT stay (at least 90 days)	0.06	[0.03, 0.13]	.001
Coping	Alcohol treatment (any)	0.50	[0.24, 1.03]	.06
	Cocaine use (any)	0.34	[0.16, 0.73]	.006
Personal	Hostility (high)	2.24	[1.06, 4.73]	.04
	Injection drug use (ever)	2.19	[1.07, 4.47]	.03
	Psychiatric hospitalization (any)	2.58	[1.22, 5.46]	.01
	Positive social support (yes)	1.10	[1.00, 1.21]	.04

Note. $N = 345$. CI = confidence interval; *OR* = odds ratio; PC = peer coaching; PC-NCM = peer coaching-nursing case management; RDT = residential drug treatment. [a]Reference class is usual care. [b]Reference class is White.

On the other hand, incarceration location (prison vs. jail) and contract type had no relationship with vaccine completion, as shown in Table 2.

Table 3 presents the findings of logistic regression analysis. Asian/Pacific Islander ethnicity (compared to White), higher levels of hostility, higher levels of positive social support, and history of IDU were related to vaccine noncompletion. Moreover, having been admitted for a psychiatric illness was related to noncompletion of the HAV/HBV vaccine. Alternatively, reporting six or more friends was a protective factor. Recent cocaine use was also found to be related to vaccine completion. Being part of postrealignment was related to vaccine noncompletion, whereas having been in RDT for at least 90 days was a strong predictor of completion. Although there were no multicollinearity problems and the zero-order correlation between having six or more friends and positive social support was low (.23), we performed sensitivity analyses alternatively dropping one and then the other variable from the regression model. The direction of the effect of the social support variable that remained in the model did not change, but the significance was no longer below the $p < .05$ level.

DISCUSSION

Although homeless men on parole from California jails and prisons are at high risk for hepatitis A and B infection (Weinbaum et al., 2005), few studies have focused on improving HAV/HBV vaccination completion for this population. This article presents findings of varying levels of PC and nurse-delivered intervention that encouraged all participants—regardless of intervention condition assignment—to complete the three-series HAV/HBV accelerated Twinrix vaccine among those eligible. Although no treatment differences were found in terms of vaccine completion rates—because of the bundled nature of the programs—it is not possible to say whether the PC or nurse-delivered intervention resulted in the overall successful

73% completion rate of the three-series vaccine. Clearly, an intensive nurse case management approach did not necessarily result in a greater vaccine completion rate for the PC-NCM intervention condition. Furthermore, regardless of level of interaction by peer coaches or nurses, encouragement of vaccine completion was helpful across all intervention conditions (PC-NCM vs. PC vs. UC). However, we must acknowledge that more than one quarter (27%) did not complete the vaccine series, despite being informed of their risk for HBV infection.

The fact that Asian American/Pacific Islander (AA/PI) ethnicity was found to be related to noncompletion of the HAV/HBV vaccine is novel. Minimal work has been done understanding vaccination compliance among various races and ethnicities within homeless populations. AA/PIs are a large umbrella group composed of many subgroups; thus, it is somewhat challenging to decipher why AA/PIs had a higher level of noncompletion. However, in one study focused on ethnic-specific influences and barriers among AA/PI children, speaking limited English at home, length of time in the U.S., and not discussing HBV vaccination with a healthcare provider were found to be barriers to vaccination (Pulido, Alvarado, Berger, Nelson, & Todoroff, 2001). Despite these findings, the authors contended that greater understanding of nuances between groups is necessary to understand barriers (Pulido et al., 2001).

Interestingly, this was not the case for African Americans or Hispanics. In one study, understanding psychosocial predictors of HAV/HBV vaccination among young African American men in the south (n = 143), data reveal that increased vaccination was related to decreased barrier perception, increased perceived medical severity, and perceived barriers of HBV infection (Rhodes & Diclemente, 2003).

High levels of hostility and having a history of psychiatric hospitalization were likewise related to noncompletion of the HAV/HBV vaccine series. Adequate assessment of psychiatric comorbidity may be necessary to improve HAV/HBV vaccine completion by helping individuals to contend with hostility. Furthermore, adequate mental health referral may enable homeless ex-offenders to improve vaccine receipt. Future intervention work should focus on reducing hostility by providing additional group sessions that may aid in managing the hostility and, ultimately, increasing vaccine receptivity. Furthermore, anger management has been shown to likewise result in improved outcomes such as sustained reduction in feeling of anger and physical aggression (Wilson et al., 2013) and improved behavioral and cognitive coping mechanisms (Tang, 2001).

A history of IDU was also related to vaccine noncompliance. For those struggling with drug and alcohol addiction, prevention of infection may not be a high priority as meeting the challenges of overcoming addiction becomes paramount. Despite these findings, recent cocaine use was found to be related to vaccine completion. It may be that cocaine was not used heavily or that it served as a proxy for unmeasured variables associated with vaccine completion. Daily crack users were less likely to initiate the HBV vaccine series (Ompad et al., 2004). In this study, however, men who refused the vaccine were counted as not having completed it.

Increased social support in terms of self-report of having six or more friends was a protective factor for noncompletion, whereas the positive social support subscale predicted noncompletion. Another study found that partner support was predictive of vaccine completion (Nyamathi et al., 2012); therefore, social support does appear to play a role in vaccine compliance. When either six or more friends or positive social support was dropped from the model, the effect of the remaining measure was reduced. Thus, more information related to the individuals providing social support and the nature of their support is needed to understand how social support influences HAV/HBV vaccine completion.

However, it seems likely that vaccine completion would be enhanced by interventions aimed at improving positive social support networks. There was also a trend for those who had any alcohol treatment to be more likely to complete the vaccine series, perhaps because of increased access to health education and care. However, drug treatment was unrelated.

Length of time at the RDT site was positively associated with vaccine completion. In fact, in our sample, homeless men on parole who spent at least 3 months in RDT programs were far more likely to complete the vaccination series. Other studies have found that those who complete RDT are less likely to relapse and use drugs; in addition, they may be less likely to recidivate (Condelli & Hubbard, 1994; Conner, Hampton, Hunter, & Urada, 2011). Preventive care, such as vaccination, may be further improved by RDT sites with access to healthcare practitioners such as public health nurses.

Policies enacted in the California state prison system, in particular, realignment (or reducing state prison population by transferring inmates to county jails), may affect vaccination completion. Realignment has shifted responsibility for the custody, treatment, and supervision of individuals convicted of nonviolent, nonserious, nonsex crimes from the state to counties (California Realignment, 2013). Our study sample included individual's pre- and postrealignment, and our findings show that, following realignment, vaccination completion dropped markedly. As this is a relatively new policy enacted in California, it is challenging to ascertain the possible causes; however, contract types may have been altered for some individuals at the RDT site, whereas others may have been shifted from RDT to community supervision. Thus, the long-term impact of realignment will need to be assessed in the near future. Findings in this study point to the need for greater understanding of the ramifications of major criminal justice policies and their effect on preventive care.

This study provides preliminary evidence of the need to incorporate public health nurses along with peer coaches at RDT sites to improve health promotion, education, and prevention and, in particular, HAV/HBV vaccination. In fact, RDT facilities are in a prime position to address the healthcare needs of homeless ex-offenders who are exiting prison and jail. Partnering with nurses may improve HAV/HBV vaccination rates but may also promote health in general. In particular, it would be important for nurses to understand predictors of vaccine completion in this targeted population and to promote greater attention and focus in the screening process to those individuals less likely to complete.

Equally important, future studies need to incorporate more therapeutic resources and medical resources for a population that emerges from penitentiaries having experienced abuse, victimization, and a history of drug use and dependency issues. This study points to the need for a greater awareness of the needs of IDUs and of the efficacy of tailored programs focused on these issues. Likewise, we propose that more effort be spent on understanding the thought process of IDU users regarding their beliefs of HAV/HBV prevention.

Limitations

Homeless men on parole constitute a population with unique health concerns and life issues affected by the laws and penal practices in their areas. The degree to which findings from Los Angeles County generalize to other jurisdictions is unknown. Furthermore, self-report is liable to distortion and impression management. To enhance the vaccination efforts of ex-offenders, more research is needed to better understand how homeless men on parole perceive their health, report their health behaviors, and access healthcare.

Conclusions

Vaccine completion rates were similar to those reported by others and did not differ according to level of intervention delivered. Asian/Pacific Islander ethnicity, having been admitted for a psychiatric illness, having higher levels of hostility, having higher levels of positive social support, having a history of IDU, and being part of post realignment were independently associated with noncompletion, whereas recent cocaine use, having six or more friends, and RDT stay of at least 90 days were predictive of completion. Findings advocate for special attention to screening and enhanced intervention focused among these high-risk individuals.

Accepted for publication January 13, 2015.

The authors acknowledge this study was funded by the National Institute on Drug Abuse (1R01DA27213–01). This protocol was registered at ClinicalTrials.gov (NCT 01844414).

The authors have no conflicts of interest to report.

Corresponding author: Adeline Nyamathi, ANP, PhD, FAAN, School of Nursing, University of California, Los Angeles, Room 2–250, Factor Building, Los Angeles, CA 90095–1702 (e-mail: anyamath@sonnet.ucla.edu).

REFERENCES

Amity Foundation. (2014). *Amity experience and expertise.* Retrieved from http://www.amityfdn.org/About%20Amity/index.php.

Anglin, M. D., Longshore, D., Turner, S., et al. (1996). *Studies of the functioning and effectiveness of Treatment Alternatives to Street Crime (TASC) programs.* Los Angeles, CA: UCLA Drug Abuse Research Center. Retrieved from https://www.ncjrs.gov/App/Publications/abstract.aspx?ID=l69780.

Assem. Bill 109. (2011). Chapter 15, 2011 Cal. Stat. Retrieved from http:// www.leginfo.ca.gov/pub/11-12/bill/asm/ab_0101-0150/ab_109_bill_ 20110404_chaptered.html.

California Department of Corrections and Rehabilitation. (2011). *Public safety realignment.* Retrieved from http://www.cdcr.ca.gov/About_CDCR/docs/Realignment-Fact-Sheet.pdf.

California Department of Corrections and Rehabilitation. (2013a). *Realignment report: A one-year examination of offenders released from state prison in the first six months of public safety realignment.* Sacramento, CA: CDCR, Office of Research. Retrieved from http://www.cdcr.ca.gov/realignment/docs/Realignment%206%20Month%20Report%20Final_5%2016%2013%20v1.pdf.

California Department of Corrections and Rehabilitation. (2013b). *Spring 2013: Adult population projections fiscal years 2012/13-2017/18.* Sacramento, CA: CDCR, Office of Research. Retrieved from http://www.cdcr.ca.gov/Reports_Research/Offender_Information_Services_-Branch/Projections/S13 Pub.pdf.

California Realignment. (2013). *About California Realignment.org.* Sacramento, CA: Californians for Safety and Justice. Retrieved from http://www.safeandjust.org/CalRealignment/About-Realignment.

Carver, C. S. (1997). You want to measure coping but your protocol's too long: Consider the brief COPE. *International Journal of Behavioral Medicine, 4*, 92–100. doi:10.1207/s15327558ijbm0401_6.

Centers for Disease Control and Prevention. (2004). *Transmission of hepatitis B virus in correctional facilities—Georgia January 1999-June 2002.* Atlanta, GA: Morbidity and Mortality Weekly Report. Retrieved from http://www.cdc.gov/mmwr/preview/ mmwrhtml/mm5330a2.htm.

Centers for Disease Control and Prevention. (2010). *Table 2.1 reported cases of acute hepatitis A by state—United States, 2006–2010.* Atlanta, GA: U.S. Department of Health and Human Services. Retrieved from http://www.cdc.gov/hepatitis/Statistics/2010Surveillance/Table2.1.htm.

Centers for Disease Control and Prevention. (2012). *Hepatitis B epidemiology and prevention of vaccine-preventable diseases. The pink book: Course textbook—12th edition*. Retrieved from http://www.cdc.gov/vaccines/pubs/pinkbook/hepb.html.

Christensen, P. B., Fisker, N., Krarup, H. B., et al. (2004). Hepatitis B vaccination in prison with a 3-week schedule is more efficient than the standard 6-month schedule. *Vaccine, 22*, 3897–3901. doi:10.10l6/j.vaccine .2004.04.011.

Condelli, W. S., & Hubbard, R. L. (1994). Relationship between time spent in treatment and client outcomes from therapeutic communities. *Journal of Substance Abuse Treatment, 11*, 25–33. doi:10 .1016/0740–5472(94)90061–2.

Conner, B.T., Hampton, A. S., Hunter, J., & Urada, D. (2011). Treating opioid use under California's Proposition 36: Differential outcomes by treatment modality. *Journal of Psychoactive Drugs, 43*, 77–83. doi:10.1080/02791072.2011.602281.

Derogatis, L. R., & Melisaratos, N. (1983). The brief symptom inventory: An introductory report. *Psychological Medicine, 13*, 595–605. doi:10.1017/S0033291700048017.

Diamond, C., Thiede, H., Perdue, T., et al. (2003). Viral hepatitis among young men who have sex with men: Prevalence of infection, risk behaviors, and vaccination. *Sexually Transmitted Diseases, 30*, 425–432.

GlaxoSmithKline. (2011). Highlights of prescribing information. Retrieved from https://www.gsksource.com/gskprm/htdocs/documents/ TWINRIX.PDF.

Greenberg, G. A., & Rosenheck, R. A. (2008). Jail incarceration, homelessness, and mental health: A national study. *Psychiatric Services, 59*, 170–177. doi:10.1176/appi.ps.59.2.170.

Hennessey, K. A., Bangsberg, D. R., Weinbaum, C., & Hahn, J. A. (2009). Hepatitis A seroprevalence and risk factors among homeless adults in San Francisco: Should homelessness be included in the risk-based strategy for vaccination? *Public Health Reports, 124*, 813–817.

Hennessey, K. A., Kim, A. A., Griffin, V., et al. (2009). Prevalence of infection with hepatitis B and C viruses and co-infection with HIV in three jails: A case for viral hepatitis prevention in jails in the United States. *Journal of Urban Health, 86*, 93–105. doi:10.1007/s11524-008-9305-8.

Hunt, D. R., & Saab, S. (2009). Viral hepatitis in incarcerated adults: A medical and public health concern. *American Journal of Gastroenterology, 104*, 1024–1031. doi:10.1038/ajg.2008.143.

Immunization Action Coalition. (2013). *Vaccine-preventable diseases Hepatitis B*. Saint Paul, MN: Immunization Action Coalition. Retrieved from http://www.vaccineinformation.org/hepatitis-b.

Khan, A. J., Simard, E. P., Bower, W. A., et al. (2005). Ongoing transmission of hepatitis B virus infection among inmates at a state correctional facility. *American Journal of Public Health, 95*, 1793–1799. doi:10.2105/ ajph.2004.047753.

Lazarus, R. S., & Folkman, S. (1984). *Stress, appraisal, and coping*. New York, NY: Springer.

Maher, L., Chant, K., Jalaludin, B., & Sargent, P. (2004). Risk behaviors and antibody hepatitis B and C prevalence among injecting drug users in south-western Sydney, Australia. *Journal of Gastroenterology Hepatology, 19*, 1114–1120. doi:10.1111/j.1440–1746.2004.03438x.

McNeil, R., & Guirguis-Younger, M. (2012). Illicit drug use as a challenge to the delivery of end-of-life care services to homeless persons: Perceptions of health and social services professionals. *Palliative Medicine, 26*, 350–359. doi:10.1177/0269216311402713.

National Health Care for the Homeless Council. (2014). *What is the official definition of homelessness?* Nashville, TN: National Health Care for the Homeless Council. Retrieved from http://www.nhchc.org/faq/official-definition-homelessness/.

Center, N. V. I. (2014). *Vaccine laws*. Retrieved from http://www.nvic.org/vaccine-laws.aspx#.

Nyamathi, A. (1989). Comprehensive health seeking and coping paradigm. *Journal of Advanced Nursing, 14*, 281–290. doi:10.1111/ j. 1365-2648.1989tb03415.x.

Nyamathi, A., Christiani, A., Nahid, P., et al. (2006). A randomized controlled trial of two treatment programs for homeless adults with latent tuberculosis infection. *International Journal of Tuberculosis and Lung Disease, 10*, 775–782.

Nyamathi, A., Leake, B., Albarran, C., et al. (2011). Correlates of depressive symptoms among homeless men on parole. *Issues in Mental Health Nursing, 32*, 501–511. doi:10.3109/01612840.2011.569111.

Nyamathi, A., Liu, Y., Marfisee, M., et al. (2009). Effects of a nurse-managed program on hepatitis A and B vaccine completion among homeless adults. *Nursing Research, 58*, 13–22. doi:10.1097/NNR.0b013e3181902b93.

Nyamathi, A., Marlow, E., Branson, C., et al. (2012). Hepatitis A/B vaccine completion among homeless adults with a history of incarceration. *Journal of Forensic Nursing, 8*, 13–22. doi:10.1111/j.1939-3938.2011.01123.x.

Nyamathi, A., Nahid, P., Berg, J., et al. (2008). Efficacy of nurse case-managed intervention for latent tuberculosis among homeless subsamples. *Nursing Research, 57*, 33–39. doi:10.1097/01.NNR.0000280660.26879.38.

Nyamathi, A., Salem, B. E. S., Farabee, D., et al. (2014). Predictors of high level of hostility among homeless men on parole. *Journal of Offender Rehabilitation, 53*, 95–115. doi:10.1080/10509674.2013.868388.

Nyamathi, A., Shoptaw, S., Cohen, A., et al. (2010). Effect of motivational interviewing on reduction of alcohol use. *Drug & Alcohol Dependence, 107*, 23–30. doi:10.1016/j.drugalcdep.2009.08.021.

Nyamathi, A., Sinha, K., Greengold, B., et al. (2010). Predictors of HAV/HBV vaccination completion among methadone maintenance clients. *Research in Nursing & Health, 33*, 120–132. doi:10.1002/nur.20371.

Nyamathi, A. M., Stein, J. A., Dixon, E., et al. (2003). Predicting positive attitudes about quitting drug and alcohol use among homeless women. *Psychology of Addictive Behaviors, 17*, 32–41. doi:10.1037/0893-164X.17.1.32.

Ompad, D. C., Galea, S., Wu, Y., et al. (2004). Acceptance and completion of hepatitis B vaccination among drug users in New York City. In *Communicable Disease and Public Health, 7*, 294–300. Retrieved from http://deepblue.lib.umich.edu/bitstream/handle/2027.42/40386/Ompad_Acceptance%20and%20Completion%20of%20Hepatitis%20B%20Vaccination_2004.pdf?sequence=1&isAllowed=y.

Pew Charitable Trusts. (2008). *One in 100: Behind bars in America in 2008*. Washington, D.C.: Pew Center for the States. Retrieved from http://www.pewstates.org/research/reports/one-in-100–85899374411.

Pulido, M. J., Alvarado, E. A., Berger, W., et al. (2001). Vaccinating Asian Pacific Islander children against hepatitis B: Ethnic-specific influences and barriers. *Asian American and Pacific Islander Journal of Health, 9*, 211–220.

Radloff, L. S. (1977). The CES-D scale: A self-report depression scale for research in the general population. *Applied Psychological Measurement, 1*, 385–401. doi:10.1177/014662167700100306.

Rhodes, S. D., & Diclemente, R. J. (2003). Psychosocial predictors of hepatitis B vaccination among young African-American gay men in the deep south. *Sexually Transmitted Diseases, 30*, 449–454.

Rich, J. D., Ching, C. G., Lally, M. A., et al. (2003). A review of the case for hepatitis B vaccination of high-risk adults. *American Journal of Medicine, 114*, 316–318. doi:10.10l6/S0002-9343(02)01560-7.

Salem, B. E., Nyamathi, A., Keenan, C., et al. (2013). Correlates of risky alcohol and methamphetamine use among currently homeless male parolees. *Journal of Addictive Diseases, 32*, 365–376. doi:10.1080/10550887.2013 .849973.

Schlotfeldt, R. (1981). Nursing in the future. *Nursing Outlook, 29*, 295–301.

Seiter, R. P., & Kadela, K. R. (2003). Prisoner reentry: What works, what does not, and what is promising. *Crime & Delinquency, 49*, 360–388. doi:10.1177/0011128703049003002.

Sherbourne, C. D., & Stewart, A. L. (1991). The MOS social support survey. *Social Science & Medicine, 32*, 705–714. doi:10.1016/ 0277-9536(91)90150-B.

Simpson, D., & Chatham, L. (1995). *TCU/DATARforms manual.Ft.* Worth, TX: Institute of Behavioral Research, Texas Christian University.

Stein, J. A., Andersen, R. M., Robertson, M., & Gelberg, L. (2012). Impact of hepatitis B and C infection on health services utilization in homeless adults: A test of the Gelberg-Andersen behavioral model for vulnerable populations. *Health Psychology, 31*, 20–30. doi:10 .1037/a0023643.

Stewart, A. L., Hays, R. D., & Ware, J. E. Jr. (1988). The MOS short-form general health survey. Reliability and validity in a patient population. *Medical Care, 26*, 724–735.

Stout, R. L., Wirtz, P. W., Carbonari, J. P., & Del Boca, F. K. (1994). Ensuring balanced distribution of prognostic factors in treatment outcome research. *Journal of Studies on Alcohol and Drugs, 12*, 70.

Tang, M. (2001). Clinical outcome and client satisfaction of an anger management group program. *Canadian Journal of Occupational Therapy, 68*, 228–236. doi:10.1177/000841740106800406.

Tsai, J., Kasprow, W. J., & Rosenheck, R. A. (2014). Alcohol and drug use disorders among homeless veterans: Prevalence and association with supported housing outcomes. *Addictive Behaviors, 39*, 455–460. doi:10.1016/j.addbeh.2013.02.002.

Weinbaum, C. M., Sabin, K. M., & Santibanez, S. S. (2005). Hepatitis B, hepatitis C, and HIV in correctional populations: A review of epidemiology and prevention. *AIDS, 19*, S41–S46.

Wilson, C., Gandolfi, S., Dudley, A., et al. (2013). Evaluation of anger management groups in a high-security hospital. *Criminal Behavior and Mental Health, 23*, 356–371. doi:10.1002/ cbm.1873.

World Health Organization. (2014). *Hepatitis A: Key facts.* Geneva, Switzerland: WHO Press. Retrieved from http://www.who.int/mediacentre/factsheets/fs328/en/.

Zuckerman, A. J. (1996). Chapter 70: Hepatitis viruses. In S. Baron (Ed.), *Medical microbiology* (4th ed.). Galveston, TX: University of Texas Medical Branch.

Example of a Longitudinal/ Cohort Study (Hawthorne et al., 2016)

Parent Spirituality, Grief, and Mental Health at 1 and 3 Months After Their Infant's/Child's Death in an Intensive Care Unit

Dawn M. Hawthorne PhD, RN[a,], JoAnne M. Youngblut PhD, RN, FAAN[b], Dorothy Brooten PhD, RN, FAAN[c]*

Problem: The death of an infant/child is one of the most devastating experiences for parents and immediately throws them into crisis. Research on the use of spiritual/religious coping strategies is limited, especially with Black and Hispanic parents after a neonatal (NICU) or pediatric intensive care unit (PICU) death.

Purpose: The purpose of this longitudinal study was to test the relationships between spiritual/religious coping strategies and grief, mental health (depression and post-traumatic stress disorder) and personal growth for mothers and fathers at 1 (T1) and 3 (T2) months after the infant's/child's death in the NICU/PICU, with and without control for race/ethnicity and religion.

Results: Bereaved parents' greater use of spiritual activities was associated with lower symptoms of grief, mental health (depression and post-traumatic stress), but not post-traumatic stress in fathers. Use of religious activities was significantly related to greater personal growth for mothers, but not fathers.

Conclusion: Spiritual strategies and activities helped parents cope with their grief and helped bereaved mothers maintain their mental health and experience personal growth.

IN 2008 IN the United States, 28,033 infants (0–1 year old) and 22,844 children and adolescents under the age of 18 died (Matthews, Minino, Osterman, Strobino, & Guyer, 2011). Most died in an intensive care unit (Fontana, Farrell, Gauvin, Lacroix, & Janvier, 2013). The death of an infant/child is unimaginable and one of the most devastating events that parents can experience. The resulting stress disrupts their mental and physical health (Youngblut, Brooten, Cantwell, del Moral, & Totapally, 2013). While parents' symptoms of depression and

[a]Christine E. Lynn College of Nursing, Florida Atlantic University, Boca Raton, FL

[b]Dr. Herbert & Nicole Wertheim Professor in Prevention and Family Health, Nicole Wertheim College of Nursing & Health Sciences, Florida International University, Miami, FL

[c]Nicole Wertheim College of Nursing & Health Sciences, Florida International University, Miami, FL

PTSD diminished over the first 13 months post-death, about one-third continued to have symptoms indicative of clinical depression and/or PTSD. The number of chronic health conditions parents reported at 13 months post-death was more than double that before the ICU death (Youngblut et al., 2013). Physical and emotional symptoms occur during the early phase of grieving and continue for years afterwards (Werthmann, Smits, & Li, 2010).

Some parents turn to spirituality and religion to cope with their loss. Although often used interchangeably, spirituality involves caring for the human spirit; achieving a state of wholeness; connecting with oneself, others, nature and God/life forces; and an attempt to understand the meaning and purpose of life (O'Brien, 2014) even in the most difficult circumstances. In contrast, religion is an organized system of faith with a set of rules that individuals may use in guiding their lives (Koenig, 2009). Religion may be an explicit expression of spirituality. Therefore an individual may be spiritual without espousing a specific religion or very religious without having a well-developed sense of spirituality (Subone & Baider, 2010).

Research about bereaved parents' use of spiritual coping strategies and its effects on their psychological adjustment after their child's NICU/PICU death is limited. Most studies in this area have focused on religious coping neglecting the potential effect of non-religious spiritual coping strategies in helping bereaved parents (primarily White) cope with their grief. There is minimal research on whether bereaved parents use religious and/or spiritual coping strategies in early grief and on the differences between mothers' and fathers' coping strategies. Additionally, most studies on spirituality as a coping strategy in the grieving process have examined spirituality at one time point with very little research on the use of spirituality over time. The purpose of this longitudinal study with a sample of Hispanic, Black non-Hispanic, and White non-Hispanic bereaved parents was to test the relationships between spiritual/religious coping strategies and grief, mental health, (depression and post-traumatic stress disorder) and personal growth for mothers and fathers at 1 (T1) and 3 (T2) months after the infant's/child's death in the NICU/PICU, with and without control for race/ethnicity and religion.

Use of Spirituality/Religion as a Coping Strategy

The few studies on the use of spiritual/religious coping strategies by bereaved parents whose infants/children died in the NICU/PICU have described using rituals, sacred text, and prayer; putting their trust in God; having access to their clergy/pastor; connecting with others and remaining connected to the deceased child as spiritual strategies that help to alleviate the parents' pain, provide inner strength and comfort, and give meaning and purpose to their child's death (Ganzevoort & Falkenburg, 2012; Meert, Thurston, & Briller, 2005).

Bereaved parents may find solace (Klass, 1999) in using spiritual and/or religious coping strategies. Parents who believe in a heaven or an afterlife find comfort in believing that their deceased child is in a better place and close to God and that when they die they will be reunited with their child (Armentrout, 2009; Ganzevoort & Falkenburg, 2012; Klass, 1999). Similar beliefs were identified by Lichtenhal, Currier, Neimeyer, and Keese (2010) who found that bereaved parents' reliance on spiritual or religious beliefs proved helpful in coping with their grief. In that study, 28 (18%) of 156 bereaved parents believed that their child's death was God's will and 25 parents (16%) believed that their child was safe in heaven. Bereaved parents also can find healing or bring meaning to their own lives through spirituality, independent of religion, with meditation, inspirational writings, poetry, nature walks, listening to or creating music, painting or sculpting, and therapeutic touch, among others (Klass, 1999; Meert et al., 2005).

Research has found that some bereaved parents expressed anger with God for their infant's/child's death. Some felt that God was punishing them; others questioned or abandoned their belief in a perfect omniscient and omnipotent God, instead choosing to believe in a higher power that can make mistakes (Armentrout, 2009; Bakker & Paris, 2013). Meert et al. (2005) found that 30 to 60% of bereaved parents expressed anger and blame at themselves and God for their infant's/child's death.

An infant's/child's admission, stay and subsequent death in the NICU/PICU is overwhelming and painful for parents. Many are faced with the difficult decision of limiting treatment or withdrawing life support from their very sick infant/child (Buchi et al., 2007). Researchers have found that bereaved parents described their grief as feelings of emptiness, sadness, deep suffering, emotional devastation and being nonfunctional following the death of their infant/child in the ICU (Armentrout, 2009; Meert, Briller, Myers-Shim, Thurston, & Karbel, 2009).

Parent Mental Health and Personal Growth

Research on the effects of an infant's/child's death on parents' mental health and personal growth has found symptoms of PTSD, depression, and anxiety; lower quality of life; and minimal involvement in social activities up to 6 years after the loss (Werthmann et al., 2010). However few studies have examined parent mental health and personal growth following an infant's/child's death in the NICU/PICU. In bereaved parents 13 months after the death of their infant/child in the NICU/PICU, Youngblut et al. (2013) found that 30% of parents had scores indicative of depression and 35% of PTSD.

Personal growth is described by bereaved parents as a positive change in themselves, their family and social life (Armentrout, 2009; Buchi et al., 2007). These changes included beginning to find meaning and purpose in their lives, moving forward with their lives and becoming emotionally stronger (Armentrout, 2009; Buchi et al., 2007). They describe their values and priorities as being redefined, often finding material things less important and a greater appreciation for family relationships (Armentrout, 2009). Parents often became involved in community activities that transformed their lives and honored the memory of the deceased infant/child; some joined organizations whose goals were to help others (Armentrout, 2009).

In summary, parents have difficulty dealing with their infant's or child's death, even when studied years after the death. Youngblut et al. (2013) found that bereaved parents had symptoms of depression, panic attacks, anxiety, chest pain, hypertension, and headaches after the child's death. Religion and spirituality have been used interchangeably in research, so it is unclear whether religious and spiritual activities are equally effective or have differing effects. Most of the research on bereaved parents has been after a child's death due to cancer or trauma in primarily White families (Youngblut & Brooten, 2012). The study reported here is part of a racially/ethnically diverse sample of parents in a larger longitudinal study of parent health and family functioning through the first 13 months after an infant's or child's death in a NICU or PICU.

Conceptual Framework

Hogan, Morse, and Tason (1996) defines grief as "a process of coping, learning and adapting" (p. 44) irrespective of the relationship of the bereaved person to the deceased with six phases. The first phase is "Getting the news" that a loved one has a terminal diagnosis, or "Finding out" their loved one has died. The bereaved person responds to the news with shock, especially if the death was sudden. "Facing reality" is the second phase where the bereaved person experiences intense feelings of grief. In the third phase, "Becoming engulfed in the suffering," the bereaved person longs for the deceased and often experiences feelings of sadness, loneliness, guilt, and reliving the past. As the bereaved person gradually "Emerges from the suffering" in the fourth phase, they begin to experience some good days and by the fifth phase, "Getting on with their lives," hope and happiness gradually begin to return. In the final phase "Experiencing personal growth," the bereaved person develops a new perspective on life. They often reorganize and re-prioritize aspects of their lives, making it more purposeful and meaningful. These stages are hypothesized to be cyclical, not linear (Hogan et al., 1996). Greater parent use of spiritual/religious coping activities is expected to help parents through this process, resulting in less severe parent grief (despair, detachment and disorganization) and better parent mental health (depression, post-traumatic stress) and personal growth at 1 and 3 months post-death.

Methods

The sample for this study consisted of 165 bereaved parents (114 mothers, 51 fathers) of 124 deceased infants/children (69 NICU and 55 PICU) recruited for the larger study from four level III NICUs and four tertiary care PICUs. Death records from the Office of Vital Statistics, Florida Department of Health, were used to identify infants and children who died in other NICUs or PICUs in South Florida. Parents were eligible for the study if their deceased newborn was from a singleton pregnancy and lived for more than 2 hours in the NICU or their deceased infant/child was 18 years or younger and a patient in the PICU for at least 2 hours. Parents had to understand spoken English or Spanish. Exclusion criteria were multiple gestation pregnancy if the deceased was a newborn, being in a foster home before hospitalization, injuries suspected to be due to child abuse, and death of a parent in the illness/injury event.

Measures of Dependent Variables

Grief was measured with four of the six subscales in the Hogan Grief Reaction Checklist (HGRC; Hogan, Greenfield, & Schmidt, 2001): despair (hopelessness, sadness and loneliness), detachment (detached from others, avoidance of intimacy), disorganization (difficulty in concentrating and/or retaining new information), and personal growth (personal transformation; becoming more compassionate, tolerant and hopeful). Bereaved parents rated each of the 61 items on a 5-point scale from 1 "does not describe me at all" to 5 "describes me very well" with higher summative scores indicating higher grief symptoms or personal growth in the previous two weeks. Hogan et al. (2001) reported internal consistencies for the 4 subscales of .82 to .89 and test-retest reliabilities from .77 to .85. In this study, Cronbach's alphas for the four subscales at T1 and T2 were .84–.93 for mothers and .79–.89 for fathers.

Depression was measured with the Beck Depression Inventory (BDI-II) (Beck, Steer, & Brown, 1996). Parents rated each of the 21 items on a scale from 0 to 3 with higher summative scores indicating greater severity of depressive symptoms. Beck et al. reported an internal consistency of .92 and test-retest reliability of .93. In this study, internal consistencies were .89–.93 for mothers and fathers at T1 andT2.

Post-traumatic stress disorder (PTSD) was measured with the Impact of Events Scale-Revised (IES-R; Weiss & Marmar, 1997). Bereaved parents rated each of the 22 items from 0 "not at all" to 4 "extremely" to indicate how distressing each item had been during the past 1 weeks with respect to the death of their infant/child. Higher summative scores indicate greater severity of PTSD symptoms. Weiss and Marmar reported internal consistencies for the three subscales as .79–.92. In this study, Cronbach's alphas for the subscales at T1 and T2 were .76–.86 for mothers and .71–.91 for fathers.

Measures of Independent Variables

Spiritual coping was measured with the Spiritual Coping Strategies Scale (SCS) (Baldacchino & Bulhagiar, 2003). The SCS contains two subscales: religious strategies/activities (9 items) and spiritual strategies/activities (11 items). Activities on the religious subscale are oriented toward religion and belief in God (attending church, praying, and trusting in God). Activities on the spiritual subscale are oriented toward relationship with self (reflection), others (relating to relatives and friends by confiding in them) and the environment (appreciating nature and the arts). Parents rated each activity on a 4–point scale ranging from 0 "never used" to 3 "used often" with higher scores indicating greater use of religious and spiritual activities. Baldacchino and Bulhagiar reported Cronbach's alphas of .82 for the religious and .74 for the spiritual strategies/activities subscales. Construct validity of the SCS subscales is supported by correlations of .40 with the well-established Spiritual Well Being instrument (Baldacchino & Bulhagiar, 2003). In this study, parents' subscales internal consistencies at T1 and T2 were .87 to .90 for religious activities and .80 to .82 for spiritual activities.

Race/ethnicity was categorized as "White, non-Hispanic," "Black non-Hispanic," or "Hispanic/Latino(a)" based on parent self-identified race (White, Black, Asian, Native American) and Ethnicity (Hispanic-yes/no). Two dummy- coded variables were created to represent race/ethnicity in the regression analyses: Black non-Hispanic (yes/no) and Hispanic/Latino (yes/no). White non-Hispanic was coded as the comparison group.

Religion indicated by the parent was categorized as Protestant, Catholic, none (atheists, agnostics) and other (Jewish, Buddhist, Muslim, Santeria/Espiritismo, Mormon and Rastafarian). Three dummy-coded variables were created to represent religion in the regression analyses: "Protestant" (yes/no), "Catholic" (yes/no), and "other" (yes/no). The "none" group was coded as the comparison group.

Procedure

The study was approved by the Institutional Review Boards (IRB) from the University, the 4 recruitment facilities, and the State Department of Health prior to recruitment of study participants. A clinical co-investigator from each NICU/PICU identified eligible families. The project director sent a letter to each family (Spanish on one side and English on the other) describing the study and called the family to explain the study. Of the 348 families contacted for the larger study, 188 (54%) families signed consent forms for their participation and review of their deceased child's medical record. The SCS was added to the study after 64 families were recruited. The remaining 124 families completed the SCS. Data were collected in the family's home or another place of their choosing at 1 (T1) and 3 (T2) months post-death. Data were collected from mothers and fathers separately.

Data Analysis

Analyses were conducted separately for mothers and fathers for each time point. Correlations were used to test the relationships of the SCS subscales with bereaved mothers' and fathers' grief (despair, detachment, disorganization), mental health (depression and PTSD) and personal growth at T1 and T2. Multiple regression analyses were used to test whether these relationships changed when the influence of race/ethnicity and religion were controlled. A priori power analysis showed that a sample size of 115 would provide sufficient power (≥80%) to detect an adjusted R^2 of 0.02 representing a medium effect and with alpha set at .05.

Results

In this sample of 114 mothers and 51 fathers from 124 families, fathers were older than mothers on average. Most parents were married or living with a partner, Hispanic (38%) or Black non-Hispanic (40%), high school graduates, employed, and Protestant (53%) or Catholic (27%). Of the 93 families who provided income data, 39% had annual incomes less than $30,000 (Table 1).

More infants/children died in the NICU (n = 69, 56%) than the PICU (n = 55, 44%); 70 (56%) were boys. The average infant/child age was 34.9 (SD = 60.38) months at death. More than half were infants (n = 95, 76%), followed by toddlers/preschoolers (n = 5, 4%), school age children (n = 12, 10%) and adolescents (n = 12, 10%). Mean length of stay was 32 days (SD = 63.10). Causes of death were respiratory conditions (n = 36, 29%), prematurity (n = 27, 22%), congenital anomalies (n = 20, 16%), infection (n = 13, 10%), accidents (n = 11, 9%), neurological disorders (n = 6, 5%), cardiac arrest (n = 5, 4%), cancer (n = 4, 3%), and complications of surgery (n = 2, 2%).

TABLE 1 Description of the Sample.

Characteristic	Mothers (n = 114)	Fathers (n = 51)
Age [*M* (SD)]	31.1 (7.73)	36.8 (9.32)
Race [*n* (%)]		
White non-Hispanic	22 (19%)	14 (28%)
Black non-Hispanic	50 (44%)	16 (31%)
Hispanic	42 (37%)	21 (41%)
Education [*n* (%)]		
<High school	12 (11%)	7 (14%)
High school graduate	31 (27%)	13 (25%)
Some college	36 (32%)	12 (24%)
College degree	35 (30%)	19 (37%)
Partnered [*n* (%)]	84 (74%)	43 (84%)
Employed [*n* (%)]	63 (55%)	32 (78%)
Religion [*n* (%)]		
Protestant	62 (54%)	26 (51%)
Catholic	33 (29%)	11 (22%)
Jewish	4 (4%)	2 (4%)
Other	1 (1%)	2 (4%)
None	14 (12%)	10 (20%)
Total family annual income [*n* (%)]	*N* =93 families	
<$3000	4 (4%)	
$3000–29,999	33 (35%)	
$30,000–49,999	22 (24%)	
≥$50,000	34 (37%)	

Grief and Mental Health

Use of spiritual activities was more strongly related to all outcomes for mothers and fathers than use of religious activities. Bereaved mothers' greater use of spiritual activities, but not religious activities, was significantly related to lower symptoms of grief (despair, detachment and disorganization), depression, and PTSD at T1 and T2 (Table 2). Controlling for race/ethnicity and religion, spiritual activities continued to have a significant influence on mothers' grief and mental health outcomes, except for disorganization at T2 (Table 3). The influence of religious activities remained non-significant when race/ethnicity and religion were controlled.

Bereaved fathers' greater use of spiritual activities was significantly related to lower symptoms of grief (despair, detachment and disorganization) and depression at T1 and T2 (Table 2). Fathers' greater use of religious activities was related to lower symptoms of grief and depression at T1 but not at T2 (Table 2). Controlling for race/ethnicity and religion, the influence of spiritual activities on fathers' grief, but not depression or PTSD, remained statistically significant at T1, but not at T2 (Table 4). The influence of religious activities was no longer significant for any of the fathers' T1 and T2 outcomes when race/ethnicity and religion were controlled.

Personal Growth

For mothers, use of spiritual and religious activities was significantly related to greater personal growth at both T1 and T2, with (T1: adjusted $R^2 = .10, \beta = .34$, T2: $R^2 = .10, \beta = .33$, $p < .01$) and without control for race/ethnicity and religion (Table 2) For fathers, spiritual activities were related to greater personal growth at T1 and T2, but the positive effects of religious activities on fathers' personal growth was significant at T2 only (Table 2). Fathers'

TABLE 2 Correlations of Parents' Use of Spiritual and Religious Activities with Grief, Mental Health and Personal Growth at 1 (T1) and 3 (T2) Months Post-Death.

		SPIRITUAL ACTIVITIES		RELIGIOUS ACTIVITIES	
Parent Outcome	Time Point	Mothers (n = 108)	Fathers (n = 50)	Mothers (n = 108)	Fathers (n = 50)
Grief					
Despair	T1	−.54**	−.47**	−.18	−.32**
	T2	−.51**	−.29*	−.11	−.15
Detachment	T1	−.56**	−.61**	−.19	−.26*
	T2	−.53**	−.35**	−.02	−.10
Disorganization	T1	−.41**	−.43**	−.02	−.25*
	T2	−.55**	−.23*	−.02	−.10
Depression	T1	−.54**	−.46**	−.19	−.27*
	T2	−.55**	−.39**	−.14	−.01
PTSD	T1	−.30**	−.29	−.10	−.12
	T2	−.35**	−.07	−.08	−.03
Personal Growth	T1	.51**	.51**	.42**	.10
	T2	.64**	.49**	.37**	.31**

* $p < .05$.
** $p < .01$.

TABLE 3 Effects of Mothers' Use of Spiritual Activities at T1 on Outcomes at 1 and 3 Months After their Infant's/Child's Death, Controlling for Race/Ethnicity and Religion.

	GRIEF											
	DESPAIR		DETACHMENT		DISORGANIZATION		DEPRESSION		PTSD		PERSONAL GROWTH	
	1 mo	3 mo	1 mo	3 mo	1 mo	3 mo	1 mo	3 mo	1 mo	3 mo	1 mo	3 mo
	β	β	β	β	β	β	β	β	β	β	β	β
Black non–Hispanic [a]	.12	.03	.14	.15	−.23	−.04	.09	.15	.25	.25	.04	.09
Hispanic [a]	.10	.10	.18	.33*	.04	.15	.18	.24	.35**	.33	−.12	−.07
Protestant religion [a]	.13	.21	.27	.47*	.45*	.42	.15	.26	.04	.07	.30	.23
Catholic religion [a]	.01	.12	.21	.30	.19	.22	.08	.11	−.05	−.02	.13	.14
Other religion [a]	.01	.06	.09	.26	.15	.24	.10	.15	.03	.03	−.04	.02
Spiritual activities	−.55*	−.53*	−.58*	−.59*	−.41*	−.29	−.56*	−.59*	−.33*	−.37*	.46*	.62*
F	6.29*	4.90*	7.34*	7.51*	3.69*	.54	5.86*	6.61*	2.62*	2.90*	7.65*	10.74*
Adj R^2	.27	.23	.31	.33	.16	.04	.26	.30	.10	.13	.32	.43

[a] Scored yes = 1, no= 0.
* $p < .05$.
** $p < .01$.

TABLE 4 Effects of Fathers' Use of Spiritual Activities on Grief at 1 and 3 Months After their Infant's/Child's Death, Controlling for Race/Ethnicity and Religion.

	GRIEF DESPAIR		GRIEF DETACHMENT		GRIEF DISORGANIZATION	
	1 mo	3 mo	1 mo	3 mo	1 mo	3 mo
	β	β	β	β	β	β
Black non-Hispanic [a]	−.06	.19	−.03	.12	−.12	−.13
Hispanic [a]	.34	.35	.19	.18	.16	.01
Protestant religion [a]	−.23	−.27	−.15	−.02	−.17	.03
Catholic religion [a]	−.19	−.13	−.12	−.01	.11	.14
Other religion [a]	−.26	.02	−.21	.35	−.13	.24
Spiritual activities	−.58**	−.28	−.69**	−.25	−.50**	−.19
F	3.06*	1.25	4.30*	1.81	2.45*	1.06
Adj R^2	.24	−.04	.34	.11	.18	.01

[a] Scored yes = 1, no = 0.
* $p < .05$.
** $p < .01$.

spiritual and religious activities were not related to their personal growth when race/ethnicity and religion were controlled.

DISCUSSION

Loss of an infant or child is devastating for mothers and fathers and it is often associated with increased morbidity (Youngblut et al., 2013) and mortality (Espinosa & Evans, 2013). Youngblut et al. reported that about one third of the bereaved parents in their sample had clinical depression and/or PTSD at 13 months after their infant's or child's death in the NICU/PICU. Identifying strategies that help parents cope with the death of their child may mitigate some of these negative health effects.

Spiritual coping strategies may be helpful to parents at this time of very high stress. In this study, mothers' and fathers' spiritual activities at 1 month post-death were related to less severe symptoms of grief at both 1 and 3 months. Use of religious activities was helpful in reducing fathers' grief at 1 month, but not at 3 months; these activities were not related to mothers' grief at either time point. These findings suggest that fathers may find more solace in religious activities than mothers. If so, use of both spiritual and religious activities may help fathers move through the grieving process faster, allowing them to return to their previous routines such as returning to work earlier than bereaved mothers (Aho, Tarkka, Kurki, & Kaunonen, 2006; Armentrout, 2009).

Mothers' use of spiritual activities, but not religious activities, was related to less severe symptoms of depression and PTSD at 1 and 3 months. Fathers' use of spiritual activities was related to less severe symptoms of depression at both 1 and 3 months. Use of religious activities was related to less severe symptoms of depression at 1 month for fathers' after their infant's/child's death.

Gender differences in coping with grief are supported in the literature. Bereaved mothers need to talk more about the death than bereaved fathers (Barrera et al., 2007; Buchi et al., 2007), whereas bereaved fathers were found to cope with their grief by isolating themselves from family and friends (Aho et al., 2006). Religious activities such as praying privately or watching religious programs may allow fathers periods of solitude grieving, not requiring discussion of the infant/child and their feelings about the death. These activities also may serve to limit the opportunities for mothers and others to engage fathers in conversation about the deceased infant/child.

In contrast, spiritual activities involve engaging with others, discussing difficulties with others who have endured similar circumstances, spending time with and confiding in relatives and/or friend. These activities provide the mothers with the discussion they reportedly want and need. This suggests that bereaved mothers valued the social support received from family and friends and used non-religious activities to relieve feelings of hopelessness, sadness and loneliness, to connect with their inner self, to acknowledge their strengths and ultimately find peace (Bakker & Paris, 2013). Additionally, studies of gender differences in bereaved couples' grief reaction have found mothers to have a longer recovery time in adjusting to their grief than fathers (Armentrout, 2009; Lang, Gottlieb, & Amsel, 1996). Perhaps it reflects societal expectations that men should be stoic which is reinforced in the workplace and social gatherings.

Personal growth at 1 and 3 months was greater for mothers using greater spiritual and religious activities. Fathers had greater personal growth at 1 and 3 months with greater use of spiritual activities and at 3 months with religious activities. This is consistent with other studies in which bereaved parents describe a transformation in their lives. Personal growth was identified as becoming more compassionate, caring, and sensitive to the needs of others and becoming more giving of themselves by reaching out to other bereaved parents (Armentrout, 2009; Lichtenhal et al., 2010).

Stronger associations were found between greater use of spiritual activities as compared to religious activities and positive bereavement outcomes over time. A possible explanation for this relationship may be that in times of crisis bereaved parents engaged in coping activities that are based on their personal beliefs and values to buffer their grief. Spiritual practices can be characterized as being more personal, individualistic and include secular terms that are free from religious rules or regulations. Religious coping gives indirect control to God/the sacred and reduces the need for personal control (Koenig, 2009).

Additionally, some research studies found that bereaved parents expressed negative feelings such as anger at God for their infant's/child's death; some felt that God was punishing them and others questioned God their faith (Armentrout, 2009; Ganzevoort & Falkenburg, 2012). Meert et al. (2005) found that 30 to 60% of bereaved parents expressed anger and blame at themselves and God for their infant's/child's death and this may result in using less religious coping activities to cope with early grief.

Controlling for race/ethnicity and religion made little difference in the influence of spiritual activities on mothers' and fathers' grief and mothers' mental health. However, most of the bivariate relationships with religious activities did not remain when race/ethnicity and religion were controlled

Limitations of the Study

There are several additional limitations of the study. At 1 and 3 months post-death, parents were in early stages of grieving. Thus, these findings may not be applicable to parents who are later in the grieving process. In this study most of the bereaved parents reported spiritual activities, not religious activities as effective in helping them to cope with their grief and mental health for a longer period of time. The average age for these bereaved parents was early to mid-thirties and it is possible that individuals of this age may not be strongly affiliated to a religious group (Fowler, 1995).

Additionally, the use of religious and spiritual strategies was not significantly related to bereaved fathers' PTSD at both T1 and T2 and personal growth at T1. This is possibly related to the small number of men who participated in this study, which is a common occurrence in these studies (Lichtenhal et al., 2010) and is a limitation of this study.

Conclusion

Research studies have found that bereaved parents experience many emotional benefits associated with the use of religious coping to deal with their grief and mental health (Lichtenhal et al., 2010; Meert et al., 2005). In this study, religious activities were not effective in lowering symptoms of grief, depression, and PTSD for bereaved mothers at 1 month and fathers at 3 months post-death. This suggests that spiritual activities may assist bereaved mothers to reduce their symptoms of grief, depression, PTSD and increase personal growth over a longer period of time than religious activities. While religious activities might be helpful in the first month after the child's death, maybe religious activities come into play later when their anger with God has diminished. The use of spiritual activities such as self-refection, confiding in others and cultivating friendships may be more helpful to parents over time.

The findings when race/ethnicity and religion were controlled suggested that the use of spiritual, and not religious activities helped both mothers and fathers cope with their grief but the use and/or effect of using spiritual activities was helpful for bereaved mothers with their mental health and personal growth for a longer time.

Clinical Relevance

The results from this longitudinal study with a racially and ethnically diverse sample provide evidence for healthcare professionals about the importance of spiritual coping activities for bereaved mothers and fathers. Dissemination of this information in the clinical areas to nurses and other healthcare team members will enable bereaved parents to receive relevant and appropriate support following the death of their infant/child.

The study findings suggest that nurses may encourage bereaved parents, especially mothers to identify and use an array of spiritual activities, such as self-reflection, relating to family and friends by confiding in them; finding meaning and purpose to live through their situation may help parents cope with their infant's or child's death, decreasing their symptoms of grief and improving their mental health. Intervening in this manner may enable bereaved parents to receive relevant and appropriate support following the death of their infant/child.

Future Research

Findings from this research study provide implications for future research. The responses obtained from bereaved parents at 1 month and 3 months are applicable to parents in the early stages of bereavement. Further research is needed to determine if any changes, whether negative or positive, occurred in bereaved parents' use of religious and spiritual activities to cope and the effect on their grief response, mental health and personal growth in the later stage of bereavement.

Additionally, future research that specifically examines differences in bereaved mothers' and fathers' use of religious and spiritual activities, with a larger sample of fathers, can determine the specific supportive spiritual coping activities that may be used to help bereaved mothers and fathers cope with their grief.

Acknowledgments

This research was supported by a grant from the National Institutes of Health, National Institute for Nursing Research, R01 NR009120 (Youngblut/Brooten) & Diversity Supplement R01 NR009120–S1 (Hawthorne).

REFERENCES

Aho, A. L., Tarkka, M. T., Kurki, P. A., & Kaunonen, M. (2006). Father's grief after the death of a child. *Issues in Mental Health and Nursing, 27*, 647–663.

Armentrout, D. C. (2009). Living with grief following removal of infant life support: Parent's perspective. *Critical Care Nursing Clinics of North America, 21*, 253–265.

Bakker, J. J., & Paris, J. (2013). Bereavement and religion online: Stillbirth, neonatal loss, and parental religiosity. *Journal for the Scientific Studies of Religion, 52*, 657–674.

Baldacchino, D. R., & Bulhagiar, A. (2003). Psychometric evaluation of the spiritual coping strategies scale in English, Maltese: Back translation and bilingual versions. *Journal of Advanced Nursing, 42*, 558–570.

Barrera, M., O'Connor, K., D'Agostino, N. M., et al. (2007). Patters of parental bereavement following the loss of a child and related factors. *Omega: Journal of Death and Dying, 55*, 145–167.

Beck, A. T., Steer, R. A., & Brown, G. K. (1996). *Beck Depression Inventory-II*. San Antonio, TX: The Psychological Corporation.

Buchi, S., Morgeli, H., Schnyder, U., et al. (2007). Grief and post-traumatic growth in parents 2–6 years after the death of their extremely premature baby. *Psychotherapy and Psychosomatics, 76*, 106–114.

Espinosa, J., & Evans, W. N. (2013). Maternal bereavement: The heightened mortality of mothers after the death of a child. *Economics in Human Biology, 11*, 371–381.

Fontana, M. S., Farrell, C., Gauvin, F., et al. (2013). Modes of death in pediatrics: Differences in the ethical approach in neonatal and pediatric patients. *Journal of Pediatrics, 162*, 1107–1111.

Fowler, J. W. (1995). *Stages of faith development: The psychology of human development and the quest for meaning*. San Francisco: Harper & Row.

Ganzevoort, R. R., & Falkenburg (2012). Stories beyond life and death: Spiritual experiences of continuity and discontinuity among parents who loose a child. *Journal of Empirical Theology*, 189–204.

Hogan, N. S., Greenfield, D. B., & Schmidt, L. A. (2001). Development and validation of the Hogan grief reaction checklist. *Death Studies, 25*, 1–32.

Hogan, N. S., Morse, J. M., & Tason, M. C. (1996). Toward an experiential theory of bereavement. *Omega: Journal of Death and Dying, 33*, 43–65.

Klass, D. (1999). *The spiritual lives of bereaved parents*. Ann Arbor, MI: Edwards Brothers.

Koenig, H. G. (2009). Research on religion, spirituality, and mental health: A review. *The Canadian Journal of Psychiatry, 54*, 283–289.

Lang, A., Gottlieb, L. N., & Amsel, R. (1996). Predictors of husband's and wives' grief reactions following infant death: The role of marital intimacy. *Death Studies, 20*, 33–57.

Lichtenhal, W. G., Currier, J. M., Neimeyer, R. A., & Keese, N. J. (2010). Sense and significance: A mixed methods examinations of meaning making after the loss of a one's child. *Journal of Clinical Psychology, 66*, 791–812.

Matthews, T. J., Minino, A. M., Osterman, M. J. K., et al. (2011). Annual summary of vital statistics: 2008. *Pediatrics, 127*, 146–157.

Meert, K. L., Briller, S. H., Myers-Shim, S., et al. (2009). Examining the needs of bereaved parents in the pediatric intensive care unit: A qualitative study. *Death Studies, 33*, 712–740.

Meert, K. L., Thurston, C. S., & Briller, S. H. (2005). The spiritual needs of parents at the time of their child's death in the pediatric intensive care unit and during bereavement: A qualitative study. *Pediatric Critical Care, 6*, 420–427.

O'Brien, E. M. (2014). *Spirituality in nursing* (5th ed.). Sudbury, MA: Jones and Bartlett.

Subone, A., & Baider, L. (2010). The spiritual dimension of cancer care. *Critical Reviews in Oncology Nursing, 73*, 228–235.

Weiss, D. S., & Marmar, C. R. (1997). The impact of event scale—Revised. In J. Wilson, & T. Keane (Eds.), *Assessing Psychological Trauma and PTSD* (pp. 399–411). New York: Guildford.

Werthmann, J., Smits, L. J. M., & Li, J. (2010). Parental mortality rates in a western country after the death of a child: Assessment of the role of the child's sex. *Gender Medicine, 7*, 39–46.

Youngblut, J. M., & Brooten, D. (2012). Perinatal and pediatric issues in palliative and end-of-life care from the 2011 Summit on the Science of Compassion. *Nursing Outlook, 60*, 343–350.

Youngblut, J. M., Brooten, D., Cantwell, G. P., et al. (2013). Parent health and functioning 13 months after infant or child NICU/PICU death. *Pediatrics, 132*, e1295–e1301. http://dx.doi.org/10.1542/peds.2013–1194 (Epub 2013 Oct 7, PMC3813397).

Example of a Qualitative Study (van Dijk et al., 2015)

Postoperative Patients' Perspectives on Rating Pain: A Qualitative Study

Jacqueline F.M. van Dijk[a,], Sigrid C.J.M. Vervoort[b], Albert J.M. van Wijck[a], Cor J. Kalkman[c], Marieke J. Schuurmans[d]*

ABSTRACT

Background: In postoperative pain treatment patients are asked to rate their pain experience on a single uni-dimensional pain scale. Such pain scores are also used as indicator to assess the quality of pain treatment. However, patients may differ in how they interpret the Numeric Rating Scale (NRS) score.

Objectives: This study examines how patients assign a number to their currently experienced postoperative pain and which considerations influence this process.

Methods: A qualitative approach according to grounded theory was used. Twenty-seven patients were interviewed one day after surgery.

Results: Three main themes emerged that influenced the Numeric Rating Scale scores (0–10) that patients actually reported to professionals: score-related factors, intrapersonal factors, and the anticipated consequences of a given pain score. Anticipated consequences were analgesic administration—which could be desired or undesired—and possible judgements by professionals. We also propose a conceptual model for the relationship between factors that influence the pain rating process. Based on patients' score-related and intrapersonal factors, a preliminary pain score was "internally" set. Before reporting the pain score to the healthcare professional, patients considered the anticipated consequences (i.e., expected judgements by professionals and anticipation of analgesic administration) of current Numeric Rating Scale scores.

Conclusions: This study provides insight into the process of how patients translate their current postoperative pain into a numeric rating score. The proposed model may help professionals to understand the factors that influence a given Numeric Rating Scale score and suggest the most appropriate questions for clarification. In this way, patients and professionals may arrive

[a] Pain Clinic, Department of Anesthesiology, University Medical Center Utrecht, The Netherlands

[b] Department of Internal Medicine & Infectious Diseases, University Medical Center Utrecht, The Netherlands

[c] Department of Anesthesiology, University Medical Center Utrecht, The Netherlands

[d] Department of Nursing Science, University Medical Center Utrecht, The Netherlands

at a shared understanding of the pain score, resulting in a tailored decision regarding the most appropriate treatment of current postoperative pain, particularly the dosing and timing of opioid administration.

What is already known about the topic?

- Patients are asked to rate their pain experience on a single uni-dimensional pain scale.
- Patients' pain scores are the leading indicator in postoperative pain treatment.
- It is unknown how patients interpret the NRS scores.

What this paper adds

- Three main themes emerged that influenced patients' NRS scores actually reported to professionals: score-related factors, intrapersonal factors and the anticipated consequences of assigning a particular NRS score.
- A conceptual model emerged for the relationship between factors that influence the pain rating process. When assigning an NRS score to their pain, patients process the first two themes in stages: They first weigh score-related factors and intrapersonal factors. Some patients go through a last stage before telling the professional: weighing the judgements by healthcare professionals and the anticipated consequences of reporting a particular NRS score against their actual desire for more or less analgesics.
- The proposed model could help professionals to better understand the complex process by which patients assign pain scores and could serve as a basis for a dialogue beyond the given pain scores.

1. Introduction

The adequacy of pain treatment is an important healthcare quality indicator. Many patients still experience severe pain after surgery, suggesting that there is considerable room for improvement in postoperative pain management (Apfelbaum et al., 2003; Sommer et al., 2008). The quality of pain management is in many quality systems operationalized in terms of measuring patients' pain scores.

Pain is subjective, and nociception cannot be measured directly. In clinical practice, patients are asked to rate their (sometimes complex) pain experience on a single unidimensional pain scale. However, in contrast to the high number of quantitative studies using the Numeric Rating Scale (NRS), only one study is found how chronic pain patients use the NRS (Williams et al., 2000) but no study has explored how postoperative patients interpret the NRS, how they assign a number from 0 to 10 to their pain, and what considerations come into play when translating a highly subjective pain experience into a single number.

Patients' pain scores are the leading indicator in postoperative pain treatment (Aubrun et al., 2003; Idvall et al., 2008; Gordon et al., 2005; Max et al., 1995; VMS, 2009). Clinical observations and physiological parameters used in pain treatment should be considered with caution. Nurses often underestimate patients' pain (Idvall et al., 2005; Sloman et al., 2005) and vital signs can be influenced by other factors besides pain (Arbour and Gelinas, 2010; Gelinas and Arbour, 2009). Several guidelines advise healthcare professionals to administer additional analgesics when patients report an NRS score greater than 3 or 4 (Gordon et al., 2005; Hartrick et al., 2003; Max et al., 1995; VMS, 2009). In a previous study, we reported that patients with NRS scores of 4, 5, or 6 vary in the interpretation of their score (Van Dijk et al., 2012). In that study, we observed that some patients reporting NRS scores between 4 and 6 considered their pain "bearable" and refused opioids, while other patients with identical NRS scores considered their pain "unbearable" and requested more opioids. This raises the question of whether simple thresholds such as "NRS $>$ 3 or 4" are the most appropriate cut-off points upon which professionals should base their decisions regarding administering additional analgesics. In postoperative pain management, both undertreatment and overtreatment are undesirable. Unrelieved pain has adverse psychological and physiological consequences, including increased rates of postoperative complications and prolonged hospital stays (Watt-Watson, 1999). Conversely, unnecessary use of analgesics, especially opioids, increases the patient's discomfort due to the side effects (e.g., nausea, vomiting, and pruritus) and potentially harmful adverse effects (e.g., oversedation and respiratory depression) (Cashman and Dolin, 2004; Taylor et al., 2005). For optimal pain treatment, patients and professionals must communicate effectively and have a shared understanding of the burden of the patient's currently experienced pain.

The aim of this qualitative study was to explore how patients assign a number on the basis of the NRS to their currently experienced postoperative pain and which considerations influence this process.

2. Methods

2.1. Study Design

The study was descriptive and qualitative in nature. The method used was based on grounded theory (Charmaz, 2014), a qualitative research method designed to aid in the systematic collection and analysis of data and the construction of a model. Individual interviews were used as the data-collection method. Guidelines for conducting qualitative studies established by the Consolidated Criteria for Reporting Qualitative Research (COREQ) were followed (Tong et al., 2007).

2.2. Participants

The study was conducted between November 2012 and July 2013 in a university hospital. Patients were eligible for selection if they had surgery the day before and currently experienced postoperative pain with a reported NRS score of at least 4. Patients were selected purposively by the researcher (JvD) and to create a diverse sample patients were selected with regard to sex, age, ethnicity, previous pain experiences, and previous experience with rating an NRS score. Theoretical sampling was used as much as possible; we started with a homogeneous sample of patients, and as the data collection proceeded and themes emerged, we turned to a more heterogeneous sample to see under what conditions the themes hold (Charmaz, 2014).

The researcher was not involved in the patients' care. Exclusion criteria were as follows: younger than 18 years, unable to read and understand Dutch, cognitive impairment, having impaired hearing, or not being well enough to be interviewed. The researcher identified eligible patients by consulting the Electronic Patient Dossiers (EPDs) and asked the nurse on the ward whether identified eligible patients could be interviewed. None of the eligible patients were unable to be interviewed. Thereafter, the researcher approached the patients, provided information about the study, and handed over an information letter. After reading the letter, patients were asked to consider participation in the study. All 27 patients who were asked agreed to participate, and written informed consent was obtained. The study was approved by the medical ethics committee of the University Medical Centre Utrecht in which the study took place.

2.3. Data Collection

Data were collected using semi-structured, in-depth interviews on the day after surgery. The researcher's (JvD) interview technique (validity and reliability of the interview style) during the first two interviews was discussed with experts). The questions were open-ended, and all interviews started with, "The nurse regularly asks you to assign a number from 0 to 10 to your pain, where 0 is no pain and 10 is the 'worst imaginable' pain. We heard from some patients that they perceived it as difficult to assign a number to their pain. How is that for you? Can you tell me how you assign a number to your pain?" A topic guide for the interviews based on the literature, the knowledge of nursing experts, and preliminary studies of the research group was used (Table 1). The Dutch school grades were chosen as a topic because the meaning of these grades (where 1 is insufficient and 10 is excellent) are the opposite of meaning of the pain scores. Therefore, Dutch patients could be confused when they were asked to score their pain on the NRS.

Insights from the interim analyses were incorporated in the interview guidelines used in subsequent interviews. Interviews were conducted in a private room on the ward, digitally recorded and transcribed verbatim. Identifying details were removed from the transcripts. The interviews lasted between 5 and 32 min (mean 12 min). Information concerning age, gender, ethnicity, surgical procedure, presence of chronic pain, and education was obtained using a structured questionnaire.

During data collection, memos were made containing impressions and thoughts about the themes and their relationships. Data collection stopped after saturation was reached (i.e., interviewees were selected until the new information obtained did not provide further insight into the themes or no further new themes emerged) (Charmaz, 2014).

2.4. Data Analysis

The data analysis was conducted by two researchers (SV and JvD) and supported by NVivo 10 software (QSR International, Cambridge, MA, USA). Data were analysed applying constant comparison analysis. First the texts were read out in full to obtain an overall picture and then reread to elucidate the details. During open coding meaningful paragraphs were analysed and initial concepts identified leading to fragmentation of the data. Axial coding enabled the concepts to be aggregated according to their similarities leading to categories (themes). New data were compared with the evolved categories. Throughout selective coding relations between the categories were defined and a preliminary model was described (Boeije, 2010). The theoretical model in development was compared with the interview transcripts to verify the interpretation into the original interview texts. During the coding process, the researchers discussed the concepts and categories. When their opinions differed, they discussed the issue until consensus was reached. A third researcher (CK, an expert in the field of pain treatment with a different

TABLE 1 **The Topic Guide for the Interviews.**
The value of the numbers from 0 to 10
Pain score at that moment
Bearable or unbearable pain
Assigning scores at the upper extreme of the scale
Previous experiences with pain
Upbringing
The role of the healthcare professional
Analgesics: when desiring light or strong analgesics fear of addiction and side effects
Grades at school from 1 to 10

background), read the transcripts, checked the coding, and discussed his opinion if different, allowing us to verify the themes and the preliminary model. The research team reviewed the main categories and its relations and worked towards consensus about the interpretations and finally the theoretical model was developed.

2.5. Trustworthiness

The trustworthiness of the study was enhanced by the use of different techniques (Lincoln and Guba, 1985). The credibility was established by generating a non-judgemental atmosphere during interviews ensuring to learn from patients. Transcribing the interviews verbatim reduces the chances for bias. During data collection and data analysis memos were written supporting the research process and the creation of theoretical ideas and hypothesis. Researcher triangulation during data analysis and peer debriefing by the researchers team enhanced both the credibility and conformability of the interpretation. By means of peer debriefing broader perspectives and possible meanings were uncovered and reflexivity, guaranteed by the critical stance to the interview style and feedback of other researchers led to more depth which enhanced accurateness. To guarantee the transferability as much as possible, thick description was pursued by the amount of respondents, diversity of the sample, duration of interviews and describing the details for imitability.

3. Results

The age of the 14 men and 13 women who participated in the study was between 18 and 79 years old (mean 51). The severity of surgery varied from minor (e.g., thyroidectomy) to major (e.g., spinal fusion). Demographic and medical data are presented in Table 2.

Translating currently experienced pain into an NRS score between 0 and 10 appeared to be a complex process for the patients. From the analysis, three main themes emerged regarding the process of scoring one's pain experience: score-related factors, intrapersonal factors, and the anticipated consequences of rating one's pain with an NRS score. The latter theme comprised two subthemes: expected judgements by professionals and anticipation

TABLE 2 **Demographic Data.**

N	27
Male, *n*	14
Age, mean (range)	51 (18–79)
Ethnicity, *n*	
Caucasian	23
Other	4
Surgical type, *n*	
Orthopaedic	16
General	5
Gynaecologic	3
Plastic surgery	2
Vascular surgery	1
Education, *n*	
Low	10
Median	10
High	7
Patients with chronic pain, *n*	6

TABLE 3 **Three Main Themes and Associated Factors that Emerged from the Interview Analyses.**

		ANTICIPATED CONSEQUENCES OF ASSIGNING A PARTICULAR NRS SCORE	
Score-related Factors	**Intrapersonal Patient Factors**	**Judgements by Professionals**	**Analgesic Administration**
• Unique pain experience	• Previous pain experiences	• Being seen as a bother	• Encounter ambivalence
• Distinction between bearable and unbearable pain	• Being tough on oneself	• Experiencing basic mistrust	• Suffering side effects
• Avoiding high extremes	• Pain threshold	• Wish to meet the expectations of professionals	• Variation on timing of opioids
• Different pain level at rest and movement	• Holding oneself to one's own standards		• Nurses have own point of view
	• Desiring confirmation from professionals		

of analgesic administration, particularly opioids. Factors that were reported to influence the rating of pain using an NRS score are shown in Table 3.

A model emerged of the interrelation between the themes clarifying what underlies patients' rating of their pain on the NRS (Fig. 1). Patients went through consecutive stages wherein the themes were at play. However, not all patients were affected by the themes in the same way. Based on the patients' score-related and intrapersonal patient factors, a preliminary pain score was "internally" set. Before reporting the pain score to the healthcare professional, the patient considered the anticipated consequences of the current NRS score. Based on these expectations, this preliminary pain score was sometimes adjusted to a definitive pain score that was reported to the professional. First, patients expected that professionals would judge them regarding the magnitude of the reported pain score. Second, patients considered what pain treatment would likely be administered as a result of their reported pain score. Some patients wanted to meet the expectations of the professional and considered what would be the most socially acceptable pain score. Based on these considerations, the "adjusted" pain score was then communicated to the healthcare professional.

3.1. Score-related Factors

Unique pain experience: Patients found it difficult to rate their pain using an NRS score, because they felt they had an "unique" pain experience. They said it was difficult to explain

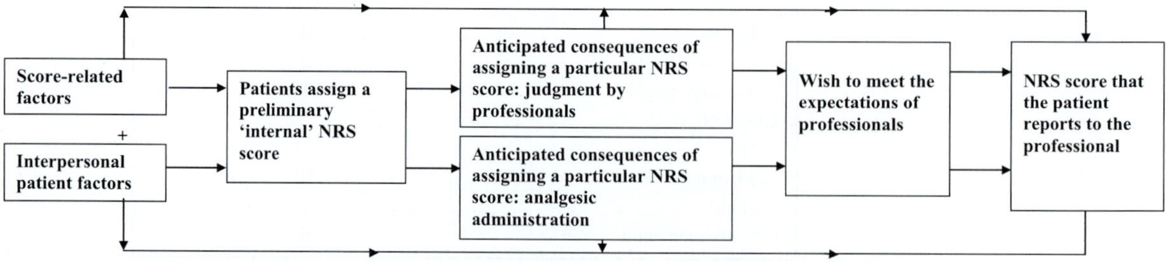

FIG 1 The model for the patients' underlying process of rating an NRS score to their pain.

to another person exactly what they felt or what their pain level was in relation to what they felt. Several patients said that everyone experiences pain differently and therefore will assign their own value from 0 to 10.

> "It's difficult to measure. You've got your interpretation and I've got mine" (male, age 51).
>
> "I think about worst pain as something I've never felt before and zero is no pain. I always find it a very difficult question to assign a number" (female, age 51).

Many patients perceived it as difficult to assign a number from 0 to 10 to their experienced pain, especially when it concerned the intermediate pain scores (NRS scores of 4 to 6). For some patients who had chronic pain in addition to acute postoperative pain, it was even more difficult to rate their current pain experience, because they often experienced different types of pain that differed in intensity.

Distinction between "bearable" and "unbearable" pain: To make it easier to rate their pain, some patients first created a cut-off point between bearable and unbearable pain, the latter often expressed as an NRS score of 6 or higher.

> "I balance between bearable and severe. If it is bearable then it is a six, it is not good, but I can bear it. But when I feel it with any movement and it's really painful, then it is eight or sometimes nine"(female, age 79).

The number 5 was seen by many patients as a natural midpoint of the pain scale. Therefore, patients themselves often used an NRS score of 5 as a cut-off point: At 5 and below, the pain was considered bearable, and at above 5, the pain was called "real pain."

> "'Five' I would consider the average, that is bearable. Over five, then I'd say: give me something. That is not really bearable I think. So, as long it is up to five, I'd say I am doing OK" (female, age 45).

Patients concluded that there clearly was a difference between their interpretation of bearable and unbearable pain and that of professionals. In the patients' opinion, many professionals considered only NRS scores below 4 as representing bearable pain, while many patients considered an NRS score of 6 as indicating bearable pain. In the Netherlands school system, a grade system from 1 to 10 is traditionally used, where 1 means completely insufficient and 10 denotes excellent. In this system, a score of 6 is sufficient to pass an exam. One patient mentioned that this had an effect on how she used the NRS.

> "The grades at school that is something you are familiar with, that is also a validation, that has an effect, because that's what you grew up with. Because it is also a kind of validation, when you give the pain a number then you also validate something, you know? Yes, I think so" (male, age 77).

Most patients said that they were not confused when rating their pain experience in relation to scores they were used to getting at Dutch schools.

Avoiding high extremes: Most patients assign an extreme score on the NRS as follows: 0 and 1 meaning no or light pain and 9 and 10 meaning the worst imaginable pain. Some patients explained that they would never use the highest pain score, because "10" is so extreme that they could not imagine having so much pain.

> "If it hurts a little, then it is often two or three. Higher than five, then it has to hurt a lot. I would never give a ten. Yeah, 'unbearable' wouldn't cross my mind" (male, age 36).

Other patients said that they would never assign a very high number to their pain, because they mentally compared their current situation to a more severe imagined situation.

Different pain level at rest and movement: When patients were asked how they assigned a number to their pain, many patients said they experienced a difference between pain at rest and pain at movement. Patients mostly assigned two different numbers to their pain: an NRS score below four at rest and an NRS score above six or seven at movement.

> "If I lie very still and I have used the PCA pump then it is a three or four, and when I move it goes up to a seven, eight" (male, age 41).

Some patients consider their pain at rest as bearable and only move if necessary. Patients accepted a brief moment of pain at movement and did not want additional analgesics for such short severe pain episodes.

3.2. Intrapersonal Patient Factors

Previous pain experiences: When rating their current pain using an NRS score, patients used past pain experiences as a benchmark to judge their current pain level. Patients who had experienced severe pain in the past tended to consider their current pain as less severe than patients who had not experienced severe pain before. They explained that they understood what "worst imaginable" pain was and accordingly recalibrated the NRS.

> "I now rate it a three, almost no pain, but I've had surgery before and then they asked it as well. I've had a tonsillectomy and then you're actually constantly in pain, so I had an eight or something, that's really very painful, that's not normal anymore" (female, age 18).

> "My neuropathic pain was severe and then you know how 'worst imaginable' pain can be. And that's quite irritating because I've had a lot of pain and if you have to compare then I say, 'it's a four' and you compare it with a ten that is not as high as someone else's, I always find it difficult to distinguish. And then they (the nurses) say, 'oh, then it's okay'. But they don't know with what I'm comparing it" (female, age 26).

Being tough on oneself: Regarding their postoperative pain experience, many patients said that they were tough on themselves.

> "They have often told me that I am very hard on myself. I didn't allow myself to complain. I was very hard on myself" (male, age 41).

Patients said that they expected pain after surgery and that they could bear some pain. Moreover, patients indicated that postoperative pain is temporary. Sometimes, high NRS scores were given, yet patients considered the experienced pain bearable and did not want additional analgesic treatment. Several patients said that they thought it was appropriate to be tough on themselves, and they often traced that back to their own upbringing and the way they were taught to handle pain during childhood.

> "I don't moan quickly. I don't often visit the doctor. I get that from my upbringing. Yeah, it has to be really necessary before I make a fuss" (female, age 45).

Pain threshold: Many patients thought they had a high pain threshold, because they could bear a lot of pain.

> "My pain threshold is quite high because I've been through a lot. My knees had to be bent three years ago. So, I can take quite a lot because that was very severe" (male, age 41).

One patient said that the individual pain threshold depends on the degree of resilience that one has and that this differs between people. Patients who also had chronic pain considered their postoperative pain intermediate but bearable, explaining that they were used to having pain. They explained that because they were accustomed to pain, they had a high pain threshold and could handle more pain than patients without chronic pain.

> "You learn to live with it, but there are limits. Anyone else would already be screaming because of the pain, but my pain threshold is a bit higher" (male, age 45).

Few patients said they had a low pain threshold because they could not bear a lot of pain. One patient told the interviewer that after giving birth to her children, she could not bear pain anymore.

Holding oneself to one's own standards: Many patients considered NRS scores of 4 and higher, especially scores between 4 and 6, still bearable. During the interviews, the researcher explained to the patients how professionals are taught that NRS scores of 4 and higher are unacceptable and require intervention. Even after this explanation, patients continued to maintain their own point of view (i.e., that NRS scores between 4 and 6 were bearable). They said they had their own standards about the meaning of the different numbers of the pain scale.

> Interviewer: "You told me a six, seven is bearable. Would you alter it if I told you that nurses consider zero to four as bearable pain?"
>
> Patient: "No, because I have got my own norm, I am more used to pain and I think it is bearable. If I'm in pain and I can handle it, it is bearable for me" (male, age 47).

Desiring confirmation from professionals: Patients sometimes doubt about the NRS score they assign to their pain. Patients appreciated it when the professional confirmed their assignment of a high number to their pain. They were more convinced that they had correctly assigned a number to their pain experience if the doctor or nurse had said that a high level of pain was expected or normal.

> "When I actually told him (the doctor), he said 'yes I can imagine, because it's all bruised'. So then I thought 'see, I'm not exaggerating!'. I have the idea that they will then think I'm being a wimp" (female, age 63).

3.3. Anticipated Consequences of Assigning a Particular NRS Score

Patients appeared to take the anticipated consequences of a given NRS score into account before telling the professional a number. They sometimes purposefully assigned a lower NRS score than the pain actually experienced in anticipation of the reaction of healthcare professionals. Patients were sometimes reluctant to provide an NRS score, fearing it is "too high" or "too low" that possibly lead to a reaction of the professional they did not expect. With giving a particular score, patients tried to anticipate whether professionals will administrate analgesics or not. Therefore, this distinction led to two subthemes: "judgment by care professionals" and "analgesic administration."

3.3.1 Judgements by healthcare professionals. Being seen as a bother: Patients were worried that healthcare professionals would consider them being a bother if they reported high NRS scores.

> "That is not because I want to be tough or anything, that is not the issue, but I just don't want to be a bother. That's the point, I just don't want to be bothersome" (male, age 47).
>
> "In the past, you didn't complain, you just got on with it. That's what's in me and always will be" (female, age 63).

Patients fear that professionals think that they exaggerate pain. Consequently patients anticipated on the risk of being judged as bothersome by the professional and therefore do not want to complain. Many patients said they were afraid of being seen as troublesome while hospitalized. To avoid being seen as troublesome, they did not ask for analgesics, especially when they observed that the nurses were busy.

> Interviewer: "Why did you wait two hours before you requested any analgesics?"
>
> Patient: "Because I didn't want to be troublesome" (male, age 70).

Experiencing basic mistrust: The expression of pain using a number from 0 to 10 was influenced by patients' perception of professionals; some patients hesitated to report a high NRS score, thinking that healthcare professionals would not believe that they were really in so much pain.

> "This week I gave a high pain score and I noticed that they (the nurses) looked at me as if to say, 'mmm, that is a very high score'. They almost don't believe you. Probably because it is rare that the pain score is that high. Like they can't handle it that the pain is so severe, I think, I noticed that" (male, age 45).

This basic mistrust, patients said, led them to intentionally report lower NRS scores than they actually perceived.

> "Well, there are interpretation differences between people. You're not allowed to complain. So, you lessen your pain score because you feel that no-one will accept if you say 'I feel so awful. I'm in so much pain', then you minimize your pain" (female, age 65).

One patient defined basic mistrust as "mental pain": "It hurt when someone said to me, 'Nothing is wrong with you!'" Patients thought that this disbelief was due to a lack of visible tissue damage. Patients felt they were not taken seriously by healthcare professionals when reporting an NRS score. They perceived that the professionals did not consider their pain serious. Patients clearly indicated that they wanted to be taken seriously, even when professionals thought that the reported NRS score was (too) high. Some patients indicated that it was important that the professional just listened to them, without judging.

> "Being taken seriously is pleasant for a patient. Knowing that you are being taken seriously, even though from an objective point of view it (the pain score) is not quite the right number on the scale" (female, age 65).

Wish to meet the expectations of professionals: Some patients wanted to meet the expectations of the professional in what pain score fits best on the experienced pain, considering what would be the most socially acceptable pain score. They adjusted their pain score to the estimated level of which they thought the professional will find it logical.

> "Then I think I will lower my score, otherwise they (the nurses) will think 'do you really have so much pain?' (female, age 63).
>
> "I am just going to give my usual scores and for now, I just not take my neuralgia into account. When my neuralgia gets worse again, then I will give it a score of 20 because adjusting my measure to even worse pain has been proven not efficacious to give a clear explanation of my experienced pain (to the nurses)" (female, age 26).

3.3.2 Analgesic administration. *Encounter ambivalence*: Many patients were ambivalent towards analgesics. On the one hand, they needed analgesics after surgery to recover, but on the other hand, they actually thought analgesics were not good for them because of toxicity.

"If it really hurts, after surgery for example, then I think it's necessary. But if it's not necessary, then preferably no painkiller, because ultimately it's junk what you're putting in your body" (female, age 18).

Some patients accepted analgesics and other patients said that most pain is transient, and therefore, refused analgesics. The different negative terms for analgesics given by patients, like "junk" or "rubbish," supported this opinion.

"There is so much rubbish in and I think every time 'O my God, it's morphine and it's better if I can do without.' They (the nurses) have explicitly told me that it's okay, but it plays on my mind" (female, age 71).

Suffering side effects: Some patients said that they refused opioids because they had previously experienced typical opioid side effects, such as sedation and nausea, even when the nausea had been treated appropriately. Once they are no longer opioid naive, patients often consciously weigh the desired analgesic effects of opioids against the negative side effects." One patient expressed this eloquently as follows:

"But as soon as I use too much morphine then I become very nauseous. You are constantly trying to find a balance between bearable pain and bearable nausea, shall we say" (female, age 65).

Variation on timing of opioids: There was significant variation in the pain levels at which patients wanted opioids to be administered. Some patients said they could bear the pain and did not need any analgesics. Other patients wanted light analgesics to be administered at NRS scores of 4–6. However, a large variability was seen when patients needed opioids: Some patients said they needed opioids at NRS scores from 6 onwards, while some only required opioids from NRS 7 or even higher:

"I want painkillers from a four and above and morphine, no, then I would say: eight or above" (male, age 36).

Patients gave different reasons for not wanting opioids (e.g., they had heard terrifying stories about opioids from family and friends, they had previously suffered from the side effects of opioids, they wanted to bear their own pain, they believed that pain was a signal telling the body it needed to rest or that they had to get used to pain).

Nurses have own point of view: Patients said that nurses had their own point of view about the meaning of the numbers from 0 to 10 and do not use the score to communicate about pain with the patient:

"As far as I can remember nobody asked me a question like that if the pain was mild because if it is severe, six or seven, then they (the nurses) say, 'what can we do about it?' But when it is three or four then they immediately say, 'okay' and write it down. I would prefer if they said, 'do you want us to do something about it or can you handle it', instead of saying, 'so, you're okay then'" (female, age 26).

Patients said that there was no agreement in terms of the NRS score at which nurses administered analgesics. One patient describes this as follows:

"Well I thought, the pain is easing, so I said five or four, one of those I said and then she (the nurse) said, 'well then you don't need any more painkillers.' And then I said no, then it is a six because it hurt and I needed them. Now I assume with five I won't get any painkillers so I think ok, with five no painkillers and I want some so I give a six and then I get them" (female, age 32).

In contrast, some patients who rated their pain as NRS 6 or 7 did not want additional analgesic medication, but nurses insisted that they accept additional pain medication according to acute pain treatment guidelines.

4. Discussion

The qualitative approach in this study identifies several elements underlying the process of a patient translating his/her currently experienced postoperative pain into a reported rating on the NRS. A model of this decision-making process is proposed made of the interrelationship between the factors that influence this rating process. The model may help healthcare professionals to better understand this process and the factors that possibly influence the NRS score that is actually reported to them. When assigning an NRS score to their pain, patients process the first two themes in stages: They first weigh score-related factors and intrapersonal factors. Some patients go through a last stage before telling the professional: weighing the anticipated consequences of reporting a particular NRS score against their actual desire for more or less analgesics. Patients can be aware of these factors, but most often, the entire process appears to be implicit and subconscious.

Quantifying pain through the self-reported NRS score from 0 to 10 is often referred to as the gold standard for pain assessment (Schiavenato and Craig, 2010). However, for a gold standard, self-report is fraught with limitations. Nowadays, pain professionals develop guidelines for pain treatment including the manner for instructing and informing patients how they should interpret NRS scores from 0 to 10. Our data suggest that this single number does not tell the whole story. Instead, healthcare professionals should listen to the patient's story about the experienced pain rather than simply administering analgesics as soon as a single pain score exceeds a numeric threshold. Without a pain assessment beyond the NRS by healthcare professionals, postoperative patients may be at risk of both undertreatment and overtreatment of their pain. The scores on the NRS are only important to detect change in postoperative pain treatment. Knowledge of the factors in this study that influence a patient's pain scoring can help professionals use simple questions to explore patients' unique pain experiences and consequently titrate analgesic treatment in dialogue with the patient, improving the quality and safety of care.

The current study also confirmed that patients find it especially difficult to rate their unique pain experience on the NRS when their score is in the middle of the sequence (i.e., 4 to 6) (Eriksson et al., 2014; Williams et al., 2000). Therefore, many patients considered an NRS score of 7 as the limit of pain acceptance, and at 7 or above, opioids were desired. This is clearly a much higher pain threshold than currently taught to professionals based on guidelines for acute pain management. There is no agreement on the optimal NRS cut-off score in guidelines for pain treatment and there is no agreement on how to identify an optimal NRS cut-off score for pain treatment (Gerbershagen et al., 2011). Rigid cut-off scores in guidelines for pain treatment should not be used with individual patients to prevent a risk of over- or undertreatment. Therefore, patients should be asked what their individual cut-off score is when they require a particular intervention.

Many factors are known to affect the experience of pain, including gender, age, culture, previous experiences, types of surgery, the meaning the pain has to the individual experiencing it, and psychological factors (e.g., coping skills) (Gerbershagen et al., 2013; Mackintosh, 2007). Patients often arrived at a new NRS score by comparing their worst previous pain experience with the current pain sensation (Dionne et al., 2005; Manias et al., 2004). In the current study, we found that the NRS scores from 0 to 10 can conceal real differences in pain intensity across patients, because previous pain experiences differ between patients.

In line with this finding, a previous study concluded that it is impossible to compare pain scores between patients, because we cannot share pain experiences (Bartoshuk et al., 2003).

Subjective norms influence the social pressure on the individual to exhibit (or not exhibit) a particular behaviour (Rhodes and Courneya, 2003). Our findings confirmed the idea that patients do not want to deviate from perceived social norms and be known as an individual who complains a lot (Eriksson et al., 2014; Hansson et al., 2011). Patients are afraid of being judged by healthcare professionals when the NRS score they report is perceived as "too high." This exact situation, called basic mistrust, is described in a phenomenological study in which nurses did not believe the patients (Söderhamn and Idvall, 2003). Only when there is confirmation by the professional does the patient feel empowered to assign a high NRS score.

Patients also envision what their reported pain scores will mean regarding the subsequent administration of analgesics, especially opioids. There appears to be a wide variation in how patients interpret NRS scores in relation to if, when, and how much analgesia needs to be given. The NRS cut-off points used in guidelines for acute pain are often lower than those of patients; patients tend to use the midpoint of the scale as the NRS cut-off value for additional analgesia. Therefore, most patients with NRS scores of 4, 5, and even 6 consider their pain "bearable" and do not want opioid analgesics. It seems that many professionals have learned this from patients and do not administer analgesics when patients' NRS pain scores are in the middle of the scale. In turn, patients have learned from previous reactions of professionals at what NRS score they will be administered a certain analgesic. A study of chronic pain patients also showed that patients have to give an NRS score higher than 5 in order to receive more analgesics from the nurse (Hansson et al., 2011).

Understanding the process by which patients make decisions is important to understand the decisions they make. In previous studies several factors are described that influence patients' decision-making process, e.g., past experiences, cognitive biases, age, and belief in personal relevance (Dietrich, 2010; Juliusson et al., 2005; Sagi and Frieland, 2007). Once the decision is made, levels of regret or satisfaction will impact future decisions (Juliusson et al., 2005; Sagi and Frieland, 2007). In the current study, patients anticipate on the consequences on reporting a particular pain score whether professionals will administrate analgesics or not depending on their past experiences in pain treatment. Additionally, patients anticipate on the judgement by healthcare professionals; some patients hesitated to report a high NRS score, thinking that healthcare professionals would not believe that they were really in so much pain (Idvall et al., 2008).

When the NRS score is used, a shared understanding of patients and professionals is crucial to the adequate treatment of pain. However, this seems difficult to realize, because the interpretation of pain scores differs between individuals. Everyone has its own standards and values that are impossible to change in favour of looking the same way to the pain scores from 0 to 10. Culture influences how each person experiences and responds to pain. Some cultures value stoicism and tend to avoid saying that there is pain and other cultural groups tend to be more expressive about pain (Narayan, 2010). Patients' diverse cultural patterns are not right or wrong, just different. The purpose is to achieve individualized pain assessment and pain treatment. Professionals evaluate patients' pain and make judgements that are required for prescribing pain treatment. Therefore, healthcare professionals must learn to think about analgesic administration in a more "patient- oriented" way: a patient has to be seen as a whole person in his/her social context, and his/her feelings, wishes, expectations, norms, and experiences have to be taken into account (Ouwens et al., 2012). Patients want to participate in the treatment of their pain and tell the healthcare professionals if and when they need analgesics because patients know what pain they have (Idvall et al., 2008; McTier et al., 2014; Joelsson et al., 2010).

Many patients could tolerate short bouts of severe pain during movement as well and did not desire additional opioids. For some patients, the pain can be so severe as to preclude adequate coughing. In these cases, it is important that patients accept additional analgesia to prevent pneumonia. In a previous study, we educated patients about the principles in postoperative pain management (Van Dijk et al., 2015). Patients' knowledge and beliefs changed, moreover, their behaviour did not change. Postoperative patients still gave high pain scores and considered this as bearable and did not want (extra) analgesics. Changing patients' habits is very difficult, as patients in the current qualitative study say that they want to hold their own standards and remain having their own point of view about pain management.

Although our study was restricted to only one university hospital, the richness of the data makes us confident that our analysis has captured the most typical aspects of patients' underlying processes for rating their pain on the NRS. Moreover, the current study is strengthened by the number of interviews and the fact that the new insights that emerged during data collection were incorporated into the interview topic list. In this qualitative study, only Dutch patients were interviewed, and the results are, therefore, not immediately generalizable to other countries and cultures. While we believe that many of the themes that we elicited (e.g., fear of being judged) will also emerge when repeated in other countries in the Western world, ideally a cross-cultural international study should be conducted to expand on the themes and to validate or extend our conceptual model of how patients arrive at their reported NRS scores. Such a study would possibly give interesting and important insights into crosscultural differences in the pain experience and responses to pharmacologic and non-pharmacologic pain treatments offered.

5. Conclusions

In postoperative pain management, NRS cut-off scores are widely used as a basis for administering or withholding opioid analgesics. Patients however, have a different view on these NRS cut-off scores; many patients consider NRS scores 4, 5 and 6 as bearable and do not need analgesics. Therefore, it is necessary to communicate with patients beyond the NRS score. The current qualitative study identified several elements of the underlying process (e.g., previous pain experiences, being tough on oneself, basic mistrust by healthcare professionals, and variation on timing of opioids) by which patients translate acute postoperative pain into a rating on the NRS. The factors in the model are subsumed under three main themes: score-related factors, intrapersonal factors, and the anticipated consequences of reporting a particular NRS score. Knowing these factors could help healthcare professionals to better understand the complex process by which patients assign pain scores and the factors that influence the scores that are ultimately reported to them. This could serve as basis for a dialogue aimed at clarifying the patient's current needs and result in more patient-centred, shared decision making regarding (opioid) analgesic administration improving the quality and safety of care.

6. Relevance to Clinical Practice

Pain assessment is the foundation of pain management when a patient is experiencing postoperative pain. Frequent and thorough assessment of patients' pain provides information to achieve optimal pain relief. We recommend assessing patients' pain on the NRS. Asking patients to score their pain on the NRS ensures that all professionals assess pain in the same way and with adequate treatment of postoperative pain, subsequent NRS scores are expected to be lower. Nevertheless, the NRS score is not an absolute number. Once the patient has reported an NRS score, the professional is not finished. Rather, the professional should communicate with the patient to understand the meaning of this particular score without being judgemental. Healthcare professionals should understand that patients can have their own interpretation of the pain scale and might have different ideas regarding the particular NRS score that signifies the need for additional analgesics. Rigid cut-off scores in guidelines for postoperative pain treatment should not be used with individual patients; patients should be asked what their individual cut-off score is when requiring a particular intervention.

Acknowledgments

The authors would like to thank all the participants for their contribution to this study.
Conflict of interest: None declared.
Funding: Support was provided solely by departmental sources.
Ethical approval: This study was approved by the Medical Ethics Committee of the University Medical Center Utrecht.

Appendix A. Supplementary Data

Supplementary material related to this article can be found, in the online version, at http://dx.doi.org/10.1016/j. ijnurstu.2015.08.007.

REFERENCES

Apfelbaum, J. L., Chen, C., Mehta, S. S., & Gan, T. J. (2003). Postoperative pain experience: results from a national survey suggest postoperative pain continues to be undermanaged. *Anesth. Analg*, *97*(2), 534–540.

Arbour, C., & Gelinas, C. (2010). Are vital signs valid indicators for the assessment of pain in post-operative cardiac surgery ICU adults? *Intens. Crit. Care Nurs*, *26*(2), 83–90.

Aubrun, F., Paqueron, X., Langeron, O., et al. (2003). What pain scales do nurses use in the postanaesthesia care unit? *Eur. J. Anaesthesiol*, *20*(9), 745–749.

Bartoshuk, L. M., Duffy, V. B., Fast, K., et al. (2003). Labeled scales (e.g., category, Likert, VAS) and invalid across-group comparisons: what we have learned from genetic variation in taste. *Food Qual. Prefer*, *14*(2), 125–138.

Boeije, H. (2010). *Analysis in Qualitative Research*. London: SAGE.

Cashman, J. N., & Dolin, S. J. (2004). Respiratory and haemodynamic effects of acute postoperative pain management: evidence from published data. *Br. J. Anaesth*, *93*(2), 212–223.

Charmaz, K. (2014). *Constructing Grounded Theory* (2nd ed.). London: SAGE Publications.

Dietrich, C. (2010). Decision making: factors that influence decision making, heuristics used, and decision outcomes. *Stud. Pulse*, *2*(2), 1–3.

Dionne, R. A., Bartoshuk, L., Mogil, J., & Witter, J. (2005). Individual responder analyses for pain: does one pain scale fit all? *Trends Pharmacol. Sci*, *26*(3), 125–130.

Eriksson, K., Wikström, L., Årestedt, K., et al. (2014). Numeric rating scale: patients' perceptions of its use in postoperative pain assessments. *Appl. Nurs. Res*, *27*(1), 41–46.

Gelinas, C., & Arbour, C. (2009). Behavioral and physiologic indicators during a nociceptive procedure in conscious and unconscious mechanically ventilated adults: similar or different? *J. Crit. Care*, *24*(4), 628.e7–628.17.

Gerbershagen, H. J., Rothaug, J., Kalkman, C. J., & Meissner, W. (2011). Determination of moderate-to-severe postoperative pain on the numeric rating scale: a cut-off point analysis applying four different methods. *Br. J. Anaesth*, *107*(4), 619–626.

Gerbershagen, H. J., Aduckathil, S., van Wijck, A. J., et al. (2013). Pain intensity on the first day after surgery: a prospective cohort study comparing 179 surgical procedures. *Anesthesiology*, *118*(4), 934–944.

Gordon, D. B., Dahl, J. L., Miaskowski, C., et al. (2005). American Pain Society recommendations for improving the quality of acute and cancer pain management: American Pain Society quality of care task force. *Arch. Intern. Med*, *165*(14), 1574–1580.

Hansson, K. S., Fridlund, B., Brunt, D., et al. (2011). The meaning of the experiences of persons with chronic pain in their encounters with the health service. *Scand. J. Caring Sci*, *25*(3), 444–450.

Hartrick, C., Kovan, J., & Shapiro, S. (2003). The numeric rating scale for clinical pain measurement: a ratio measure? *Pain Pract*, *3*(4), 310.

Idvall, E., Berg, K., Unosson, M., & Brudin, L. (2005). Differences between nurse and patient assessments on postoperative pain management in two hospitals. *J. Eval. Clin. Pract*, *11*(5), 444–451.

Idvall, E., Bergqvist, A., Silverhjelm, J., & Unosson, M. (2008). Perspectives of Swedish patients on postoperative pain management. *Nurs. Health Sci*, *10*(2), 131–136.

Joelsson, M., Olsson, L. E., & Jakobsson, E. (2010). Patients' experience of pain and pain relief following hip replacement surgery. *J. Clin. Nurs*, *19*(19–20), 2832–2838.

Juliusson, E., Karlsson, N., & Garling, T. (2005). Weighing the past and the future in decision making. *Eur. J. Cogn. Psychol*, *17*(4), 561–575.

Lincoln, Y., & Guba, E. (Eds.), (1985). *Naturalistic Inquiry*. Newbury Park: Saga Publication.

Mackintosh, C. (2007). Assessment and management of patients with postoperative pain. *Nurs. Stand*, *22*(5), 49–55.

Manias, E., Bucknall, T., & Botti, M. (2004). Assessment of patient pain in the postoperative context. *West. J. Nurs. Res*, *26*(7), 751–769.

Max, M. B., Donovan, M., Miaskowski, C. A., et al. (1995). Quality improvement guidelines for the treatment of acute pain and cancer pain. *J. Am. Med. Assoc*, *274*(23), 1874–1880.

McTier, L., Botti, M., & Duke, M. (2014). Patient participation in quality pain management during an acute care admission. *Clin. J. Pain*, *30*(4), 316–323.

Narayan, M. C. (2010). Culture's effects on pain assessment and management. *Am. J. Nurs*, *110*(4), 38–47, quiz 48–9.

Ouwens, M., van der Burg, S., Faber, M., & van der Weijden, T. (2012). *Shared Decision Making and Self-management, in Dutch*. Nijmegen: Scientific Institute for Quality of Healthcare.

Rhodes, R. E., & Courneya, K. S. (2003). Investigating multiple components of attitude, subjective norm, and perceived control: an examination of the theory of planned behaviour in the exercise domain. *Br. J. Social Psychol*, *42*(1), 129–146.

Sagi, A., & Frieland, N. (2007). The cost of richness: the effect of the size and diversity of decision sets on post-decision regret. *J. Personal. Social Psychol*, *93*(4), 515–524.

Schiavenato, M., & Craig, K. D. (2010). Pain assessment as a social transaction: beyond the "gold standard". *Clin. J. Pain*, *26*(8), 667–676.

Sloman, R., Rosen, G., Rom, M., & Shir, Y. (2005). Nurses' assessment of pain in surgical patients. *J. Adv. Nurs*, *52*(2), 125–132.

Söderhamn, O., & Idvall, E. (2003). Nurses' influence on quality of care in postoperative pain management: a phenomenological study. *Int. J. Nurs. Pract*, *9*(1), 26–32.

Sommer, M., de Rijke, J. M., van Kleef, M., et al. (2008). The prevalence of postoperative pain in a sample of 1490 surgical inpatients. *Eur. J. Anaesthesiol*, *25*(4), 267–274.

Taylor, S., Kirton, O. C., Staff, I., & Kozol, R. A. (2005). Postoperative day one: a high risk period for respiratory events. *Am. J. Surg*, *190*(5), 752–756.

Tong, A., Sainsbury, P., & Craig, J. (2007). Consolidated criteria for reporting qualitative research (COREQ): a 32-item checklist for interviews and focus groups. *Int. J. Qual. Health Care*, *19*(6), 349–357.

Van Dijk, J. F. M., Van Wijck, A. J. M., Kappen, T. H., et al. (2012). Postoperative pain assessment based on numeric ratings is not the same for patients and professionals: a cross-sectional study. *Int. J. Nurs. Stud*, *49*(1), 65–71.

Van Dijk, J. F., van Wijck, A. J., Kappen, T. H., et al. (2015). The effect of a preoperative educational film on patients' postoperative pain in relation to their request for opioids. *Pain Manag. Nurs*, *16*(2), 137–145.

VMS Safety Program. (2009). "Early recognition and treatment of pain". (in Dutch), www.vmszorg.nl.

Watt-Watson, J. H. (1999). Canadian pain society position statement on pain relief. *Pain Res. Manag*, *4*(2), 75–78.

Williams, A. C. D. C., Davies, H. T. O., & Chadury, Y. (2000). Simple pain rating scales hide complex idiosyncratic meanings. *Pain*, *85*(3), 457–463.

APPENDIX D

Example of a Correlational Study (Turner et al., 2016)

Psychological Functioning, Post-Traumatic Growth, and Coping in Parents and Siblings of Adolescent Cancer Survivors

Andrea M. Turner-Sack, PhD, Rosanne Menna, PhD, Sarah R. Setchell, PhD, Cathy Maan, PhD, and Danielle Cataudella, PsyD

Purpose/Objectives: To examine psychological functioning, post-traumatic growth (PTG), coping, and cancer-related characteristics of adolescent cancer survivors' parents and siblings.

Design: Descriptive, correlational.

Setting: Children's Hospital of Western Ontario in London, Ontario, Canada.

Sample: Adolescents who finished cancer treatment 2–10 years prior (n = 31), as well as their parents (n = 30) and siblings (n = 18).

Methods: Participants completed self-report measures of psychological distress, PTG, life satisfaction, coping, and cancer-related characteristics.

Main Research Variables: Psychological functioning, PTG, and coping.

Findings: Parents' and siblings' PTG levels were similar to survivors' PTG levels; however, parents reported higher PTG than siblings. Parents who used less avoidant coping, were younger, and had higher life satisfaction experienced less psychological distress. Parents whose survivor children used more active coping reported less psychological distress. Siblings who were older used more active coping, and the longer it had been since their brother or sister was diagnosed, the less avoidant coping they used.

Conclusions: Childhood and adolescent cancer affects survivors' siblings and parents in unique ways.

Implications for Nursing: Relationship to the survivor, use of coping strategies, life satisfaction, and time since diagnosis affect family members' postcancer experiences.

Since the 1980s, the incidence rates of childhood and adolescent cancer have increased and the mortality rates have decreased in the United States and Canada (National Cancer Institute, n.d.; National Cancer Institute of Canada, 2008). This has resulted in a growing population of young cancer survivors with a unique set of psychological issues. Researchers have explored some of these issues, including survivors' moods, anxieties, and coping strategies (Dejong & Fombonne, 2006; Schultz et al., 2007; Turner-Sack, Menna, Setchell, Mann, & Cataudella, 2012). However, the focus is often on the negative aspects of childhood cancer, such as depression, with fewer studies addressing a more positive aspect, such as positive changes in perspectives, life priorities, and interpersonal relationships (Kamibeppu et al., 2010; Seitz, Besier, & Goldbeck, 2009). In addition, the experiences of young cancer survivors' families often are ignored.

The diagnosis and treatment of cancer in childhood or adolescence can be exceptionally stressful not only for the young patients with cancer, but also for members of their family. Several studies suggest that parents of children and adolescents with cancer experience psychological distress, post-traumatic stress, and poor quality of life (Brown, Madan-Swain, & Lambert, 2003; Kazak et al., 1997, 2004; Witt et al., 2010). Other studies indicate that parents of cancer survivors appear to function just as well as parents of healthy controls or in accordance with standardized norms (Dahlquist, Czyzewski, & Jones, 1996; Greenberg, Kazak, & Meadows, 1989; Radcliffe, Bennett, Kazak, Foley, & Phillips, 1996).

Similar to research on parents of young cancer survivors, studies of the psychological impact on siblings within these families are scarce. Several studies have found that siblings of young cancer survivors have more negative emotional reactions (e.g., fear, worry, anger), more post-traumatic stress, and poorer quality of life than controls (Alderfer et al., 2010; Alderfer, La-bay, & Kazak, 2003). Other studies found that siblings of survivors function similarly to their peers whose siblings are healthy (Dolgin et al., 1997; Kamibeppu et al., 2010). Together, these findings suggest that family members of young cancer survivors experience a range of psychological responses to cancer and that additional research could provide some clarification.

Although understanding how survivors' cancer affects their parents and siblings is important, equally important is understanding the associations among family members' psychological functioning. In accordance with a family systems perspective, a person's wellbeing is related to other family members' wellbeing (Nichols & Schwartz, 2001). In support of this perspective, research generally has found that most young cancer survivors' psychological functioning is related to their parents' psychological functioning (Barakat et al., 1997; Brown et al., 2003; Phipps, Long, Hudson, & Rai, 2005). Few studies have examined the relations between young cancer survivors' psychological distress and their siblings' psychological distress.

Although coping with a traumatic experience, such as cancer, tends to be distressing, it also may provide individuals with the opportunity to achieve positive change, such as post-traumatic growth (PTG). PTG is defined as mastering a previously experienced trauma, perceiving benefits from it, and developing beyond the original level of psychological functioning (Tedeschi, Park, & Calhoun, 1998). Similar to the literature concerning young cancer survivors, PTG in parents of young survivors has received little attention. The few studies that exist suggest that parents of young survivors may experience at least some degree of PTG (Best, Streisand, Catania, & Kazak, 2001; Yaskowich, 2003). Research of PTG in other family members of patients with cancer also is limited. Kamibeppu et al. (2010) found that young adult sisters of young adult childhood cancer survivors reported experiencing greater PTG than female controls. Other studies identified some positive changes that siblings experienced (e.g., feeling more mature, independent, and empathic; valuing life more) (Barbarin et al., 1995; Chesler, Allswede, & Barbarin, 1992; Havermans & Eiser, 1994), but the researchers did not determine whether the siblings perceived as much benefit from the trauma or developed beyond their original level of functioning enough to be consistent with PTG. In keeping with the familial model of illness-related stress and growth, the current study examined PTG in parents and siblings of adolescent cancer survivors.

The lack of research examining the relations among family members' levels of PTG is not surprising given the limited research examining PTG in parents and siblings of young cancer survivors. Two studies have found that parents' PTG was not correlated with adolescent cancer survivors' overall PTG (Michel, Taylor, Absolom, & Eiser, 2010; Yaskowich, 2003). However, parents' PTG accounted for as much as 10% of the variance in two aspects of survivors' PTG: improved relationships and appreciation for life (Yaskowich, 2003). These results suggest that the association between survivor PTG and PTG among other family members warrants further investigation. The current study fills a notable gap in the literature by examining the associations between adolescent cancer survivors' PTG and PTG in parents and siblings of survivors.

An additional goal of the current study was to examine whether coping strategies were related to psychological functioning and PTG in parents and siblings of adolescent cancer survivors. Available studies suggest that parents of young patients with cancer and survivors who use more self-directed and active coping report lower levels of psychological distress, and those who use more emotion-focused and avoidant coping report higher levels of psychological distress (Fuemmeler, Mullins, & Marx, 2001; Norberg, Lindblad, & Boman, 2005). Other studies indicate that siblings of adolescent cancer survivors who have high emotional social support tend to be less depressed, be less anxious, and have fewer behavioral problems than siblings with low emotional social support (Barrera, Fleming, & Khan, 2004). To the researchers' knowledge, no studies have examined the associations between parents' and siblings' coping strategies and their levels of PTG, but Calhoun and Tedeschi's (1998) model of PTG suggests that active social support and acceptance coping are most closely associated with PTG.

Examining demographic and cancer-related variables, such as age of parents and siblings, survivors' age at diagnosis, time since diagnosis, and time since treatment completion, can provide insight into the experiences of young cancer survivors and their families. Little is known about the relations between age and psychological functioning, PTG, and coping in siblings of cancer survivors (Alderfer et al., 2003). Several studies have found that adolescent cancer survivors' age at diagnosis was unrelated to parents' posttraumatic stress symptoms (Brown et al., 2003; Kazak et al., 1997) and PTG (Barakat, Alderfer, & Kazak, 2006). In terms of PTG, theorists have suggested that, although positive consequences of life crises can happen shortly after the crisis, they are more likely to occur after a long process of crisis resolution and personal recovery (Schaefer & Moos, 1992). However, the only known study to examine the relation between time since cancer treatment and parental PTG found that a shorter time since the end of young cancer survivors' treatment was associated with more PTG in fathers but not mothers (Barakat et al., 2006).

The goals of the current study were to (a) examine psychological functioning (defined as level of distress and life dissatisfaction), PTG, and coping in parents and siblings of adolescent cancer survivors; (b) compare adolescent cancer survivors, parents, and siblings on those same variables; and (c) examine psychological functioning, PTG, and coping in parents and siblings in relation to age, time, and cancer-related variables.

METHODS

Sample

English-speaking Canadian families with an adolescent (aged 13–20 years) who completed treatment for a solid tumor, leukemia, or lymphoma 2–10 years earlier at a children's hospital were eligible to participate in the study (see Table 1). They were not eligible if they had a cancer relapse, an organ transplantation, a brain tumor that required only surgery, or

TABLE 1 Characteristics of Study Participants

Characteristic	ADOLESCENT CANCER SURVIVORS (N = 31)		PARENTS (N = 30)		SIBLINGS (N = 18)	
	$\bar{X}$	SD	$\bar{X}$	SD	$\bar{X}$	SD
Age (years)	15.74	2.25	45.07	5.64	15.67	2.74
Age at diagnosis (years)	7.45	4.75	–	–	6.83	3.97
Time since diagnosis (years)	8.28	3.02	–	–	–	–
Time since treatment completion (years)	6.47	2.67	–	–	–	–
Treatment duration (months)	21.31	12.1	–	–	–	–
Characteristic	**n**		**n**		**n**	
Gender						
Female	20		29		9	
Male	11		1		9	
Ethnicity						
European/Canadian	27		27		16	
Not reported	4		3		2	
Education						
Graduated college or university	–		20		–	
Graduated high school	–		7		–	
Not reported	–		3		–	
Diagnosis						
Acute lymphoblastic leukemia	18		–		–	
Hodgkin lymphoma	4		–		–	
Acute myelogenous leukemia	3		–		–	
Ewing's sarcoma	2		–		–	
Osteosarcoma	2		–		–	
Non-Hodgkin lymphoma	1		–		–	
Wilms' tumor	1		–		–	
Treatment[a]						
Chemotherapy	31		–		–	
Radiation	4		–		–	
Surgery	3		–		–	

[a] Several respondents had multiple types of treatment.

significant cognitive or neurologic impairments. All siblings reported living with the survivor while he or she was receiving treatment.

Procedure

Following institutional ethics approvals from the University of Windsor in Ontario, Canada and the University of Western Ontario in London, Ontario, Canada, data were collected from the pediatric oncology population at Children's Hospital of Western Ontario in London, Ontario, Canada. Questionnaires were mailed to 89 families that met criteria for the study. They were informed that participants' names would be entered into a drawing for a $50 gift certificate from a local store. Thirty-one adolescents, 30 parents, and 18 siblings returned completed packages. In total, 35 families had at least one member participate in the study. Fourteen families had an adolescent, parent, and sibling participate. The remaining 21 families had various combinations of family member participation, and, as such, the adolescent, parent, and sibling groups represent different sets of families in the current study.

Measures

Demographics and cancer variables: Participants completed a background questionnaire that asked about age, gender, ethnicity, education, type of cancer, age at diagnosis, time since diagnosis, time since treatment completion, and length and type of treatment.

Psychological distress: The Brief Symptom Inventory (BSI) (Derogatis & Melisaratos, 1983) was used to assess psychological distress. Participants used this 53-item questionnaire to self-report to what extent they experienced psychological symptoms. Participants rated their symptoms in a number of areas (e.g., somatization, depression, anxiety) on a five-point scale ranging from 0–4, with 0 indicating not at all and 4 indicating extremely. The BSI generates scores on three overall indices of distress: General Severity Index (GSI), Positive Symptom Distress Index, and Positive Symptom Total. Analyses used GSI t scores, with low scores indicating low psychological distress. The internal consistency in the current study was 0.97 for survivors and siblings and 0.98 for parents.

Life satisfaction: Survivors and siblings completed the Students' Life Satisfaction Scale (SLSS) (Huebner, 1991), a self-report questionnaire that assesses global life satisfaction in children and adolescents. Participants used a six-point scale ranging from 1 (strongly disagree) to 6 (strongly agree) to respond to seven statements about their lives. The average score per SLSS item was used in the analyses, with high scores indicating more life satisfaction. The internal consistency in the current study was 0.87 for survivors and siblings.

Parents completed the Satisfaction With Life Scale (SWLS) (Diener, Emmons, Larsen, & Griffin, 1985), a self-report questionnaire that assesses adult global life satisfaction. Parents used a seven-point scale ranging from 1 (strongly disagree) to 7 (strongly agree) to respond to five statements about their life. The average score per SWLS item was used in the analyses, with high scores indicating more life satisfaction. In the current study, the internal consistency was 0.91 for parents.

Post-traumatic growth: The PTG Inventory (PTGI) (Tedeschi & Calhoun, 1996) assesses the experience of positive changes following a traumatic event. Participants used the 21-item self-report questionnaire to indicate the extent to which they experienced various positive changes. Participants used a six-point scale ranging from 0–5, with 0 indicating "I did not experience this change as a result of my crisis," and 5 indicating "I experienced this change to a very great degree as a result of my crisis." The PTGI wording was modified to refer specifically to changes resulting from having had a family member with cancer. In addition, the language used in the PTGI given to siblings was modified to better suit a younger population (similar to modifications used by Yaskowich [2003]). The average score per PTGI item was used in the analyses, with high scores indicating more PTG. Tedeschi and Calhoun (1996) reported an internal consistency coefficient of 0.9 for the full scale and a test-retest reliability of 0.71 after two months. Yaskowich (2003) reported an internal consistency of 0.94 for the full scale of the modified PTGI in a sample of 35 adolescent cancer survivors. The internal consistency of the modified PTGI was 0.94 for survivors and siblings and 0.96 for parents in the current study.

Coping strategies: The COPE (Carver, Scheier, & Weintraub, 1989) assesses coping strategies in adolescents and adults. Participants used this 60-item self-report questionnaire to rate the way they respond to stressful events. Participants used a four-point scale ranging from 1–4, with 1 indicating "I usually do not do this at all," and 4 indicating

"I usually do this a lot." The COPE yields scores on 15 different scales. Factor analyses have revealed slightly different factor structures for adolescents and adults. Phelps and Jarvis (1994) proposed a four-factor structure for adolescents: active coping, emotion-focused coping, avoidant coping, and acceptance coping.

Similarly, Carver et al. (1989) proposed a four-factor structure for adults: active coping, social support and emotion-focused coping, avoidant coping, and acceptance coping. The current study used the four factors proposed by Phelps and Jarvis (1994) for the survivors and siblings and the four factors proposed by Carver et al. (1989) for the parents. The religious coping scale was not associated with any of the factors but was included for all groups. High scores on a particular factor or scale reflect a greater use of that type of coping strategy. In the current study, internal consistency ranged from 0.74 (acceptance coping) to 0.94 (religious coping) for survivors and siblings, and from 0.52 (avoidant coping) to 0.94 (religious coping) for parents.

Data Analyses

All tests of significance were two-tailed with an alpha level of 0.01 to correct for the number of analyses performed and type I errors. Analyses were completed separately for parents and siblings. Pearson product-moment correlations and standard regressions with forward entry were conducted to examine parents' and siblings' reports of demographic and cancer-related variables in relation to their reported levels of psychological distress, life satisfaction, PTG, and coping strategies. Independent sample t tests were conducted to compare the survivors, parents, and siblings on measures of psychological distress, life satisfaction, PTG, and coping strategies. To examine the associations between survivors' coping, psychological distress, and PTG and that of their matched parents, Pearson product-moment correlations were used.

RESULTS

The focus of this article is family members of adolescent cancer survivors, particularly their parents and siblings. Detailed information on the psychological functioning, PTG, and coping of adolescent cancer survivors in the current study are provided in Turner-Sack et al. (2012).

Parents' psychological distress was positively associated with age ($r = 0.53$, $p < 0.01$) and avoidant coping (e.g., denial, disengagement) ($r = 0.52$, $p < 0.01$), and it was negatively associated with life satisfaction ($r = -0.62$, $p < 0.001$) and active coping (e.g., focusing on, planning, and actively dealing with problems; seeking helpful social support) ($r = -0.57$, $p < 0.001$). Life satisfaction was also positively correlated with active coping ($r = 0.56$, $p < 0.001$). Time since treatment completion was positively associated with parents' social support and emotion-focused coping ($r = 0.5$, $p < 0.01$).

A standard regression analysis was performed to predict parents' psychological distress using parent variables correlated with it: active coping, avoidant coping, life satisfaction, and age. The overall regression model for psychological distress was significant ($R^2 = 0.51$; $F[3, 22] = 7.69$, $p < 0.001$). Examination of the squared semipartial correlation coefficients indicated that avoidant coping ($\beta = 0.37$, $t[25] = 2.42$, $p < 0.05$; $sr^2 = 0.13$), age ($\beta = 0.35$, $t[25] = -2.26$, $p < 0.05$; $sr^2 = 0.11$), and life satisfaction ($\beta = -0.33$, $t[25] = 2.14$, $p < 0.05$; $sr^2 = 0.1$) made significant unique contributions to the prediction of psychological distress. Therefore, parents who used less avoidant coping, were younger, and had higher life satisfaction were likely to experience less psychological distress. Parents' PTG was not significantly associated with any of the study variables.

Siblings' age was positively associated with active coping ($r = 0.73, p < 0.001$). Avoidant coping was negatively associated with time since diagnosis ($r = -0.67, p < 0.01$) and life satisfaction ($r = -0.71, p < 0.001$). None of the variables correlated with siblings' psychological distress or PTG at the 0.01 significance level.

For each measure, the mean scores, standard deviations, and ranges of scores are presented for adolescent cancer survivors and siblings (see Table 2) and parents (see Table 3). Survivors, parents, and siblings reported similar levels of psychological distress but significantly different levels of PTG ($F[2, 75] = 5.32, p < 0.01$). Parents' PTG was significantly higher than that of siblings ($t[46] = 2.91, p < 0.01$), and survivors' PTG was similar to that

TABLE 2 Scores on Measures of Psychological Distress, Coping, Post-Traumatic Growth, and Life Satisfaction for Adolescent Cancer Survivors and Siblings

	ADOLESCENT CANCER SURVIVORS (N = 31)			SIBLINGS (N = 18)		
Measure	**$\bar{X}$**	**SD**	**Range**	**$\bar{X}$**	**SD**	**Range**
Brief Symptom Inventory[a] COPE[b]	47.31	13.59	25–79	48.94	10.83	27–72
• Acceptance coping	2.58	0.42	1.63–3.53	2.53	0.46	1.81–3.19
• Active coping	2.23	0.58	1.38–3.38	2.17	0.49	1.38–3.13
• Avoidant coping	1.33	0.3	1–2.05	1.41	0.3	1.08–2.15
• Emotion-focused coping	2.08	0.77	1.13–3.63	1.99	0.73	1–3.5
• Religious coping	2.24	1	1–4	1.88	1.13	1–4
Post-Traumatic Growth Inventory[c]	2.15	1.01	0–3.62	1.84	1.14	0–3.33
Students' Life Satisfaction Scale [d]	4.77	0.86	2.3–5.9	4.43	0.79	2.4–5.3

[a] Possible scores range from 1 (low psychological distress) to 100 (high psychological distress).
[b] Possible scores range from 1 (lesser use of the coping strategy) to 4 (greater use of the coping strategy).
[c] Possible scores range from 0 (low post-traumatic growth) to 5 (high post-traumatic growth).
[d] Possible scores range from 1 (low life satisfaction) to 6 (high life satisfaction).

TABLE 3 Scores on Measures of Psychological Distress, Coping, Post-Traumatic Growth, and Life Satisfaction for Parents (N = 30)

Measure	**$\bar{X}$**	**SD**	**Range**
Brief Symptom Inventory[a]	53.72	11.94	33–80
COPE[b]			
• Acceptance coping	3.01	0.42	1.98–3.75
• Active coping	2.81	0.54	1.58–3.91
• Avoidant coping	1.55	0.25	1.17–2.17
• Religious coping	2.64	1.01	1–4
• Social support and emotion-focused coping	2.61	0.52	1.58–3.55
Post-Traumatic Growth Inventory[c]	2.83	1.13	0.05–4.67
Satisfaction With Life Scale[d]	5.21	1.2	1.8–7

[a] Possible scores range from 1 (low psychological distress) to 100 (high psychological distress).
[b] Possible scores range from 1 (lesser use of the coping strategy) to 4 (greater use of the coping strategy).
[c] Possible scores range from 0 (low post-traumatic growth) to 5 (high post-traumatic growth).
[d] Possible scores range from 1 (low life satisfaction) to 6 (high life satisfaction).

TABLE 4 Correlations Between Adolescent Cancer Survivors' and Matched Parents' Psychological Distress, Post-Traumatic Growth, and Coping (N = 28)

Variable	PD	PTG	ACT	AVD	SSEF	ACP	RLG
PD	−0.11	0.09	0.08	0.06	0.13	0.05	−0.041
PTG	−0.45*	0.05	0.39*	−0.04	−0.12	0.31	0.02
ACT	−0.53**	0.04	0.14	−0.07	−0.38*	0.18	0.08
AVD	−0.2	−0.05	0.23	0.02	0.02	0.1	0.01
EF	−0.19	0.14	0.08	0.04	−0.08	−0.15	−0.43*
ACP	−0.14	−0.24	−0.01	0.19	−0.11	0.03	−0.13
RLG	−0.05	0.04	0.2	0.02	0.15	−0.14	−0.15

* $p < 0.05$; ** $p < 0.001$

ACP—acceptance coping; ACT—active coping; AVD—avoidant coping; EF—emotion-focused coping; PD—psychological distress; PTG—post-traumatic growth; SSEF—social support and emotion-focused coping; RLG—religious coping

of parents (t[58] = −2.43, not significant [NS]) and siblings (t[47] = −0.98, NS). No significant differences were seen between survivors and siblings on their levels of life satisfaction (t[47] = 1.16, NS) or active (t[47] = 0.3, NS), avoidant (t[46] = −0.93, NS), emotion-focused (t[47] = 0.39, NS), acceptance (t[47] = 0.38, NS), or religious (t[47] = 1.14, NS) coping strategies. Parents' coping levels were not compared with survivor or sibling coping levels because the adult COPE factor structure differed from the adolescent COPE factor structure.

In 28 of the 35 participating families, the survivor and one of his or her parents participated, resulting in 28 matched survivor-parent dyads. Correlations for matched dyads are presented in Table 4. Parents' psychological distress was negatively correlated with their survivor child's active coping ($r = -0.53$, $p < 0.01$).

DISCUSSION

The current study revealed that younger age, higher life satisfaction, and less avoidant coping were strong predictors of lower psychological distress in parents of adolescent cancer survivors. As parents get older, they may have a greater awareness of the difficulties and possible limitations that their adolescent cancer survivors may face. Younger parents may pay less attention to these difficulties or be more naive about them and, as such, report experiencing less psychological distress. Parents who are more satisfied with their lives (e.g., feel their lives are good, have what they want in life, would change little about their lives) may have fewer concerns and feel assured and grounded, which could contribute to lower levels of psychological distress. This finding is consistent with previous studies that found that parents' reports of external attributions about cause, rather than self-blame and family satisfaction, are associated with better psychological adjustment (Kazak et al., 1997; Vrijmoet-Wiersma et al., 2008). Finally, parents who face their difficulties to a greater degree are likely less troubled or burdened by neglected ongoing difficulties and, therefore, experience less psychological distress.

Research on how family members of young cancer survivors cope is scarce. The current study found that the longer ago that the adolescent cancer survivors completed treatment, the more social support and emotion-focused coping the parents used. As time passes after treatment is completed, parents may feel that they have more time in their daily lives to use the social support available to them and feel better able to face and deal with their emotions. The findings also suggest that older siblings were likely to use more active coping strategies. When a brother or sister was receiving cancer treatment, parents were occupied with the child with cancer, so older siblings likely had to attend to their own needs (Alderfer et al., 2010). In addition, during this period of time, siblings may have learned about the use of self-reliance, active coping, and problem solving.

Overall, siblings used similar coping strategies to survivors. Siblings whose brother or sister was diagnosed longer ago tended to use less avoidant coping. Siblings may use avoidant coping to deal with the stressors they experience soon after their brother or sister is diagnosed. As time passes, they may experience fewer cancer-related stressors, better adapt to such stressors, and find more effective ways of coping with them, using less avoidant coping strategies. The current study also found that siblings with greater life satisfaction used less avoidant coping. Those who are more satisfied with their lives may feel that they have fewer problems or difficult situations to avoid and, therefore, use less avoidant coping.

The researchers' results indicate that adolescent cancer survivors, parents, and siblings had average levels of psychological distress compared to reported norms. This finding is consistent with previous research that reported that most young cancer survivors have average or above-average levels of global adjustment (Fritz & Williams, 1988; Greenberg et al., 1989; Kazak et al., 1997), and parents of young patients with cancer and survivors have levels of anxiety, depression, and overall distress comparable to reported norms (Dahlquist et al., 1996; Greenberg et al., 1989; Radcliffe et al., 1996). These findings also fit with Van Dongen-Melman, De Groof, Hählen, and Verhulst (1995), who suggested that young siblings of child and adolescent cancer survivors and young siblings of healthy children and adolescents have similar levels of psychological distress.

Knowledge Translation

- Parents and adolescent siblings of young cancer survivors can experience post-traumatic growth.
- Healthcare providers can help identify family members of young cancer survivors who are experiencing psychological difficulties by being aware of the risk factors.
- Healthcare providers can educate family members about healthy, effective coping strategies; helping parents learn how to deal with their stressors more directly may enhance their psychological functioning.

In the current study, parents experienced a level of PTG that was similar to survivors, as well as to adult cancer survivors in other research (Cordova, Cunningham, Carlson, & Andrykowski, 2001; Weiss, 2002) and parents of child and adolescent cancer survivors in other research (Yaskowich, 2003). However, their level of PTG was higher than husbands of breast cancer survivors (Weiss, 2002) and lower than siblings in the current study. Although their own lives are not at risk, parents of young cancer survivors may be as affected by, and likely to experience PTG in response to, the trauma of cancer as if their own lives were at risk. Because of the close and dependent nature of the child-parent relationship, parents may feel closer to the trauma of cancer and experience a stronger reaction than siblings or husbands of cancer survivors. However, the latter may be related, at least in part, to gender differences.

Siblings experienced less PTG than parents in the current study and less PTG than adult cancer survivors in other research (Cordova et al., 2001). However, they experienced similar levels of PTG to the survivors in the current study, adolescent cancer survivors in other research (Yaskowich, 2003), and husbands of breast cancer survivors in other research (Weiss, 2002). Therefore, proximity to the trauma may influence PTG, as may cognitive maturation. The current study also indicates that even siblings in early adolescence have the capacity to experience PTG in response to their brother or sister having had cancer. To the researchers' knowledge, this is the first study to report the status of PTG in siblings and parents of adolescent cancer survivors.

Parents' psychological distress was associated with survivors using less active coping. Active coping involves actively planning and dealing with problems, focusing on problems without getting distracted, and seeking helpful social support. Parents whose survivor children actively address and cope with their challenges may feel relieved and proud that the survivors are capable of dealing with life's difficulties. In contrast, parents whose survivor children use little active coping may feel the need to plan for them and actively encourage them to solve their problems. These parents may feel burdened by such added responsibilities and more worried about the survivors, which could result in higher levels of psychological distress.

Limitations

The sample size was small, which could have limited the power and obscured significant effects that may have been revealed with a larger sample. The sample consisted primarily of middle-class European/Canadians who chose to participate in the study; therefore, the results may not generalize to more diverse populations and to family members who chose not to participate. All but one of the parents in the current study were mothers; therefore, the results may not generalize to fathers. Finally, the survivors, parents, and siblings represented different sets of families.

IMPLICATIONS FOR NURSING

Healthcare providers have contact not only with their patients, but also with their patients' family members. These findings demonstrate the need to be aware of the potential impact of cancer on all family members. Parents and siblings of survivors can experience PTG, which suggests that they experience the adolescents' cancer as personally traumatic. Older parents of adolescent cancer survivors, as well as those who are less satisfied with their lives, are at greater risk for experiencing psychological distress. Family members who are at risk can be provided with education about, and support in developing, healthy and effective coping strategies. Professional consultation may be useful for parents already demonstrating signs of psychological distress. For some parents, using avoidant coping strategies may be self-protective as they deal with extreme stressors. However, others may benefit from learning alternate coping strategies to help them more directly address their needs and struggles.

CONCLUSION

The findings support the need to continue examining the effects of childhood and adolescent cancer on the entire family. Additional studies would benefit from having all members of each family participate to obtain a true family systems perspective on the impact of childhood and adolescent cancer. In addition, studies should continue attempting to identify factors that contribute to PTG in family members of young cancer survivors.

REFERENCES

Alderfer, M. A., Labay, L. E., & Kazak, A. E. (2003). Brief report: Does posttraumatic stress apply to siblings of childhood cancer survivors? *Journal of Pediatric Psychology, 28*, 281–286. doi:10.1093/jpepsy/jsg016.

Alderfer, M. A., Long, K. A., Lown, E. A., et al. (2010). Psychosocial adjustment of siblings of children with cancer: A systematic review. *Psycho-Oncology, 19*, 789–805. doi:10.1002/pon.1638.

Barakat, L. P., Alderfer, M. A., & Kazak, A. E. (2006). Posttraumatic growth in adolescent cancer survivors and their mothers and fathers. *Journal of Pediatric Psychology, 31*, 413–419. doi:10.1093/jpepsy/jsj058.

Barakat, L. P., Kazak, A. E., Meadows, A. T., et al. (1997). Families surviving childhood cancer: A comparison of posttraumatic stress symptoms with families of healthy children. *Journal of Pediatric Psychiatry, 22*, 843–859. doi:10.1093/jpepsy/22.6.843.

Barbarin, O. A., Sargent, J. R., Sahler, O. J., et al. (1995). Sibling adaptation to childhood cancer collaborative study. *Journal of Psychosocial Oncology, 13*, 1–20. doi:10.1300/J077V13N03_01.

Barrera, M., Fleming, C. F., & Khan, F. S. (2004). The role of emotional social support in the psychological adjustment of siblings of children with cancer. *Child: Care, Health, and Development, 30*, 103–111. doi:10.1111/j.1365–2214.2003.00396.x.

Best, M., Streisand, R., Catania, L., & Kazak, A. E. (2001). Parental distress during pediatric leukemia and posttraumatic stress symptoms (PTSS) after treatment ends. *Journal of Pediatric Psychology, 26*, 299–307. doi:10.1093/jpepsy/26.5.299.

Brown, R. T., Madan-Swain, A., & Lambert, R. (2003). Posttraumatic stress symptoms in adolescent survivors of childhood cancer and their mothers. *Journal of Traumatic Stress, 16*, 309–318. doi:10.1023/A:1024465415620.

Calhoun, L., & Tedeschi, R. G. (1998). Posttraumatic growth: Future directions. In R. G. Tedeschi & C. L. Park (Eds.), *Posttraumatic growth: Positive changes in the aftermath of crisis* (pp. 215–240). Mahwah, NJ: Lawrence Erlbaum Associates.

Carver, C. S., Scheier, M. F., & Weintraub, J. K. (1989). Assessing coping strategies: A theoretically based approach. *Journal of Personality and Social Psychology, 56*, 267–283. doi:10.1037/0022–3514.56.2.267.

Chesler, M. A., Allswede, J., & Barbarin, O. O. (1992). Voices from the margin of the family: Siblings of children with cancer. *Journal of Psychosocial Oncology, 9*, 19–42. doi:10.1300/J077v09n04_02.

Cordova, M. J., Cunningham, L. L., Carlson, C. R., & Andrykowski, M. A. (2001). Posttraumatic growth following breast cancer: A controlled comparison study. *Health Psychology, 20*, 176–185. doi:10.1037/0278-6133.20.3.176.

Dahlquist, L. M., Czyzewski, D. I., & Jones, C. L. (1996). Parents of children with cancer: A longitudinal study of emotional distress, coping style, and marital adjustment two and twenty months after diagnosis. *Journal of Pediatric Psychology, 21*, 541–554. doi:10.1093/jpepsy/21.4.541.

Dejong, M., & Fombonne, E. (2006). Depression in paediatric cancer: An overview. *Psycho-Oncology, 15*, 533–566. doi:10.1002/pon.1002.

Derogatis, L. R., & Melisaratos, N. (1983). The Brief Symptom Inventory: An introductory report. *Psychological Medicine, 13*, 595–605.

Diener, E., Emmons, R. A., Larsen, R. J., & Griffin, S. (1985). The Satisfaction with Life Scale. *Journal of Personality Assessment, 49*, 71–75. doi:10.1207/s15327752jpa4901_13.

Dolgin, M. J., Blumensohn, R., Mulhern, R. K., et al. (1997). Sibling adaptation to childhood cancer collaborative study: Cross-cultural aspects. *Journal of Psychosocial Oncology, 15*, 1–14.

Fritz, G. K., & Williams, J. R. (1988). Issues of adolescent development for survivors of childhood cancer. *Journal of the American Academy of Child and Adolescent Psychiatry, 27*, 712–715. doi:10.1097/00004583-198811000-00008.

Fuemmeler, B. F., Mullins, L. L., & Marx, B. P. (2001). Posttraumatic stress and general distress among parents of children surviving a brain tumor. *Children's Health Care, 30*, 169–182. doi:10.1207/S15326888CHC3003_1.

Greenberg, H. S., Kazak, A. E., & Meadows, A. T. (1989). Psychological functioning in 8–16-year-old cancer survivors and their parents. *Journal of Pediatrics, 114*, 488–493. doi:10.1016/S0022-3476(89)80581-5.

Havermans, T., & Eiser, C. (1994). Sibling of a child with cancer. *Child: Care, Health, and Development, 20*, 309–322. doi:10.1111/j.1365-2214.1994.tb00393.x.

Huebner, E. S. (1991). Initial development of the Student's Life Satisfaction Scale. *School Psychology International, 12*, 231–240. doi:10.1177/0143034391123010.

Kamibeppu, K., Sato, I., Honda, M., et al. (2010). Mental health among young adult survivors of childhood cancer and their siblings including posttraumatic growth. *Journal of Cancer Survivorship, 4*, 303–312. doi:10.1007/s11764-010-0124-z.

Kazak, A. E., Alderfer, M., Rourke, M. T., et al. (2004). Posttraumatic stress disorder (PTSD) and posttraumatic stress symptoms (PTSS) in families of adolescent childhood cancer survivors. *Journal of Pediatric Psychology, 29*, 211–219. doi:10.1093/jpepsy/jsh022.

Kazak, A. E., Barakat, L. P., Meeske, K., et al. (1997). Posttraumatic stress, family functioning, and social support in survivors of childhood leukemia and their mothers and fathers. *Journal of Consulting and Clinical Psychology, 65*, 120–129. doi:10.1037/0022-006X.65.1.120.

Michel, G., Taylor, N., Absolom, K., & Eiser, C. (2010). Benefit finding in survivors of childhood cancer and their parents: Further empirical support for the Benefit Finding Scale for Children. *Child: Care, Health, and Development, 36*, 123–129. doi:10.1111/j.1365-2214.2009.01034.x.

National Cancer Institute. (n.d.). *SEER cancer statistics review 1975–2003*. Retrieved from http://seer.cancer.gov/csr/1975_2003/ results_merged/sect_28_childhood_ cancer.pdf.

National Cancer Institute of Canada. (2008). *Canadian cancer statistics*. Retrieved from http://www.cancer.gov/aboutnci/servingpeople/aya-snapshot.pdf.

Nichols, M. P., & Schwartz, R. C. (2001). *Family therapy: Concepts and methods* (5th ed.). Boston: Allyn and Bacon.

Norberg, A. L., Lindblad, F., & Boman, K. K. (2005). Coping strategies in parents of children with cancer. *Social Science and Medicine, 60*, 965–975. doi:10.1016/j.socscimed.2004.06.030.

Phelps, S. B., & Jarvis, P. A. (1994). Coping In adolescence: Empirical evidence for a theoretical based approach to assessing coping. *Journal of Youth and Adolescence, 23*, 359–371.

Phipps, S., Long, A., Hudson, M., & Rai, S. N. (2005). Symptoms of post-traumatic stress in children with cancer and their parents: Effects of informant and time from diagnosis. *Pediatric Blood Cancer, 45*, 952–959. doi:10.1002/pbc.20373.

Radcliffe, J., Bennett, D., Kazak, A. E., et al. (1996). Adjustment in childhood brain tumor survival: Child, mother, and teacher report. *Journal of Pediatric Psychology, 21*, 529–539. doi:10.1093/jpepsy/21.4.529.

Schaefer, J. A., & Moos, R. H. (1992). Life crises and personal growth. In B.N. Carpenter (Ed.), *Personal coping: Theory, research, and applications* (pp. 149–170). New York, NY: Praeger.

Schultz, K. A., Ness, K. K., Whitton, J., et al. (2007). Behavioral and social outcomes in adolescent cancer survivors of childhood cancer: A report from the childhood cancer survivor study. *Journal of Clinical Oncology, 25*, 3649–3656. doi:10.1200/JCO.2006.09.2486.

Seitz, D. C., Besier, T., & Goldbeck, L. (2009). Psychosocial interventions for adolescent cancer patients: A systematic review of the literature. *Psycho-Oncology, 18*, 683–690. doi:10.1002/pon.1473.

Tedeschi, R., Park, C. L., & Calhoun, L. G. (1998). *Posttraumatic growth: Positive changes in the aftermath of crisis*. Mahwah, NJ: Lawrence Erlbaum Associates.

Tedeschi, R. G., & Calhoun, L. G. (1996). The Post-Traumatic Growth Inventory: Measuring the positive legacy of trauma. *Journal of Traumatic Stress, 9*, 455–471. doi:10.1002/jts.2490090305.

Turner-Sack, A. M., Menna, R., Setchell, S. R., et al. (2012). Posttraumatic growth, coping strategies, and psychological distress in adolescent survivors of cancer. *Journal of Pediatric Oncology Nursing, 29*, 70–79. doi:10.1177/1043454212439472.

Van Dongen-Melman, J.E., De Groot, A., Hählen, K., & Verhulst, F.C. (1995). Siblings of childhood cancer survivors: How does this "forgotten" group of children adjust after cessation of successful cancer treatment? *European Journal of Cancer*, *31*, 2277–2283. doi:10.1016/0959-8049(95)00475-0.

Vrijmoet-Wiersma, C. M., van Klink, J. M., Kolk, A. M., et al. (2008). Assessment of parental psychological stress in pediatric cancer: A review. *Journal of Pediatric Psychology*, *33*, 694–706. doi:10.1093/jpepsy/jsn007.

Weiss, T. (2002). Posttraumatic growth in women with breast cancer and their husbands: An intersubjective validation study. *Journal of Psychosocial Oncology*, *20*, 65–80. doi:10.1300/J077v20n02_04.

Witt, W. P., Litzelman, K., Wisk, L. E., et al. (2010). Stress-mediated quality of life outcomes in parents of childhood cancer and brain tumor survivors: A case-control study. *Quality of Life Research*, *19*, 995–1005.

Yaskowich, K. (2003). Posttraumatic growth in children and adolescents with cancer. *Digital Dissertations*, *63*, 3948.

E APPENDIX

Example of a Systematic Review/ Meta-Analysis (Al-Mallah et al., 2015)

The Impact of Nurse-Led Clinics on the Mortality and Morbidity of Patients With Cardiovascular Diseases

Mouaz H. Al-Mallah, MD, MSc, FACC, FAHA, FESC; Iyad Farah, RN; Wedad Al-Madani, MSc; Bassam Bdeir, MD; Samia Al Habib, MD, PhD; Maureen L. Bigelow, RN; Mohammad Hassan Murad, MD, MPH; Mazen Ferwana, MD, PhD

Background: Nurse-led clinics (NLCs) have been developed in several health specialties in recent years. The aim of this analysis is to summarize and appraise the available evidence about the effectiveness of NLCs on the morbidity and mortality outcomes in patients with cardiovascular diseases (CVDs).

Methods: We searched Cochrane databases, MEDLINE, Web of Science, PubMed, EMBASE, Google Scholar, BIOSIS, and bibliography of secondary sources from inception through February 20, 2013. Studies were selected and data were extracted independently by 2 investigators. Eligible studies were randomized trials of NLCs of patients with CVD. Of 56 potentially relevant articles screened initially, 12 trials met the inclusion criteria. The outcomes of interest were all-cause mortality, cardiovascular mortality, nonfatal myocardial infarction, major adverse cardiac events, revascularization, lipids control, and adherence to antiplatelet medications. We performed random-effects meta-analysis to estimate summary risk ratios and quantified between-studies heterogeneity with the I^2 statistic.

Results: The 12 trials allocated 4886 patients to NLCs and 4954 patients to usual care. The NLC patients had decreased all-cause mortality (odds ratio, 0.78; 95% confidence interval [CI], 0.65–0.95; $P < .01$) and myocardial infarction (odds ratio, 0.63; 95% CI, 0.39–1.00; $P = .05$) and had higher adherence to lipid-lowering medication (odds ratio, 1.57; 95% CI, 1.14–2.17; P = .006) compared with controls. They also had increased adherence to antiplatelet therapy compared with controls (odds ratio, 1.42; 95% CI, 1.01–1.98; $P = .04$). There was no statistically significant difference in the risk of cardiovascular death (odds ratio, 0.68; 95% CI, 0.40–1.15; $P = .68$), major adverse cardiac events (odds ratio, 0.79; 95% CI, 0.55–1.14; $P = .21$), or revascularization (odds ratio, 0.87; 95% CI, 0.66–1.16; $P = .36$) between NLC patients and controls.

Conclusions: The available evidence suggests a favorable effect of NLCs on all-cause mortality, rate of major adverse cardiac events, and adherence to medications in patients with CVD.

Nurse-led clinics (NLCs) have been developed in several health specialties in recent years. This intervention involves monitoring of patients with chronic diseases, managing their medications, providing health education and psychological support, and prescribing medications when permittable by jurisdiction. Therefore, there has been a growing literature regarding the evidence of the effectiveness of NLCs in a variety of chronic diseases including cancer, rheumatoid arthritis, inflammatory bowel disease, preoperative setting, and cardiac disease.[1–6]

Cardiovascular diseases (CVDs) constitute a leading cause of morbidity and mortality in many countries. The World Health Organization has projected that by 2030, almost 23.6 million people will die of CVD.[7] Several systematic reviews have suggested that NLCs improve some of the outcomes of patients with CVD, including hypertension and coronary heart disease.[5,6,8] However, the focus of these reports was on short-term outcomes (patient satisfaction, patient education, risk factor assessment, and continuity of care). These short-term process outcomes are of importance; however, the long-term efficacy of these clinics has not been sufficiently investigated and is critical. Specifically, what is the impact on all-cause mortality, CVD mortality, myocardial infarction incidence, and adherence to medications known to impact other patient-important outcomes? Hence, we conducted this systematic review and metaanalysis to summarize and appraise the available evidence supporting the use of NLCs in the setting of CVD.

SPECIFIC REVIEW QUESTION

What is the effectiveness of NLCs in terms of morbidity and mortality in patients with CVD in outpatient settings?

METHOD

Eligibility Criteria

We included randomized controlled trials that enrolled patients with CVD at the beginning of the study who were followed up by NLCs in outpatients settings. Evaluation of the following outcomes was conducted: all-cause mortality, cardiovascular mortality, myocardial infarction, major adverse cardiac events (MACEs), revascularization rate, adherence to lipid-lowering and antiplatelet medications, and achieving cholesterol and low-density lipoprotein targets, all defined according to the protocols of the included studies.

Cardiovascular disease was defined as previous myocardial infarction, percutaneous or surgical coronary revascularization, angiographic evidence of atherosclerosis in 1 or more major coronary arteries, or a positive stress electrocardiogram, echocardiogram, or nuclear stress test result. Trials that enrolled patients with recent revascularization were included. We included studies in which patients with multiple diseases were enrolled if the outcomes for patients with coronary heart disease were reported separately or if these patients comprised at least half of the study participants.

We excluded studies if they were not randomized, were primary prevention studies, evaluated single modality interventions (such as exercise programs or telephone follow up), or tested inpatient interventions. We excluded noncomparative trials (eg, did not have a control arm). Trials that had a follow-up duration of less than 9 months were excluded.

Search Strategy

A comprehensive literature search was conducted by an expert reference librarian with input from study investigators with experience in systematic reviews (M.F, M.A.M., and M.H.M.). We used a 2-level search strategy. First, we searched public domain databases including MEDLINE, EMBASE, the Cochrane Central Register of Controlled Trials CENTRAL, Database of Abstracts of Reviews of Effects, Cochrane Database of Systematic Reviews, Web of Science, BIOSIS, and Google Scholar. Searches included MeSH and text words terms, with combinations of "AND and OR" Boolean operator. We used many terms, including, but not limited to, *nurse led clinics, secondary prevention, cardiac disease, coronary artery disease*, and *myocardial infarction*. Other relevant studies were also identified through a manual search of secondary sources, including references of initially identified articles; we hand-searched the bibliographies of all identified studies to identify any studies missed by the literature searches. Specialized journals were also searched, such as the *Journal of Clinical Nursing* and *Canadian Journal of Cardiology*. The search was performed without any language restrictions. When an abstract from a meeting and a full article referred to the same trial, only the full article was included in the analysis. When there were multiple reports from the same trial, we used the most complete and/or recent. The last search update was run on February 20, 2013.

Study Identification and Data Abstraction

Two investigators (F.I. and W.A.M.) independently reviewed the titles and abstracts of all citations to identify eligible studies. Both investigators used prestandardized data abstraction forms to extract data from relevant articles. Discrepancies were resolved by consensus. The number of events in each eligible trial was extracted, when available, on the basis of the intention-to-treat approach.

Quality of Included Studies

Two reviewers independently assessed quality of the included studies by examining components derived from the Cochrane risk of bias tool, including generation of allocation sequence (classified as adequate if based on computer-generated random numbers, tables of random numbers, or similar), concealment of allocation (classified as adequate if based on central randomization, sealed envelopes, or similar), blinding (patients, caregivers outcome assessors, and data analysts), adequacy of follow-up, and the use of intention-to-treat analysis. Disagreements between the reviewers were resolved by discussion or arbitrated with a third reviewer.

Statistical Analysis

We calculated the odds ratio and 95% confidence intervals (CIs) from each study and pooled across studies using the DerSimonian random-effects models. The number needed to treat to prevent 1 event was calculated by using the inverse of the pooled absolute risk reduction. To assess heterogeneity of treatment effect among trials, we used the I^2 statistic. The I^2 statistic represents the proportion of heterogeneity of effects across trials that is not attributable to chance or random error. Hence, a value greater than 50% reflects large or substantial heterogeneity that is due to real differences in study populations, protocols, interventions, and outcomes.[9] Publication bias was assessed graphically using a funnel plot. The *P* value threshold for statistical significance was set at 0.05 for effect sizes. Analyses were conducted using RevMan software (version 5.1).[10] This systematic review is reported according to the recommendations set forth by the Preferred Reporting Items for Systematic Reviews and Meta-analyses work groups.[11]

RESULTS

Search Results and Study Description

A total of 302 abstracts were identified by the electronic search strategy, of which 56 full-text articles met the eligibility for assessment. A total of 12 trials fulfilled the inclusion criteria of prospective randomized controlled trials evaluating the impact of NCLs in patients with CVD.[12–23] Figure 1 shows the results of the search strategy and Table 1 summarizes the included studies.

There were 9840 patients enrolled in the 12 trials, 4886 in the treatment arm (NLCs) and 4954 in the usual care arm. The mean follow-up duration was 2 years. Seven studies were conducted in the United Kingdom, of which 1 was a multicenter study (Europe); 4 were in the United States; and 1 was in Canada. The studies varied in the frequency of follow-up of their participants; 8 studies saw their patients in 2 to 6 months, and in 2 studies, participants were followed up every week for the first 6 weeks and then assessed after 1 year. Only 1 study in the United States involved a nurse practitioner who was authorized to prescribe, and in the rest of the studies, nurses in the intervention arm were not. Studies varied in their intervention modalities; nurses in 6 studies provided lifestyle advice and medications management, and 3 used only lifestyle, counseling, and educational interventions.[14,17,21] The NLCs were managed by nurses, case manager, and/or dietician, as well as supervised by physicians. In terms of communication types between the nurses in charge

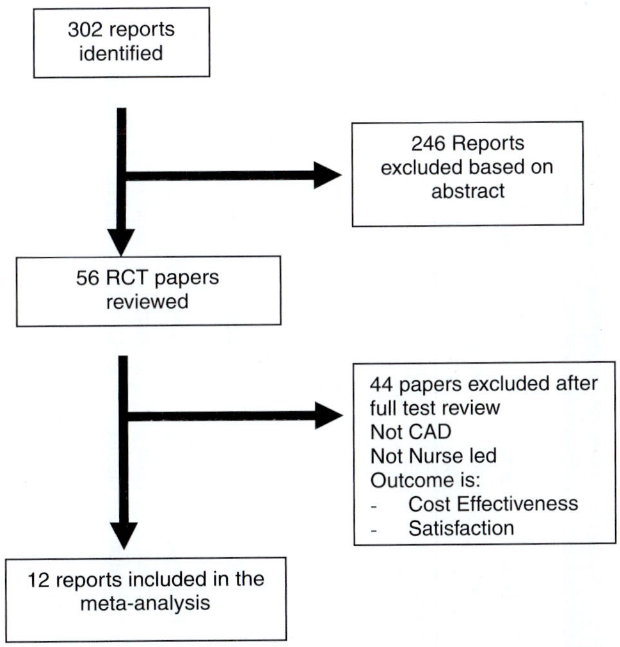

FIG 1 Flowchart of the study. RCT indicates randomized clinical trial; CAD, coronary artery disease.

TABLE 1 Characteristics of the Trials Included in the Meta-analysis

	Allen et al, 2002	Campbell et al, 1998	Cupples et al, 1994	Debusk et al, 1994	Delany et al, 2008	Goodman et al, 2008	Haskell et al, 1994	Jolly et al, 1999	Khanal et al, 2006	Lapointe et al, 2006	Murchi et al, 2003	Wood et al, 2008
Enrollment period	NA	NA	NA	NA	1995/2005	NA	Feb 1984–Mar 1987	April 1995–Sep 1996	April 2002 and Feb 2004	Jan 2001/ Sep 2002	NA	NA
Publication year	2002	1998	1994	1994	2008	2007	1994	1999	2007	2006	2003	2008
Enrolling sites	United States/ Canada	United Kingdom	United Kingdom	United States	United Kingdom	United Kingdom	United States	United Kingdom	United States	Canada	United Kingdom	United Kingdom
CAD definition	Postcoronary revascularization	Coronary heart disease	Angina for at least 6 mo	Acute myocardial infarction	Coronary heart disease	CAD waiting for CABG	By angiography	Myocardial infarction with angina	Angiography	MI based on lab and EKG	NA	Coronary heart disease
Sample size	228	1173	688	585	1343	188	300	597	1233	127	1343	1940
Mean follow-up, y	1	1	2	1	10	NA	4	1	2	1.5	4.7	1
Age, mean (SD), y	60.3 ± 9.9	66.1	63.1 ± 7	57 ± 8	NA	NA	NA	NA	NA	57.4 ± 9.2	NA	62.7 ± 10
Females, %	29	41.6	40.6	21.2	NA	19	15	29	38	16.50	42	30
Previous MI, %	54	45	30	15.2	NA	36	48	71	20	CAD 35	45	50.5

NA is used to show that these data were not reported in the original studies
Abbreviations: CABG, coronary artery bypass graft; CAD, coronary artery disease; EKG, electrocardiogram; MI, myocardial infarction; NA, not applicable.

and the physicians, in 4 of the studies, nurses followed up participants, and if medications were needed or the targets were not obtained, they either telephoned the physicians or referred the patients to them.[12,21,23] However, there was no clear description of how nurses communicated with physicians in charge in 5 studies.[14,16–18,22]

Of the 12 trials, 9 reported all-cause mortality outcomes [13–21] and included 6319 patients, 3,146 in the NLC group and 3173 in usual care. Five studies reported cardiovascular death results [14–16,18,21]; 2973 patients were included, 1,492 in the NLC arm and 1481 in usual care.

Meta-analysis

Patients in the NLC group had decreased all-cause mortality (odds ratio, 0.78; 95% CI, 0.65–0.95; $P < .01$) and myocardial infarction (odds ratio, 0.63; 95% CI, 0.39–1.00; $P = .05$) and had higher adherence to lipid-lowering medication (odds ratio, 1.57; 95% CI, 1.14–2.17; $P = .006$) compared with controls. They also had increased adherence to antiplatelet therapy compared with controls (odds ratio, 1.42; 95% CI, 1.01–1.98; $P = .04$). There was no statistically significant difference in the risk of cardiovascular death (odds ratio, 0.68; 95% CI, 0.40–1.15; $P = .68$), major adverse cardiac events (odds ratio, 0.79; 95% CI, 0.55–1.14; $P = .21$), or revascularization (odds ratio, 0.87; 95% CI, 0.66–1.16; $P = .36$) between NLC patients and controls. Results are depicted in Figure 2.

There was no heterogeneity in the analyses of all-cause mortality, cardiovascular mortality, myocardial infarction, and revascularization ($I^2 < 50\%$). However, there was large heterogeneity ($I^2 > 50\%$) for all the remaining outcomes. The small number of included trials precluded statistical testing for publication bias; however, visual inspection of funnel plot is consistent with symmetry (Figure 3).

Methodological Quality

Overall, the trials had moderate risk of bias (Figure 4). Generation of allocation was adequate in all trials, and allocation of concealment was adequate in only 4 studies. Blinding of caregivers, outcome assessment, and data analyst was not clear in all trials. Almost all included trials reported the proportion of patients who were lost to follow-up, ranging from 1.9% to 31%. All trials used an intention-to-treat analysis. Table 2 describes the methodological quality of the 9 randomized controlled trials included in this systematic review.

DISCUSSION

This systematic review and meta-analysis provided evidence supporting the effectiveness of NLCs in lowering the risk of all-cause mortality and myocardial infarction and adherence to medications in patients with CVD.

We found that NLCs significantly increase the likelihood of use of lipid-lowering medication adherence. This is consistent with 3 previous systematic reviews that showed a significant reduction in cholesterol level among patients managed by NLCs compared with the usual care clinics.[5,24] One review investigated interventions related to education, assessment of risk factors, consultations, and/or follow-up.[5] The second review search was conducted from 2002 to 2008, and the main outcomes were smoking cessation, diet adherence, quality of life, and general health status,[6] whereas our review's main objective is to assess hard endpoints. The third review was on the effect of the clinical nurse specialist practice in acute setting; the main outcomes are length of stay, cost, and functional status. Finally,

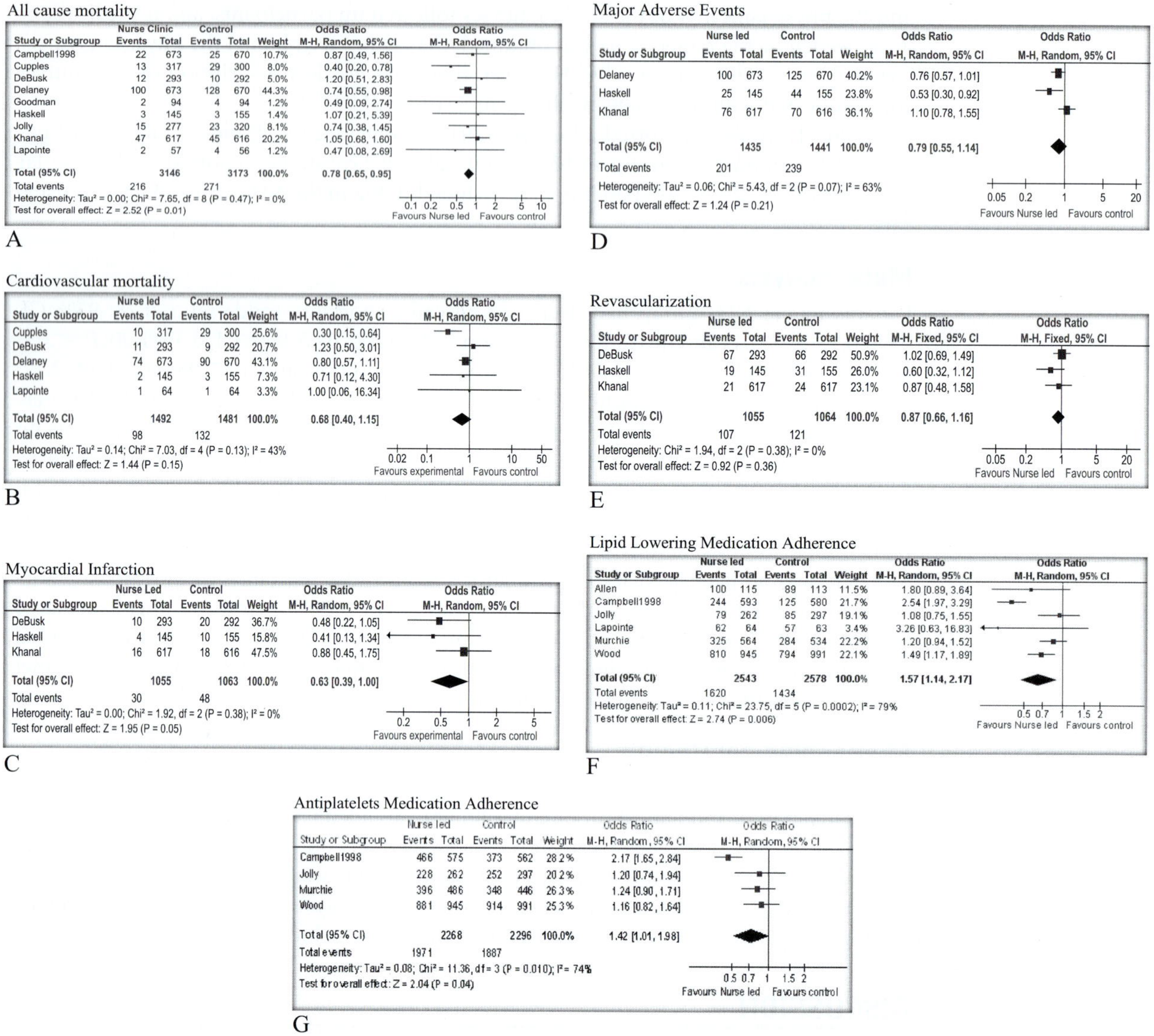

FIG 2 Forest plot of the outcomes analyzed in this study. **A,** All-cause mortality; **B,** cardiovascular mortality; **C,** myocardial infarction; **D,** major adverse events; **E,** revascularization; **F,** lipid-lowering medication adherence; and **G,** antiplatelet medication adherence. CI indicates confidence interval.

their search was from 1990 to 2008 and restricted to trials conducted in the United States. It included not only randomized controlled trials but also observational studies.[24] In addition, our review was specifically designed to include only randomized controlled trials and studies that used lifestyle advise, assessment, as well as drug interventions by nurses.

On the other hand, the patients included in the trials are relatively young and most often men. This was also seen in a recent non randomized study by Bdeir et al.[25] Although the included trials did not report the outcomes stratified by age and gender, it is possible that

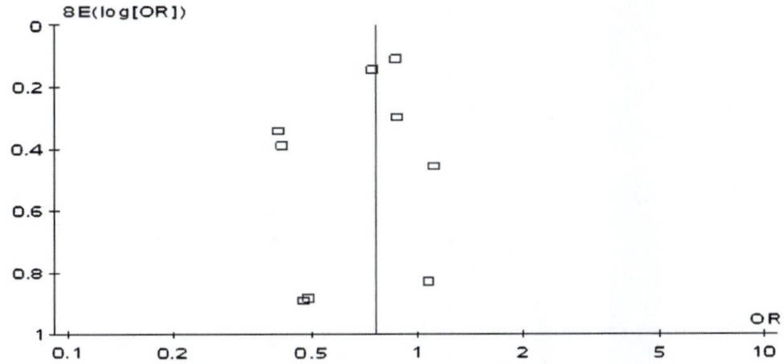

FIG 3 Funnel plot. No indication of publication bias was seen.

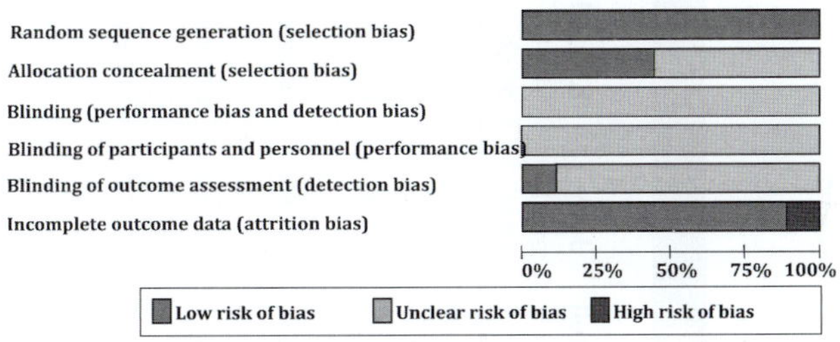

FIG 4 Study quality assessment.

the benefit of these clinics is more notable in this age group. Further studies are needed to assess the potential benefit of NLCs in an older population.

The studies included in this review seemed to have fair quality and moderate risk of bias. As blinding participants and researchers is challenging in this context, blinding data analysts and outcome assessors is possible but was not explicitly performed in these trials. Many of the studies followed up patients for a relatively short period; 3 studies were for 1 year,[12,13,23] 1 study was for 18 months,[21] 1 study was for 2 years,[14] 2 studies were for 4 years,[18,22] and 1 study was for 10 years.[16] Hence, although our intention was to evaluate long-term outcomes, the available evidence is of relatively short-term. Lastly, applying this evidence to different settings (managed care, private payers, United States, Europe, developing countries, etc) will be challenging and should be considered a limitation of this evidence. The infrastructure, legislation, insurance coverage, and range of services delegated to nurses vary widely across these settings.

Many of the included outcomes had significant heterogeneity. An obvious potential explanation for heterogeneity is the variation in the intensity of the intervention and the nature of nurses' expertise, background, and involvement in the care of the patients, as well as differences in the conditions and complexity of the patients. One other possible cause of heterogeneity, however, is the variation in the care provided to the control group. Previous studies of case management in patients with CVD suggested that when the "usual care" arm of studies receives minimal management, the benefits seen in these studies may be larger.[15,20] Such benefit may not be observed if the control arm received better secondary prevention measures.[23] Considering the observed unexplained heterogeneity, the pooled estimates we provide should be considered an average estimate of NLC effect that is expected when these clinics are implemented across various settings. Variations in these settings will affect the

TABLE 2 **Quality Assessment of the Trials Included in the Meta-analysis**

	Allen et al, 2002	Campbell et al, 1998	Cupples et al, 1994	Debusk et al, 1994	Delany et al, 2008	Goodman et al, 2008	Haskell et al, 1994	Jolly et al, 1999	Khanal et al, 2006	Lapointe et al, 2006	Murchl et al, 2003	Wood et al, 2008
Generation of allocation	Adequate	Adequate	Adequate	Adequate	Adequate	Adequate	Adequate	Adequate	Adequate	Adequate	Adequate	Adequate
Allocation concealment	Unclear	Unclear	Adequate	Adequate	Unclear	Adequate	Adequate	Unclear	Unclear	Unclear	Adequate	Unclear
Blinding of participants	Unclear	Unclear	Unclear	Unclear	Unclear	Unclear	Unclear	Unclear	Unclear	Unclear	Unclear	Unclear
Blinding of caregivers	Unclear	Unclear	Unclear	Unclear	Unclear	Unclear	Unclear	Unclear	Unclear	Unclear	Unclear	Unclear
Blinding of outcome assessment	Unclear	Unclear	Adequate	Unclear	Unclear	Unclear	Unclear	Unclear	Unclear	Unclear	Unclear	Unclear
Blinding of data analyst	Unclear	Unclear	Unclear	Unclear	Unclear	Unclear	Unclear	Unclear	Unclear	Unclear	Unclear	Unclear
% Loss to follow-up	31	7	4.20	13.50	1.90	0	8.70	10	6	12.60	4.40	20
Intention-to-treat analysis	Yes	No	No	Yes	Yes	Yes	No	Yes	Yes	Yes	Yes	Yes

expected benefit. This average effect is helpful, nevertheless, from a public health or policy level perspective.

Limitations

Our study has several limitations. We included only studies that reported hard endpoints. The mechanism for the decrease in these hard endpoints could be due to better adherence to guidelines recommended medical therapies (as seen in the use of the lipid-lowering and antiplatelet medications). However, there were no data reported on the control of hypertension, diabetes, smoking cessation, and other risk factors. These factors may have contributed to the lower mortality and better outcomes. In addition, the interventions used in each NLC may be different in each clinic. Being nurse led is the main common characteristic of this intervention. Further data may be needed to determine the impact of other interventions in each clinic on outcomes.

Implications for Clinical Practice and Research

Our findings suggest that NLCs can have an important role and should be considered when delivering care to patients with CVD. Translating this evidence into effective models of care may be challenging, but the reduction in mortality is compelling. Structured models of care should be developed and tested locally. Patient and community engagement is paramount to develop such programs. Partnership with patients and communities is essential not only for the NLC program development but also for conducting research in these programs, particularly when testing the cultural and ethnic appropriateness of these interventions. Future research is also needed on the cost-effectiveness of NLCs and perhaps on better stratification to determine which patients are most appropriate to receive this care. For example, which stages of CVD are the most amenable or most responsive to NLCs? What type or level of training should be required of a nurse undertaking extended roles in NLCs? A systematic review of worldwide conducted research demonstrates wide variation in nurses' job titles, duties, and qualifications.[26]

What's New and Important

- A meta-analysis of 12 randomized trials and more than 9000 patients evaluating the role of NLC in management of cardiac patients was conducted.
- Nurse-led clinic is associated with better adherence to medical therapy and better survival compared with usual care.
- This model would be ideal to reduce cost and improves outcomes in the current era.

CONCLUSION

The available evidence suggests a favorable effect of NLCs on all-cause mortality, rate of major adverse cardiac events, and adherence to medications in patients with CVD.

REFERENCES

1. Lewis, R., Neal, R. D., Williams, N. H., et al. (2009). Nurse-led vs. conventional physician-led follow-up for patients with cancer: systematic review. *J Adv Nurs*, *65*(4), 706–723.

2. Ndosi, M., Vinall, K., Hale, C., et al. (2011). The effectiveness of nurse-led care in people with rheumatoid arthritis: a systematic review. *Int J Nurs Stud*, *48*(5), 642–654.
3. Belling, R. M. S., & Woods, L. (2009). Specialist nursing interventions for inflammatory bowel disease. *Cochrane Database Syst Rev*, (4), CD006597. doi: 10.1002/14651858.CD006597.pub2.
4. Craig, S. E. (2005). Does nurse-led pre-operative assessment reduce the cancellation rate of elective surgical in-patient procedures: a systematic review of the research literature. *Br J Anaesthetic Recovery Nurs*, *6*(3), 41–47.
5. Page, T., Lockwood, C., & Conroy-Hiller, T. (2005). Effectiveness of nurse-led cardiac clinics in adult patients with a diagnosis of coronary heart disease. *International Journal of Evidence-Based Healthcare*, *3*(1), 2–26.
6. Schadewaldt, V., & Schultz, T. (2011). Nurse-led clinics as an effective service for cardiac patients: results from a systematic review. *Int J Evid Based Healthc*, *9*(3), 199–214.
7. WHO. (September 2012). *Cardiovascular diseases (CVDs). Fact sheet no. 317*. http://www.who.int/cardiovascular_diseases/en/. Accessed 22.11.12.
8. Clark, C. E., Lindsay, F. P. S., Rod, S. T., & John, L. C. (2010). Nurse led interventions to improve control of blood pressure in people with hypertension: systematic review and meta-analysis. *BMJ*, *341*, c3995.
9. Higgins, J. P., Thompson, S. G., Deeks, J. J., & Altman, D. G. (2003). Measuring inconsistency in meta-analyses. *BMJ*, *327*(7414), 557–560.
10. RevMan [computer program]. Version 5.1. Copenhagen, Denmark: The Nordic Cochrane Center. http://ims.cochrane .org/revman/download. Accessed 08.01.15.
11. Liberati, A., Altman, D. G., Tetzlaff, J., et al. (2009). The PRISMA statement for reporting systematic reviews and meta-analyses of studies that evaluate health care interventions: explanation and elaboration. *J Clin Epidemiol*, *62*(10), e1–e34.
12. Allen, J. K., Blumenthal, R. S., Margolis, S., et al. (2002). Nurse case management of hypercholesterolemia in patients with coronary heart disease: results of a randomized clinical trial. *Am Heart J*, *144*(4), 678–686.
13. Campbell, N. C., Ritchie, L. D., Thain, J., et al. (1998). Secondary prevention in coronary heart disease: a randomised trial of nurse led clinics in primary care. *Heart*, *80*(5), 447–452.
14. Cupples, M. E., & McKnight, A. (1994). Randomised controlled trial of health promotion in general practice for patients with high cardiovascular risk. *Br Med J*, *309*, 993–996.
15. DeBusk, R., Charles, A. D., Robert, S. H., et al. (1994). A case-management system for coronary risk factor modification after acute myocardial infarction. *Ann Intern Med*, *120*(9), 721–729.
16. Delaney, E. K., Murchie, P., Lee, A. J., et al. (2008). Secondary prevention clinics for coronary heart disease: a 10-year follow-up of a randomised controlled trial in primary care. *Heart*, *94*(11), 1419–1423.
17. Goodman, H., Parsons, A., Davison, J., et al. (2008). A randomised controlled trial to evaluate a nurse-led programme of support and lifestyle management for patients awaiting cardiac surgery: 'Fit for Surgery: Fit for Life' Study. *Eur J Cardiovasc Nurs*, *7*(3), 189–195.
18. Haskell, W. L., Alderman, E. L., Fair, J. M., et al. (1994). Effects of intensive multiple risk factor reduction on coronary atherosclerosis and clinical cardiac events in men and women with coronary artery disease. The Stanford Coronary Risk Intervention Project (SCRIP). *Circulation*, *89*(3), 975–990.
19. Jolly, K., Bradley, F., Sharp, S., et al. (1999). Randomised controlled trial of follow up care in general practice of patients with myocardial infarction and angina: final results of the Southampton Heart Integrated Care Project (SHIP). The SHIP Collaborative Group. *BMJ*, *318*(7185), 706–711.
20. Khanal, S., Omar, O., Michael, P. H., et al. (2007). Active Lipid Management In Coronary Artery Disease (ALMICAD) Study. *Am J Med*, *120*(8), 734.e711–734.e717.
21. Lapointe, F., Lepage, S., Larrivee, L., & Maheux, P. (2006). Surveillance and treatment of dyslipidemia in the post-infarct patient: can a nurse led management approach make a difference? *Can J Cardiol*, *22*(9), 761–767.

22. Murchie, P. C. N., Ritchie, L. D., Simpson, J. A., & Thain, J. (2003). Secondary prevention clinics for coronary heart disease: four year follow up of a randomised controlled trial in primary care. *BMJ*, *326*, 84–87.
23. Wood, D. A., Kotseva, K., & Connolly, S. (2008). Nurse-coordinated multidisciplinary, family-based cardiovascular disease prevention programme (EUROACTION) for patients with coronary heart disease and asymptomatic individuals at high risk of cardiovascular disease: a paired, cluster-randomised controlled trial. *Lancet*, *371*, 1999–2012.
24. Newhouse, R., Stanik-Hutt, J., & White, K. (2011). Advanced practice nurse outcomes 1990–2008. *Nurs Econ*, *29*(5), 230–250.
25. Bdeir, B., Conboy, T., Mukhtar, A., et al. (2014). Impact of a nurseled heart failure program on all-cause mortality [published online ahead of print]. *J Cardiovasc Nurs*.
26. Laurant, M. R. D., Hermens, R., et al. (2005). Substitution of doctors by nurses in primary care. *Cochrane Database Syst Rev*, *5*, CD001271.

GLOSSARY

A

A Priori From Latin: *the former*; before the study or analysis.

Absolute Risk Reduction (ARR) A value that gives reduction of risk in absolute terms. The ARR is considered the "real" reduction because it is the difference between the risk observed in those who did and did not experience the event.

Abstract A short, comprehensive synopsis or summary of a study at the beginning of an article.

Accessible Population A population that meets the population criteria and is available.

Accreditation A process in which an organization demonstrates attainment of predetermined standards set by an external nongovernmental organization responsible for setting and monitoring compliance in a particular industry sector.

After-Only Design An experimental design with two randomly assigned groups—a treatment group and a control group. This design differs from the true experiment in that both groups are measured only after the experimental treatment.

After-Only Nonequivalent Control Group Design A quasi-experimental design similar to the after-only experimental design, but subjects are not randomly assigned to the treatment or control groups.

AGREE II Guideline A widely used instrument to evaluate the applicability of a guideline to practice. The AGREE II was developed to assist in evaluating guideline quality, provide a methodological strategy for guideline development, and inform practitioners about what information should be reported in guidelines and how it should be reported.

Analysis of Covariance (ANCOVA) A statistic that measures differences among group means and uses a statistical technique to equate the groups under study in relation to an important variable.

Analysis of Variance (ANOVA) A statistic that tests whether group means differ from each other, rather than testing each pair of means separately. ANOVA considers the variation among all groups.

Anecdotes Summaries of an observation that records a behavior of interest.

Anonymity A research participant's protection of identity in a study so that no one, not even the researcher, can link the subject with the information given.

Antecedent Variable A variable that affects the dependent variable but occurs before the introduction of the independent variable.

Assent An aspect of informed consent that pertains to protecting the rights of children as research subjects.

Attention Control Operationalized as the control group receiving the same amount of "attention" as the experimental group.

Auditability The researcher's development of the research process in a qualitative study that allows a researcher or reader to follow the thinking or conclusions of the researcher.

B

Benchmarking A systematic approach for gathering information about process or product performance and then analyzing why and how performance differs between business units.

Beneficence An obligation to act to benefit others and to maximize possible benefits.

Bias A distortion in the data-analysis results.

Boolean Operator Words used to define the relationships between words or groups of words in literature searches. Examples of Boolean operators are words such as "AND," "OR," "NOT," and "NEAR."

Bracketing A process during which the researcher identifies personal biases about the phenomenon of interest to clarify how personal experience and beliefs may color what is heard and reported.

C

Case Control Study See *ex post facto study*.

Case Study Method The study of a selected contemporary phenomenon over time to provide an in-depth description of essential dimensions and processes of the phenomenon.

CASP Tools Checklists that provide an evidence-based approach for assessing the quality, quantity, and consistency of specific study designs.

Categorical Variable A variable that has mutually exclusive categories but has more than two values.

Chance Error Attributable to fluctuations in subject characteristics that occur at a specific point in time and are often beyond the awareness and control of the examiner. Also called *random error*.

Chi-Square (χ^2) A nonparametric statistic that is used to determine whether the frequency found in each category is different from the frequency that would be expected by chance.

Citation Management Software Software that formats citations.

Clinical Guidelines Systematically developed practice statements designed to assist clinicians about health care decisions for specific conditions or situations.

Clinical Microsystems A QI model developed specifically for health care. It is considered the building block of any health care system and is the smallest replicable unit in an organization. Members of a clinical microsystem are interdependent and work together toward a common aim.

Clinical Question The first step in development of an evidence-based practice project.

Closed-Ended Question Question that the respondent may answer with only one of a fixed number of choices.

Cluster Sampling A probability sampling strategy that involves a successive random sampling of units. The units sampled progress from large to small. Also known as *multistage sampling*.

Cohort The subjects of a specific group that are being studied.

Cohort Study See *longitudinal/prospective studies*.

Common Cause Variation Variation that occurs at random and is considered a characteristic of the system.

Community-Based Participatory Research Qualitative method that systematically accesses the voice of a community to plan context-appropriate action.

Concealment Refers to whether the subjects know that they are being observed.

Concept An image or symbolic representation of an abstract idea.

Conceptual Definition General meaning of a concept.

Conceptual Framework A structure of concepts and/or theories pulled together as a map for the study. This set of interrelated concepts symbolically represents how a group of variables relates to each other.

Conceptual Literature Published and unpublished non–data-based material, such as reports of theories, concepts, synthesis of research on concepts, or professional issues, some of which underlie reported research, as well as other nonresearch material.

Concurrent Validity The degree of correlation of two measures of the same concept that are administered at the same time.

Conduct of Research The analysis of data collected from a homogeneous group of subjects who meet study inclusion and exclusion criteria for the purpose of answering specific research questions or testing specified hypotheses.

Confidence Interval Quantifies the uncertainty of a statistic or the probable value range within which a population parameter is expected to lie.

Confidentiality Assurance that a research participant's identity cannot be linked to the information that was provided to the researcher.

Consent See *informed consent*.

Consistency Data are collected from each subject in the study in exactly the same way or as close to the same way as possible.

Constancy Methods and procedures of data collection are the same for all subjects.

Constant Comparative Method A process of continuously comparing data as they are acquired during research with the grounded theory method.

Construct An abstraction that is adapted for scientific purpose.

Construct Validity The extent to which an instrument is said to measure a theoretical construct or trait.

Consumer One who actively uses and applies research findings in nursing practice.

Content Analysis A technique for the objective, systematic, and quantitative description of communications and documentary evidence.

Content Validity The degree to which the content of the measure represents the universe of content or the domain of a given behavior.

Content Validity Index A calculation that gives a researcher more confidence or evidence that the instrument truly reflects the concept or construct.

Context Environment where event(s) occur(s).

Context Dependent An observation as defined by its circumstance or context.

Continuous Variable (Data) A variable that can take on any value between two specified points (e.g., weight).

Contrasted-Group Approach A method used to assess construct validity. A researcher identifies two groups of individuals who are suspected to have an extremely high or low score on a characteristic. Scores from the groups are obtained and examined for sensitivity to the differences. Also called *known-group approach*.

Control Measures used to hold uniform or constant the conditions under which an investigation occurs.

Control Chart Used to track system performance over time. It includes information on the average performance level for the system depicted by a center line displaying the system's average performance (the mean value) and the upper and lower limits depicting one to three standard deviations from average performance level.

Control Event Rate (CER) Proportion of patients in a control group in which an event is observed.

Control Group The group in an experimental investigation that does not receive an intervention or treatment; the comparison group.

Controlled Vocabulary The terms that indexers have assigned to the articles in a database. When possible, it is helpful to match the words that you use in your search to those specifically used in the database.

Convenience Sampling A nonprobability sampling strategy that uses the most readily accessible persons or objects as subjects in a study.

Convergent Validity A strategy for assessing construct validity in which two or more tools that theoretically measure the same construct are administered to subjects. If the measures are positively correlated, convergent validity is said to be supported.

Correlation The degree of association between two variables.

Correlational Study A type of nonexperimental research design that examines the relationship between two or more variables.

Credibility Steps in qualitative research to ensure accuracy, validity, or soundness of data.

Criterion-Related Validity Indicates the degree of relationship between performance on the measure and actual behavior either in the present (concurrent) or in the future (predictive).

Critical Appraisal Appraisal by a nurse who is a knowledgeable consumer of research and who can appraise research evidence and use existing standards to determine the merit and readiness of research for use in clinical practice.

Critical Reading An active interpretation and objective assessment of an article during which the reader is looking for key concepts, ideas, and justifications.

Critique The process of critical appraisal that objectively and critically evaluates a research report's content for scientific merit and application to practice.

Cronbach's Alpha Test of internal consistency that simultaneously compares each item in a scale to all others.

Cross-Sectional Study A nonexperimental research design that looks at data at one point in time—that is, in the immediate present.

Culture The system of knowledge and linguistic expressions used by social groups that allows the researcher to interpret or make sense of the world.

Cumulative Index to Nursing and Allied Health Literature (CINAHL) A print or computerized database; computerized CINAHL is available on CD-ROM and online.

D

Data Information systematically collected in the course of a study; the plural of *datum.*

Data-Based Literature Reports of completed research.

Data Saturation A point when data collection can cease. It occurs when the information being shared with the researcher becomes repetitive. Ideas conveyed by the participant have been shared before by other participants; inclusion of additional participants does not result in new ideas.

Database A compilation of information about a topic organized in a systematic way.

Debriefing The opportunity for researchers to discuss the study with the participants; participants may refuse to have their data included in the study at this time.

Deductive A logical thought process in which hypotheses are derived from theory; reasoning moves from the general to the particular.

Degrees of Freedom The number of quantities that are unknown minus the number of independent equations linking these unknowns; a function of the number in the sample.

Delimitations Those characteristics that restrict the population to a homogeneous group of subjects.

Delphi Technique The technique of gaining expert opinion on a subject. It uses rounds or multiple stages of data collection, with each round using data from the previous round.

Demographic Data Data that includes information that describes important characteristics about the subjects in a study (e.g., age, gender, race, ethnicity, education, marital status).

Dependent Variable In experimental studies, the presumed effect of the independent or experimental variable on the outcome.

Descriptive Statistics Statistical methods used to describe and summarize sample data.

Design The plan or blueprint for conduct of a study.

Developmental Study A type of nonexperimental research design that is concerned not only with the existing status and interrelationship of phenomena, but also with changes that take place as a function of time.

Dichotomous Variable A nominal variable that has two categories (e.g., male/female).

Directional Hypothesis A hypothesis that specifies the expected direction of the relationship between the independent and dependent variables.

Dissemination The communication of research findings.

Divergent Validity/Discriminant Validity A strategy for assessing construct validity in which two or more tools that theoretically measure the opposite of the construct are administered to subjects. If the measures are negatively correlated, divergent validity is said to be supported.

Domains Symbolic categories that include the smaller categories of an ethnographic study.

E

Effect Size An estimate of how large of a difference there is between intervention and control groups in summarized studies.

Electronic Database A database that can be accessed by computers or electronic information services.

Electronic Index The electronic means by which journal sources (periodicals) of data-based and conceptual articles on a variety of topics (e.g., doctoral dissertations) are found, as well as the publications of professional organizations and various governmental agencies.

Element The most basic unit about which information is collected.

Eligibility Criteria The characteristics that restrict the population to a homogeneous group of subjects.

Emic View A native's or insider's view of the world.

Empirical The obtaining of evidence or objective data.

Empirical Literature A synonym for data-based literature; see *data-based literature.*

Equivalence Consistency or agreement among observers using the same measurement tool or agreement among alternate forms of a tool.

Error Variance The extent to which the variance in test scores is attributable to error rather than a true measure of the behaviors.

Ethics The theory or discipline dealing with principles of moral values and moral conduct.

Ethnographic Method A method that scientifically describes cultural groups. The goal of the ethnographer is to understand the native's view of their world.

Ethnography/Ethnographic Method A qualitative research approach designed to produce cultural theory.

Etic View An outsider's view of another's world.

Evaluation Research The use of scientific research methods and procedures to evaluate a program, treatment, practice, or policy outcomes; analytical means are used to document the worth of an activity.

Evidence-Based Clinical Guidelines A set of guidelines that allows the researcher to better understand the evidence base of certain practices.

Evidence-Based Practice The conscious and judicious use of the current "best" evidence in the care of patients and delivery of health care services.

Evidence-Based Practice Guidelines Practice guidelines developed based on research findings.

Ex Post Facto Study A type of nonexperimental research design that examines the relationships among the variables after the variations have occurred.

Exclusion Criteria Those characteristics that restrict the population to a homogeneous group of subjects.

Existing Data Data gathered from records (e.g., medical records, care plans, hospital records, death certificates) and databases (e.g., US Census, National Cancer Database, Minimum Data Set for Nursing Home Resident Assessment and Care Screening).

Experiment A scientific investigation in which observations are made and data are collected by means of the characteristics of control, randomization, and manipulation.

Experimental Design A research design that has the following properties: randomization, control, and manipulation.

Experimental Event Rate (EER) The proportion of patients in experimental treatment groups in which an event is observed.

Experimental Group The group in an experimental investigation that receives an intervention or treatment.

Expert-Based Clinical Guidelines Guidelines developed from the combination of opinions from known experts in the field, along with current research evidence.

Exploratory Survey A type of nonexperimental research design that collects descriptions of existing phenomena for the purpose of using the data to justify or assess current conditions or to make plans for improvement of conditions.

External Validity The degree to which findings of a study can be generalized to other populations or environments.

Extraneous Variable Variable that interferes with the operations of the phenomena being studied. Also called *mediating variable.*

F

Face Validity A type of content validity that uses an expert's opinion to judge the accuracy of an instrument. (Some would say that face validity verifies that the instrument gives the subject or expert the appearance of measuring the concept.)

Factor Analysis A type of validity that uses a statistical procedure for determining the underlying dimensions or components of a variable.

Field Notes Descriptions kept by a researcher that detail the environment and nonverbal communications observed by a researcher that enrich data collected.

Findings Statistical results of a study.

Fisher Exact Probability Test A test used to compare frequencies when samples are small and expected frequencies are less than six in each cell.

Fittingness Answers the following questions: Are the findings applicable outside the study situation? Are the results meaningful to the individuals not involved in the research?

Flowchart Depicts how a process works, detailing the sequence of steps from the beginning to the end of a process.

Forest Plot Also known as a *blobbogram,* a forest plot graphically depicts the results of analyzing a number of studies.

Frequency Distribution Descriptive statistical method for summarizing the occurrences of events under study.

G

Generalizability (Generalize) The inferences that the data are representative of similar phenomena in a population beyond the studied sample.

Grand Nursing Theories Sometimes referred to as nursing conceptual models, these include the theories/models that were developed to describe the discipline of nursing as a whole.

Grand Theory All-inclusive conceptual structures that tend to include views on people, health, and the environment to create a perspective of nursing.

Grand Tour Question A broad overview question.

Grounded Theory Theory that is constructed inductively from a base of observations of the world as it is lived by a selected group of people.

Grounded Theory Method An inductive approach that uses a systematic set of procedures to arrive at a theory about basic social processes.

H

Hazard Ratio A weighted relative risk based on the analysis of survival curves over the whole course of the study period.

History The internal validity threat that refers to events outside of the experimental setting that may affect the dependent variable.

Homogeneity Similarity of conditions. Also called *internal consistency.*

Hypothesis A prediction about the relationship between two or more variables.

Hypothesis-Testing Approach The method used when an investigator uses the theory or concept underlying the measurement instruments to validate the instrument.

Hypothesis-Testing Validity A strategy for assessing construct validity, in which the theory or concept underlying a measurement instrument's design is used to develop hypotheses that are tested. Inferences are made based on the findings about whether the rationale underlying the instrument's construction is adequate to explain the findings.

I

Inclusion Criteria See *eligibility criteria.*

Independent Variable The antecedent or the variable that has the presumed effect on the dependent variable.

Inductive Reasoning A logical thought process in which generalizations are developed from specific observations; reasoning moves from the particular to the general.

Inferential Statistics Procedures that combine mathematical processes and logic to test hypotheses about a population with the help of sample data.

Information Literacy The skills needed to consult the literature and answer a clinical question.

Informed Consent An ethical principle that requires a researcher to obtain the voluntary participation of subjects after informing them of potential benefits and risks.

Institutional Review Boards (IRBs) Boards established in agencies to review biomedical and behavioral research involving human subjects within the agency or in programs sponsored by the agency.

Instrumental Case Study Research that is done when the researcher pursues insight into an issue or wants to challenge a generalization.

Instrumentation Changes in the measurement of the variables that may account for changes in the obtained measurement.

Integrative Review Synthesis review of the literature on a specific concept or topic.

Internal Consistency The extent to which items within a scale reflect or measure the same concept.

Internal Validity The degree to which it can be inferred that the experimental treatment, rather than an uncontrolled condition, resulted in the observed effects.

Interpretive Phenomenology An approach to research that "seeks to reveal and convey deep insight and understanding of the concealed meanings of everyday life experiences" (deWitt & Ploeg, 2006, pp. 216–217).

Interrater Reliability The consistency of observations between two or more observers, often expressed as a percentage of agreement between raters or observers or a coefficient of agreement that takes into account the element of chance. This usually is used with the direct observation method.

Interval Measurement Level used to show rankings of events or objects on a scale with equal intervals between numbers but with an arbitrary zero (e.g., centigrade temperature).

Intervening Variable A variable that occurs during an experimental or quasi-experimental study that affects the dependent variable.

Intervention Deals with whether or not the observer provokes actions from those who are being observed.

Intervention Fidelity The process of enhancing the study's internal validity by ensuring that the intervention is delivered systematically to all subjects.

Interview Guide A list of questions and probes used by interviews that use open-ended questions.

Interviews A method of data collection in which a data collector questions a subject verbally. Interviews may be in person or performed over the telephone, and they may consist of open-ended or close-ended questions.

Intrinsic Case Study Research that is undertaken to gain a better understanding of the essential nature of the case.

Item to Total Correlation The relationship between each of the items on a scale and the total scale.

J

Justice The principle that human subjects should be treated fairly.

K

Kappa Expresses the level of agreement observed beyond the level that would be expected by chance alone. Kappa (K) ranges from +1 (total agreement) to 0 (no agreement). K greater than 0.80 generally indicates good reliability. K between 0.68 and 0.80 is considered acceptable/substantial agreement. Levels lower than 0.68 may allow tentative conclusions to be drawn when lower levels are accepted.

Key Informants Individuals who have special knowledge, status, or communication skills, and who are willing to teach the ethnographer about the phenomenon.

Knowledge-Focused Triggers Ideas that are generated when staff read research, listen to scientific papers at research conferences, or encounter evidence-based practice guidelines published by government agencies or specialty organizations.

Kuder-Richardson (KR-20) Coefficient The estimate of homogeneity used for instruments that use a dichotomous response pattern.

L

Lean A QI model that focuses on eliminating waste from the production system by designing the most efficient and effective system. It is sometimes referred to as the Toyota Quality Model.

Level of Significance (Alpha Level) The risk of making a type I error, set by the researcher before the study begins.

Levels of Evidence A rating system for judging the strength of a study's design.

Levels of Measurement Categorization of the precision with which an event can be measured (nominal, ordinal, interval, and ratio).

Likelihood Ratios Provide the nurse with information about the accuracy of a diagnostic test and can also help the nurse to be a more efficient decision maker by allowing the clinician to quantify the probability of disease for any individual patient.

Likert-Type Scales Lists of statements for which respondents indicate whether they "strongly agree," "agree," "disagree," or "strongly disagree."

Limitation Weakness of a study.

Literature Review A systematic and critical appraisal of the most important literature on a topic.

Lived Experience In phenomenological research, a term used to refer to the focus on living through events and circumstances (prelingual), rather than thinking about these events and circumstances (conceptualized experience).

Longitudinal Study A nonexperimental research design in which a researcher collects data from the same group at different points in time.

M

Manipulation The provision of some experimental treatment, in one or varying degrees, to some of the subjects in the study.

Matching A special sampling strategy used to construct an equivalent comparison sample group by filling it with subjects who are similar to each subject in another sample group in terms of preestablished variables, such as age and gender.

Maturation Developmental, biological, or psychological processes that operate within an individual as a function of time and are external to the events of the investigation.

Mean A measure of central tendency; the arithmetic average of all scores.

Measurement The standardized method of collecting data.

Measurement Effects Administration of a pretest in a study that affects the generalizability of the findings to other populations.

Measurement Error The difference between what really exists and what is measured in a given study.

Measures of Central Tendency A descriptive statistical procedure that describes the average member of a sample (mean, median, and mode).

Measures of Variability Descriptive statistical procedure that describes how much dispersion there is in sample data.

Median A measure of central tendency; the middle score.

Mediating Variable A variable that intervenes between the independent and dependent variable.

Meta-Analysis A research method that takes the results of multiple studies in a specific area and synthesizes the findings to make conclusions regarding the area of focus.

Meta-Summary Integrations that are approximately equal to the sum of parts, or the sum of findings across reports in a target domain of research.

Meta-Synthesis Integrates qualitative research findings on a topic and is based on comparative analysis and interpretative synthesis.

Methodological Research The controlled investigation and measurement of the means of gathering and analyzing data.

Microrange Theory The linking of concrete concepts into a statement that can be examined in practice and research.

Middle Range Nursing Theories Theories that contain a limited number of concepts and are focused on a limited aspect of reality.

Modality The number of peaks in a frequency distribution.

Mode A measure of central tendency; the most frequent score or result.

Model A symbolic representation of a set of concepts that is created to depict relationships.

Mortality The loss of subjects from time 1 data collection to time 2 data collection.

Multiple Analysis of Variance (MANOVA) A test used to determine differences in group means; used when there is more than one dependent variable.

Multiple Regression A measure of the relationship between one interval level dependent variable and several independent variables. Canonical correlation is used when there is more than one dependent variable.

Multistage Sampling (Cluster Sampling) Involves a successive random sampling of units (clusters) that programs from large to small and meets sample eligibility criteria.

Multitrait–Multimethod Approach A type of validity that uses more than one method to assess the accuracy of an instrument (e.g., observation and interview of anxiety).

Multivariate Statistics A statistical procedure that involves two or more variables.

N

Naturalistic Setting An environment of familiar "day-to-day" surroundings.

Negative Likelihood Ratio (LR) The LR of a negative test indicates the accuracy of a negative test result by comparing its performance when the disease is absent to that when the disease is present. The better test to use to rule out disease is the one with the smaller likelihood ratio of a negative test.

Negative Predictive Value Expresses the proportion of those with negative test results who truly do not have the disease.

Network Sampling (Snowball Effect Sample) A strategy used for locating samples that are difficult to locate. It uses social networks and the fact that friends tend to have characteristics in common; subjects who meet the eligibility criteria are asked for assistance in getting in touch with others who meet the same criteria.

Nominal The level of measurement that simply assigns data into categories that are mutually exclusive.

Nominal Measurement Level used to classify objects or events into categories without any relative ranking (e.g., gender, hair color).

Nondirectional Hypothesis Indicates the existence of a relationship between the variables but does not specify the anticipated direction of the relationship.

Nonequivalent Control Group Design A quasi-experimental design that is similar to the true experiment, but subjects are not randomly assigned to the treatment or control groups.

Nonexperimental Research Design Research design in which an investigator observes a phenomenon without manipulating the independent variable(s).

Nonparametric Statistics Statistics that are usually used when variables are measured at the nominal or ordinal level because they do not estimate population parameters and involve less restrictive assumptions about the underlying distribution.

Nonprobability Sampling A procedure in which elements are chosen by nonrandom methods.

Normal Curve A curve that is symmetrical about the mean and is unimodal.

Null Hypothesis A statement that there is no relationship between the variables and that any relationship observed is a function of chance or fluctuations in sampling.

Null Value In an experiment, when a value is obtained that indicates that there is no difference between the treatment and control groups.

Number Needed to Treat The number of people who need to receive a treatment (or intervention) in order for one patient to receive any benefit.

O

Objective Data that are not influenced by anyone who collects the information.

Objectivity The use of facts without distortion by personal feelings or bias.

Observation A method for measuring psychological and physiological behaviors for the purpose of evaluating change and facilitating recovery.

Observed Score The actual score obtained in a measurement.

Observed Test Score Derived from a set of items; actually consists of the true score plus error.

Odds Ratio (OR) An estimate of relative risk used in logistic regression as a measure of association; describes the probability of an event.

One-Group (Pretest–Posttest) Design Design used by researchers when only one group is available for study. Data are collected before and after an experimental treatment on one group of subjects. In this type of design, there is no control group and no randomization.

Open-Ended Question Question that the respondent may answer in his or her own words.

Operational Definition The measurements used to observe or measure a variable; delineates the procedures or operations required to measure a concept.

Opinion Leaders From the local peer group, viewed as a respected source of influence, considered by associates as technically competent, and trusted to judge the fit between the innovation and the local situation.

Ordinal The level of measurement that systematically categorizes data in an ordered or ranked manner. Ordinal measures do not permit a high level of differentiation among subjects.

Ordinal Measurement Level used to show rankings of events or objects; numbers are not equidistant, and zero is arbitrary (e.g., class ranking).

P

Paradigm From Greek: *pattern*; it has been applied to science to describe the way people in society think about the world.

Parallel Form Reliability See *alternate form reliability*.

Parameter A characteristic of a population.

Parametric Statistics Inferential statistics that involve the estimation of at least one parameter, require measurement at the interval level or above, and involve assumptions about the variables being studied. These assumptions usually include the fact that the variable is normally distributed.

Participant Observation When the observer keeps field notes (a short summary of observations) to record the activities, as well as the observer's interpretations of these activities.

Pearson Correlation Coefficient (Pearson *r*) A statistic that is calculated to reflect the degree of relationship between two interval level variables. Also called the *Pearson Product Moment Correlation Coefficient.*

Percentile Represents the percentage of cases a given score exceeds.

Performance Measurement A tool that tracks an organization's performance using standardized measures to document and manage quality.

Phenomena Those things that are perceived by our senses (e.g., pain, losing a loved one).

Phenomenological Method A process of learning and constructing the meaning of human experience through intensive dialogue with persons who are living the experience.

Phenomenological Research Phenomenological research is based on phenomenological philosophy and is research aimed at obtaining a description of an experience as it is lived in order to understand the meaning of that experience for those who have it.

Phenomenology A qualitative research approach that aims to describe experience as it is lived through, before it is conceptualized.

Philosophical Beliefs The system of motivating values; concepts; principles; and the nature of human knowledge of an individual, group, or culture.

Philosophical Research Based on the investigation of the truths and principles of existence, knowledge, and conduct.

Pilot Study A small, simple study conducted as a prelude to a larger-scale study that is often called the "parent study."

Plan-Do-Study-Act (PDSA) Improvement Cycle The last step of the Improvement Model.

Population A well-defined set that has certain specified properties.

Positive Likelihood Ratio (LR) The LR of a positive test indicates the accuracy of a positive test result by comparing its performance when the disease is present to that when the disease is absent. The best test to use for ruling in a disease is the one with the largest likelihood ratio of a positive test.

Positive Predictive Value Expresses the proportion of those with positive test results who truly have disease.

Power Analysis The mathematical procedure to determine the number for each arm (group) of a study.

Predictive Validity The degree of correlation between the measure of the concept and some future measure of the same concept.

Prefiltered Evidence Evidence for which an editorial team has already read and summarized articles on a topic and appraised its relevance to clinical care.

Primary Source Scholarly literature that is written by the person(s) who developed the theory or conducted the research. Primary sources include eyewitness accounts of historic events, provided by original documents, films, letters, diaries, records, artifacts, periodicals, or audio/video recordings.

Probability The probability of an event is the event's long-run relative frequency in repeated trials under similar conditions.

Probability Sampling A procedure that uses some form of random selection when the sample units are chosen.

Problem-Focused Triggers Those that are identified by staff through quality improvement, risk surveillance, benchmarking data, financial data, or recurrent clinical problems.

Program A list of instructions in a machine-readable language written so that a computer's hardware can carry out an operation; software.

Prospective Study A nonexperimental study that begins with an exploration of assumed causes and then moves forward in time to the presumed effect.

Psychometrics The theory and development of measurement instruments.

Public Reporting Provides objective information to promote consumer choice, guide QI efforts, and promote accountability for performance among providers and delivery organizations. It also allows organizations to compare their performance across standard measures against their peer organizations locally and nationally.

Purpose That which encompasses the aims or objectives the investigator hopes to achieve with the research, not the question to be answered.

Purposive Sampling A nonprobability sampling strategy in which the researcher selects subjects who are considered to be representative of the population.

Q

Qualitative Measurement The items or observed behaviors are assigned to mutually exclusive categories that are representative of the kinds of behavior exhibited by the subjects.

Qualitative Research The study of research questions about human experiences. It is often conducted in natural settings and uses data that are words or text, rather than numerical, in order to describe the experiences that are being studied.

Quality Health Care Care that is safe, effective, patient-centered, timely, efficient, and equitable.

Quality Improvement (QI) The systematic use of data to monitor the outcomes of care processes, as well as the use of improvement methods to design and test changes in practice for the purpose of continuously improving the quality and safety of health care systems.

Quantitative Measurement The assignment of items or behaviors to categories that represent the amount of a possessed characteristic.

Quantitative Research The process of testing relationships, differences, and cause and effect interactions among and between variables. These processes are tested with either hypotheses and/or research questions.

Quasi-Experiment Research designs in which the researcher initiates an experimental treatment, but some characteristic of a true experiment is lacking.

Quasi-Experimental Design A study design in which random assignment is not used, but the independent variable is manipulated and certain mechanisms of control are used.

Questionnaires Paper-and-pencil instruments designed to gather data from individuals about knowledge, attitudes, beliefs, and feelings.

Quota Sampling A nonprobability sampling strategy that identifies the strata of the population and proportionately represents the strata in the sample.

R

Random Error An error that occurs when scores vary in a random way. Random error occurs when data collectors do not use standard procedures to collect data consistently among all subjects in a study.

Random Selection A selection process in which each element of the population has an equal and independent chance of being included in the sample.

Randomization A sampling selection procedure in which each person or element in a population has an equal chance of being selected to either the experimental group or the control group.

Randomized Controlled Trial (RCT) A research study using a true experimental design.

Range A measure of variability; difference between the highest and lowest scores in a set of sample data.

Ratio The highest level of measurement that possesses the characteristics of categorizing, ordering, and ranking, and also has an absolute or natural zero that has empirical meaning.

Ratio Measurement Level that ranks the order of events or objects, and that has equal intervals and an absolute zero (e.g., height, weight).

Reactivity The distortion created when those who are being observed change their behavior because they know that they are being observed.

Recommendation Application of a study to practice, theory, and future research.

Refereed Journal or Peer-Reviewed Journal A scholarly journal that has a panel of external and internal reviewers or editors; the panel reviews submitted manuscripts for possible publication. The review panels use the same set of scholarly criteria to judge if the manuscripts are worthy of publication.

Relationship/Difference Studies Studies that trace the relationships or differences between variables that can provide a deeper insight into a phenomenon.

Relative Risk (RR) Risk of event after experimental treatment as a percentage of original risk.

Relative Risk Reduction (RRR) A helpful tool to indicate how much of the baseline risk (the control group event rate) is removed as a result of having the intervention.

Reliability The consistency or constancy of a measuring instrument.

Reliability Coefficient A number between 0 and 1 that expresses the relationship between the error variance, the true variance, and the observed score. A zero correlation indicates no relationship. The closer to 1 the coefficient is, the more reliable the tool.

Repeated Measures Studies See *longitudinal study*.

Representative Sample A sample whose key characteristics closely approximate those of the population.

Research The systematic, logical, and empirical inquiry into the possible relationships among particular phenomena to produce verifiable knowledge.

Research Hypothesis A statement about the expected relationship between the variables; also known as a *scientific hypothesis*.

Research Literature A synonym for data-based literature.

Research Problem Presents the question that is to be asked in a research study.

Research Question A key preliminary step wherein the foundation for a study is developed from the research problem and results in the research hypothesis.

Research Utilization A systematic method of implementing sound research-based innovations in clinical practice, evaluating the outcome, and sharing the knowledge through the process of research dissemination.

Research-Based Protocols Practice standards that are formulated from findings of several studies.

Respect for Persons The principle that people have the right to self-determination and to treatment as autonomous agents; that is, they have the freedom to participate or not participate in research.

Respondent Burden Occurs when the length of the questionnaire or interview is too long or the questions are too difficult for respondents to answer in a reasonable amount of time considering their age, health condition, or mental status.

Retrospective Data Data that have been manifested, such as scores on a standard examination.

Retrospective Study A nonexperimental research design that begins with the phenomenon of interest (dependent variable) in the present and examines its relationship to another variable (independent variable) in the past.

Review of the Literature An extensive, systematic, and critical review of the most important published scholarly literature on a particular topic. In most cases it is not considered exhaustive.

Risk Potential negative outcome(s) of participation in a research study.

Risk/Benefit Ratio The extent to which the benefits of the study are maximized and the risks are minimized such that the subjects are protected from harm during the study.

Root Cause Analysis (RCA) A structured method used to understand sources of system variation that lead to errors or mistakes, including sentinel events, with the goal of learning from mistakes and mitigating hazards that arise as a characteristic of the system design.

Run Chart A graphical data display that shows trends in a measure of interest; trends reveal what is occurring over time.

S

Sample A subset of sampling units from a population.

Sampling A process in which representative units of a population are selected for study in a research investigation.

Sampling Error The tendency for statistics to fluctuate from one sample to another.

Sampling Frame A list of all units of the population.

Sampling Interval The standard distance between the elements chosen for the sample.

Sampling Unit The element or set of elements used for selecting the sample.

Saturation See *data saturation.*

Scale A self-report inventory that provides a set of response symbols for each item. A rating or score is assigned to each response.

Scientific Approach A logical, orderly, and objective means of generating and testing ideas.

Scientific Hypothesis The researcher's expectation about the outcome of a study; also known as the *research hypothesis.*

Scientific Literature A synonym for data-based literature; see *data-based literature.*

Scientific Observation Collecting data about the environment and subjects. Data collection has specific objectives to guide it, is systematically planned and recorded, is checked and controlled, and is related to scientific concepts and theories.

Secondary Analysis A form of research in which the researcher takes previously collected and analyzed data from one study and reanalyzes the data for a secondary purpose.

Secondary Source Scholarly material written by a person(s) other than the individual who developed the theory or conducted the research. Most are usually published. Often a secondary source represents a response to or a summary and critique of a theorist's or researcher's work. Examples are documents, films, letters, diaries, records, artifacts, periodicals, or tapes that provide a view of the phenomenon from another's perspective.

Selection The generalizability of the results to other populations.

Selection Bias The internal validity threat that arises when pretreatment differences between the experimental group and the control group are present.

Self-Report Data collection methods that require subjects to respond directly to either interviews or structured questionnaires about their experiences, behaviors, feelings, or attitudes. These are commonly used in nursing research and are most useful for collecting data on variables that cannot be directly observed or measured by physiological instruments.

Semiquartile Range A measure of variability; range of the middle 50% of the scores. Also known as *semi-interquartile range.*

Sensitivity The proportion of those with disease who test positive.

Simple Random Sampling A probability sampling strategy in which the population is defined, a sampling frame is listed, and a subset from which the sample will be chosen; members are randomly selected.

Situation-Specific Theories More specific theories than middle range theories, they are composed of a limited number of concepts. They are narrow in scope, explain a small aspect of phenomena and processes of interest to nurses, and are usually limited to specific populations or field of practice.

Snowball Effect Sampling (Network Sampling) A strategy used for locating samples difficult to locate. It uses the social network and the fact that friends tend to have characteristics in common; subjects who meet the eligibility criteria are asked for assistance in getting in touch with others who meet the same criteria.

Solomon Four-Group Design An experimental design with four randomly assigned groups: the pretest–posttest intervention group, the pretest–posttest control group, a treatment or intervention group with only posttest measurement, and a control group with only posttest measurement.

Specificity The proportion of those without disease who test negative. It measures how well the test rules out disease when it is really absent; a specific test has few false positive results.

Split-Half Reliability An index of the comparison between the scores on one half of a test with those on the other half to determine the consistency in response to items that reflect specific content.

Stability An instrument's ability to produce the same results with repeated testing.

Standard Deviation (SD) A measure of variability; measure of average deviation of scores from the mean.

Statistic A descriptive index for a sample such as a sample mean or a standard deviation.

Statistical Hypothesis States that there is no relationship between the independent and dependent variables. The statistical hypothesis is also known as the null hypothesis.

Stratified Random Sampling A probability sampling strategy in which the population is divided into strata or subgroups. An appropriate number of elements from each subgroup are randomly selected based on their proportion in the population.

Survey Studies Descriptive, exploratory, or comparative studies that collect detailed descriptions of existing variables and use the data to justify and assess current conditions and practices, or to make more plans for improving health care practices.

Survival Curve A graph that shows the probability that a patient "survives" in a given state for at least a specified time (or longer).

Systematic Data collection carried out in the same manner with all subjects.

Systematic Error Attributable to lasting characteristics of the subject that do not tend to fluctuate from one time to another. Also called *constant error.*

Systematic Review The process whereby investigators find all relevant studies, published and unpublished, on the topic or question; at least two members of the review team independently assess the quality of each study, include or exclude studies based on preestablished criteria, statistically combine the results of individual studies, and present a balanced and impartial evidence summary of the findings that represents a "state of the science" conclusion about the evidence, supporting benefits and risks of a given health care practice.

Systematic Sampling A probability sampling strategy that involves the selection of subjects randomly drawn from a population list at fixed intervals.

T

***t* Statistic** Commonly used in research; it tests whether two group means are more different than would be expected by chance. Groups may be related or independent.

Target Population A population or group of individuals that meet the sampling criteria.

Test A self-report inventory that provides for one response to each item that the examiner assigns a rating or score. Inferences are made from the total score about the degree to which a subject possesses whatever trait, emotion, attitude, or behavior the test is supposed to measure.

Test–Retest Reliability Administration of the same instrument twice to the same subjects under the same conditions within a prescribed time interval, with a comparison of the paired scores to determine the stability of the measure.

Testability Variables of proposed study that lend themselves to observation, measurement, and analysis.

Testing The effects of taking a pretest on the scores of a posttest.

Text Data in a contextual form; that is, narrative or words that are written and transcribed.

Theme A label that represents a way of describing large quantities of data in a condensed format.

Theoretical Framework Theoretical rationale for the development of hypotheses.

Theoretical Literature A synonym for conceptual literature; see *conceptual literature.*

Theory Set of interrelated concepts, definitions, and propositions that present a systematic view of phenomena for the purpose of explaining and making predictions about those phenomena.

Time Series Design A quasi-experimental design used to determine trends before and after an experimental treatment. Measurements are taken several times before the introduction of the experimental treatment; the treatment is introduced, and measurements are taken again at specified times afterward.

Transferability See *fittingness.*

Treatment Effect The impact of the independent variable/intervention on the dependent variable.

Triangulation The expansion of research methods in a single study or multiple studies to enhance diversity, enrich understanding, and accomplish specific goals.

True (Classic) Experiment Also known as the *pretest–posttest control group design.* In this design, subjects are randomly assigned to an experimental or control group, pretest measurements are performed, an intervention or treatment occurs in the experimental group, and posttest measurements are performed.

Trustworthiness The rigor of the research in a qualitative research study.

Type I Error The rejection of a null hypothesis that is actually true.

Type II Error The acceptance of a null hypothesis that is actually false.

V

Validity The determination of whether a measurement instrument actually measures what it is purported to measure.

Variable A defined concept.

W

Web Browser Software program used to connect to or "read" the World Wide Web.

INDEX

F

J

K

L

Q

S

T